BIOCHEMISTRY OF EXERCISE

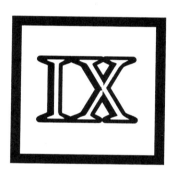

Ronald J. Maughan, PhD
Susan M. Shirreffs, BSc
University of Aberdeen, Scotland

Editors

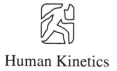

Human Kinetics

Library of Congress Cataloging-in-Publication Data

International Biochemistry of Exercise Conference (9th : 1994 :
  Aberdeen, Scotland)
    Biochemistry of exercise IX / Ron J. Maughan, Susan M. Shirreffs,
  editors.
        p. cm.
    "Proceedings of the 9th International Biochemistry of Exercise
  Conference, held on July 21-26, 1994 in Aberdeen, Scotland"--Copr.
  p.
    Includes bibliographical references.
    ISBN 0-88011-486-X
    1. Exercise--Physiological aspects--Congresses.   2. Muscles-
  -Metabolism--Congresses.   3. Biochemistry--Congresses.   I. Maughan,
  Ron J., 1951-   . II. Shirreffs, Susan M., 1971-   . III. Title.
  QP301.I536   1994
  612'.044--dc20   96-10897

ISBN: 0-88011-486-X

Copyright © 1996 by Human Kinetics Publishers, Inc.

Proceedings of the 9th International Biochemistry of Exercise Conference held on July 21-
26, 1994 in Aberdeen, Scotland.

Permission notices for material reprinted in this book from other sources can be found on
pp. xxiii-xxv.

Acquisitions Editors: Richard Washburn, PhD, and Rick Frey, PhD; **Developmental Editor:**
Julia Anderson; **Assistant Editor:** Jacqueline Eaton Blakley; **Editorial Assistant:** Coree
Schutter; **Copyeditor:** Karen Bojda; **Proofreader:** Pam Johnson; **Graphic Artists:** Yvonne
Winsor and Sandra Meier; **Graphic Designer:** Keith Blomberg; **Cover Designer:** Jack Davis;
Printer: Edwards Brothers

Printed in the United States of America   10 9 8 7 6 5 4 3 2 1

Human Kinetics
Web site: http://www.humankinetics.com/

United States: Human Kinetics
P.O. Box 5076
Champaign, IL 61825-5076
1-800-747-4457
e-mail: humank@hkusa.com

Canada: Human Kinetics, Box 24040
Windsor, ON N8Y 4Y9
1-800-465-7301 (in Canada only)
e-mail: humank@hkcanada.com

Europe: Human Kinetics, P.O. Box IW14
Leeds LS16 6TR United Kingdom
(44) 1132 781708
e-mail: humank@hkeurope.com

Australia: Human Kinetics
57A Price Avenue
Lower Mitcham, South Australia 5062
(08) 277 1555
e-mail: humank@hkaustralia.com

New Zealand: Human Kinetics
P.O. Box 105-231, Auckland 1
(09) 523 3462
e-mail: humank@hknewz.com

This book is dedicated in memory of John Sutton.

Contents

Conference Organization

Organizing Committee
Ron Maughan, Aberdeen, Scotland
Eric Newsholme, Oxford, England
Jacques Poortmans, Brussels, Belgium
Clyde Williams, Loughborough, England

Local Organization
Stuart Galloway
John Leiper
Yannis Pitsiladis
Susan Shirreffs

Research Group on the Biochemistry of Exercise
J.R. Poortmans, Belgium, Chairman
H. Galbo, Denmark, Vice-Chairman
F.W. Booth, U.S.A.
J.D. Chen, China
P. di Prampero, Italy
C. Guezennec, France
J. Henriksson, Sweden
J.O. Holloszy, U.S.A.
R.J. Maughan, U.K.
K. Nazar, Poland
E.A. Newsholme, U.K.
D. Pette, Germany
V. Rogozkin, Russia
Y. Sato, Japan
T. Takala, Finland
A.W. Taylor, Canada
A. Tsopanakis, Greece

Contributors

Peter Arner
Department of Medicine
Karolinska Institute, Huddinge
   University Hospital
Huddinge, Sweden

John R. Arthur
Rowett Research Institute
Aberdeen, Scotland

Jens Bangsbo
Copenhagen Muscle Research Centre
August Krogh Institute
University of Copenhagen
Copenhagen, Denmark

Daniela Barbieri
Department of Biomedical Sciences
University of Modena School of
   Medicine
Modena, Italy

Eva E. Blomstrand
Pripps Bryggerier
Research Laboratories
Stockholm, Sweden

Kristina Bodin
Department of Clinical Chemistry
Huddinge University Hospital
Karolinska Institute
Huddinge, Sweden

Gregory C. Bogdanis
Department of Physical Education,
   Sports Sciences, and Recreation
   Management
Loughborough University
Loughborough, England

Leslie H. Boobis
Sunderland District Hospital
Sunderland, England

Frank W. Booth
Department of Physiology and Cell
   Biology
University of Texas-Houston Health
   Science Center
Houston, TX, U.S.A.

Joseph G. Cannon
Noll Physiological Research Center
Pennsylvania State University
University Park, PA, U.S.A.

James A. Carson
University of Texas-Houston Health
   Science Center
Houston, TX, U.S.A.

Anna Casey
Department of Physiology and
   Pharmacology
University Medical School
Queens Medical Centre
Nottingham, England

Andrew R. Coggan
Metabolism Unit
Shriners Burn Institute
Galveston, TX, U.S.A.

Dumitru Constantin-Teodosiu
Department of Physiology and
   Pharmacology
University Medical School
Queens Medical Centre
Nottingham, England

Andrea Cossarizza
Department of Biomedical Sciences
University of Modena School of
   Medicine
Modena, Italy

J. Mark Davis
Department of Exercise Science
University of South Carolina
Columbia, SC, U.S.A.

Flemming Dela
Department of Medical Physiology
The Panum Institute
Copenhagen, Denmark

Garry G. Duthie
Rowett Research Institute
Aberdeen, Scotland

David J. Dyck
School of Human Biology
University of Guelph
Guelph, ON, Canada

Karyn Esser
University of Illinois at Chicago
Chicago, IL, U.S.A.

William J. Evans
Noll Physiological Research Center
Pennsylvania State University
University Park, PA, U.S.A.

Maria A. Fiatarone
Human Nutrition Research Center on
  Aging
Tufts University
Boston, MA, U.S.A.

Claudio Franceschi
Department of Biomedical Sciences
University of Modena School of
  Medicine
Modena, Italy

Keith N. Frayn
Oxford Lipid Metabolism Group,
  Sheikh Rashid Laboratory
Radcliffe Infirmary
Oxford, England

Henrik Galbo
Department of Medical Physiology
The Panum Institute
Copenhagen, Denmark

Liying Gao
Department of Physiology and
  Biophysics
University of Illinois at
  Urbana-Champaign
Urbana, IL, U.S.A.

Emanuela Grassilli
Department of Biomedical Sciences
University of Modena School of
  Medicine
Modena, Italy

Allison Green
Department of Physiology and
  Pharmacology
University Medical School
Queens Medical Centre
Nottingham, England

Howard J. Green
Department of Kinesiology
University of Waterloo
Waterloo, ON, Canada

Paul L. Greenhaff
Department of Physiology and
  Pharmacology
University Medical School
Queens Medical Centre
Nottingham, England

A. John Griffiths
Endocrine Unit, Department of
  Medicine
Hammersmith Hospital
London, England

Mark Hargreaves
Department of Physiology
The University of Melbourne
Parkville, Australia

Jan Henriksson
Department of Physiology and
  Pharmacology
The Karolinska Institute
Stockholm, Sweden

Peter Hespel
Department of Kinesiology
Catholic University of Leuven
Leuven, Belgium

Vanessa Hodgetts
DRA Centre for Human Sciences
Gosport, Hampshire, England

Laurie Hoffman-Goetz
University of Waterloo
Waterloo, ON, Canada

John O. Holloszy
Washington University School of
  Medicine
St. Louis, MO, U.S.A.

Eric Hultman
Department of Clinical Chemistry
Huddinge University Hospital
Karolinska Institute
Huddinge, Sweden

John L. Ivy
Department of Kinesiology and Health
  Education
University of Texas
Austin, TX, U.S.A.

Malcolm J. Jackson
Muscle Research Centre, Department
  of Medicine
University of Liverpool
Liverpool, England

Eva Jansson
Department of Medical Laboratory
  Sciences and Technology
Huddinge University Hospital
Huddinge, Sweden

Robert R. Jenkins
Biology Department
Ithaca College
Ithaca, NY, U.S.A.

Alison McE. Jenkinson
Rowett Research Institute
Aberdeen, Scotland

David Jones
Department of Experimental
  Orthopaedics and Biomechanics
Phillips University
Marburg, Germany

Galina Kalachnikova
Department of Biomedical Sciences
University of Modena School of
  Medicine
Modena, Italy

Bente Kiens
University of Copenhagen
Copenhagen, Denmark

Zhu Ku
University of Tennessee Health
  Science Center
Memphis, TN, U.S.A.

Henryk K.A. Lakomy
Department of Physical Education,
  Sports Science, and Recreation
  Management
Loughborough University
Loughborough, England

Gunnar Leivseth
Department of Physiology
University of Tromso
Tromso, Norway

Vandana Menon
University of Tennessee Health
  Science Center
Memphis, TN, U.S.A.

Daniela Monti
Department of Biomedical Sciences
University of Modena School of
  Medicine
Modena, Italy

Philip C. Morrice
Rowett Research Institute
Aberdeen, Scotland

N. Nakai
Division of Health Promotion Science,
   Graduate School of Medicine
Nagoya University
Nagoya, Japan

Mary E. Nevill
Department of Physical Education,
   Sports Science, and Recreation
   Management
Loughborough University
Loughborough, England

Eric A. Newsholme
Department of Biochemistry
University of Oxford
Oxford, England

Earl G. Noble
Faculty of Kinesiology and Department
   of Physiology, Faculty of Medicine
University of Western Ontario
London, ON, Canada

David C. Nieman
Department of Health and Exercise
   Science
Appalachian State University
Boone, NC, U.S.A.

H. Ohno
Department of Hygiene
National Defense Medical College
Tokolozawa, Japan

N. Ohsaki
Division of Health Promotion Science,
   Graduate School of Medicine
Nagoya University
Nagoya, Japan

I. Ohsawa
Research Center of Health, Physical
   Fitness, and Sports
Nagoya University
Nagoya, Japan

Lawrence B. Oscai
School of Kinesiology
University of Illinois at Chicago
Chicago, IL, U.S.A.

Y. Oshida
Nagoya University
Nagoya, Japan

Bente Klarlund Pedersen
Department of Infectious Diseases
Copenhagen Muscle Research Centre
Copenhagen, Denmark

Diane M. Raab-Cullen
Osteoporosis Research Center
Creighton University
Omaha, NE, U.S.A.

Erik A. Richter
Copenhagen Muscle Research Centre,
   August Krogh Institute
University of Copenhagen
Copenhagen, Denmark

Richard L. Sabina
Department of Biochemistry
Medical College of Wisconsin
Milwaukee, WI, U.S.A.

Kent Sahlin
Department of Physiology and
   Pharmacology, Physiology III
Karolinska Institute and University
   College of Physical Education and
   Sports
Stockholm, Sweden

Paolo Salomoni
Department of Biomedical Sciences
University of Modena School of
   Medicine
Modena, Italy

Stefano Salvioli
Department of Biomedical Sciences
University of Modena School of
   Medicine
Modena, Italy

J. Sato
Department of Internal Medicine III
Nagoya University School of
   Medicine
Nagoya, Japan

Y. Sato
Research Center of Health, Physical
   Fitness, and Sports
Nagoya University
Nagoya, Japan

Y. Shimomura
Department of Bioscience
Nagoya Institute of Technology
Nagoya, Japan

Timothy M. Skerry
Department of Anatomy
University of Bristol
Bristol, United Kingdom

Everett L. Smith
Department of Preventive Medicine
University of Wisconsin
Madison, WI, U.S.A.

Karin Söderlund
Department of Clinical Chemistry
Huddinge University Hospital
Karolinska Institute
Huddinge, Sweden

Lawrence L. Spriet
School of Human Biology
University of Guelph
Guelph, ON, Canada

Bente Stallknecht
Department of Medical Physiology
The Panum Institute
Copenhagen, Denmark

Albert W. Taylor
Faculty of Kinesiology and
    Department of Physiology, Faculty
    of Medicine
University of Western Ontario
London, ON, Canada

Ronald L. Terjung
Department of Physiology
State University of New York Health
    Science Center
Syracuse, NY, U.S.A.

Donald B. Thomason
Department of Physiology and Biophysics
University of Tennessee Health
    Science Center
Memphis, TN, U.S.A.

Jamie Timmons
Department of Physiology and
    Pharmacology
University Medical School
Queens Medical Centre
Nottingham, England

Leonarda Troiano
Department of Biomedical Sciences
University of Modena School of
    Medicine
Modena, Italy

Franco Tropea
Department of Biomedical Sciences
University of Modena School of
    Medicine
Modena, Italy

Richard W. Tsika
Department of Physiology and
    Biophysics
University of Illinois at
    Urbana-Champaign
Urbana, IL, U.S.A.

Peter C. Tullson
Department of Physiology
State University of New York Health
    Science Center
Syracuse, NY, U.S.A.

Lorraine Turcotte
Department of Exercise Sciences
University of Southern California
Los Angeles, CA, U.S.A.

Gerrit van Hall
University of Limburg
Maastricht, The Netherlands

Anton J.M. Wagenmakers
Department of Human Biology
University of Limburg
Maastricht, The Netherlands

Clyde Williams
Department of Physical Education,
    Sports Science, and Recreation
    Management
Loughborough University
Loughborough, England

William W. Winder
Zoology Department
Brigham Young University
Provo, UT, U.S.A.

K. Yamanouchi
Department of Internal Medicine I
Aichi Medical University
Nagakute, Japan

Zhen Yan
University of Texas-Houston Health
  Science Center
Houston, TX, U.S.A.

Jiwei Yang
University of Tennessee Health
  Science Center
Memphis, TN, U.S.A.

Preface

The conference on which this volume is based was the ninth in a series organized by the Research Group on the Biochemistry of Exercise. The quality of the previous meetings, which have been held triennially since 1968, set a high standard and established this as the most prestigious meeting in the field of exercise biochemistry.

The Ninth International Conference on the Biochemistry of Exercise was held in Aberdeen, Scotland, on 21-26 July 1994, and was the first in the series to be held in the United Kingdom. The meeting was truly international, attracting a total of 340 delegates from 36 different countries: 257 participants came from outside the British Isles.

The aim of the Scientific Committee was to provide a forum for reviews of recent progress and presentation of new findings in exercise biochemistry, covering both the basic mechanisms involved and also some applied topics. The degree to which this objective was achieved can be judged by the contents of this volume.

The conference opened with a keynote address by Sir Andrew Huxley, winner of the 1964 Nobel Prize in physiology for his work on the sliding filament theory of muscle contraction. The format of the meeting included plenary sessions held each morning and two parallel symposia, which took place in the afternoon. The conference concluded with a closing lecture by Professor Bengt Saltin. Poster sessions were held on the first three days of the conference, and the abstracts of these presentations are published as a supplement to *Clinical Science* (vol. 87, 1994). These proceedings contain the manuscripts prepared by the participants in the plenary sessions and symposia.

Acknowledgments

This conference was made possible by the generous financial support of a number of organizations, and their contribution to the success of the meeting is gratefully acknowledged.

The Organizing Committee is pleased to record our gratitude to the following major sponsors:

Gatorade Sports Science Institute
International Science Foundation
Mars Inc.
Mars U.K. Ltd.
SmithKline Beecham
The Isostar Sports Nutrition Foundation

We also wish to acknowledge the contributions of Shaklee U.S., Inc.

We would also like to thank the U.S. Air Force European Office of Aerospace Research and Development for its contribution toward the success of this conference.

Conference Welcome

From 1968 onward, the Research Group on Biochemistry of Exercise has traveled to three continents (Europe, America, Asia), increasing the number of participants from 100 to 400. Three years ago, the board of our research group agreed to hold its next meeting in Great Britain, having in mind the aphorism by A.V. Hill, British Nobel Prize winner:

> Some of the most consistent physiological data available are contained, not in books on physiology, not even in books on medicine, but in the world's records of running different horizontal distances. (*Muscular Activity,* 1926)

Originally, we planned to organize our ninth conference in the oldest university in the United Kingdom. Due to technical difficulties, we had to leave the romance of Oxford for the spirits of the glens and the granite city of Aberdeen.

In 1994, the scientific community commemorated the 200th anniversary of the death of Antoine Lavoisier, beheaded by stupid French revolutionists. This aristocrat may be regarded as a founder of physiological chemistry, who carried out experiments on respiration of subjects performing work. Generations of chemists and physiologists worked to refine the analytical methods Lavoisier invented. Nowadays we are switching to molecular biology, but let us not forget all those who, like Antoine Lavoisier, Claude Bernard, Otto Warburg, and Hans Krebs, drove us toward a general understanding of the elements of scientific creativity.

Ron Maughan and his local team were highly efficient in organizing the practical details of this meeting. The delegates of 36 different countries enjoyed the scientific program, and it is the sincere hope of the Research Group that the numerous readers of these proceedings will share the same satisfaction.

In order to recognize the high level of scientific research made by some contributors in our growing field of interest, two awards were delivered during the conference. The Wander Award, dedicated to a young scientist, was handed over to Dr. Ylva R.K. Hellsten (Karolinska Institute, Stockholm, Sweden) for her work on the "Exchange of Purines in Human Liver and Skeletal Muscle With Short-Term Exercise." An Honor Award, allocated to a senior investigator, was attributed to Professor John O. Holloszy (Washington University School of Medicine, St. Louis, Missouri, United States), who received a golden-covered medal in recognition of his outstanding achievement in the field of biochemistry of exercise.

Jacques R. Poortmans
Chairman of the Research Group on Biochemistry of Exercise

Credits

Figure 3.1 Reprinted, by permission, from A.R. Coggan, W.M. Kohrt, R.J. Spina, D.M. Bier, and J.O. Holloszy, 1990, "Endurance training decreases plasma glucose turnover and oxidation during moderate intensity exercise in men," *Journal of Applied Physiology* 68:990-996.

Figure 3.2 Adapted, by permission, from A.R. Coggan, R.J. Spina, W.M. Kohrt, J.P. Kirwan, D.M. Bier, and J.O. Holloszy, 1992, "Plasma glucose kinetics during exercise in subjects with high and low lactate thresholds," *Journal of Applied Physiology* 78:1873-1880.

Figure 3.3 Reprinted, by permission, from L.A. Mendenhall, S.C. Swanson, D.L. Habash, and A.R. Coggan, 1994, "Ten days of exercise training reduces glucose production and utilization during moderate-intensity exercise," *American Journal of Physiology* 266:E136-E143.

Figure 4.2 Reprinted, by permission, from G.I. Bell et al., 1990, "Molecular biology of mammalian glucose transporters," *Diabetes Care* 13:198-208.

Figure 4.3 Reprinted, by permission, from E. Karnieli et al., 1981, "Insulin-stimulated translocation of glucose transport systems in the rat adipose cell," *Journal of Biological Chemistry* 256:4772-4777.

Table 4.1 Reprinted, by permission, from G.I. Bell et al., 1990, "Molecular biology of mammalian glucose transporters," *Diabetes Care* 13:198-208.

Figure 5.1 Reprinted, by permission, from M. Kjaer, B. Kiens, M. Hargreaves, and E.A. Richter, 1991, "Influence of active muscle mass on glucose homeostasis during exercise in humans," *Journal of Applied Physiology* 71:552-557.

Figure 5.2 Reprinted, by permission, from J. Wahren, P. Felig, and L. Hagenfeldt, 1978, "Physical exercise and fuel homeostasis in diabetes mellitus," *Diabetologia* 14:213-222. Copyright 1978 by Springer-Verlag.

Figure 5.3 Reproduced from *The Journal of Clinical Investigation*, 1994, vol. 93, pp. 974-981 by copyright permission of the American Society for Clinical Investigation.

Figure 6.1 Reprinted, by permission, from H. Galbo, 1992, "Exercise physiology: Humoral function," *Sport Science Review* 1(1):72.

Figure 7.2 Reprinted, by permission, from V. Hodgetts, S.W. Coppack, K.N. Frayn, and T.D.R. Hockaday, 1991, "Factors controlling fat mobilization from human subcutaneous adipose tissue during exercise," *Journal of Applied Physiology* 71:445-451.

Figure 7.5   Reprinted, by permission, from A.J. Griffiths, S.M. Humphreys, M.L. Clark, and K.N. Frayn, 1994, "Forearm substrate utilization during exercise after a meal containing both fat and carbohydrate," *Clinical Science* 86:169-175.

Figure 9.1   Reprinted, by permission, from B. Kiens, B. Essen-Gustavsson, N.J. Christensen, and B. Saltin, 1993, "Skeletal muscle substrate utilization during submaximal exercises in man: Effect of endurance training," *Journal of Physiology (London)* 469:459-478.

Figure 9.2   Reprinted, by permission, from L.P. Turcotte, E.A. Richter, and B. Kiens, 1992, "Increased plasma FFA uptake and oxidation during prolonged exercise in trained vs. untrained humans," *American Journal of Physiology* 262:E791-E799.

Figure 9.3   Reprinted, by permission, from L.P. Turcotte, B. Kiens, and E.A. Richter, 1991, "Saturation kinetics of palmitate uptake in perfused skeletal muscle," *FEBS Letters* 279:327-329.

Figure 14.3   Adapted, by permission, from W.W. Winder, J. Arogyasami, I.M. Elayan, and D. Cartmill, 1990, "Time course of exercise-induced decline in malonyl-CoA in different muscle types," *American Journal of Physiology* 259:E266-E271.

Figure 14.4   Reprinted, by permission, from C. Duan and W.W. Winder, 1993, "Control of malonyl-CoA by glucose and insulin in perfused skeletal muscle," *Journal of Applied Physiology* 74:2543-2547.

Figure 19.5   Reprinted, by permission, from G. Bogdanis, M.E. Nevill, L.H. Boobis, H.K.A. Lakomy, and A.M. Nevill, 1995, "Recovery of power output and muscle metabolites following 30 s of maximal sprint cycling in man," *Journal of Physiology* 482(2):467-480.

Figure 19.6   Reprinted, by permission, from G. Bogdanis, M.E. Nevill, L.H. Boobis, H.K.A. Lakomy, and A.M. Nevill, 1995, "Recovery of power output and muscle metabolites following 30 s of maximal sprint cycling in man," *Journal of Physiology* 482(2):467-480.

Figure 20.3   Adapted, by permission, from J. Bangsbo et al., 1992, "Elevated muscle acidity and energy production during exhaustive exercise in man," *American Journal of Physiology* 263:R891-R899.

Figure 20.5   Adapted, by permission, from J. Bangsbo et al., 1992, "Elevated muscle acidity and energy production during exhaustive exercise in man," *American Journal of Physiology* 263:R891-R899.

Figure 20.6   Adapted, by permission, from J. Bangsbo, T.E. Graham, B. Kiens, and B. Saltin, 1992, "Elevated muscle glycogen and anaerobic energy production during exhaustive exercise in man," *Journal of Physiology* 451:205-222.

Table 22.1   Reprinted, by permission, from W.R. Frontera, V.A. Hughes, and W.J. Evans, 1991, ''A cross-sectional study of upper and lower extremity muscle strength in 45-78 year old men and women,'' *Journal of Applied Physiology* 71:646.

Figure 35.1   Adapted, by permission, from J.D. Fernstrom, 1994, ''Dietary amino acids and brain function,'' *Journal of the American Dietetic Association* 94:71-77.

PART I

Regulation of Carbohydrate Metabolism in Exercise

Regulation of Carbohydrate Metabolism During Exercise: New Insights and Remaining Puzzles

John O. Holloszy

Washington University School of Medicine, St. Louis, Missouri, U.S.A.

Muscle glycogen and blood glucose are essential for performance of prolonged, strenuous exercise. Depletion of glycogen in the working muscles or development of hypoglycemia due to depletion of liver glycogen makes continued performance of vigorous exercise impossible. A number of acute and chronic adaptations have evolved to conserve glycogen during exercise. This overview will deal with the regulation of carbohydrate metabolism during exercise, with emphasis on the adaptive responses to training. It is not meant to be a review of the extensive literature on this topic nor to provide a balanced picture of different viewpoints. Rather, its purpose is to summarize the author's views, and to highlight some of the major gaps in our knowledge.

Regulation of Blood Glucose Concentration During Exercise

Blood glucose concentration in the postabsorptive state is determined by the balance between the rate of glucose production by the liver and the rate of glucose utilization by the other tissues. The large increase in glucose removal from the blood during exercise is mediated by increased utilization by the working muscles. During very strenuous exercise, blood glucose concentration may rise as the result of a rapid increase in hepatic glucose production (20), which, as reviewed by Kjær (42), results from a feedforward control mechanism probably mediated by motor center activity stimulation (central command) of sympathoadrenergic activity.

During more moderate exercise of an intensity that can be maintained for 60 min or longer, blood glucose concentration is maintained at a remarkably constant level (2, 11, 22) until liver glycogen depletion occurs, at which time hypoglycemia starts to develop (2, 10, 21). It appears well documented that increases in glucagon and catecholamines and a decrease in insulin level are responsible for protection against the development of hypoglycemia during prolonged exercise (43, 55-57). There is also evidence suggesting that afferent neural feedback from the working muscles plays a major role in the increase in glucose production during exercise (42). However, the mechanisms by which these factors are precisely regulated so as to result in an increase in the rate of glucose production that exactly matches the rate of glucose utilization is one of the major unsolved mysteries in the regulation of carbohydrate metabolism.

Factors Affecting the Regulation of Blood Glucose

There appear to be considerable, probably genetically determined, interindividual differences in the ability to preserve carbohydrate stores and to delay the onset of hypoglycemia during exercise (10). In an individual, the two major factors that determine the rate of blood glucose turnover and how long submaximal exercise of a given intensity can be performed before development of hypoglycemia are nutritional state and level of adaptation to endurance training.

Nutritional State.   In an individual who has been fasting and has a low hepatic glycogen concentration, hypoglycemia develops rapidly during moderately intense exercise, despite a reduced rate of glucose (and an increased rate of fatty acid) utilization, because gluconeogenesis cannot keep pace with the rate of glucose utilization (8, 9, 45). The reverse is true in the postprandial state after assimilation of a high carbohydrate meal in which hypoglycemia is delayed, despite an increased rate of glucose utilization, as the result of a high hepatic glycogen concentration (8, 9, 45).

Effects of Endurance Exercise Training on Blood Glucose Turnover.   The adaptations induced by endurance exercise training interact to result in a sparing of both liver (2) and skeletal muscle (41) glycogen. The magnitude of this sparing effect appears to be a function of the level of the adaptation to exercise in skeletal muscle respiratory capacity, that is, content of mitochondria (30). Because depletion of muscle or liver glycogen results in the inability to continue to exercise vigorously (4, 21, 45), this carbohydrate-sparing effect is one of the most important mechanisms by which training increases the ability to perform prolonged strenuous exercise.

Liver glycogen is the primary source of blood glucose during exercise in the postabsorptive (i.e., no carbohydrate in the gastrointestinal tract) state, while skeletal muscle glycogen, which provides most of the lactate and alanine for hepatic gluconeogenesis via the Cori and alanine cycles, serves as the major secondary source. Endurance exercise training–induced adaptations result in an increase in the proportion of energy derived from fat oxidation during prolonged exercise, resulting in a sparing of glycogen. In a study in which plasma glucose turnover was measured with [^{13}C]glucose in the same individuals before and after endurance exercise training, the rates of plasma glucose appearance (R_a), disposal (R_d), and oxidation were all approximately 33% lower during the same exercise test after training (11).

The same absolute exercise intensity represents a lower relative exercise intensity after a training-induced increase in $\dot{V}O_2$max. The proportion of energy derived from carbohydrate generally increases as exercise intensity is raised, and carbohydrate becomes the predominant fuel during strenuous exercise. Brooks and Mercier have termed the relative exercise intensity at which energy derived from carbohydrate predominates over that derived from fat as the "crossover point" (5). Viewed in this light, the decreased glucose turnover at the same absolute exercise intensity after training can, at least in part, be explained on the basis of a lower relative exercise intensity and, therefore, a smaller metabolic stress. However, well-trained athletes train and compete at relatively high exercise intensities. This raises the question of whether or not the adaptations to exercise training also result in a sparing of carbohydrate at the same relative exercise intensity. Such a comparison is, of course, complicated by the greater total energy requirement and by the recruitment of a larger muscle mass, probably including additional fibers of a different type (fast vs. slow), at the same relative, higher absolute, work rate after training.

There is not much information currently available regarding this question, and more research is needed. However, the information that is available suggests that there is a powerful carbohydrate-sparing effect of training even at the same relative exercise intensity (12, 13, 39). For example, in a study in which endurance exercise training increased $\dot{V}O_2$max from 43.2 ml · kg^{-1} · min^{-1} to 54.9 ml · kg^{-1} · min^{-1}, the respiratory exchange ratio (RER) during exercise requiring 75% of $\dot{V}O_2$max was 0.94 ± 0.1 before training and 0.91 ± 0.01 at the same relative (27% higher absolute) exercise intensity after training (39). This indicates that, whereas carbohydrate oxidation accounted for approximately 79% of the energy utilized at 75% of $\dot{V}O_2$max before training, carbohydrate oxidation accounted for only approximately 69% of the energy utilized after training and that nearly all of the 27% increase in energy expenditure was accounted for by fat oxidation. Furthermore, highly trained endurance athletes with a $\dot{V}O_2$max of 70 ml · kg^{-1} · min^{-1} had a RER of 0.88 ± 0.01 during exercise that required 75% of their $\dot{V}O_2$max, indicating that they were obtaining only approximately 58% of their energy from carbohydrate oxidation (39).

The mechanisms responsible for the slower uptake of glucose by the working muscles and for the closely matched decrease in the rate of hepatic glucose production at the same absolute exercise intensity in the trained state are poorly understood. Particularly remarkable is the still unexplained finding that glucose uptake by the working muscles during exercise at the same absolute intensity is lower after training (11) despite the fact that training increases the number of glucose transporters (GLUT4) in skeletal muscle (37). In studies on rat muscles incubated in vitro, an increase in GLUT4 is associated with increased rates of insulin- and contraction-stimulated glucose transport (48, 51).

Although the mechanisms have not been elucidated, it seems probable that the slower rate of glucose utilization is mediated by the endurance training–induced skeletal muscle adaptations that are responsible for the increased reliance on fat oxidation for energy (36). It seems clear, however, that the reduction in glucose uptake is not mediated by the classical glucose–fatty acid cycle (14). It appears likely that the effects of these adaptations on intramuscular metabolic homeostasis during exercise are responsible for the slower hepatic glucose production via a feedback mechanism that probably involves decreased catecholamine and glucagon production (42). It is of interest in this regard that, in a study of subjects who had similar $\dot{V}O_2$max but different levels of citrate synthase (which was used as a mitochondrial marker) in their vastus lateralis muscles, there was a significant inverse relationship between citrate synthase activity and the rates of plasma glucose turnover and oxidation (12). Along the same line, in a study comparing groups of rats at different levels of training, there were significant correlations between muscle respiratory capacity and the amounts of glycogen remaining in liver, in skeletal muscle, and in liver plus skeletal muscle after a 30-min exercise test (30).

Regulation of Glycogenolysis in Skeletal Muscle During Exercise

During strenuous sustained exercise or stimulation of muscles to contract in situ at intensities at which a near steady state can be attained, there is an initial burst of glycogenolysis followed by a slowing, or in some cases even a cessation, of net glycogen depletion (3, 16, 18, 41). During prolonged moderate intensity exercise, there can even be net muscle glycogen synthesis if glucose is provided (19, 38). The initial burst of glycogenolysis results in an increase in muscle lactate, which is followed by a decline despite continued contractile activity (18, 28, 35, 40). The magnitude of the initial burst of glycogenolysis and of the associated increase in muscle lactate is determined by a variety of factors, including the relative intensity of the exercise, the type of muscle involved, the initial glycogen concentration, and, very importantly, the level of endurance training. The burst of glycogenolysis and increase in lactate are smaller in trained than in untrained muscles at the same work rate (18, 26, 28).

These findings cannot be explained in terms of the classical textbook concepts regarding the regulation of glycogenolysis in skeletal muscle during exercise. Briefly summarized, glycogen phosphorylase, which catalyzes the phosphorolysis of the α-1,4–linked residues in glycogen to form glucose-1-phosphate, exists in two molecular forms. Phosphorylase b is inactive in the absence of AMP, while phosphorylase a is active in the absence of AMP or other effectors (29, 33).

The Role of Calcium

Phosphorylase b is converted to the a form by phosphorylase kinase, which requires calcium (Ca^{2+}) for catalytic activity (6, 29, 33). Phosphorylase kinase exists in a dephosphorylated, less active b form that is converted to the more active a form by protein kinase a, which is activated by increases in cAMP in response to catecholamines (15, 29, 33). Phosphorylase kinase a can activate phosphorylase at the low Ca^{2+} concentration found in the cytosol of resting muscle, while phosphorylase kinase b is inactive in resting muscle but becomes active at the Ca^{2+} concentration attained in contracting muscle (6, 29, 33). Phosphorylase b is inactive in the absence of AMP, and although the concentration of AMP in resting muscle appears to be above the K_m for its activation, phosphorylase b is thought to remain inactive because most of the AMP is protein bound (31, 44) and because of the inhibitory effects of the relatively high ATP and glucose-6-phosphate concentrations (29).

The classical picture of the regulation of glycogenolysis in skeletal muscle is based on the premise that glycogenolysis does not occur in resting muscle, because phosphorylase is essentially completely in the inactive b form (24, 29, 33). This belief persisted despite the rather consistent finding of a significant fraction, in the range of 5% to 15%, of phosphorylase in the a form in muscle under physiological conditions. The presence of phosphorylase a in resting muscle was attributed to a preparation artifact (i.e., activation during freezing or muscle homogenization). However, despite improvements in the procedures for freezing and extraction of muscle, there has been no tendency for the reported values of the proportion of phosphorylase in the *a* form in resting muscle to decline over the past 30 years, and the weight of evidence indicates that a significant proportion of phosphorylase is in the *a* form in resting muscles under physiological conditions (31, 47).

The generally accepted picture of the regulation of glycogenolysis in skeletal muscle during exercise, which is still presented in textbooks, was that muscle contraction and glycogen breakdown are coordinated by the transient increases in cytosolic Ca^{2+} concentration. In this context, it was thought that the rate of glycogenolysis is determined by the frequency of muscle contraction, with each stimulus resulting in release of Ca^{2+}, activation of phosphorylase kinase *b*, conversion of phosphorylase *b* to *a*, and a burst of glycogenolysis. This concept was based on studies on purified enzymes, on glycogen-enzyme particles, and on muscles subjected to brief tetanic stimulation (6, 23, 25, 29, 34, 53).

This picture has had to be modified because of the discovery that phosphorylase activation reverses within a few minutes during more prolonged contractile activity and that this reversal occurs despite continued contractile activity, even in the absence of muscle fatigue (i.e., during normal excitation-contraction coupling [16]). This finding was soon confirmed in other studies on rat muscles stimulated to contract in situ (1, 49, 50) and also in human skeletal muscle biopsied during exercise (7). The reversal of phosphorylase activation after a short time is important because it makes prolonged exercise possible. The activation of phosphorylase by the Ca^{2+} mechanism at the onset of exercise results in an overshoot of glycogen breakdown, far in excess of the muscles' energy requirement, with accumulation of lactate. If, as was originally thought, glycogenolysis was geared to contraction frequency, with activation by the Ca^{2+} released from the sarcoplasmic reticulum (SR) during each excitation-contraction cycle, prolonged exercise would be impossible because of fatigue caused either by lactate accumulation or by glycogen depletion.

It is now evident from the studies showing that phosphorylase activation rapidly reverses during continuous exercise that stimulation of glycogenolysis by the Ca^{2+} mechanism is transient and shuts off after making a large supply of pyruvate available to the mitochondria. Most of this pyruvate accumulates as lactate, which is in equilibrium with pyruvate in the cytosol. The mechanisms responsible for the reversal of phosphorylase activation despite continued contractile activity are not yet well understood.

The Glycogen-Enzyme-SR Complex

One process that may be involved is release of phosphorylase from glycogen (27). Most of the phosphorylase in skeletal muscle is bound to a glycogen-enzyme-SR complex that also contains phosphorylase kinase (27, 34). It seems possible that reversal of phosphorylase activation during exercise is mediated, in part, by glycogen breakdown, which releases phosphorylase and thus uncouples it from phosphorylase kinase and the Ca^{2+}-activating mechanism, and also exposes it to the inactivating enzyme phosphorylase phosphatase.

In support of this possibility, it has been shown that activation of phosphorylase by both epinephrine treatment and stimulation of contraction is severely inhibited in glycogen-depleted muscles after exercise (17). This finding can be explained by the glycogen breakdown–phosphorylase release hypothesis if, as seems probable (32), the stearic relationship between phosphorylase kinase and phosphorylase plays a crucial role in phosphorylase activation. Factors other than glycogen depletion are, however, also involved, as evidenced by the finding that phosphorylase activation is more severely inhibited after a long- than after a short-duration run to exhaustion despite a similar degree of muscle glycogen depletion (nicotinic acid was used to accelerate glycogen depletion and development of exhaustion in the short-duration exercise group) (17).

While net muscle glycogen breakdown can stop or markedly slow during moderate intensity exercise (3, 19) and during stimulation of muscles to contract in situ (16, 49), it is well documented that strenuous exercise to the point of exhaustion can result in progressive, almost complete glycogen depletion (4, 54). If the Ca^{2+} mechanism for activating phosphorylase becomes inhibited during exercise, how is this muscle glycogen depletion brought about? One possibility that has been suggested is that phosphorylase may be reactivated by a β-adrenergic stimulation–mediated increase in cAMP (49, 50, 52). Another is that during prolonged exercise a relatively small number of muscle fibers are recruited to contract at any one time, so that intermittent recruitment of motor units might allow sufficient recovery of the activation process to make possible another burst of glycogenolysis when fibers that have not been contracting are again recruited (17). Although both of these mechanisms seem reasonable and could play a role, there is currently no evidence that a reactivation of phosphorylase actually occurs during continuous exercise. Furthermore, during prolonged exercise at a given work rate, after the initial burst of glycogenolysis the rate of glycogen breakdown appears to be a function of the exercise intensity, and neither of these mechanisms involve regulatory processes for controlling the rate of glycogenolysis to match the energy requirement.

The Role of Inorganic Phosphate

A new explanation for continuous glycogen depletion during strenuous prolonged exercise that does provide a mechanism for gearing the rate of glycogenolysis to exercise intensity is based on two concepts that seemed heretical when first proposed. One is that a physiologically significant proportion of phosphorylase is in the *a* form in resting muscles in vivo (31, 47). This is in contrast to the classical model of glycogenolysis, which was built on the premise that essentially all of the phosphorylase in relaxed muscle is in the inactive *b* form and that the phosphorylase *a* activity found in resting muscle samples is a freezing or extraction artifact (24, 29, 33). The other is that availability of inorganic phosphate (Pi) rather than phosphorylase activity limits glycogenolysis in resting muscle (7, 31). This concept has been used to explain continued glycogenolysis during exercise after phosphorylase activation has reversed with a return of phosphorylase *a* percentage to or below the baseline, resting value (46).

A recent study of the effects of hypoxia and epinephrine on rat epitrochlearis muscle incubated in vitro has provided direct evidence that the concentration of Pi does limit glycogenolysis in muscle (46). Under conditions that caused no decrease in muscle glycogen in oxygenated muscle, hypoxia caused sustained glycogenolysis, with a 70% decrease in glycogen concentration over 80 min in the absence of any increase in phosphorylase in the *a* form above the basal level of about 10%. The hypoxia resulted in a large increase in muscle Pi concentration. Incubation of muscles with epinephrine in oxygenated medium resulted in an approximately sixfold increase in phosphorylase *a* percentage, but no increase in Pi, and only minimal glycogenolysis over 20 min. Despite a sixfold higher phosphorylase *a* percentage in the epinephrine-treated muscles, there was a fivefold greater glycogen depletion in the hypoxic muscles over 20 min.

Activation of phosphorylase by epinephrine in hypoxic muscles accelerated the rate of glycogenolysis about twofold. Inhibition of phosphorylase *b* had a negligible effect on the rate of glycogenolysis in hypoxic muscle (46). These findings provide direct evidence that the phosphorylase *a* activity present in unstimulated muscle is sufficient to mediate rapid glycogenolysis, that the low concentration of Pi prevents net glycogenolysis in resting, oxygenated muscle, and that an increase in Pi can cause glycogenolysis in muscle in the absence of an increase in % phosphorylase *a*. These findings also explain how continuing glycogen breakdown is mediated in contracting muscles in which phosphorylase activation has reversed and % phosphorylase *a* has returned to the level found in resting muscle.

One of the major physiological manifestations of the adaptation to endurance exercise training is a sparing of muscle glycogen. This effect is manifested both as a smaller initial burst of glycogenolysis and a slower rate of glycogen utilization during prolonged exercise (18, 28, 30, 41). The effect of training on the initial, Ca^{2+}-mediated burst of glycogenolysis has been studied in rat skeletal muscles stimulated to contract in situ (18, 28). The initial, rapid phase of glycogenolysis is markedly attenuated in endurance-trained skeletal muscles, despite no difference in the extent of phosphorylase activation as reflected in the increase in % phosphorylase *a* (28). However, as the result of the adaptive increase in mitochondria in the trained muscles (36), the decrease in phosphocreatine and, therefore, the increase in Pi concentration is markedly attenuated in response to the same contractile activity (18, 28). The steady-state concentration of Pi maintained in the muscles during continued contractile activity is also lower in the trained muscles. It seems likely that the lower level of Pi in trained muscles plays a major role in accounting for both the smaller initial burst of glycogenolysis and the slower rate of glycogen depletion during sustained contractile activity (18, 28).

In conclusion, there are still a number of major unanswered questions regarding the mechanisms involved in the regulation of carbohydrate metabolism during exercise. These include the mechanisms involved in (a) regulating hepatic glucose production to accurately match the rate of glucose uptake by the working muscles and (b) bringing about a slower rate of glucose uptake by the working muscles at the same absolute work rate in the trained than in the untrained state despite increases in GLUT4 and insulin sensitivity. On a more positive note, we now have at least a partial understanding of the mechanisms involved in gearing muscle glycogenolysis to work rate and in bringing about a slower rate of muscle glycogen depletion during exercise in the trained state.

Acknowledgments

The author's research was supported by NIH grants DK18986 and AG00425.

References

1. Aragón, J.J.; Tornheim, K.; Lowenstein, J.M. On a possible role of IMP in the regulation of phosphorylase activity in skeletal muscle. FEBS Lett. 117:K56-K64; 1980.

2. Baldwin, K.M.; Fitts, R.H.; Booth, F.W.; Winder, W.W.; Holloszy, J.O. Depletion of muscle and liver glycogen during exercise: Protective effect of training. Pflügers Arch. 354:203-212; 1975.

3. Baldwin, K.M.; Reitman, J.S.; Terjung, R.L.; Winder, W.W.; Holloszy, J.O. Substrate depletion in different types of muscle and in liver during prolonged running. Am. J. Physiol. 225:1045-1050; 1973.

4. Bergström, J.; Hermansen, L.; Hultman, E.; Saltin, B. Diet, muscle glycogen and physical performance. Acta Physiol. Scand. 71:140-150; 1967.

5. Brooks, G.A.; Mercier, J. Balance of carbohydrate and lipid utilization during exercise: The "crossover" concept. J. Appl. Physiol. 76:2253-2261; 1994.

6. Brostrom, C.O.; Hunkeler, F.L.; Krebs, E.G. The regulation of skeletal muscle phosphorylase kinase by Ca^{2+}. J. Biol. Chem. 246:1961-1967; 1971.

7. Chasiotis, D. The regulation of glycogen phosphorylase and glycogen breakdown in human skeletal muscle. Acta Physiol. Scand. (suppl. 518):1-68; 1983.

8. Christensen, E.H.; Hansen, O. Arbeitsfahigkeit und Ernährung. Skand. Arch. Physiol. 81:160-171; 1939a.

9. Christensen, E.H.; Hansen, O. Hypoglykame, arbeitsfahigkeit und ermudung. Skand. Arch. Physiol. 81:172-179; 1939b.

10. Coggan, A.R.; Coyle, E.F. Carbohydrate ingestion during prolonged exercise: Effects on metabolism and performance. Exercise Sport Sci. Rev. 19:1-40; 1991.

11. Coggan, A.R.; Kohrt, W.M.; Spina, R.J.; Bier, D.M.; Holloszy, J.O. Endurance training decreases plasma glucose turnover and oxidation during moderate-intensity exercise in men. J. Appl. Physiol. 68:990-996; 1990.

12. Coggan, A.R.; Kohrt, W.M.; Spina, R.J.; Kirwan, J.P.; Bier, D.M.; Holloszy, J.O. Plasma glucose kinetics during exercise in subjects with high and low lactate thresholds. J. Appl. Physiol. 73:1873-1880; 1992.

13. Coggan, A.R.; Raguso, C.A.; Williams, B.D.; Sidossis, L.S. Endurance training reduces plasma glucose utilization during exercise at 80% of $\dot{V}O_2$max. Med. Sci. Sports Exercise 26 (suppl.):S89; 1994. (Abstract.)

14. Coggan, A.R.; Spina, R.J.; Kohrt, W.M.; Holloszy, J.O. Effect of prolonged exercise on muscle citrate concentration before and after endurance training in men. Am. J. Physiol. 264:E215-E220; 1993.

15. Cohen, P. The role of calmodulin, troponin, and cyclic AMP in the regulation of glycogen metabolism in mammalian skeletal muscle. In: Dumont, J.E.; Greengard, P.; Robinson, G.A., eds. Advances in cyclic nucleotide research. New York: Raven; 1981:345-359.

16. Conlee, R.K.; McLane, J.A.; Rennie, M.J.; Winder, W.W.; Holloszy, J.O. Reversal of phosphorylase activation in muscle despite continued contractile activity. Am. J. Physiol. 237:R291-R296; 1979.

17. Constable, S.H.; Favier, R.J.; Holloszy, J.O. Exercise and glycogen depletion: Effects on ability to activate muscle phosphorylase. J. Appl. Physiol. 60:1518-1523; 1986.

18. Constable, S.H.; Favier, R.J.; McLane, J.A.; Fell, R.D.; Chen, M.; Holloszy, J.O. Energy metabolism in contracting rat skeletal muscle: Adaptation to exercise training. Am. J. Physiol. 253:C316-C322; 1987.

19. Constable, S.H.; Young, J.C.; Higuchi, M.; Holloszy, J.O. Glycogen resynthesis in leg muscles of rats during exercise. Am. J. Physiol. 247:R880-R883; 1984.

20. Cooper, D.M.; Barstow, T.J.; Bergner, A.; Lee, W.N.P. Blood glucose turnover during high- and low-intensity exercise. Am. J. Physiol. 257:E405-E412; 1989.

21. Coyle, E.F.; Hagberg, J.M.; Martin, W.H.; Hurley, B.; Holloszy, J.O. Carbohydrate feeding during prolonged strenuous exercise can delay fatigue. J. Appl. Physiol. 55:320-325; 1983.

22. Cryer, P.E. Glucose counterregulation in man. Diabetes 30:261-264; 1981.

23. Danforth, W.H.; Helmreich, E. Regulation of glycolysis in muscle. I. The conversion of phosphorylase b to phosphorylase a in frog sartorius muscle. J. Biol. Chem. 239:3133-3138; 1964.

24. Danforth, W.H.; Helmreich, E.; Cori, C.F. The effect of contraction and of epinephrine on the phosphorylase activity of frog sartorius muscle. Proc. Natl. Acad. Sci. USA 48:1191-1199; 1962.

25. Drummond, G.I.; Harwood, J.P.; Powell, C.A. Studies on the activation of phosphorylase in skeletal muscle by contraction and epinephrine. J. Biol. Chem. 244:4235-4240; 1969.

26. Dudley, G.A.; Tullson, P.C.; Terjung, R.L. Influence of mitochondrial content on the sensitivity of respiratory control. J. Biol. Chem. 262:9109-9114; 1987.

27. Entman, M.L.; Keslensky, S.S.; Chu, A.; Van Winkle, W.B. The sarcoplasmic reticulum-glycogenolytic complex in mammalian fast twitch skeletal muscle. J. Biol. Chem. 255:6245-6252; 1980.

28. Favier, R.J.; Constable, S.H.; Chen, M.; Holloszy, J.O. Endurance exercise training reduces lactate production. J. Appl. Physiol. 61:885-889; 1986.

29. Fischer, E.H.; Heilmeyer, L.M.G.; Haschke, R.H. Phosphorylase and the control of glycogen degradation. Curr. Top. Cell. Regul. 4:211-251; 1971.

30. Fitts, R.H.; Booth, F.W.; Winder, W.W.; Holloszy, J.O. Skeletal muscle respiratory capacity, endurance and glycogen utilization. Am. J. Physiol. 228:1029-1033; 1975.

31. Griffiths, J.R. A fresh look at glycogenolysis in skeletal muscle. Biosci. Rep. 1:595-610; 1981a.

32. Griffiths, J.R. Non-covalent control of glycogenolysis in muscle. In: Hue, L.; Van de Werve, G., eds. Short-term regulation of liver metabolism. Amsterdam: Elsevier; 1981b:77-91.

33. Gross, S.R.; Mayer, S.E. Regulation of phosphorylase b to a conversion in muscle. Life Sci. 14:401-414; 1974.

34. Heilmeyer, L.M.G., Jr.; Meyer, F.; Haschke, R.H.; Fischer, E.H. Control of phosphorylase activity in muscle glycogen particle. II. Activation by calcium. J. Biol. Chem. 245:6649-6656; 1970.

35. Hirche, H.; Wacker, U.; Langohr, H.D. Lactic acid formation in the working gastrocnemius of the dog. Int. Z. Angew. Physiol. 30:52-64; 1971.

36. Holloszy, J.O.; Coyle, E.F. Adaptations of skeletal muscle to endurance exercise and their metabolic consequences. J. Appl. Physiol. 56:831-839; 1984.

37. Houmard, J.A.; Shinebarger, M.H.; Dolan, P.L.; Leggett-Frazier, N.; Bruner, R.K.; McCammon, M.R.; Israel, R.G.; Dohm, G.L. Exercise training increases GLUT-4 protein concentration in previously sedentary middle-aged men. Am. J. Physiol. 264:E896-E901; 1993.

38. Hultman, E.; Bergström, J.; Roche-Norlund, A.E. Glycogen storage in human skeletal muscle. In: Pernow, B.; Saltin, B., eds. Muscle metabolism during exercise. New York: Plenum Press; 1971:273-288.

39. Hurley, B.F.; Hagberg, J.M.; Allen, W.K.; Seals, D.R.; Young, J.C.; Cudihee, R.W.; Holloszy, J.O. The effects of training on blood lactate levels during submaximal exercise. J. Appl. Physiol. 56:1260-1264; 1984.

40. Jorfeldt, L.; Juhlin-Dannfelt, A.; Karlsson, J. Lactate release in relation to tissue lactate in human skeletal muscle during exercise. J. Appl. Physiol. 44:350-352; 1978.

41. Karlsson, J.; Nordesjo, L.; Saltin, B. Muscle glycogen utilization during exercise after physical training. Acta Physiol. Scand. 90:210-217; 1974.

42. Kjær, M. Regulation of hormonal and metabolic responses during exercise in humans. Exercise Sport Sci. Rev. 20:161-184; 1992.

43. Marker, J.C.; Hirsch, I.B.; Smith, L.J.; Parvin, C.A.; Holloszy, J.O.; Cryer, P.E. Catecholamines in prevention of hypoglycemia during exercise in humans. Am. J. Physiol. 23:E705-E712; 1991.

44. McGilvery, R.W.; Murray, T.W. Calculated equilibria of phosphocreatine and adenosine phosphates during utilization of high energy phosphate by muscle. J. Biol. Chem. 249:5845-5849; 1974.

45. Pruett, E.D.R. Glucose and insulin during prolonged work stress in men living on different diets. J. Appl. Physiol. 28:199-208; 1970.

46. Ren, J.M.; Gulve, E.A.; Cartee, G.D.; Holloszy, J.O. Hypoxia causes glycogenolysis without an increase in percent phosphorylase a in rat skeletal muscle. Am. J. Physiol. 263:E1086-E1091; 1993.

47. Ren, J.M.; Hultman, E. Phosphorylase activity in needle biopsy samples: Factors influencing transformation. Acta Physiol. Scand. 133:109-114; 1988.

48. Ren, J.; Semenkovich, C.F.; Gulve, E.A.; Gao, J.; Holloszy, J.O. Exercise induces rapid increases in GLUT4 expression, glucose transport capacity, and insulin-stimulated glycogen storage in muscle. J. Biol. Chem. 269:14396-14401; 1994.

49. Rennie, M.J.; Fell, R.D.; Ivy, J.L.; Holloszy, J.O. Adrenaline reactivation of muscle phosphorylase after deactivation during phasic contractile activity. Biosci. Rep. 2:323-331; 1982.

50. Richter, E.A.; Ruderman, N.B.; Gavras, H.; Belur, E.R.; Galbo, H. Muscle glycogenolysis during exercise: Dual control by epinephrine and contractions. Am. J. Physiol. 242:E25-E32; 1982.

51. Rodnick, K.J.; Henriksen, E.J.; James, D.E.; Holloszy, J.O. Exercise-training, glucose transporters and glucose transport in rat skeletal muscles. Am. J. Physiol. 262:C9-C14; 1992.

52. Spriet, L.L.; Ren, J.M.; Hultman, E. Epinephrine infusion enhances muscle glycogenolysis during prolonged electrical stimulation. J. Appl. Physiol. 64:1439-1444; 1988.

53. Stull, J.T.; Meyer, S.T. Regulation of phosphorylase activation in skeletal muscle in vivo. J. Biol. Chem. 246:5716-5723; 1971.

54. Terjung, R.L.; Baldwin, K.M.; Molé, P.A.; Klinkerfuss, G.H.; Holloszy, J.O. Effect of running to exhaustion on skeletal muscle mitochondria: A biochemical study. Am. J. Physiol. 223:549-554; 1972.

55. Vranic, M.; Kawamori, R.; Pek, S.; Kovacevic, N.; Wrenshall, G.A. The essentiality of insulin and the role of glucagon in regulating glucose utilization and production during strenuous exercise in dogs. J. Clin. Invest. 57:245-255; 1976.

56. Wasserman, D.H.; Lickley, H.L.A.; Vranic, M. Interactions between glucagon and other counterregulatory hormones during normoglycemic and hypoglycemic exercise in dogs. J. Clin. Invest. 74:1404-1413; 1984.

57. Wolfe, R.R.; Nadel, E.R.; Shaw, J.H.F.; Stephenson, L.A.; Wolfe, M.H. Role of changes in insulin and glucagon in glucose homeostasis in exercise. J. Clin. Invest. 77:900-907; 1986.

CHAPTER 2

Carbohydrate Metabolism in Human Muscle Studied With the Glycemic Clamp Technique: The Influence of Physical Training

Flemming Dela

Department of Medical Physiology, The Panum Institute, Copenhagen, Denmark

This review discusses the effect of physical training on insulin-stimulated glucose uptake and carbohydrate metabolism in human skeletal muscle. The significance of aging and type 2 diabetes mellitus (NIDDM) on these parameters will be considered. Data from studies performed in three groups of subjects will be discussed; the characteristics of these subjects are shown in table 2.1. All subjects participated in the same training program, which consisted of one-legged ergometer-bicycle training for 10 wk, 6 d/wk, 30 min/d. Insulin-stimulated glucose uptake was measured in the legs by the glucose clamp technique combined with catheterization of both femoral veins and an artery. In the elderly and in the NIDDM subjects, this was done before the training started and again 16 h after the last one-legged training bout. In these two groups, data on limb substrate balances from the two legs at the first clamp are pooled (untrained legs [UT]) and will be compared with data obtained from measurements on the trained leg (T) during the second clamp. In the young subjects, however, no clamp was carried out before the training started, and comparisons of limb substrate balances are made between the two legs (one untrained [UT] and one trained [T]) from data obtained on the same clamp day 16 h after the last one-legged training bout. This means that if cotraining of the nontraining leg took place, the effect of training on the measured parameters will tend to be underestimated in the young subjects. In addition, in all groups an identical clamp was carried out after 6 d of detraining the trained leg, whereas on the fifth day, the nontraining leg performed a 30-min bout of acute exercise.

The Glucose Clamp and Arteriovenous Catheterization Technique

The principles behind the hyperinsulinemic glucose clamp technique were first outlined in 1966 (2), later refined (14), and have since been extensively used in

Table 2.1   Characteristics of Study Subjects

	$n =$	Age (yrs)	Weight (kg)	BMI (kg/m^2)	Body fat (%)	$\dot{V}O_2max$ (ml · min^{-1} · kg^{-1})	Fasting plasma glucose (mM)	Fasting plasma insulin (pmol · L^{-1})
Young								
Before training	7	23 ± 1	69 ± 2	21 ± 1	9 ± 1	46 ± 3*	ND	ND
After training	—	—	70 ± 1	21 ± 1	8 ± 1	52 ± 2*	5.3 ± .01	65 ± 7
Elderly								
Before training	8	59 ± 1	83 ± 3	26 ± 1	21 ± 2	31 ± 2	5.8 ± 0.2	72 ± 7
After training	—	—	83 ± 2	26 ± 1	21 ± 2	35 ± 2	5.6 ± 0.1	65 ± 7
NIDDM								
Before training	8	58 ± 2	86 ± 4	29 ± 1	26 ± 2	28 ± 2	10.2 ± 1.4	187 ± 22
After training	—	—	85 ± 4	29 ± 1	25 ± 2	31 ± 2	9.6 ± 1.5	144 ± 14

*Obtained during one-legged bicycle test.

ND, not determined.

measurements of whole-body insulin action. In short, plasma insulin concentrations are elevated to a desired level by infusion of exogenous insulin, while the plasma glucose concentration is maintained by a variable glucose infusion based on frequent measurements of plasma glucose concentrations. Plasma glucose concentrations can be kept within (euglycemic clamp) or below (hypoglycemic clamp) the normal range, or at any glycemic level (isoglycemic clamp).

The induced hyperinsulinemia decreases endogenous insulin secretion (as judged from measurements of C-peptide [14, 36]) and increases glucose utilization, and at high insulin concentrations (> approximately 700 pmol · L^{-1}) hepatic glucose production (HGP) ceases.

Glucose infusion rates (GIR), necessary to maintain the chosen glycemic level, increase during the clamp. However, after approximately 90 min of hyperinsulinemia and glucose infusion, a leveling off in GIR is seen, and GIR now equals the sum of the decrease in HGP and the increase in glucose utilization. It has been questioned whether a steady-state situation is actually present after 90 min, since an increase in GIR has been found even after 5 and 6 h of hyperinsulinemia (≈ 650 pmol · L^{-1}) (20, 33). In the studies presented here, however, GIR did not increase significantly from 90 to 120 min, and the average GIR during these 30 min (corrected for loss of glucose in urine) is taken as an index of whole-body insulin action.

In these studies insulin was infused in order to achieve plasma insulin concentrations of approximately 350, 1,200, and 16,000 pmol · L^{-1} in both healthy subjects and in patients with NIDDM. The highest insulin concentration is a true maximal insulin stimulus for glucose uptake, as increasing plasma insulin concentrations to approximately 70,000 pmol · L^{-1} does not increase glucose uptake rates further (6).

By the use of the hyperinsulinemic glucose clamp technique, whole-body insulin action is estimated, but no distinction between the various insulin-sensitive tissues can be made. Skeletal muscle accounts for the major part of glucose utilization during hyperinsulinemia, and by combining the hyperinsulinemic glucose clamp technique with arteriovenous catheterization of a leg or a forearm, the influence of hyperinsulinemia on skeletal muscle glucose metabolism can be estimated. Net uptake and release of hormones, substrates, and metabolites are calculated as measured arteriovenous (a-v) differences times blood flow in the limb. Furthermore, by measurement of oxygen (O_2) and carbon dioxide (CO_2) concentrations in the arterial and venous blood, local RQ values can be calculated, and local carbohydrate and lipid metabolism can be estimated according to the principles of indirect calorimetry (23, 41). However, to calculate these parameters, protein oxidation in the limb must also be considered. A constant value can be used (26), or the protein oxidation in the limb can be estimated by assuming that limb protein oxidation constitutes the same fraction of whole-body protein oxidation as limb oxygen uptake of whole-body oxygen uptake: protein oxidation$_{limb}$ = protein oxidation$_{whole\ body}$ × $\dot{V}O_{2(limb)}$/ $\dot{V}O_{2(whole\ body)}$ (17). Second, as most automatic analyzers measure CO_2 in the plasma phase, it is important to convert to whole blood CO_2 content (21).

Anatomically, muscle mass in the leg is approximately 64% of leg weight (43), but from a metabolic point of view much more (approximately 95%) than that (39). Thus, the leg serves well as a perfused muscle preparation in analogy to the perfused rat hindquarter (39), and the balances measured across the leg are attributed to skeletal muscle. The model has been used to assess the influence of acute exercise (3) and of decreased physical activity (34, 37) on insulin-stimulated glucose uptake. In numerous studies, in both healthy subjects and in patients with NIDDM, the model has been used to characterize insulin-stimulated blood flow and glucose metabolism in skeletal muscle during rest and during exercise, but until recently (17, 18) the model had not been used to evaluate the effect of training on insulin-stimulated glucose metabolism in skeletal muscle.

The forearm has also been used as a perfused muscle preparation (22, 32). In this model the venous catheter is inserted into an antecubital vein in the retrograde direction (deep venous catheter), and the blood flow is mostly measured by venous occlusion plethysmography (44), but the dye dilution technique has also been used (32). However, using the forearm presents no advantage compared with using the legs. On the contrary, the muscle mass in the forearm is very small compared to that in the leg, demanding highly sensitive techniques in order to detect the smaller differences in the measured parameters. Furthermore, although the venous blood sampling technique is essential, withdrawal of large blood samples (> 10 ml) can lead to admixture of blood from superficial veins or to retrograde mixing (40).

The Effect of Insulin on Blood Flow

Where limb blood flow was measured by dye or thermodilution techniques, most studies (16, 17, 30, 34) but not all (12, 13) have reported an increase in blood flow with insulin in a dose-dependent manner.

The mechanism by which insulin stimulates leg blood flow and thereby increases glucose delivery to the muscles is unknown. Most likely, the vasodilatory effect of insulin is secondary to an insulin-mediated increase in local metabolism (1, 16, 30), but a direct or nerve-mediated effect on smooth muscle in the arterioles is also possible (1, 10).

It has been suggested that the skeletal muscle insulin resistance seen in patients with NIDDM could be explained to a great extent by an impaired effect of insulin to increase glucose delivery to the muscles (31). However, this conclusion was reached based on clamp studies carried out at euglycemia (31), which is by definition not the normal condition for patients with NIDDM. During euglycemia, patients with NIDDM have a diminished metabolic rate, since no glucose is taken up by mass action. The euglycemic situation is artificial, and the patients are not investigated in their habitual state. In contrast, if insulin-stimulated blood flow is measured during isoglycemic conditions (i.e., glucose clamp at fasting glucose concentrations), the metabolic rate is similar to that in matched healthy controls, and so is the blood flow response to increasing insulin concentrations (figure 2.1; 16). Therefore, the insulin resistance seen in skeletal muscle of NIDDM patients cannot be attributed to a defect in glucose delivery.

An increase in insulin concentration from approximately 350 to approximately 1,200 pmol · L^{-1} resulted in an increase in blood flow by $32 \pm 14\%$ (UT and T legs pooled) in young subjects, while the increase was less pronounced ($21 \pm 3\%$; $p <$ .05) in the elderly subjects (figure 2.1). Thus, a decreased ability to increase blood flow in response to insulin seems to develop with age.

The Effect of Training on Insulin-Stimulated Leg Blood Flow

During glucose clamps, the highest blood flow rates are seen in young, healthy subjects (figure 2.1). This is only partly explained by increased muscle mass in younger subjects, as leg blood flow per kilogram was still higher in young than in elderly or NIDDM subjects (data not shown). At all insulin concentrations, blood

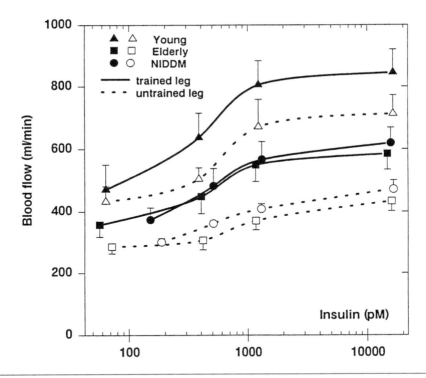

Figure 2.1   Insulin-stimulated blood flow in trained and untrained legs in seven young (23 ± 1 yr) and eight elderly (59 ± 1 yr) healthy subjects and in seven patients with NIDDM (58 ± 1 yr), all of whom had performed one-legged endurance training for 10 wk. Blood flow was measured at rest by thermodilution technique during a three-step hyperinsulinemic glucose clamp, in which fasting plasma glucose concentrations were maintained, in combination with catheterization of both femoral veins and an artery. Blood flow always increased in response to insulin infusions ($p < .05$) and was higher ($p < .05$) in the young subjects than in the elderly or in NIDDM patients, with no difference between the latter two groups. The increase in blood flow from insulin concentrations at approximately 350 to 1,200 pmol · L^{-1} was higher ($p < .05$) in young than in elderly subjects (32 ± 14% and 21 ± 3%, respectively; T and UT leg pooled).

flow was higher in trained (T) than in untrained (UT) legs (figure 2.1). However, in young subjects no difference ($p > .05$) between T and UT legs was seen when flow was corrected for the increased muscle mass in the T leg. In contrast to the young subjects, the difference between T and UT legs still existed in the NIDDM ($p = .06$) and elderly ($p = .006$; two-way ANOVA for repeated measures) subjects after correction for increased muscle mass in the T leg.

Leg Muscle Glucose Extraction

Arteriovenous glucose concentration differences in the legs are expressed relative to the prevailing arterial glycemic level (i.e., as glucose extraction ratios [artery-venous/venous]; figure 2.2). This permits comparisons between groups

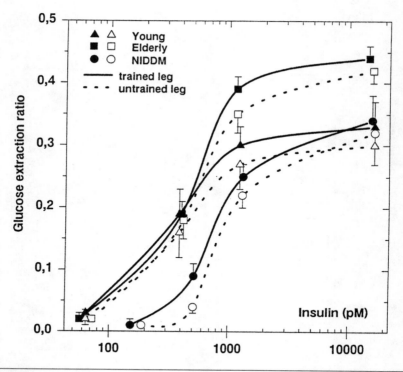

Figure 2.2 Glucose extraction ratio during insulin stimulation in trained and untrained legs in seven young (23 ± 1 yr) and eight elderly (59 ± 1 yr) healthy subjects and in seven patients with NIDDM (58 ± 3 yr), all of whom had performed one-legged endurance training for 10 wk. Glucose extraction ratio was measured during a three-step hyperinsulinemic glucose clamp, in which fasting plasma glucose concentrations were maintained, in combination with catheterization of both femoral veins and an artery. Glucose extraction ratios were calculated as arteriovenous glucose concentration differences divided by arterial glucose concentration [(a − v)/v]. Glucose extraction ratios were always higher during insulin infusion in T than in UT legs in young subjects ($p < .05$), whereas the difference between T and UT legs did not attain statistical significance in the elderly subjects or in the NIDDM patients. During insulin infusion, glucose extraction ratios were always higher ($p < .05$) in elderly subjects than in NIDDM patients. At the two highest insulin concentrations, glucose extraction ratios were higher ($p < .05$) in elderly than in young subjects.

clamped at different glucose concentrations. In the young subjects, the glucose extraction ratio was higher in T than in UT legs at basal ($p < .1$) and subsequent ($p < .05$) insulin concentrations (figure 2.2). In contrast, the difference in glucose extraction ratios between T and UT legs did not reach statistical significance at any insulin concentration in either the elderly or the NIDDM subjects (figure 2.2). This quantitative discrepancy between young and older subjects is probably due to the fact that, although the content of the insulin-sensitive glucose transporter in skeletal muscle (GLUT4) increased ($p < .05$) in all three groups in

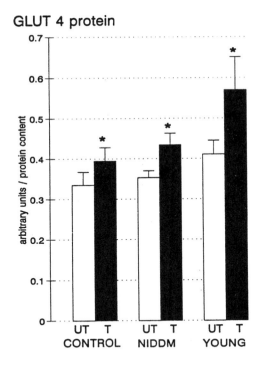

GLUT 4 protein

Figure 2.3   Total content of GLUT4 protein in muscle biopsies from vastus lateralis taken after an overnight fast, before (untrained leg [UT]) and at the end (trained leg [T]) of a one-legged endurance training program in elderly, healthy subjects (control; 59 ± 1 yr; $n = 8$); in patients with NIDDM (NIDDM; 58 ± 3 yr; $n = 7$); and in young, healthy subjects (young; 23 ± 1 yr; $n = 5$). Asterisks (*) denote significant difference from UT leg ($p < .05$). The increase in response to training was higher ($p < .05$) in young than in elderly or NIDDM groups.

response to the training (15, 19), the increase was higher ($p < .05$) in young compared with elderly and NIDDM subjects (figure 2.3).

Glucose extraction ratio is lower in NIDDM patients than in elderly subjects matched for age and lean body mass (figure 2.2). This difference in glucose extraction ratio is important in the face of identical blood flow (figure 2.1), and it cannot be ascribed to lower total GLUT4 content in the muscles in NIDDM subjects (figure 2.3). Possible explanations include hampered diffusion of glucose from the capillaries into the interstitial space or defect(s) in the translocation process or in the intrinsic activity of the glucose transporters. In addition, decreased oxidative and nonoxidative glucose metabolism would, in turn, be reflected by a decreased glucose extraction from the capillaries.

At the first clamp step (insulin concentrations ≈ 350 pmol · L^{-1}), glucose extraction ratios were similar in healthy elderly and young subjects (figure 2.2). However, as insulin concentrations were increased, the glucose extraction ratio increased more in the elderly than in the young subjects (figure 2.2). Thus, at maximal insulin concentrations, glucose extraction ratios were 42 ± 2% (UT) and 44 ± 2% (T) in the elderly subjects, while in the young subjects the ratios were lower ($p < .05$): 30 ± 3% (UT) and 33 ± 4% (T). Considering that the insulin-sensitive GLUT4 has a K_m value of 2 to 5 mM (5, 25), it seems expedient that glucose extraction in the young subjects at insulin concentrations of approximately 1,200 and 16,000 pmol · L^{-1} were not increased to a greater extent. This is so because venous glucose concentrations (being representative of glucose concentrations in the interstitial space) were approximately 3.30 mM (maximum insulin concentrations; T and UT pooled). A further decrease would mean that the glucose transporter would operate far from its V_{max}. As a consequence, glucose transport across the sarcolemma would be less effective. Therefore, instead of increasing the glucose extraction, glucose delivery (blood flow) is increased, leading to a higher average glucose concentration in the capillaries and an increased diffusion rate from the capillary to the interstitial space. The higher glucose extraction ratio in the elderly than in the young subjects (figure 2.2) might therefore be a compensating event due to an inability to increase blood flow sufficiently.

Leg Muscle Glucose Clearance

Leg muscle glucose clearance is calculated as the glucose extraction ratio × blood flow. In the untrained state (figure 2.4, dotted lines, open symbols), a clear distinction between insulin-stimulated glucose clearance in three groups can be made: young > elderly > NIDDM.

Although almost 40 yr older, the elderly, healthy subjects improved insulin action in skeletal muscle to the same extent after training as the young subjects (figure 2.4). In fact, at the two highest insulin concentrations, the increases due to training were even higher ($p < .05$) than in the younger subjects. It follows that glucose clearance after training was similar in the young and elderly subjects. This is remarkable but in line with the finding that elderly people retain the ability to adapt to training (8), having the same muscle fiber type distribution, capillary density, and mitochondrial enzyme activity as comparably trained young people (9). Thus, these findings strongly support the notion that aging per se does not result in skeletal muscle insulin resistance. The deterioration of glucose tolerance often seen with aging is probably more a result of changes in lifestyle (e.g., decreased daily physical activity and obesity). Maximal insulin-stimulated glucose clearance after training differed by approximately 10% in the elderly compared with the young subjects ($p > .05$), while total content of skeletal muscle GLUT4 protein was significantly higher (approximately 30%) after training in the young than in the elderly subjects. This finding emphasizes that the total content of GLUT4 may not be related to the membrane-bound fraction in a linear fashion, and that other factors (e.g., glucose supply or diffusion conditions) are involved in the glucose clearance process. In the young subjects, a significant correlation ($r = .84$, $p < .05$) between total content of GLUT4 and maximal insulin-stimulated leg glucose uptake rates was found (15; figure 2.5).

Detraining and Acute Exercise

After 6 d of detraining, glucose clearance in the trained legs was not significantly different from that of untrained legs in young subjects (17) or in the elderly and NIDDM subjects (data not shown). Thus, the effect of training on insulin-stimulated skeletal muscle glucose clearance is short-lived (17), a finding that extends similar, previous findings in the whole body (36) and is in line with findings after 7 d of

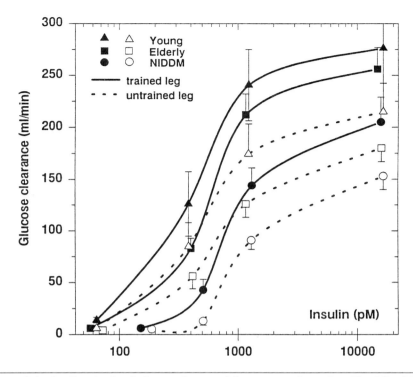

Figure 2.4 Insulin-stimulated glucose clearance (glucose extraction ratio × blood flow) in trained and untrained legs in seven young (23 ± 1 yr) and eight elderly (59 ± 1 yr) healthy subjects and in seven patients with NIDDM (58 ± 3 yr), all of whom had performed one-legged endurance training for 10 wk. NIDDM patients were insulin resistant compared with elderly subjects ($p < .05$), who were insulin resistant compared with young subjects ($p < .05$). In all three groups, insulin-stimulated glucose clearance increased with training ($p < .05$). No difference was seen between trained legs of young and elderly subjects ($p > .05$).

bed rest (34). No effect of acute exercise on skeletal muscle glucose clearance was found (data not shown; 17). Previous studies of the effect of acute exercise on insulin-stimulated glucose uptake have shown both an increase (35, 38) and no effect (7), and a single exercise bout has been shown to have no effect on muscle GLUT4 content (29). It is possible that the single 30-min bout of bicycle exercise performed with the nontraining leg caused some degree of muscle damage, which could lead to decreased insulin action, in line with the findings of decreased insulin action (27, 28) and GLUT4 content (4) after eccentric exercise.

Fuel Metabolism and Fate of Glucose in Trained and Untrained Legs During Hyperinsulinemia

In response to the training, glucose clearance rates increase in both young and elderly healthy subjects as well as in NIDDM patients (figure 2.4). The improvement in insulin action is predominantly reflected in an increase in glucose storage

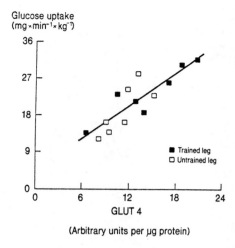

Glucose uptake
(mg × min⁻¹ × kg⁻¹)

GLUT 4

(Arbitrary units per µg protein)

Figure 2.5   The relationship between maximal (16,669 ± 574 pmol · L^{-1}) insulin-stimulated glucose uptake in trained and untrained legs and total content of the insulin-sensitive glucose transporter (GLUT4) in vastus lateralis muscle ($r = .84$, $p < .05$). Seven young (23 ± 1 yr) healthy subjects who had performed one-legged endurance training for 10 wk were studied during a hyperinsulinemic, euglycemic clamp with catheterization of the femoral veins and an artery. Biopsies were obtained in the basal state.

(glycogen formation), estimated from indirect calorimetry. Thus, at maximal insulin concentration (approximately 16,000 pmol · L^{-1}), estimated glycogen formation was increased approximately 25% in T compared with UT legs in all three groups (all $p < .05$). It is also interesting that in young, elderly, and NIDDM subjects the release of lactate as a percentage of the glucose taken up was always higher ($p < .05$) in T compared with UT legs (at maximal insulin concentrations: 11 ± 2% vs. 7 ± 2% [young]; 8 ± 1% vs. 5 ± 1% [elderly]; 10 ± 2% vs. 7 ± 1% [NIDDM], respectively).

Whole-Body Glucose Clearance

In the elderly and in the NIDDM subjects, clamps were carried out both before and after completion of the one-legged training program, allowing an evaluation of the effect of training on whole-body glucose clearance. In spite of the fact that only one leg had been trained, whole-body glucose clearance was increased after completion of the training program (figure 2.6). In figure 2.6 is also shown whole-body glucose clearance for the young subjects after training (no clamp was performed before the training began). Clearly, young subjects have increased insulin action compared with older individuals. The difference in insulin action between the young and the elderly subjects after training is less in skeletal muscle (figure 2.4) than in the whole body (figure 2.6), probably reflecting the differences in percentage of body fat (table 2.1).

An estimate of the possible maximal effect of training in these subjects can be calculated by assuming that muscle mass of the whole body and of the legs are

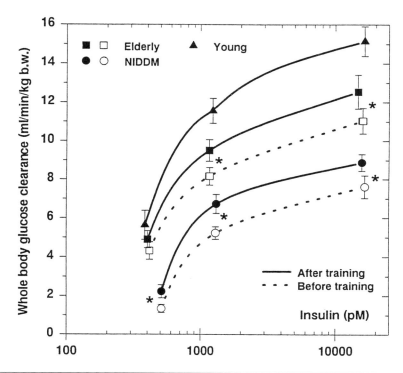

Figure 2.6   Whole-body insulin-stimulated glucose clearance in seven young (23 ± 1 yr) and eight elderly (59 ± 1 yr) healthy subjects and in seven patients with NIDDM (58 ± 3 yr), all of whom had performed one-legged endurance training for 10 wk. Before (elderly subjects and NIDDM patients) and after (all subjects) the training program, a hyperinsulinemic glucose clamp was performed. Glucose was clamped at fasting plasma glucose concentrations. Whole-body glucose clearance was calculated as steady-state glucose infusion rates divided by arterial plasma glucose concentrations. At insulin concentrations of approximately 1,200 and 16,500 pmol · L^{-1}, whole-body glucose clearance was always higher ($p < .05$) in young subjects than in elderly subjects or NIDDM patients. Asterisks (*) denote significant ($p < .05$) difference between before and after training.

approximately 40% and 64%, respectively (43). If all the muscles in the body were trained to the same extent as the leg muscles, whole-body glucose clearance would be 3.12 ± 0.68, 8.31 ± 0.94, and 10.63 ± 1.48 ml · min^{-1} · kg^{-1} in NIDDM subjects and 5.94 ± 0.66, 13.11 ± 1.11, and 14.98 ± 1.03 ml · min^{-1} · kg^{-1} in the elderly subjects during the three clamp steps (compare with figure 2.6).

In both elderly and NIDDM subjects, approximately 45% of the increase in whole-body glucose clearance can be accounted for by the increase in the trained leg. This reflects that the one-legged ergometer bicycle trains not only leg muscle, but also respiratory muscles, arm muscles, and to some extent the muscles in the nontraining leg. The nontraining leg cannot be kept completely relaxed while the other leg is performing the bicycling.

In summary, these studies have shown that physical training increases insulin-stimulated glucose clearance in skeletal muscle by approximately 25% in both young and elderly healthy subjects as well as in patients with NIDDM. This effect is due to a local contraction-dependent mechanism that is invoked by repeated exercise, because a single exercise bout is insufficient to bring about these adaptations of the skeletal muscle. The training effect is short-lived (< 6 d). Furthermore, physical training increases the total content of the insulin-sensitive glucose transporter in skeletal muscle, irrespective of age or NIDDM.

References

1. Anderson, E.A.; Mark, A.L. The vasodilator action of insulin. Implications for the insulin hypothesis of hypertension. Hypertension 21:136-141; 1993.
2. Andres, R.; Swerdloff, R.; Pozefsky, T.; Coleman, D. Manual feedback technique for the control of blood glucose concentration in man. In: Skeggs, L.T. Jr., ed. Automation in analytical chemistry. New York: Mediad; 1966:486-491.
3. Annuzzi, G.; Riccardi, G.; Capaldo, B.; Kaijser, L. Increased insulin-stimulated glucose uptake by exercised human muscles one day after prolonged physical exercise. Eur. J. Clin. Invest. 21:6-12; 1991.
4. Asp, S.; Daugaard, J.R.; Richter, E.A. Eccentric exercise decreases GLUT4 protein in human skeletal muscle. J. Physiol. 482(3):705-712; 1995.
5. Bell, G.I.; Burant, C.F.; Takeda, J.; Gould, G.W. Structure and function of mammalian facilitative sugar transporters. J. Biol. Chem. 268:19161-19164; 1993.
6. Bergman, R.N.; Finegood, D.T.; Ader, M. Assessment of insulin sensitivity in vivo. Endocrine Rev. 6:45-86; 1985.
7. Bourey, R.E.; Coggan, A.R.; Kohrt, W.M.; Kirwan, J.P.; King, D.S.; Holloszy, J.O. Effect of exercise on glucose disposal: Response to a maximal insulin stimulus. J. Appl. Physiol. 69(5):1689-1694; 1990.
8. Coggan, A.R.; Spina, R.J.; King, D.S.; Rogers, M.A.; Brown, M.; Nemeth, P.M.; Holloszy, J.O. Skeletal muscle adaptations to endurance training in 60- to 70-yr-old men and women. J. Appl. Physiol. 72:1780-1786; 1992.
9. Coggan, A.R.; Spina, R.J.; Rogers, M.A.; King, D.S.; Brown, M.; Nemeth, P.M.; Holloszy, J.O. Histochemical and enzymatic characteristics of skeletal muscle in master athletes. J. Appl. Physiol. 68:1896-1901; 1990.
10. Creager, M.A.; Liang, C.; Coffman, J.D. Beta adrenergic-mediated vasodilator response to insulin in the human forearm. J. Pharmacol. Exp. Therapeutics 235:709-714; 1985.
11. DeFronzo, R.A. Lilly Lecture 1987. The triumvirate: β-cell, muscle, liver. A collusion responsible for NIDDM. Diabetes 37:667-687; 1988.
12. DeFronzo, R.A.; Gunnarsson, R.; Björkman, O.; Olsson, M.; Wahren, J. Effects of insulin on peripheral and splanchnic glucose metabolism in noninsulin-dependent (type II) diabetes mellitus. J. Clin. Invest. 76:149-155; 1985.
13. DeFronzo, R.A.; Jacot, E.; Jequier, E.; Maeder, E.; Wahren, J.; Felber, J.P. The effect of insulin on the disposal of intravenous glucose. Results from indirect calorimetry and hepatic and femoral venous catheterization. Diabetes 30:1000-1007; 1981.
14. DeFronzo, R.A.; Tobin, J.D.; Andres, R. Glucose clamp technique: A method for quantifying insulin secretion and resistance. Am. J. Physiol. 237(3):E214-E223; 1979.

15. Dela, F.; Handberg, A.; Mikines, K.J.; Vinten, J.; Galbo, H. GLUT 4 and insulin receptor binding and kinase activity in trained human muscle. J. Physiol. 469:615-624; 1993.
16. Dela, F.; Larsen, J.J.; Mikines, K.J.; Galbo, H. Normal effect of insulin to stimulate leg blood flow in NIDDM. Diabetes 44:221-226; 1995.
17. Dela, F.; Mikines, K.J.; Linstow, V.M.; Secher, N.H.; Galbo, H. Effect of training on insulin mediated glucose uptake in human skeletal muscle. Am. J. Physiol. 263:E1134-E1143; 1992.
18. Dela, F.; Mikines, K.J.; Sonne, B.; Galbo, H. Effect of training on the interaction between insulin and exercise in human muscle. J. Appl. Physiol. 76(6):2386-2393; 1994.
19. Dela, F.; Ploug, T.; Handberg, A.; Petersen, L.N.; Larsen, J.J.; Mikines, K.J.; Galbo, H. Physical training increases muscle GLUT-4 protein and mRNA in patients with NIDDM. Diabetes 43:862-865; 1994.
20. Doberne, L.; Greenfield, M.S.; Schulz, B.; Reaven, G.M. Enhanced glucose utilization during prolonged glucose clamp studies. Diabetes 30:835; 1981.
21. Douglas, A.R.; Jones, N.L.; Reed, J.W. Calculation of whole blood CO_2 content. J. Appl. Physiol. 65(1):473-477; 1988.
22. Ferrannini, E.; Taddei, S.; Santoro, D.; Natali, A.; Boni, C.; Chiaro, D.D.; Buzzigoli, G. Independent stimulation of glucose metabolism and Na-K exchange by insulin in the human forearm. Am. J. Physiol. 255(18):E953-E958; 1988.
23. Frayn, K.N. Calculation of substrate oxidation rates in vivo from gaseous exchange. J. Appl. Physiol. 55(2):628-634; 1983.
24. Fraze, E.; Chiou, Y.M.; Chen, I.; Reaven, G.M. Age-related changes in postprandial plasma glucose, insulin, and free fatty acids concentrations in nondiabetic individuals. J. Am. Geriatr. Soc. 35:224-228; 1987.
25. Gould, G.W.; Holman, G.D. The glucose transporter family: Structure, function and tissue-specific expression. Biochem. J. 295:329-341; 1993.
26. Kelley, D.E.; Reilly, J.P.; Veneman, T.; Mandarino, L.J. Effects of insulin on skeletal muscle glucose storage, oxidation, and glycolysis in humans. Am. J. Physiol. 258(21):E923-E929; 1990.
27. King, D.S.; Feltmeyer, T.L.; Baldus, P.J.; Sharp, R.L.; Nespor, J. Effects of eccentric exercise on insulin secretion and action in humans. J. Appl. Physiol. 75:2151-2156; 1993.
28. Kirwan, J.P.; Hickner, R.C.; Yarasheski, K.E.; Kohrt, W.M.; Wiethop, B.V.; Holloszy, J.O. Eccentric exercise induces transient insulin resistance in healthy individuals. J. Appl. Physiol. 72:2197-2202; 1992.
29. Koivisto, V.A.; Bourey, R.E.; Vuorinen-Markkola, H.; Koranyi, L. Exercise reduces muscle glucose transport protein (GLUT-4) mRNA in type 1 diabetic patients. J. Appl. Physiol. 74(4):1755-1760; 1993.
30. Laakso, M.; Edelman, S.V.; Brechtel, G.; Baron, A.D. Decreased effect of insulin to stimulate skeletal muscle blood flow in obese man. J. Clin. Invest. 85:1844-1852; 1990.
31. Laakso, M.; Edelman, S.V.; Brechtel, G.; Baron, A.D. Impaired insulin-mediated skeletal muscle blood flow in patients with NIDDM. Diabetes 41:1076-1083; 1992.
32. Louard, R.J.; Fryburg, D.A.; Gelfand, R.A.; Barrett, E.J. Insulin sensitivity of protein and glucose metabolism in human forearm skeletal muscle. J. Clin. Invest. 90:2348-2354; 1992.

33. Lundgren, F.; Eden, E.; Arfvidsson, B.; Lundholm, K. Insulin time-dependent effects on the leg exchange of glucose and amino acids in man. Eur. J. Clin. Invest. 21:421-429; 1991.

34. Mikines, K.J.; Richter, E.A.; Dela, F.; Galbo, H. Seven days of bed rest decrease insulin action on glucose uptake in leg and whole body. J. Appl. Physiol. 70(3):1245-1254; 1991.

35. Mikines, K.J.; Sonne, B.; Farrell, P.A.; Tronier, B.; Galbo, H. Effect of physical exercise on sensitivity and responsiveness to insulin in humans. Am. J. Physiol. 254(54):E248-E259; 1988.

36. Mikines, K.J.; Sonne, B.; Tronier, B.; Galbo, H. Effects of acute exercise and detraining on insulin action in trained men. J. Appl. Physiol. 66(2):704-711; 1989.

37. Richter, E.A.; Kiens, B.; Mizuno, M.; Strange, S. Insulin action in human thighs after one-legged immobilization. J. Appl. Physiol. 67(1):19-23; 1989.

38. Richter, E.A.; Mikines, K.J.; Galbo, H.; Kiens, B. Effect of exercise on insulin action in human skeletal muscle. J. Appl. Physiol. 66(2):876-885; 1989.

39. Ruderman, N.B.; Houghton, C.R.S.; Hems, R. Evaluation of the isolated perfused rat hindquarter for the study of muscle metabolism. Biochem. J. 124:639-651; 1971.

40. Simonsen, L.; Bülow, J.; Madsen, J.; Hermansen, F.; Astrup, A. Local forearm and whole-body respiratory quotient in humans after an oral glucose load—Methodological problems. Acta Physiol. Scand. 147:69-75; 1993.

41. Simonson, D.C.; DeFronzo, R.A. Indirect calorimetry: Methodological and interpretative problems. Am. J. Physiol. 258(21):E399-E412; 1990.

42. Spence, J.C. Some observations on sugar tolerance, with special reference to variations found at different ages. Q. J. Med. 14:314-326; 1921.

43. Stolwijk, J.A.J.; Hardy, J.D. Temperature regulation in man—A theoretical study. Pflügers Arch. 291:129-162; 1966.

44. Yki-Järvinen, H.; Young, A.A.; Lamkin, C.L.; Foley, J.E. Kinetics of glucose disposal in whole body and across the forearm in man. J. Clin. Invest. 79:1713-1719; 1987.

CHAPTER 3

Effect of Endurance Training on Glucose Metabolism During Exercise: Stable Isotope Studies

Andrew R. Coggan

Metabolism Unit, Shriners Burn Institute, Galveston, Texas, U.S.A.

One of the hallmark adaptations to endurance exercise training is a reduction in the rate of carbohydrate oxidation during submaximal exercise. This decrease in carbohydrate utilization is the result, in part, of a slower rate of muscle glycogenolysis during exercise in the trained state (7, 14, 17, 24, 27). However, recent studies have demonstrated that a reduction in the production, uptake, and oxidation of plasma-borne glucose is often quantitatively just as important (5, 6, 8, 9, 17, 21, 23, 27). These recent studies are the topic of this review.

Training and Glucose Utilization During Exercise

Initial studies using the a-v balance method found no effect of one-legged training on the rate of limb glucose uptake during two-legged exercise at 70% $\dot{V}O_2$max (14, 24). More recently, Kiens et al. (18) found that one-legged training did not reduce the rate of glucose uptake during moderate-intensity knee extension exercise. However, these results probably are simply due to an inadequate training stimulus (4). In keeping with this interpretation, Jansson and Kaijser (17) found that the rate of glucose uptake was markedly lower in highly trained cyclists than in untrained men during exercise at 65% to 70% $\dot{V}O_2$max. Similar results were obtained in another recent cross-sectional investigation using knee extension exercise (27).

However, the first *longitudinal* study to show that training reduces glucose utilization during exercise relied on stable isotope tracer dilution methodology (5). In this study, a primed, constant infusion of [U-^{13}C]glucose was used to quantify the rates of appearance (R_a), disappearance (R_d), and oxidation (R_{ox}) of plasma-borne glucose in healthy but untrained men cycling for 2 h at 60% of $\dot{V}O_2$max. The men were then retested during exercise performed at the same absolute power output after they had completed 12 wk of strenuous endurance training. (The subjects were

27

retested during exercise performed at the same absolute intensity, as opposed to the same relative intensity, to avoid the confounding effect of differences in absolute energy demand during exercise.) During the final 30 min of exercise, the R_d of glucose was approximately 30% lower after training (figure 3.1). Since almost all of the glucose taken up during exercise was eventually oxidized, both before and after training, the estimated R_{ox} of glucose also fell by approximately 30% (figure 3.1). Indeed, although glucose oxidation represented only about one-third of total carbohydrate oxidation during exercise before training, the decrease in glucose oxidation with training accounted for just over one-half of the overall training-induced reduction in carbohydrate oxidation during exercise.

The aforementioned study was therefore the first to clearly demonstrate that endurance training of humans reduces reliance on plasma glucose as an energy source during moderate-intensity exercise. This finding has been confirmed in several subsequent longitudinal studies, both by the present author (9, 21) and by others (23), and as previously indicated is also supported by recent cross-sectional observations (27). These subsequent studies have also demonstrated that this adaptation is evident throughout exercise (9, 21, 23, 27), as well as very early in training (i.e., after only 5-10 d) (21, 23). Moreover, these studies have confirmed the original finding that, after the initial stages of moderate-intensity exercise, a reduction in glucose utilization is quantitatively just as important as a reduction in muscle glycogenolysis in accounting for the overall training-induced decrease in the rate of carbohydrate oxidation. This is so even though muscle glycogen remains the major source of carbohydrate energy, both before and after training (9, 21, 23, 27). Endurance training therefore results in a preferential sparing of plasma glucose

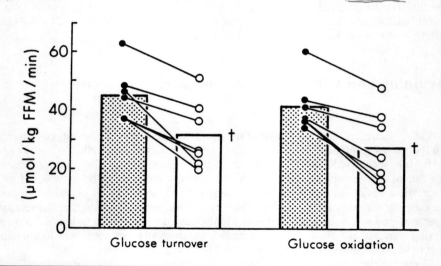

Figure 3.1   Effect of endurance training on steady-state rates of glucose appearance and disappearance (turnover) and oxidation during prolonged exercise at 60% of pretraining $\dot{V}O_2$max. FFM = fat free mass; bars = group mean values before (stippled) and after (open) training; circles and lines = responses of individual subjects; † = significantly lower than before training ($p < .001$).

Reprinted from Coggan, Kohrt, Spina, Bier, and Holloszy 1990.

during exercise. As a consequence, trained individuals are better able to maintain euglycemia during prolonged exercise (9, 21).

Mechanisms

Training-induced alterations in substrate metabolism during exercise are thought to be largely due to the well-known increase in muscle mitochondrial content, which minimizes the disturbance to cellular energy homeostasis during exercise (cf. 15). In keeping with this concept, the time course of the reduction in glucose R_d with training (21, 23) closely parallels that of the increase in muscle respiratory capacity (25). Moreover, when two groups of subjects equal in $\dot{V}O_2$max but differing in muscle citrate synthase (CS) activity (and therefore also differing in lactate threshold [LT]) were studied during 90 min of exercise at 55% of $\dot{V}O_2$max, the R_{ox} of glucose was 25% lower in the group with the higher muscle CS activity (8). The percentage of total energy derived from plasma glucose was also inversely related ($r = -.85$; $p < .01$) to muscle CS activity when the data were considered on an individual basis (figure 3.2). Along the same lines, McConnell et al. (20) recently observed an inverse relationship ($r = -.72$; $p < .05$) between glucose R_d and muscle CS activity in a heterogeneous group of men cycling at 75% of $\dot{V}O_2$max. These findings support the hypothesis that the reduction in glucose utilization with training is due to the increase in muscle respiratory enzyme activity.

Despite such data, the precise biochemical mechanism responsible for the slower rate of glucose use after training remains uncertain. However, because training increases muscle hexokinase activity (7, 22) and attenuates the rise in muscle glucose-6-phosphate concentration during exercise (7, 17), it seems unlikely that training

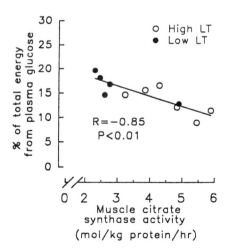

Figure 3.2   Relationship between muscle citrate synthase activity and the percentage of total energy derived from glucose oxidation during 90 min of exercise at 55% $\dot{V}O_2$max in subjects similar in $\dot{V}O_2$max but differing in blood lactate threshold (LT).
Adapted from Coggan, Spina, Kohrt, Kirwan, Bier, and Holloszy 1992.

inhibits the rate of glucose phosphorylation. It has therefore been hypothesized (4, 5, 21) that the decrease in glucose uptake and oxidation with training is the result of a reduction in the rate of glucose transport. This hypothesis may at first seem paradoxical, since the number of glucose transporters in skeletal muscle increases with training (16). An increase in total transporter number, though, does not rule out the possibility that training somehow reduces activation of the glucose transport process itself during exercise. Unfortunately, testing this hypothesis will be quite difficult, because of the technical challenge of measuring muscle glucose transport in exercising humans. Furthermore, studies of rats (26) may not be useful in this regard, since training does not consistently inhibit glucose utilization during exercise in this species (2, 11, 26).

Training and Glucose Production During Exercise

Glycogenolysis Versus Gluconeogenesis

During moderate-intensity exercise, the reduction in glucose R_d with training is matched by a quantitatively similar fall in glucose R_a, such that euglycemia is maintained (5, 21, 23). To determine whether this decrease in hepatic glucose production is due to a reduction in glycogenolysis, in gluconeogenesis, or in both processes, six men were studied during 2 h of exercise at 60% pretraining VO_2peak, both before and after endurance training (9). The overall R_a of glucose was determined using a primed, continuous infusion of $[6,6-^2H]$glucose, whereas the rate of gluconeogenesis was determined from the incorporation of ^{13}C into glucose from simultaneously infused $[^{13}C]$bicarbonate. (Although bicarbonate is not a gluconeogenic precursor in a net sense, glucose becomes labeled as a result of pyruvate carboxylation and subsequent isotopic exchange in the tricarboxylic acid cycle.) The rate of hepatic glycogenolysis was then estimated from the difference between the rate of gluconeogenesis and the total rate of glucose production. As expected based on previous studies (5, 21, 23), training markedly reduced the overall R_a of glucose during exercise (table 3.1). This decrease was due, in part, to a significant fall in the rate of gluconeogenesis (table 3.1). However, this could account for only about a third of the overall decrease in glucose production, indicating that the reduction in glucose R_a must have been mostly due to a decrease in the rate of hepatic glycogenolysis (table 3.1). Thus, in humans, reductions in glycogenolysis and in gluconeogenesis both contribute to the overall training-induced decrease in glucose R_a. This differs notably from rats, in which training reduces hepatic glycogenolysis (1, 12, 26) but apparently increases gluconeogenesis (2, 11, 26) during exercise.

Mechanisms

It is widely recognized that training alters the neuroendocrine response to exercise performed at the same absolute intensity in the untrained and trained states. In particular, plasma glucagon, epinephrine, and norepinephrine concentrations increase less and plasma insulin concentration decreases less during exercise after training (5, 9, 21). Because of the importance of these hormones in glucoregulation (cf. 10),

Table 3.1   Total Glucose Production and Estimated Rates of Hepatic Gluconeogenesis and Glycogenolysis During Prolonged Exercise Before and After Endurance Training

	Before training	After training
Total glucose R_a (μmol · min^{-1} · kg^{-1})	36.8 ± 3.8	21.5 ± 3.6*
Gluconeogenesis (μmol · min^{-1} · kg^{-1})	7.5 ± 1.6	3.1 ± 0.6*
Glycogenolysis (μmol · min^{-1} · kg^{-1})	29.2 ± 4.1	18.4 ± 3.2*

Values are mean $\pm$ *SE* for six subjects, averaged over 120 min of exercise. R_a = rate of appearance.

*Significantly lower than before training ($p < .001$). Data are from Coggan et al. (9).

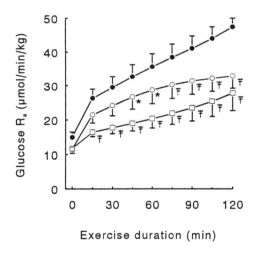

Figure 3.3   Glucose rate of appearance (R_a) at rest and during prolonged exercise at 60% of pretraining $\dot{V}O_2$max before (closed circles), after 10 d (open circles), and after 12 wk (open squares) of endurance training. Significantly lower than before training: *$p < .05$; ‡$p < .001$.

Reprinted from Mendenhall, Swanson, Habash, and Coggan 1994.

it seems likely that these adaptations play a major role in accounting for the smaller rise in glucose production during exercise in trained individuals. This is consistent with the fact that a short-term (i.e., 10 d) training program, which rapidly altered the glucoregulatory hormone response to exercise, also significantly reduced glucose R_a (21; figure 3.3). However, other factors (such as alterations in hormone action or in gluconeogenic precursor availability) must also contribute to the lesser stimulation of glucose production during exercise after training. This is so because glucose R_a was further reduced after 12 wk of training even though the neuroendocrine response to exercise was unchanged (figure 3.3). Thus, as with training-induced changes in glucose R_d, additional studies are still needed to more clearly define the exact mechanisms by which training reduces glucose R_a during exercise.

The Crossover Concept

As previously reviewed, it is now firmly established that endurance training of humans reduces glucose production and utilization during moderate-intensity exercise performed at the same absolute intensity in the untrained and trained states. However, glucose production and utilization increase exponentially with increasing exercise intensity (cf. 4), and trained individuals typically exercise at higher absolute intensities than untrained individuals. Furthermore, as previously discussed, training increases total glucose transporter number (16) and hexokinase activity (7, 22) in skeletal muscle and also reduces intramuscular glucose-6-phosphate concentrations during exercise (7, 17), all of which should theoretically enhance the capacity of muscle to take up and oxidize glucose. Brooks and Mercier (3) have therefore hypothesized that there is a crossover phenomenon, in which reduced glucose flux in trained subjects during moderate-intensity exercise converts to increased glucose flux during high-intensity exercise.

To test this hypothesis, glucose R_a and R_d were recently measured in untrained subjects and endurance-trained athletes cycling for 30 min at 80% of $\dot{V}O_2max$ (6). The rate of tracer infusion was increased at the onset of exercise and every minute thereafter to minimize the rate of change in plasma glucose enrichment. This procedure improves non-steady-state estimates of glucose kinetics by reducing the influence of the assumed glucose distribution volume on the calculation of R_a and R_d (13). In contrast to the decrease in glucose production observed during exercise performed at the same absolute intensity in the untrained and trained states (5, 9, 21, 23), during exercise at the same relative intensity glucose R_a did not differ in the untrained and trained subjects (table 3.2). This is consistent with the fact that there were no differences between the two groups in circulating norepinephrine, epinephrine, glucagon, or insulin concentrations during exercise. Notably, however, glucose R_a was not *higher* in the trained subjects, as predicted by the crossover concept (3), even though the absolute power output and $\dot{V}O_2$ during exercise were 57% and 40% higher, respectively, in the trained subjects (table 3.2). Furthermore, in direct opposition to the hypothesis of Brooks and Mercier (3), the R_d of glucose was significantly *lower* in the athletes than in the nonathletes (table 3.2). This was true even though the overall rate of carbohydrate oxidation during exercise was approximately 25% higher in the trained subjects, due to their higher absolute energy expenditure. As a result of this imbalance between R_a and R_d, plasma glucose concentration rose significantly during exercise in the trained subjects but did not change during exercise in the untrained subjects.

The preceding results do not exclude the possibility that training enhances glucose production and utilization during exercise at >80% $\dot{V}O_2max$. However, Kjær et al. (19) found that glucose R_d (measured using [3-^{3}H]glucose) tended to be lower in endurance-trained athletes than in untrained men during treadmill running at 100% to 110% $\dot{V}O_2max$. As in the study previously discussed, the rate of glucose clearance was significantly lower ($p < .05$) in the trained subjects, suggesting that training inhibits glucose utilization even during maximal or supramaximal exercise. Thus,

Table 3.2   Metabolic Responses to Intense Exercise in Untrained and Trained Subjects

	Untrained	Trained	Difference
Power (w/kg)	2.32 ± 0.19	3.65 ± 0.18*	+57%
$\dot{V}O_2$ (ml · min^{-1} · kg^{-1})	34.9 ± 2.3	49.0 ± 1.8*	+40%
$\dot{V}O_2$ (% $\dot{V}O_2$max)	78.7 ± 1.5	77.7 ± 1.4	−1%
Glucose R_a (μmol · min^{-1} · kg^{-1})	36.0 ± 1.7	34.3 ± 3.6	−2%
Glucose R_d (μmol · min^{-1} · kg^{-1})	33.2 ± 1.5	27.0 ± 2.6*	−19%
Glucose clearance (ml · min^{-1} · kg^{-1})	6.94 ± 0.57	5.31 ± 0.60*	−23%

Values are mean ± *SE* for eight subjects per group, averaged over 30 min of exercise.
$\dot{V}O_2$ = oxygen uptake; $\dot{V}O_2$max = maximal oxygen uptake; R_a = rate of apperance; R_d = rate of disappearance.
*Trained significantly different from untrained ($p < .001$). Data are from Coggan et al. (6).

the available data clearly do not support the hypothesis of a crossing-over in glucose utilization with increasing exercise intensity as proposed by Brooks and Mercier (3). This is true even though plasma glucose concentration tends to be higher in trained than in untrained subjects during intense exercise, as a result of an equal (9) or possibly even greater (19) rate of glucose production.

Summary

It has long been recognized that endurance-trained individuals rely less on carbohydrate and more on fat as an energy source during submaximal exercise. This carbohydrate-sparing effect of training has generally been attributed to a training-induced decrease in the rate of muscle glycogen utilization during exercise. However, recent studies using stable isotope tracers have demonstrated that a training-induced reduction in the rate of glucose utilization during exercise also plays a significant role. This is true not only during moderate-intensity exercise performed at the same absolute intensity before and after training, but also during exercise performed at the same relative (and therefore a higher absolute) intensity in the trained compared with the untrained state. By minimizing the possibility of hypoglycemia, this adaptation likely contributes to the increase in exercise performance that results from endurance training.

References

1. Baldwin, K.M.; Fitts, R.H.; Booth, F.W.; Winder, W.W.; Holloszy, J.O. Depletion of muscle and liver glycogen during exercise. Protective effect of training. Pflügers Arch. 354:203-212; 1975.

2. Brooks, G.A.; Donovan, C.M. Effect of endurance training on glucose kinetics during exercise. Am. J. Physiol. 244 (Endocrinol. Metab. 7):E505-E512; 1983.

3. Brooks, G.A.; Mercier, J. Balance of carbohydrate and lipid utilization during exercise: The "crossover" concept. J. Appl. Physiol. 76:2253-2261; 1994.

4. Coggan, A.R. Plasma glucose metabolism during exercise in humans. Sports Med. 11:102-124; 1991.

5. Coggan, A.R.; Kohrt, W.M.; Spina, R.J.; Bier, D.M.; Holloszy, J.O. Endurance training decreases plasma glucose turnover and oxidation during moderate intensity exercise in men. J. Appl. Physiol. 68:990-996; 1990.

6. Coggan, A.R.; Raguso, C.A.; Williams, B.D.; Sidossis, L.S.; Gastaldelli, A. Glucose kinetics during high-intensity exercise in endurance-trained and untrained humans. J. Appl. Physiol. 78:1203-1207; 1995.

7. Coggan, A.R.; Spina, R.J.; Kohrt, W.M.; Holloszy, J.O. Effect of prolonged exercise on muscle citrate concentration before and after endurance training in men. Am. J. Physiol. 264 (Endocrinol. Metab. 27):E215-E220; 1993.

8. Coggan, A.R.; Spina, R.J.; Kohrt, W.M.; Kirwan, J.P.; Bier, D.M.; Holloszy, J.O. Plasma glucose kinetics during exercise in subjects with high and low lactate thresholds. J. Appl. Physiol. 73:1873-1880; 1992.

9. Coggan, A.R.; Swanson, S.C.; Mendenhall, L.A.; Habash, D.L.; Kien, C.L. Effect of endurance training on hepatic glycogenolysis and gluconeogenesis during prolonged exercise in men. Am. J. Physiol. 268 (Endocrinol. Metab. 31):E375-E383; 1995.

10. Cryer, P.E. Glucose counterregulation: Prevention and correction of hypoglycemia in humans. Am. J. Physiol. 264 (Endocrinol. Metab. 27):E149-E155; 1993.

11. Donovan, C.M.; Sumida, K.D. Training improves glucose homeostasis in rats during exercise via glucose production. Am. J. Physiol. 258 (Regulat. Integrative Comp. Physiol. 27):R770-R776; 1990.

12. Fitts, R.H.; Booth, F.W.; Winder, W.W.; Holloszy, J.O. Skeletal muscle respiratory capacity, endurance, and glycogen utilization. Am. J. Physiol. 228:1029-1033; 1975.

13. Gastaldelli, A.; Raguso, C.A.; Coggan, A.R.; Wolfe, R.R. Changes in tracer infusion rates to minimize the structural error in Steele's model. FASEB J. 8:A699; 1994.

14. Henriksson, J. Training induced adaptation of skeletal muscle and metabolism during submaximal exercise. J. Physiol. 270:661-675; 1977.

15. Holloszy, J.O.; Coyle, E.F. Adaptations of skeletal muscle to endurance exercise and their metabolic consequences. J. Appl. Physiol. 56:831-838; 1984.

16. Houmard, J.A.; Egan, P.C.; Neufer, P.D.; Freidman, J.E.; Wheeler, W.S.; Israel, G.; Dohm, G.L. Elevated skeletal muscle glucose transporter levels in exercise-trained middle-aged men. Am. J. Physiol. 261 (Endocrinol. Metab. 24):E437-E443; 1991.

17. Jansson, E.; Kaijser, L. Substrate utilization and enzymes in skeletal muscle of extremely endurance-trained men. J. Appl. Physiol. 662:999-1005; 1987.

18. Kiens, B.; Essén-Gustavsson, B.; Christensen, N.J.; Saltin, B. Skeletal muscle substrate utilization during submaximal exercise in man: Effect of endurance training. J. Physiol. 469:459-478; 1993.

19. Kjær, M.; Farrell, P.A.; Christensen, N.J.; Galbo, H. Increased epinephrine response and inaccurate glucoregulation in exercising athletes. J. Appl. Physiol. 61:1693-1700; 1986.

20. McConnell, G.; Proietto, J.; Snow, R.J.; Hargreaves, M. Skeletal muscle GLUT4 and glucose uptake during exercise in humans. J. Appl. Physiol. 77:1565-1568; 1994.

21. Mendenhall, L.A.; Swanson, S.C.; Habash, D.L.; Coggan, A.R. Ten days of exercise training reduces glucose production and utilization during moderate-intensity exercise. Am. J. Physiol. 266 (Endocrinol. Metab. 29):E136-E143; 1994.

22. Morgan, T.E.; Short, F.A.; Cobb, L.A. Effect of long-term exercise on human muscle mitochondria. In: Pernow, B.; Saltin, B., eds. Muscle metabolism during exercise. New York: Plenum; 1971:87-95.

23. Phillips, S.M.; Green, H.J.; Tarnapolsky, M.A.; Grant, S.M. Decreased glucose turnover after short-term training is unaccompanied by changes in muscle oxidative potential. Am. J. Physiol. 269 (Endocrinol. Metab. 32): E222-E230; 1995.

24. Saltin, B.; Nazar, K.; Costill, D.L.; Stein, E.; Jansson, E.; Essén, B.; Gollnick, P.D. The nature of the training response: Peripheral and central adaptation to one-legged exercise. Acta Physiol. Scand. 96:289-305; 1976.

25. Spina, R.J.; Chi, M.M.-Y.; Hopkins, M.G.; Nemeth, P.M.; Lowry, O.H.; Holloszy, J.O. Mitochondrial enzymes increase in muscle in response to 7-10 days of cycle exercise. J. Appl. Physiol.; 1996. (In press.)

26. Sumida, K.D.; Donovan, C.M. Endurance training fails to inhibit skeletal muscle glucose uptake during exercise. J. Appl. Physiol. 76:1876-1881; 1994.

27. Turcotte, L.P.; Richter, E.A.; Kiens, B. Increased plasma FFA uptake and oxidation during prolonged exercise in trained vs. untrained humans. Am. J. Physiol. 262 (Endocrinol. Metab. 25):E791-E799; 1992.

CHAPTER 4

The Role of Glucose Transport in the Regulation of Glucose Utilization by Muscle

Y. Sato, Y. Oshida, I. Ohsawa, N. Nakai, N. Ohsaki; K. Yamanouchi; J. Sato; Y. Shimomura; H. Ohno
Nagoya University, Nagoya, Japan; Nagoya University, Nagoya, Japan; Nagoya University, Nagoya, Japan; Nagoya University, Nagoya, Japan; Nagoya University, Nagoya, Japan; Aichi Medical University, Nagakute, Japan; Nagoya University School of Medicine, Nagoya, Japan; Nagoya Institute of Technology, Nagoya, Japan; National Defense Medical College, Tokolozawa, Japan

Glucose transport has generally been considered the rate-limiting step in glucose uptake and utilization in muscle (9). Over the last few years, an explosion of information regarding the molecular structure and function of the proteins involved in the transfer of glucose across the cell membrane and their regulation in physiological and pathophysiological states has provided new insight into glucose metabolism (1, 13, 19, 23). The major focus of this monograph is the current knowledge of the molecular biology and physiology of glucose transports in the regulation of glucose utilization by muscle.

Glucose Transport at the Molecular Level

Glucose is not freely permeable across the lipid bilayer of the plasma membrane, but the cellular uptake of this important nutrient is accomplished by membrane-associated carrier proteins that bind and transfer across the lipid bilayer. Two classes of glucose carrier have been reported in mammalian cells: the sodium-glucose cotransporter, named SGLT1, and the facilitative glucose transporters (1, 23).

Na$^+$-Glucose Cotransporter (SGLT1)

The Na$^+$-glucose cotransporter is a secondary active transport system in the epithelial membranes, which utilizes the energy from an extracellular to an intracellular

Na$^+$ electrochemical gradient, generated by Na$^+$,K$^+$-ATPase, to drive intracellular accumulation of glucose. Therefore, this type of glucose transporter transports glucose against its concentration gradient by coupling its uptake with the Na$^+$ that is being transported down its concentration gradient. The Na$^+$-glucose transporter is present on the absorptive epithelial cells of the small intestine and is involved in the dietary uptake of glucose. The same or a related protein may be responsible for the reabsorption of glucose by the kidney.

The Na$^+$-glucose cotransporter is predicted to traverse the plasma membrane 11 times, with its COOH terminals located in the cytoplasmic NH$_2$ and in the extracellular sides of the plasma membrane, respectively (14; figure 4.1).

Facilitative Glucose Transporters

Facilitative glucose carriers accelerate the transport of glucose down its concentration gradient. Subtypes of facilitative glucose transporters have been identified from mammalian tissues. They are named GLUT (the gene symbol for facilitative glucose transporter) and are numbered in the order of their discovery: GLUT1, GLUT2,

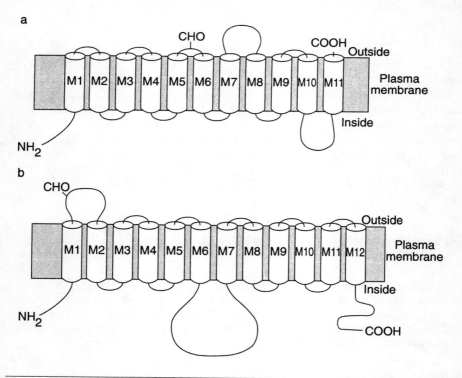

Figure 4.1 Model for orientation of glucose transporters in plasma membrane. (a) Putative membrane-spanning α-helices in Na$^+$-glucose cotransporter and (b) facilitative glucose transporter proteins are indicated and numbered M1 to M11 and M1 to M12, respectively. CHO denotes site of asparagine-linked glycosylation.

GLUT3, GLUT4, and GLUT5. These types of glucose transporters are widely distributed and are present on the surface of probably all mammalian cells. Another identifying designation for each isoform is based on the tissue in which it is abundant and that conveys a minimum of physiological information, that is, erythrocyte, liver, brain, muscle/fat, and small intestine (1, 23).

DNAs encoding the facilitative glucose transporter species isoforms have been isolated from the following species: GLUT1—human, rat, rabbit, pig, and mouse; GLUT2—human, rat, and mouse; GLUT3—human; GLUT4—human, rat, and mouse; and GLUT5—human (1).

The size of the mammalian facilitative glucose transporters varies from 492 to 524 amino acids (a polypeptide chain of about 500 amino acids; table 4.1). There is 39% to 65% individuality and 50% to 76% similarity between the amino acid sequences of the different human isoforms. The predicted topology of these transporters suggests an organization of 25 segments, with 13 largely hydrophilic segments and 12 largely hydrophobic membrane-spanning components. Both the NH_2^+ and $COOH^-$ terminals of the protein, which may vary in length or sequence among the different isoforms, are on the cytoplasmic side of the lipid bilayer (1, 23).

A large ectoplasmic loop containing an N-glycosylation site is present between the first (M1) and second (M2) transmembrane domains. A large hydrophilic intracellular segment of 65 amino acids connects transmembrane segments M6 and M7 (1, 23).

The tissue and cellular distribution of the facilitative glucose transporters is beginning to be described. The technique of RNA blotting has been used to identify human tissues expressing each transporter (1; figure 4.2). The highest levels of GLUT1 and GLUT3 mRNA are in placenta, brain, and kidney. The highest levels

Table 4.1   Human Glucose Transporters

Designation	Size (number of amino acids)	Major site of expression	Chromosomal location of gene
SGLT1 (Na⁺-glucose cotransporter)	664	Small intestine	22qll.2-qter
Facilitative glucose transporters			
GLUT1 (erythrocyte)	492	Placenta, brain, kidney, and colon	1P35-31.3
GLUT2 (liver)	524	Liver, ß-cell, kidney, and small intestine	3q26
GLUT3 (brain)	496	Many tissues, including brain, placenta, and kidney	12P13
GLUT4 (muscle/fat)	509	Skeletal muscle, heart, and brown and white fat	17P13
GLUT5 (small intestine)	501	Small intestine (jejunum)	1P31

Reprinted from Bell et al. 1990.

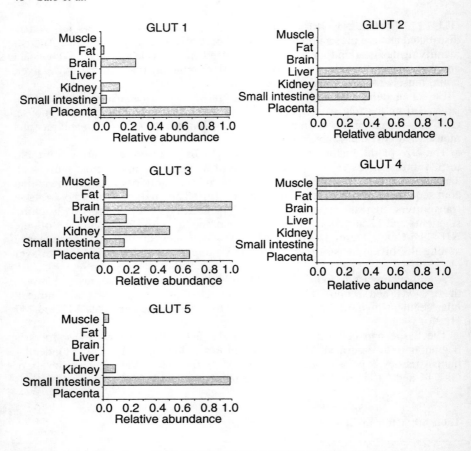

Figure 4.2   Abundance of facilitative glucose transporter mRNA in human tissues. Reprinted from Bell et al. 1990.

of GLUT2 mRNA are in the beta cells of the islets of Langerhans and liver. GLUT4 mRNA is present in insulin-responsive tissues, such as skeletal and cardiac muscle and white and brown adipose tissue; the GLUT4 isoform is responsible for insulin-stimulated glucose uptake in these tissues. The highest levels of GLUT5 mRNA are in the jejunal region of the small intestine. However, these data do not indicate the absolute amount of each isoform or its relative contribution to overall glucose uptake in each tissue. Thus, within a tissue, the cellular distribution and the absolute amount of each isoform remains to be determined (1, 13, 14, 23).

GLUT1. The human GLUT1 is located on chromosome 1 and encodes a 492-residue protein, which can be detected in most tissues. Thus, GLUT1 may be responsible for a considerable part of the constitutive non-insulin-stimulated glucose uptake. In many tissues, this glucose transporter subtype is concentrated in cells of blood-tissue barriers, suggesting a function for GLUT1 in the transport of glucose across these barriers. GLUT1 is the glucose transporter of erythrocytes (23).

GLUT2.   The human GLUT2 has been identified on chromosome 3 and encodes a glucose transporter of 524 amino acids. The tissue distribution suggests that GLUT2 mediates the uptake and release of glucose by hepatocytes and that it participates together with the Na^+-glucose cotransporter in the transepithelial transport of absorbed and reabsorbed glucose by the small intestine and kidney, respectively. Its presence in the other islet endocrine cells indicates that it may serve in the regulation of glucose-stimulated insulin secretion (23).

GLUT3.   The human GLUT3 transporter consists of 496 amino acids and is encoded by a gene on chromosome 12. GLUT3 is present at predominant levels in the brain, kidney, and placenta. Together with GLUT1, GLUT3 plays an important role in basal glucose transport activity. GLUT3 proteins in the brain are involved in glucose uptake by neurons and glial cells, while GLUT1, as already described, is chiefly responsible for the transport of glucose across the blood-brain barrier (23).

GLUT4.   The human GLUT4 polypeptide is composed of 509 amino acids and is encoded by a gene on chromosome 17. This glucose transporter subtype is present at highest levels in insulin-responsive tissues such as skeletal and cardiac muscle and fat. Within skeletal muscle, GLUT4 expression varies with muscle fiber type and occurs primarily in muscles rich in type IIa (oxidative/glycolytic) fibers, followed by muscles rich in type I (oxidative) fibers, and to a lower extent in type IIb (glycolytic) fibers.

Insulin stimulation caused a 6.4-fold greater plasma membrane GLUT4 content compared with that in the basal state, while insulin-stimulated muscles showed a 7.4-fold greater transport activity than basal muscles. Therefore, in insulin-sensitive tissues almost all the increase in glucose transport activity stimulated by insulin can be accounted for by the appearance of active GLUT4 transporters on the cell surface membrane. At present, GLUT4 is postulated to be the principal glucose transporter in muscle and adipose tissue. In the presence of insulin, the GLUT4 transporters are constantly cycling between the plasma membrane and intracellular pools of specific vesicles (19; figure 4.3).

On the other hand, under certain physiological and pathophysiological conditions, glucose transporters in muscle and adipose cells are not proportional to the measured number of glucose transporters in the plasma membrane, suggesting that additional modulation of glucose transporter activity may occur. It has been shown that catecholamines inhibit and adenosine enhances insulin-stimulated glucose transport activity in rat adipose cells without the corresponding changes in the translocation of GLUT4. Kinetic analysis of these experiments has shown changes in the turnover rate of the so-called intrinsic activity of GLUT4 (moles of glucose transported divided by transporter per unit; 23).

GLUT5.   The human GLUT5 transporter consists of 501 amino acids and is encoded by a gene on chromosome 1. GLUT5 is primarily expressed in the duodenal region of the small intestine and in the mature spermatids in testes.

Physical Exercise and Glucose Transport

Physical exercise results in increased glucose uptake by muscle. Exercise increases insulin sensitivity and responsiveness in skeletal muscle (13). DeFronzo et al. (7)

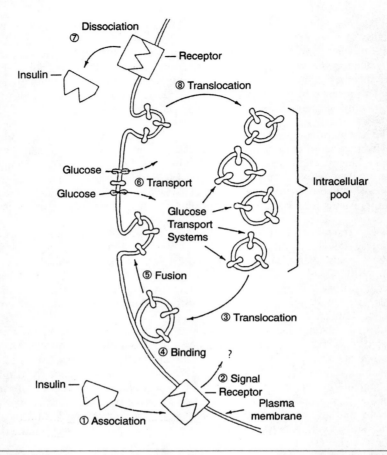

Figure 4.3   Schematic representation of a hypothetical mechanism of insulin's stimulatory action on glucose transport in the isolated rat epididymal adipose cell.
Reprinted from Karnieli et al. 1981.

have documented that exercise and insulin can act synergistically to increase glucose uptake.

Acute Exercise

The mechanism of increased glucose uptake during and after exercise is not well understood. Factors that may be involved include muscular activity factors (MAF), an increased rate of blood flow to the exercising muscle, increases in insulin binding, and changes in cytoplasmic Ca^{2+} concentrations. Since glucose transport in muscle is the major rate-limiting step in glucose utilization, regulation of this system must play an important role in exercise (20). However, some of the aforementioned factors already have been disproved (20). Cartee and Holloszy (3) provided evidence that the increased sensitivity of muscle glucose transport is not caused by insulin binding to its receptors. Another study (29) demonstrated that enhanced insulin action in muscle during the postexercise state is not related to increased kinase activity of the insulin receptor.

Recently, several studies (13, 26) have demonstrated that an acute bout of exercise can increase the number and intrinsic activity of glucose transporter proteins present in the plasma membrane of skeletal muscle. The time course of the transport-to-transporter ratio suggests that the intrinsic activity response reverses more rapidly than the response involving transporter number (11). However, the cellular signaling mechanisms that stimulate these glucose transporters are still not known.

Endurance Exercise Training

Exercise training has been shown to enhance the ability of insulin to stimulate glucose uptake in responsive tissue (13). In skeletal muscle, the GLUT4 protein constitutes the vast majority of glucose transporters. The GLUT4 protein is translocated from an intracellular location, such as low-density microsomes, to the plasma membrane in skeletal muscle in response to both insulin and contractile activity (13, 14). It has been demonstrated that the increase in the total number of GLUT4 proteins may be a major component of the increase in insulin-mediated glucose uptake that is observed with exercise training (26). Several studies have shown that exercise training increases skeletal muscle GLUT4 protein concentration in normal, healthy animals (24, 26) and also in insulin-resistant, obese Zucker rats (13). Wheel running is unique in that it stimulates hypertrophy of the soleus muscle. In one study, running was shown to increase the concentrations of enzymes involved in carbohydrate metabolism (hexokinase, citrate synthase), maximal insulin-stimulated glucose transport, and GLUT4 protein concentration by 51%. Another study demonstrated that treadmill training that does not induce soleus hypertrophy increased GLUT4 protein concentration by 47%. Thus, GLUT4 concentration is closely correlated with maximal glucose transport activity in different skeletal muscles, suggesting that GLUT4 protein concentration is an important determinant of a muscle's capacity for glucose transport (13).

Wake et al. (30) demonstrated that exercise training increases glucose transporter mRNA in muscle, which would presumably result in an increased translation of glucose transporter protein. Goodyear, Hirshman, and Horton (9) previously showed that exercise and insulin increase skeletal muscle glucose uptake both through the translocation of glucose transporters from an intracellular pool to the plasma membrane and through an increase in the average intrinsic activity of GLUT4 proteins in the plasma membrane. They suggested that increased rates of glucose uptake in endurance-trained skeletal muscle result primarily from an increase in the number of glucose transporters, especially GLUT4, present in the plasma membrane. Furthermore, these increases persist for several days after cessation of exercise training (10).

Houmard et al. (16) showed that the decrement in insulin sensitivity with the cessation of chronic muscular activity is not associated with GLUT4 protein content. The maintenance of GLUT4 levels in skeletal muscle, despite a decrease in citrate synthase activity in endurance-trained athletes, indicates that oxidative capacity and GLUT4 protein content do not always change in tandem.

Ishihara et al. (17) showed that the amount of GLUT4 was maintained under the condition of reduced weight-bearing activity of the soleus muscle through a translational or posttranslational mechanism. A more recent study (15) suggested that soleus unweighting by hindlimb suspension induces an enhancement not only in the action of insulin, but also in the action of insulinlike growth factor (IGF-I) on the glucose transport system.

Further studies are necessary to fully understand the mechanisms regulating the activation of the glucose transport system by exercise in skeletal muscle.

Physical Exercise and Syndrome X

It is known that regular physical training has beneficial effects on the prevention and treatment of so-called hypokinetic diseases such as "syndrome X," including diabetes, hypertension, and coronary artery disease (25, 27). Kaplan (18) has suggested the rather impressive term "deadly quartet" to describe the combination of upper-body obesity, insulin resistance, hypertriglyceridemia, and hypertension. The components suggested for syndrome X do not really reflect the whole spectrum of the atherosclerotic cardiovascular disease (ASCVD) risk factor cluster. Zimmet (32) provided a more comprehensive list of the components that constitute the cluster. "Syndrome X plus" (upper-body obesity, hyperuricemia, physical inactivity, and aging in addition to the risk factor cluster) was proposed as a wider representation of the actual situation. DeFronzo and Ferrannini (6) also suggested "syndrome of insulin resistance," which consists of obesity, non-insulin-dependent diabetes mellitus (NIDDM), hypertension, ASCVD, dyslipidemia, and hyperinsulinemia. All of these can predispose one to the development of atherosclerosis.

Physical exercise performed on a regular basis may be beneficial for health and longevity. The effects of exercise training may range from psychological factors to favorable changes in whole body physiology, such as enhanced aerobic capacity, to adaptive responses in cellular biochemistry (12).

Continued physical exercise improves reduced peripheral tissue sensitivity to insulin in these conditions. We have evaluated the effects of physical training in terms of the in vivo action of insulin by the multiple euglycemic clamp technique with a regular dose of 40 mU $\cdot$ m^{-2} $\cdot$ min^{-1} (insulin sensitivity–receptor defect) or a high dose of 400 mU $\cdot$ m^{-2} $\cdot$ min^{-1} (insulin responsiveness–postbinding defect) and by the microdialysis procedure (21, 27).

Both glucose infusion rate (GIR) and glucose metabolic clearance rate (MCR) provide a quantitative estimate of insulin action. Under the regular-dose condition, GIR and MCR correlated directly with maximal oxygen uptake ($\dot{V}O_2$max). MCRs in obese NIDDM patients and normal, obese subjects were significantly lower ($p < .001$) than in healthy controls, whose values were significantly lower ($p < .001$) than those in athletes. After physical training and dietary restriction for 4 to 8 wk, the decreased MCRs in obese NIDDM patients and normal, obese subjects recovered to normal levels (27). A positive correlation existed between MCR and number of steps taken per day (estimated by pedometer; $p < .01$; figure 4.4). Further, long-term, mild physical training increases insulin action despite its lack of influence on body mass index (BMI) or $\dot{V}O_2$max in young, nonobese subjects (22).

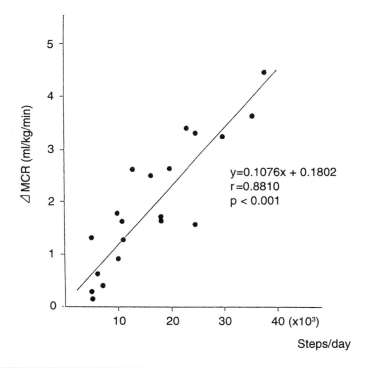

Figure 4.4   Correlation between MCR and average number of steps taken per day.

Under high-dose conditions, after physical training and dietary restriction for 4 to 8 wk, the decreased MCRs in obese NIDDM patients and normal, obese subjects were significantly increased ($p < .001$).

With the microdialysis technique, a leftward shift of the insulin dose-response curve was observed in skeletal muscle of trained rats, as compared with controls, when the lactate concentration in the dialysate was plotted against the logarithm of the mean plasma insulin concentration. On the other hand, no significant difference in the dose-response curve of the lactate concentration of the dialysate between trained and untrained rats was observed in adipose tissue (27).

These results suggest that the effects of physical training can be estimated separately from the effects of dietary factors using the euglycemic clamp and microdialysis techniques. Also, physical training in addition to dietary restriction provides a reasonable therapeutic modality for obese NIDDM and normal, obese patients from a pathophysiological point of view (27).

Physical Exercise and Aging

It is commonly known that aging is associated with glucose intolerance (28). DeFronzo (5) reported that impaired tissue sensitivity to insulin is the primary factor responsible for the decreased glucose tolerance observed with advancing age and that the site of insulin resistance must reside in peripheral tissue. It has been shown that the extensive variation previously reported in in vivo insulin-stimulated glucose disposal of aged subjects was related to differences in habitual activity. As already described (27), biochemical determination of training effects could be carried out using the euglycemic clamp technique. Consequently, the following human studies and animal experiments were performed.

Human Study

To clarify the effect of daily physical activity on the peripheral insulin action, especially with regard to insulin sensitivity and responsiveness, we carried out the following studies using the multiple euglycemic clamp technique in aged, bedridden subjects, in aged and young healthy controls, and in aged and young athletes.

At both regular- and high-dose conditions, GIR was significantly higher ($p <$ .001) in aged athletes and significantly lower ($p < .001$) in aged, bedridden subjects than in aged controls (figure 4.5). Although there was no statistical difference in GIR at high-dose clamp between young athletes and young controls, GIR at regular-dose clamp was significantly higher in young athletes than in young controls ($p < .001$).

Comparison of the aged and young groups at high-dose clamp showed there was no significant difference between the aged athletes and the young athletes, although GIR in aged controls was significantly lower ($p < .05$) than in young controls.

In order to clarify whether the decrease in insulin action in aged subjects was due to decreased insulin action in muscle itself or not, GIR per muscle was calculated. With the regular-dose condition, there was no significant difference between GIR

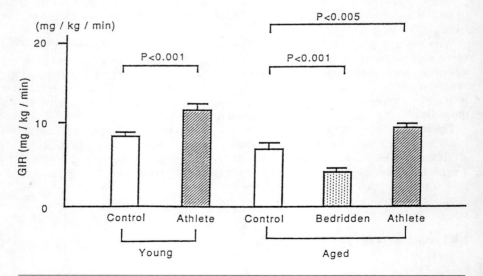

Figure 4.5   Comparison of GIR during regular-dose euglycemic clamp (insulin infusion rate = 40 mU $\cdot$ m^{-2} $\cdot$ min^{-1}).

per lean body mass (LBM) in aged athletes and that of controls. However, at the high-dose condition, MCR per lean body mass showed significant decreases in the aged controls compared with that in aged athletes and young controls.

These results might suggest that insulin responsiveness may decrease with the aging process and may be further affected by physical inactivity, whereas physical training may improve insulin responsiveness in aged individuals up to levels similar to those of young athletes. Physical training in young people may improve insulin sensitivity (31).

Coggan et al. (4) reported that endurance training was associated with 60% to 100% higher citrate synthase activity and with improved metabolic responses in young and older men but apparently could not prevent an age-related decrement in those variables or an age-related decrease in muscle mass and metabolic responses.

Animal Study

Male Wistar rats (3 wk of age) were randomly divided into three groups. In group BM (commencement of exercise before maturity), rats were kept in cages with running wheels for voluntary running for 6 mo. In group AM (commencement of exercise after maturity), rats were kept in tight cages for 2 mo and then in cages for voluntary running for 4 mo. In group NE (nonexercise), rats were kept in tight cages for 6 mo.

The two-step sequential euglycemic clamp procedure was carried out (insulin sensitivity–receptor defect: insulin infusion rate = 6 mU $\cdot$ kg^{-1} $\cdot$ min^{-1}; insulin responsiveness–postreceptor binding defect: 30 mU $\cdot$ kg^{-1} $\cdot$ min^{-1}).

Muscle GLUT4 mRNA was determined by Northern blotting analysis (30). The results obtained were as follows: (1) With the insulin infusion rate of 6 mU $\cdot$ kg^{-1} $\cdot$ min^{-1}, MCR in group BM was significantly higher ($p < .05$) than in groups AM and NE. There was no significant difference between groups AM and NE. (2) With the insulin infusion rate of 30 mU $\cdot$ kg^{-1} $\cdot$ min^{-1}, MCRs in groups BM and AM were significantly increased compared with those in group NE. (3) The concentration of GLUT4 mRNA in skeletal muscle in group AM was significantly greater than that in group NE.

These results might suggest (1) that physical exercise initiated before the onset of insulin resistance with the aging process prevents the lowering of insulin sensitivity and responsiveness in peripheral tissues; (2) that physical training after maturity improves decreased insulin responsiveness, but not insulin sensitivity; and (3) that the improvement in insulin action by physical exercise is associated, in part, with an increase in skeletal muscle GLUT4 mRNA.

Ezaki et al. (8) demonstrated that the amount of GLUT4 in some skeletal muscles decreases slightly in aged, obese rats, while exercise training increases the amount of GLUT4 more efficiently in aged rats than in young rats and ameliorates the GLUT4 decrease observed in aged rats. Another study (2) showed that although rat epitrochlearis muscle GLUT4 levels decrease early in life (between 3.5 and 13 mo), these levels are quite stable over a large portion of the adult life-span (between 13 and 25 mo) and that the increased responsiveness to insulin occurred in the absence of any increase in muscle GLUT4 levels. Further studies are necessary to clarify the more detailed molecular mechanisms in this field.

Acknowledgment

The authors thank colleagues of the diabetes research group of the First Department of Internal Medicine, Aichi Medical University, for assisting in this study and Miss K. Kawamura and Miss A. Yano for typing the manuscript. This study was supported, in part, by grants-in-aid from the Japanese Ministry of Health and Welfare.

References

1. Bell, G.I.; Kayano, T.; Buse, J.B.; Burant, C.F.; Takeda, J.; Lin, D.; Fukumoto, H.; Seino, S. Molecular biology of mammalian glucose transporters. Diabetes Care 13:198-208; 1990.
2. Cartee, G.D.; Briggs-Tung, C.; Kietzke, E.W. Persistent effects of exercise on skeletal muscle glucose transport across the life-span of rats. J. Appl. Physiol. 75:972-978; 1993.
3. Cartee, G.D.; Holloszy, J.O. Exercise increases susceptibility of muscle glucose transport to activation by various stimuli. Am. J. Physiol. 258:E390-E393; 1990.
4. Coggan, A.R.; Abduljalil, A.M.; Swanson, S.C.; Earle, M.S.; Farris, J.W.; Mendenhall, L.A.; Robitaille, P.R. Muscle metabolism during exercise in young and older untrained and endurance-trained men. J. Appl. Physiol. 75:2125-2133; 1993.
5. DeFronzo, R.A. Glucose intolerance and aging: Evidence for tissue insensitivity to insulin. Diabetes 28:1095-1101; 1979.
6. DeFronzo, R.A.; Ferrannini, E. Insulin resistance: A multifaceted syndrome responsible for NIDDM, obesity, hypertension, dyslipidemia, and atherosclerotic cardiovascular disease. Diabetes Care 14:173-194; 1991.
7. DeFronzo, R.A.; Ferrannini, E.; Sato, Y.; Felig, P.; Wahren, J. Synergistic interaction between exercise and insulin on peripheral glucose uptake. J. Clin. Invest. 68:1468-1474; 1981.
8. Ezaki, O.; Higuchi, M.; Nakatsuka, H.; Kawanaka, K.; Itakura, H. Exercise training increases more efficiently from aged obese rats than young lean rats. Diabetes 41:920-926; 1992.
9. Goodyear, L.J.; Hirshman, M.F.; Horton, E.D. The glucose transport system in skeletal muscle: Effect of exercise and insulin. Sato, Y.; Poortmans, J.; Oshida, Y., eds. Integration of medical and sports sciences. Basel: Karger; 1992:201-215.
10. Goodyear, L.J.; Hirshman, M.F.; Valyou, P.M.; Horton, E.D. Glucose transporter number, function and subcellular distribution in rat skeletal muscle after exercise training. Diabetes 41:1091-1099; 1992.
11. Goodyear, L.J.; Hirshman, M.F.; King, P.A.; Horton, E.D.; Thompson, C.H. Skeletal muscle plasma membranes glucose transport and glucose transporters after exercise. J. Appl. Physiol. 68:193-198; 1990.
12. Goodyear, L.J.; Smith, R.J. Exercise and diabetes. Kahn, C.R.; Weir, G.C., eds. Joslin's diabetes mellitus. Philadelphia: Lea & Febiger; 1994:451-459.
13. Gulve, E.A. Effects of acute and chronic exercise on insulin-stimulated glucose transport activity in skeletal muscle. Sato, Y.; Poortmans, J.; Oshida, Y., eds. Integration of medical and sports sciences. Basel: Karger; 1992:273-280.

14. Hediger, M.A.; Coady, M.J.; Ikeda, T.S.; Wright, E.M. Expression cloning and cDNA sequencing of the NA⁺/glucose co-transporter. Nature (London) 330:379-381; 1987.
15. Henriksen, E.J.; Ritter, L.S. Effect of insulin-like factors on glucose transport activity in unweighted rat skeletal muscle. J. Appl. Physiol. 75:820-824; 1993.
16. Houmard, J.A.; Hortobagy, T.; Neufer, P.D.; Johns, R.A.; Fraser, D.D.; Israel, R.G.; Dohn, G.L. Training cessation does not alter GLUT4 protein levels in human skeletal muscle. J. Appl. Physiol. 74:776-781; 1993.
17. Ishihara, H.; Asano, T.; Katagiri, H.; Lin, J.-L.; Tsukuda, K.; Inukai, K.; Yazaki, Y.; Oka, Y. Expression of GLUT4 glucose transporter in unweighted soleus muscle of normal and STZ-induced diabetic rats. Am. J. Physiol. 264:E301-E307; 1993.
18. Kaplan, N.M. The deadly quartet: Upper-body obesity, glucose intolerance, hypertriglyceridemia, and hypertension. Arch. Int. Med. 149:1514-1520; 1989.
19. Karnieli, E.; Zarnowski, M.J.; Hissin, P.J.; Simpson, I.A.; Salans, L.B.; Cushman, S.W. Insulin-stimulated translocation of glucose transport systems in the rat adipose cell. J. Biol. Chem. 256:4772-4777; 1981.
20. Koivisto, V.A.; Yki-Järvinen, H.; DeFronzo, R.A. Physical training and insulin sensitivity. Diabetes Metab. Rev. 1:445-481; 1986.
21. Oshida, Y.; Ohsawa, I.; Sato, J.; Sato, Y. Effects of adrenodemedullation on in vivo insulin-stimulated glucose utilization in relation to glycolysis in rat peripheral tissue. Endocr. J. 40:99-106; 1993.
22. Oshida, Y.; Yamanouchi, K.; Hayamizu, S.; Sato, Y. Longterm mild jogging increases insulin action despite no influence on body mass index or V̇O₂max. J. Appl. Physiol. 66:206-210; 1989.
23. Pedersen, O. Glucose transporters and diabetes mellitus. In: Marshall, S.M.; Alberti, K.G.M.M.; Krall, C.P., eds. Diabetes Ann. 7:30-54; 1993.
24. Ploug, T.; Stallknecht, B.; Pedersen, O.; Kahn, B.B.; Ohkuwa, T.; Vinten, J.; Galbo, H. Effect of endurance training on glucose transport capacity and glucose transporter expression in rat skeletal muscle. Am. J. Physiol. 259:E778-E789; 1990.
25. Reaven, G.M. Role of insulin-resistance in human disease. Diabetes 37:1595-1607; 1988.
26. Rodnick, K.J.; Holloszy, J.O.; Mondon, C.; James, D.E. Effects of exercise training on insulin-regulatable glucose-transporter protein levels in rat skeletal muscle. Diabetes 39:1425-1429; 1990.
27. Sato, Y.; Oshida, Y.; Ohsawa, I.; Sato, J.; Yamanouchi, K. Biochemical determination of training effects using insulin clamp and microdialysis techniques. In: Sato, Y.; Poortmans, J.; Oshida, Y., eds. Integration of medical and sports sciences. Basel: Karger; 1992:193-200.
28. Sato, Y.; Yamanouchi, K.; Nakajima, H.; Chikada, K.; Kato, K.; Oshida, Y.; Ohsawa, I.; Sato, J.; Sakamoto, N.; Higuchi, M.; Kobayashi, S. Improved insulin sensitivity and responsiveness after long-term physical training in aged subjects. In: Huh, K.B.; Shinn, S.H.; Kaneko, T., eds. Insulin resistance in human disease. Amsterdam: Elsevier; 1993:249-252.
29. Treadway, J.L.; James, D.E.; Burcel, E.; Ruderman, N.B. Effect of exercise on insulin receptor binding and kinase activity in skeletal muscle. Am. J. Physiol. 256:E138-E144; 1989.
30. Wake, S.A.; Sowden, J.A.; Storlien, L.H.; James, P.; Clark, W.; Shine, J.; Chisholm, D.J.; Kraegen, E.W. Effects of training and dietary manipulation on

insulin-regulatable glucose transporter mRNA in rat muscle. Diabetes 40:275-279; 1991.

31. Yamanouchi, K.; Nakajima, H.; Shinozaki, T.; Chikada, K.; Kato, K.; Oshida, Y.; Osawa, I.; Sato, J.; Sato, Y.; Higuchi, M.; Kobayashi, S. Effects of daily physical activity on insulin action in the elderly. J. Appl. Physiol. 73:2241-2245; 1992.

32. Zimmet, P.Z. Kelly West lecture 1991: Challenges in diabetes epidemiology. Diabetes Care 15:232-252; 1992.

CHAPTER 5

Determinants of Glucose Uptake in Contracting Muscle

Erik A. Richter, Peter Hespel

Copenhagen Muscle Research Centre, August Krogh Institute, University of Copenhagen, Copenhagen, Denmark; Department of Kinesiology, Faculty of Physical Education and Physiotherapy, Catholic University of Leuven, Leuven, Belgium

In a complex system such as the human body, regulation of glucose utilization is multifactorial. In muscle, like other tissues, glucose utilization is a function of three factors that usually vary in concert. These are supply (arterial concentration times blood flow), membrane glucose transport capacity, and metabolism.

The rate of transport of glucose at any given membrane permeability is dependent upon the transmembrane glucose gradient. Thus, the rate of glucose transport at a given degree of membrane transport capacity is critically dependent upon glucose supply, which delivers glucose to the outside of the muscle membrane for subsequent transmembrane transfer. Since the concentration at the outside of the muscle membrane is the interstitial glucose concentration, the transfer of glucose from the capillaries to the interstitium and diffusion through the interstitium are important. Glucose leaves muscle capillaries by simple diffusion through the capillary pores or slits (9) because the glucose molecule (molecular radius .44 nm) is much smaller than the average pore size (5-20 nm) (9). Diffusion through the interstitial space is facilitated by the aqueous environment in the interstitial space. However, a glucose gradient exists from the capillary end to the sarcolemmal end of the interstitium. The magnitude of this gradient probably varies with the diffusion distance from capillary to sarcolemma, the arterial glucose concentration, the capillary perfusion, and the actual sarcolemmal transport capacity for glucose.

The interstitial space is not easily accessible experimentally but recent developments in microdialysis techniques indicate that the average interstitial glucose concentration in adipose tissue (12, 21) and in resting rat muscle tissue (12) is very close to the venous blood glucose concentration. Similarly, recent data in human muscle during dynamic exercise suggest that the interstitial glucose concentration is close to the venous plasma glucose concentration (D. McLean and J. Bangsbo, personal communication).

Methods to Study Glucose Utilization

Whole body glucose utilization during exercise can be measured from isotopic tracer infusion studies using stable or radioactive tracers, and if the label is on carbon molecules (^{14}C or ^{13}C), it is possible to follow glucose oxidation, provided there is a steady-state labeling of the bicarbonate pool, a condition that takes time to acquire. The advantage of using tracer technology is the noninvasive nature of the technique, whereas the drawbacks are problems with lack of steady state during short-term experiments and inability to provide metabolic information in specific tissues unless combined with catheterization. The method of choice for studying local metabolism is combining arterial and venous catheterization with measurements of blood flow. A disadvantage is that a-v differences of glucose are small during exercise at euglycemia (in the range of 0.05-0.4 mmol/L) (2, 10, 23, 24, 37) and hence sometimes not easy to measure accurately. A direct comparison between isotopic turnover studies and local catheterization has been done during submaximal exercise in humans (26), and in fact a good agreement between the two measures was found (figure 5.1). Thus, when considering that the majority of glucose disposal

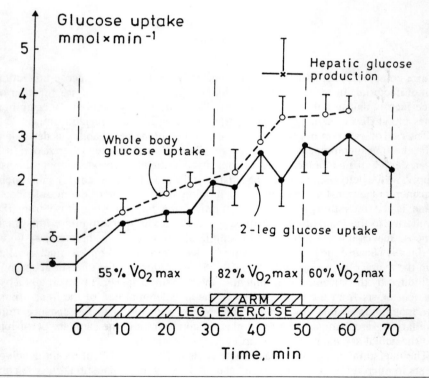

Figure 5.1   Isotopically measured whole-body glucose disappearance (dotted line) and directly measured two-leg glucose uptake (solid line) in man at rest and during ergometer cycling with legs only and with added arm cranking from 30 to 50 min of exercise. Values are means ± *SE* of seven observations.
Reprinted from Kjær, Kiens, Hargreaves, and Richter 1991.

at rest takes place in nonmuscle tissues, the rise in glucose disposal with exercise was of the same magnitude as measured with catheterization (figure 5.1).

Effect of Exercise Intensity on Muscle Glucose Uptake

In general, glucose utilization of a given muscle or muscle group increases with increasing exercise intensity (figure 5.2; 23, 47). However, at the onset of intense exercise, glucose may actually be released from contracting muscle (22), probably because rapid glycogenolysis results in significant formation of free glucose by the action of the glycogen debranching enzyme. This free glucose formation may exceed the capacity of the hexokinase reaction (which furthermore is inhibited by high intramuscular concentrations of glucose-6-phosphate that prevail during such conditions), resulting in a transient reversal of the glucose gradient and consequent net efflux of glucose. The phenomenon of glucose release only lasts a couple of minutes, after which it reverts to glucose uptake, possibly because the rate of glycogenolysis decreases. However, another possibility exists. This

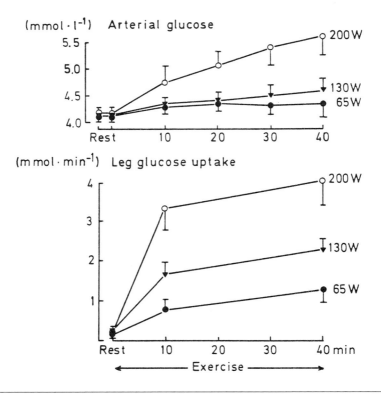

Figure 5.2   Arterial blood glucose concentration and leg glucose uptake at rest and during ergometer cycling with the legs. Open circles = 200 W; closed triangle = 130 W; closed circles = 65 W.

Reprinted from Wahren, Felig, and Hagenfeldt 1978.

relates to a possible exercise-induced increase in hexokinase activity. It has been shown in several tissues, including muscle (6, 39), that insulin induces a partial binding of hexokinase to mitochondria. Binding apparently decreases the K_m for ATP and increases the K_i for glucose-6-phosphate (31), which means that the ability of glucose-6-phosphate to inhibit the enzyme is decreased. Recently it was demonstrated that swimming exercise increases the mitochondrial-bound fraction of hexokinase in rat muscle (45), which presumably renders it less sensitive to inhibition by glucose-6-phosphate. Thus, redistribution of hexokinase during the first few minutes of exercise could alleviate inhibition of hexokinase by glucose-6-phosphate and could potentially be a mechanism involved in reverting glucose release to glucose uptake during intense exercise.

Blood flow increases linearly with increasing work load (4), and beyond 70% to 80% of $\dot{V}O_2$max, arterial glucose concentration usually also increases (25, 26, 30, 52). Together these facts mean that supply of glucose increases markedly with increasing intensity, which sets the stage for a high rate of glucose transport. When considering that glucose uptake is the product of blood flow and glucose a-v difference, it is noteworthy that the largest contributor to the exercise-induced increase in glucose uptake is the increase in flow, which may increase about 20-fold from rest to intense dynamic exercise. For instance, in the resting leg blood flow is approximately 400 to 600 ml/min (1, 2, 11, 26, 47) and increases linearly with increasing intensity to values around 5 to 7 L/min during maximal dynamic exercise (3, 23, 38). In contrast, at a constant arterial glucose concentration, the a-v difference only increases two- to three- or fourfold (23, 47). Thus, while the cellular events that increase muscle membrane glucose transport capacity with muscle contractions are very important, it should be realized that in vivo the increase in muscle perfusion accompanying exercise is of quantitatively large importance for glucose utilization.

It should at this point be mentioned that blood flow within a muscle both at rest and during electrically induced muscle contractions exhibits rather marked spatial heterogeneity (20, 33). Furthermore, glucose uptake apparently does too (20). The correlation between flow and glucose uptake within the muscle was found to be nonsignificant at rest, but during muscle contractions the correlation coefficient was .51 ($p < .05$) (20). The mechanism behind this inhomogeneity in flow and glucose uptake as well as their partial covariation is not known, and it remains to be demonstrated in humans during exercise. These findings may seem to suggest that blood flow is unimportant in regulating glucose uptake in a resting muscle, which, however, is in contrast to findings in perfused rat skeletal muscle (15, 19, 42).

At the cellular level the increase in firing frequency associated with increased exercise intensity (40) probably increases glucose uptake of the individual muscle fiber (32), and the recruitment of more fibers within the muscle is also expected to increase whole-muscle glucose utilization. However, with increasing exercise intensity, more and more type IIa and eventually type IIb fibers are recruited (40). In rats, type IIb fibers have a lower GLUT4 protein content than type IIa and type I fibers (13, 17, 29, 36) and have also been shown to have a lower rate of glucose transport during maximal electrical stimulation (8, 34). Thus, recruitment of type IIb fibers will be expected to increase glucose utilization less than recruitment of type I or type IIa fibers.

On the whole-body level, glucose utilization has also been found to increase with increasing exercise intensity. However, due to the fact that at rest most of the glucose is utilized in nonmuscle tissues, the magnitude of the increase with exercise is much smaller than when measured directly over muscle with catheters. Thus, at-rest glucose disposal (R_d) is typically around 0.8 mmol/min and may increase to maximal values of approximately 3 mmol/min during exercise at 100% $\dot{V}O_2$max (25, 30). This is in fact only about 50% of two-leg glucose uptake during exercise at 100% $\dot{V}O_2$max when measured with catheters (23) and suggests that, because of problems with steady state during the short exercise bouts at maximal exercise, isotope-derived figures on whole-body glucose utilization are inaccurate at high exercise intensities.

Another way of increasing exercise intensity on the whole-body level is by adding more active muscle mass, for example, adding arm exercise to leg exercise. The effect of adding arm exercise to leg exercise at a constant work load in one study was found to be a slight inhibition of glucose uptake without any changes in limb flow (37). In another study the interpretation was complicated by an increase in plasma glucose concentration when arm exercise was added to leg exercise (26). Teleologically, it makes sense that utilization of a limited fuel source like glucose is decreased per kilogram of active muscle when a large muscle mass is engaged in exercise. The mechanism probably involves increased sympathoadrenal activity (26, 37, 41), which, by increasing plasma FFA concentration and muscle glycogenolysis, can limit glucose uptake in muscle during exercise (7, 16, 18, 50).

Effect of Exercise Duration on Muscle Glucose Uptake

When exercising at a constant power output, within the first 4 to 5 min the blood flow to the working muscles increases to reach a plateau at which level flow is maintained remarkably constant for the duration of exercise (2, 16, 26, 44, 47). Thus, one component of glucose supply, namely blood flow, does not vary much except during the first few minutes. Therefore, glucose supply during exercise at a fixed power output varies directly with plasma glucose concentration. During most submaximal exercise, plasma glucose is quite constant until hepatic glucose production, because of glycogen depletion, cannot keep pace with peripheral glucose utilization (49, 51). Thus, during prolonged exercise, glucose supply is characterized by being fairly constant during the early stages, after which a slow decrease occurs. During exercise of intensities above approximately 70% to 80% of maximal aerobic capacity, plasma glucose may increase (25, 26, 30, 52; figure 5.2), which increases supply above that which can be accounted for by flow.

In regard to transport of glucose, the increase in permeability with onset of contractions probably occurs quite fast. In perfused rat skeletal muscle, glucose transport as measured by the uptake of radiolabeled 3-O-methylglucose was similar when measured over the first 5 min of contractions to that measured from 10 to 15 min of contractions (18), even though glucose uptake was higher in the 10- to 15-min period than in the 0- to 5-min period. This finding thus suggests that the increase in sarcolemmal permeability to glucose occurs rapidly and that other factors limit glucose uptake in the beginning of exercise. It has been suggested that such a factor may be glucose phosphorylation. Thus, during the initial stages of exercise, accumulation of glucose-6-phosphate in muscle may inhibit hexokinase and cause accumulation of free glucose in muscle (24). However, as exercise continues, glucose-6-phosphate concentrations decrease toward resting levels, which presumably gradually relieves hexokinase from inhibition and shifts the rate-limiting step in glucose utilization from metabolism back to transport (24). As mentioned earlier, another possible mechanism of relieving hexokinase from inhibition by glucose-6-phosphate may be translocation of hexokinase to mitochondria.

Not much is known about muscle glucose utilization during very prolonged exercise (> 4 h). However, it is tempting to suggest that glucose utilization might eventually decrease because of a marked increase in FFA (5, 16). In a study employing 3 h of cycling followed by 5 h of treadmill running, glucose appearance increased to a maximum after 4 h of exercise and then declined to resting values. Since plasma glucose was apparently maintained, glucose disappearance must also have decreased after 4 h of exercise (43). At the end of exercise, carbohydrate oxidation was close to resting values and was entirely accounted for by oxidation of plasma glucose (43).

Together, the changes in supply, transport, and metabolism of glucose explain the general increase in glucose utilization with increased exercise duration until glucose supply during prolonged exercise decreases. The increase in plasma concentrations of FFA during prolonged exercise is also expected to limit glucose utilization.

In regard to differences in glucose utilization by the different fiber types with exercise, no information is available in humans. Much probably depends on the specific fiber types recruited. Thus, recruitment of the more oxidative type I and type IIa fibers is expected to favor glucose utilization compared with recruitment of type IIb fibers, because, besides differences in GLUT4 protein content (13, 17, 29, 36), hexokinase activity is also higher in type I and type IIa than in type IIb fibers (40).

Role of Adenosine in Regulating Glucose Uptake

Recently it was shown that adenosine produced in contracting muscle augments the effect of insulin on glucose uptake and transport in perfused rat muscle (46; figure 5.3). Adenosine has previously been shown to be very important for insulin-stimulated glucose uptake in the heart (28). It is interesting that the effect of adenosine to increase insulin-mediated glucose transport in contracting muscle was only demonstrable in the insulin-sensitive slow-twitch and fast-twitch red fibers (46). Although the molecular mechanisms behind the effect of adenosine on insulin action are not well characterized, the demonstration of metabolic effects in addition to the known vascular effects of adenosine (14, 35) makes adenosine production in contracting muscle very interesting. Thus, adenosine might play a dual enhancing role in glucose metabolism during exercise: First, it apparently increases insulin action, and second (at least during some types of exercise [14, 27, 35]), it is also important for increasing blood flow and hence insulin and glucose delivery in contracting muscle. It remains, however, to establish the role of adenosine in glucose metabolism during exercise in humans.

Acknowledgments

The authors are supported by grants from the Danish Natural Sciences Research Council (grant no. 11-0082), the Danish Medical Research Council (grant no. 12-9535), the Novo-Nordisk Research Foundation and the Danish National Research

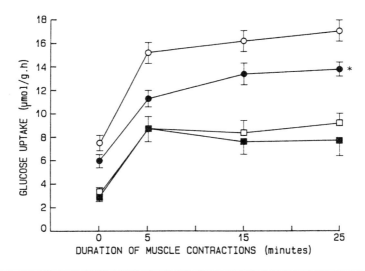

Figure 5.3   Glucose uptake at rest and during electrical stimulation in perfused rat hind-limb. Perfusate contained no insulin (squares) or insulin at 100 μU/ml (circles). Filled symbols denote addition of caffeine at 77 μM. *Values in the presence of caffeine are significantly lower than in its absence during muscle contractions. Values are means ± *SE* of 13 to 27 observations.
Reprinted from Vergauen, Hespel, and Richter 1994.

Foundation (grant no. 504-14), the Belgian National Research Foundation F.G.W.O. (grant no. 9.0031.90), and the Research Council of the Catholic University of Leuven (grant no. OT91/34).

References

1. Ahlborg, G.; Felig, P. Lactate and glucose exchange across the forearm, legs and splanchnic bed during and after prolonged leg exercise. J. Clin. Invest. 69:45-54; 1982.
2. Ahlborg, G.; Felig, P.; Hagenfeldt, L.; Hendler, R.; Wahren, J. Substrate turnover during prolonged exercise in man. Splanchnic and leg metabolism of glucose, free fatty acids and amino acids. J. Clin. Invest. 53:1080-1090; 1974.
3. Ahlborg, G.; Jensen-Urstad, M. Metabolism in exercising arm vs. leg muscle. Clin. Physiol. 11:459-468; 1991.
4. Andersen, P.; Saltin, B. Maximal perfusion of skeletal muscle in man. J. Physiol. 366:233-249; 1985.
5. Bergstrøm, J.; Hultman, E.; Jorfeldt, L.; Pernow, B.; Wahren, J. Effect of nicotinic acid on physical working capacity and on metabolism of muscle glycogen in man. J. Appl. Physiol. 26:170-176; 1969.
6. Bessman, S.P.; Geiger, P.J. Compartmentation of hexokinase and creatine phosphokinase, cellular regulation, and insulin action. Curr. Top. Cell. Regul. 16:55-86; 1980.

7. Bjørkman, O.; Milles, P.; Wasserman, D.; Lickley, L.; Vranic, M. Regulation of glucose turnover during exercise in pancreatectomized, totally insulin-deficient dogs. J. Clin. Invest. 81:1759-1767; 1988.
8. Brozinick, J.T.J.; Etgen, G.J.J.; Yaspelkis, B.B., III; Ivy, J.L. Contraction-activated glucose uptake is normal in insulin-resistant muscle of the obese Zucker rat. J. Appl. Physiol. 73:382-387; 1992.
9. Crone, C.; Levitt, D.G. Capillary permeability to small solutes. In: Renkin, E.M.; Michel, C.C., eds. Handbook of physiology: Section 2: The cardiovascular system. Bethesda, MD: American Physiological Society. 1984:411-466.
10. DeFronzo, R.; Ferrannini, E.; Sato, Y.; Felig, P.; Wahren, J. Synergistic inter-action between exercise and insulin on peripheral glucose uptake. J. Clin. Invest. 68:1468-1474; 1981.
11. DeFronzo, R.; Gunnarsson, R.; Bjørkman, O.; Olsson, M.; Wahren, J. Effects of insulin on peripheral and splanchnic glucose metabolism in noninsulin-dependent (type II) diabetes mellitus. J. Clin. Invest. 76:149-155; 1985.
12. Fuchi, T.; Rosdahl, H.; Hickner, R.C.; Ungerstedt, U.; Henriksson, J. Micro-dialysis of rat skeletal muscle and adipose tissue: Dynamics of the interstitial glucose pool. Acta Physiol. Scand. 151:249-260; 1994.
13. Goodyear, L.J.; Hirshman, M.F.; Smith, R.J.; Horton, E.S. Glucose transporter number, activity and isoform content in plasma membranes of red and white skeletal muscle. Am. J. Physiol. 261:E556-E561; 1991.
14. Goonewardene, I.P.; Karim, F. Attenuation of exercise vasodilatation by adeno-sine deaminase in anaesthetized dogs. J. Physiol. 442:65-79; 1991.
15. Grubb, B.; Snarr, J. Effect of flow rate and glucose concentration on glucose uptake rate by the rat limb. Proc. Soc. Exp. Biol. Med. 154:33-36; 1977.
16. Hargreaves, M.; Kiens, B.; Richter, E.A. Effect of increased plasma free fatty acid concentrations on muscle metabolism in exercising men. J. Appl. Physiol. 70:194-201; 1991.
17. Henriksen, E.J.; Bourey, R.E.; Rodnick, K.J.; Koranyi, L.; Permutt, M.A.; Holloszy, J.O. Glucose transporter protein content and glucose transport capacity in rat skeletal muscles. Am. J. Physiol. 259:E593-E598; 1990.
18. Hespel, P.; Richter, E.A. Glucose uptake and transport in contracting, perfused rat muscle with different pre-contraction glycogen concentrations. J. Physiol. 427:347-359; 1990.
19. Hespel, P.; Vergauen, L.; Vandenberghe, K.; Richter, E.A. Important role of insulin and flow in stimulating glucose uptake in contracting skeletal muscle. Diabetes 44:210-215; 1995.
20. Iversen, P.O.; Nicolaysen, G. Local blood flow and glucose uptake within resting and exercising rabbit skeletal muscle. Am. J. Physiol. 260:H1795-H1801; 1991.
21. Jansson, P.; Fowelin, J.; Smith, U.; Lönnroth, P. Characterization by micro-dialysis of intercellular glucose level in subcutaneous tissue in humans. Am. J. Physiol. 255:E218-E220; 1988.
22. Jorfeldt, L.; Wahren, J. Human forearm muscle metabolism during exercise: V. Quantitative aspects of glucose uptake and lactate production during exercise. Scand. J. Clin. Lab. Invest. 26:73-81; 1970.
23. Katz, A.; Broberg, S.; Sahlin, K.; Wahren, J. Leg glucose uptake during maximal dynamic exercise in humans. Am. J. Physiol. 251:E65-E70; 1986.
24. Katz, A.; Sahlin, K.; Broberg, S. Regulation of glucose utilization in human skeletal muscle during moderate dynamic exercise. Am. J. Physiol. 260:E411-E415; 1991.

25. Kjær, M.; Farrell, P.; Christensen, N.; Galbo, H. Increased epinephrine response and inaccurate glucoregulation in exercising athletes. J. Appl. Physiol. 61:1693-1700; 1986.

26. Kjær, M.; Kiens, B.; Hargreaves, M.; Richter, E.A. Influence of active muscle mass on glucose homeostasis during exercise in humans. J. Appl. Physiol. 71:552-557; 1991.

27. Koch, L.G.; Britton, S.L.; Metting, P.J. Adenosine is not essential for exercise hyperaemia in the hindlimb in conscious dogs. J. Physiol. 429:63-75; 1990.

28. Law, W.; McLane, M.; Raymond, R. Adenosine is required for myocardial insulin responsiveness in vivo. Diabetes 37:842-845; 1988.

29. Marette, A.; Richardson, J.M.; Ramlal, T.; Balon, T.W.; Vranic, M.; Pessin, J.E.; Klip, A. Abundance, localization, and insulin-induced translocation of glucose transporters in red and white muscle. Am. J. Physiol. 263:C443-C452; 1992.

30. Marliss, E.B.; Simantirakis, E.; Miles, P.D.G.; Purdon, C.; Gougeon, R.; Field, C.J.; Halter, J.B.; Vranic, M. Glucoregulatory and hormonal responses to repeated bouts of intense exercise in normal male subjects. J. Appl. Physiol. 71:924-933; 1991.

31. Mayer, S.E.; Mayfield, A.C.; Hass, J.A. Heart muscle hexokinase: Subcellular distribution and inhibition by glucose-6-phosphate. Mol. Pharmacol. 2:393-405; 1966.

32. Nesher, R.; Karl, I.; Kipnis, D. Dissociation of effects of insulin and contraction on glucose transport in rat epitrochlearis muscle. Am. J. Physiol. 249:C226-C232; 1985.

33. Piiper, J.; Pendergast, D.R.; Marconi, C.; Meyer, M.; Heisler, N.; Cerretelli, P. Blood flow distribution in dog gastrocnemius muscle at rest and during stimulation. J. Appl. Physiol. 58:2068-2074; 1985.

34. Ploug, T.; Galbo, H.; Vinten, J.; Jørgensen, M.; Richter, E.A. Kinetics of glucose transport in rat muscle: Effects of insulin and contractions. Am. J. Physiol. 253:E12-E20; 1987.

35. Poucher, S.M.; Nowell, C.G.; Collis, M.G. The role of adenosine in exercise hyperaemia of the gracilis muscle in anaesthetized cats. J. Physiol. 427:19-29; 1990.

36. Richardson, J.M.; Balon, T.W.; Treadway, J.L.; Pessin, J.E. Differential regulation of glucose transporter activity and expression in red and white skeletal muscle. J. Biol. Chem. 266:12690-12694; 1991.

37. Richter, E.A.; Kiens, B.; Saltin, B.; Christensen, N.J.; Savard, G. Skeletal muscle glucose uptake during dynamic exercise in humans: Role of muscle mass. Am. J. Physiol. 254:E555-E561; 1988.

38. Roca, J.; Agusti, A.G.N.; Alonso, A.; Poole, D.C.; Viegas, C.; Barbera, J.A.; Rodriguez-Roisin, R.; Ferrer, A.; Wagner, P.D. Effects of training on muscle O_2 transport at $\dot{V}O_2$max. J. Appl. Physiol. 73:1067-1076; 1992.

39. Russel, R.R., III; Mrys, J.M.; Mommessin, J.I.; Taegtmeyer, H. Compartmentation of hexokinase in rat heart. J. Clin. Invest. 90:1972-1977; 1992.

40. Saltin, B.; Gollnick, P. Skeletal muscle adaptability: Significance for metabolism and performance. In: Handbook of physiology: Sec. 10. Skeletal muscle. Bethesda, MD: American Physiological Society. 1983:555-631.

41. Savard, G.K.; Richter, E.A.; Strange, S.; Kiens, B.; Christensen, N.J.; Saltin, B. Norepinephrine spillover from skeletal muscle during exercise in humans: Role of muscle mass. Am. J. Physiol. 257:H1812-H1818; 1989.

42. Schultz, T.; Lewis, S.; Westbie, D.; Wallin, J.; Gerich, J. Glucose delivery: A modulator of glucose uptake in contracting skeletal muscle. Am. J. Physiol. 233:E514-E518; 1977.
43. Stein, T.; Hoyt, R.; O'Toole, M.; Leskiw, M.; Schluter, M.; Wolfe, R.; Hiller, W.D. Protein and energy metabolism during prolonged exercise in trained athletes. Int. J. Sports Med. 10:311-316; 1989.
44. Turcotte, L.P.; Richter, E.A.; Kiens, B. Increased plasma FFA uptake and oxidation during prolonged exercise in trained vs. untrained humans. Am. J. Physiol. 262:E791-E799; 1992.
45. Van Houten, D.R.; Davis, J.M.; Meyers, B.M.; Durstine, J.L. Altered cellular distribution of hexokinase in skeletal muscle after exercise. Int. J. Sports Med. 13:436-438; 1992.
46. Vergauen, L.; Hespel, P.; Richter, E.A. Adenosine receptors mediate synergistic stimulation of glucose uptake and transport by insulin and by contractions in rat skeletal muscle. J. Clin. Invest. 93:974-981; 1994.
47. Wahren, J.; Felig, P.; Ahlborg, G.; Jorfeldt, L. Glucose metabolism during leg exercise in man. J. Clin. Invest. 50:2715-2725; 1971.
48. Wahren, J.; Felig, P.; Hagenfeldt, L. Physical exercise and fuel homeostasis in diabetes mellitus. Diabetologia 14:213-222; 1978.
49. Wasserman, D.H.; Cherrington, A.D. Hepatic fuel metabolism during muscular work: Role and regulation. Am. J. Physiol. 260:E811-E824; 1991.
50. Wasserman, D.; Lacy, D.; Goldstein, R.; Williams, P.; Cherrington, A. Exercise-induced fall in insulin and increase in fat metabolism during prolonged muscular work. Diabetes 38:484-490; 1989.
51. Wasserman, D.; Lacy, D.; Green, D.; Williams, P.; Cherrington, A. Dynamics of hepatic lactate and glucose balances during prolonged exercise and recovery in the dog. J. Appl. Physiol. 63:2411-2417; 1987.
52. Yale, J.; Leiter, L.; Marliss, E. Metabolic responses to intense exercise in lean and obese subjects. J. Clin. Endocrinol. Metab. 68:438-445; 1989.

PART II

Regulation of Fat Metabolism in Exercise

CHAPTER 6

Regulation of Fat Metabolism in Exercise

Henrik Galbo, Bente Stallknecht
The Panum Institute, Copenhagen, Denmark

The understanding of fat metabolism in exercise has until recently been quite limited and did not improve much during the last two decades, although the need for more sophisticated views was emphasized (5, 6, 25). It has for a long time been known that overall fat combustion increases in response to exercise and reaches a peak at about 60% of $\dot{V}O_2$max (figure 6.1). Furthermore, it increases with exercise duration, if the exercise is not very heavy (7, 10). A fat-enriched diet as well as physical training enhances fat combustion in exercise (5, 6, 10, 16). Exercise enhances lipolysis in both adipose tissue and active muscle (5, 10, 16, 19, 25), whereas plasma triglyceride-derived FFA contributes only little to exercise metabolism in the postabsorptive state (5, 25).

Our views mostly have been based on whole-body measurements rather than on measurements on individual tissues, and they often rely on measurements that are imprecise or encumbered with many assumptions (5, 6, 19). The signals directly influencing lipolysis in exercise are also not known in detail. A decrease in plasma insulin and an increase in sympathoadrenal activity are considered the major determinants of fat cell lipolysis in exercise (5).

In recent years, however, new techniques have been introduced, and data have accumulated that represent a significant step forward in the understanding of fat metabolism in exercise. The new findings will be introduced here and will be discussed in detail in subsequent chapters by scientists who have contributed significantly to the progress.

Role of Various Fat Deposits

FFAs are produced during the lipolysis of triglyceride in many tissues, and until recently it has not been possible to directly evaluate the relative roles of these various fat depots in exercise. The size of intraabdominal fat stores correlates directly with insulin resistance and is considered an important determinant of type 2 diabetes,

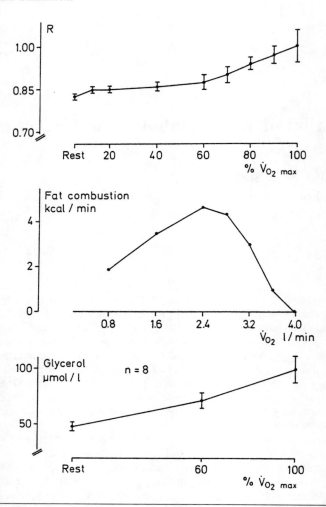

Figure 6.1   Relationship between exercise intensity, overall fat combustion, and lipolysis. R = respiratory exchange ratio.
Reprinted from Galbo 1992.

hyperlipemia, and hypertension (4). Celiac ganglion blockade selectively impairs sympathetic nerve activity to the splanchnic area. So, it is interesting that during exercise in humans glycerol and FFA concentrations in plasma have been shown to be lower in experiments with celiac ganglion blockade than in control experiments (12). The difference was not fully equalized even by infusion of epinephrine to supraphysiological concentrations (12). Albeit indirect, these findings indicate that during exercise FFAs are mobilized from splanchnic fat depots and that local sympathetic nervous activity is involved in the stimulation.

So far, metabolism of intraabdominal fat stores cannot be studied directly in humans. However, new techniques have been introduced that allow direct assessment of metabolism in more superficial adipose tissues. Catheterization of a vein that drains abdominal subcutaneous tissue makes application of Fick's principle possible (1, 9, 22). Microdialysis makes it possible to determine intercellular substrate concentrations in subcutaneous adipose tissues of different locations, and local venous concentrations may be calculated using a number of assumptions (1, 22). With both techniques, a continuous increase in lipolysis within local fat stores has been demonstrated during prolonged moderate exercise in humans (3, 9). The two techniques have different disadvantages, and it has been concluded that they should be regarded as complementary rather than alternative (1).

Signals Eliciting Lipolysis

It is possible through the microdialysis fiber to selectively deliver biologically active substances—for example, hormones and receptor-blocking agents—to the extracellular space in a given adipose tissue. In this way, regulatory mechanisms directly influencing lipolysis can be evaluated (1). Progress has also been made in the exploration of the signals eliciting these mechanisms. Focus has been on the relative importance of neural control from motor centers (central command) or via activity in afferent nerves from working muscles versus humoral feedback regulation. Most recently, attenuated increases in glycerol, FFA, and beta-hydroxybutyrate concentrations have been found during electrically induced cycling in quadriplegics and in healthy subjects with epidural anesthesia of the legs compared with findings during voluntary exercise (13, 15). This indicates that during exercise stimulation of lipolysis is normally triggered off by activity in motor centers and afferent muscle nerves.

The findings are in line with those of an earlier study, which aimed at selective enhancement of central command during a given absolute work load (14). In contrast to voluntary exercise, in both of the mentioned studies of electrically induced cycling no decrease in plasma insulin was seen (13, 15). This confirms that a reduction in insulin secretion is essential for enhancement of lipolysis in exercise.

FFA Uptake in Muscle

After release into plasma, FFA may be taken up into working muscle, and the uptake and oxidation may be directly related to FFA delivery (5, 27). Nevertheless, it has been difficult to demonstrate an enhancing effect of an artificial increase in FFA availability on fat combustion in humans (5). In agreement with this, FFA uptake in muscle has recently been found to show saturation (26). The saturation may reflect that uptake is limited by membrane transport capacity because a possible FFA carrier protein has recently been identified (5). However, evidence exists that FFAs accumulate intracellularly in exercising muscle (25). This indicates that FFA uptake is limited, at least partially, by intracellular disposal. Compatible with this, in trained compared with untrained subjects, a higher capacity to oxidize FFA in muscle is accompanied by a higher threshold for saturation of FFA uptake (27).

Determination of the uptake of FFA in muscle in vivo requires use of labeled FFA, because lipolysis in fat cells may contribute to local venous FFA concentrations.

However, uptake of FFA determined from arteriovenous differences in tracer concentrations equals gross uptake only if no efflux of tracer takes place. This assumption is inconsistent with the previously mentioned existence of an intracellular FFA pool (1, 6). In case tracer efflux exists, the measured FFA uptake equals net uptake in muscle only if no intracellular tracer dilution takes place. This assumption is inconsistent with the fact that turnover of intramuscular triglyceride is seen during exercise—at least if equilibration of intramuscular triglyceride stores has not been achieved during prolonged tracer infusion prior to exercise (6, 10). It follows that in future studies, in order to account better for intramuscular FFA kinetics, it will be necessary to determine concentrations and specific activities of protein-bound and free intracellular FFA.

Lipolysis in Muscle

In vitro, both contractions and catecholamines may enhance intramuscular lipolysis (5, 6). However, the enzymatic mechanisms involved have not been well understood. For some time it was believed that regulation of intramuscular lipolysis was mediated by intracellular lipoprotein lipase (18). However, this enzyme is synthesized as a secretory protein and has an inappropriate pH optimum (18). These objections do not apply to the adipose tissue hormone-sensitive lipase, which recently has been found also in muscle (18). Hormone-sensitive lipase from muscle can be simultaneously phosphorylated and activated by cAMP-dependent protein kinase. Therefore, a very exciting possibility, which has yet to be elucidated, exists in regard to control of muscle metabolism: Breakdown of triglyceride and glycogen in muscle may be regulated by enzymes—hormone-sensitive lipase and glycogen phosphorylase, respectively—that are activated in parallel and under dual control by Ca^{2+} and hormones.

There is evidence to suggest that muscle lipoprotein lipase (LPL) and hormone-sensitive lipase are activated simultaneously (18). Chylomicron triglyceride is a better substrate compared with very low density lipoprotein triglyceride for muscle LPL. This fact, as well as the higher plasma triglyceride concentration in the fed than in the fasting state, explains why the uptake of plasma triglycerides in exercising muscle is higher in the former than in the latter condition (8). It is interesting that, because LPL may be released from contracting muscle to plasma (18), measurements of plasma triglyceride extraction in muscle may underestimate the exercise-induced increase in plasma triglyceride turnover. Muscle LPL activity may also be increased after exercise (11), accounting for the fact that meal-induced lipemia can be reduced by prior exercise (21). This postexercise enhancement of plasma triglyceride clearance accompanies an increase in glucose clearance; these parallel events serve to replenish muscle triglyceride and glycogen stores, respectively.

FFA Recycling

Mobilization of FFA from triglyceride by lipolysis is not accurately matched with fat oxidation. Thus, during prolonged exercise FFAs accumulate extracellularly. Furthermore, animal studies have indicated that during exercise some of the FFAs mobilized by lipolysis are reesterified locally (i.e., intracellular recycling) or are reesterified elsewhere after transport within the circulation (i.e., intercellular recycling of FFA) (5, 6). The existence of triglyceride–fatty acid cycling also can be deduced in exercising humans from simple measurements (figure 6.1). Lipolysis increases with exercise intensity as indicated by the plasma glycerol concentration. Nevertheless, fat combustion decreases at high work loads and approaches zero at maximal exercise (figure 6.1). Since plasma FFA concentrations are lower at maximal exercise than at rest, it appears that in this condition all mobilized FFAs are trapped and possibly reesterified within the fat stores.

Studies of FFA cycling in humans are now carried out with more sophisticated techniques. Using the previously mentioned catheterization of a vein that drains abdominal subcutaneous tissue to obtain a-v differences in glycerol and FFA concentrations, it has been shown that fractional FFA reesterification is 20% to 30% at rest and decreases to values near zero during 1 h of exercise at 60% of $\dot{V}O_2max$ (9). The applied technique gives the overall reesterification within this particular adipose tissue and does not distinguish between the origin of reesterified FFAs, that is, between intra- and intercellular recycling (5). It is not clear why the results of the human study disagree with those of prior canine studies using similar techniques (2). In dogs the fractional reesterification of FFA in the inguinal fat pad was 66% both at rest and during prolonged running, and the total reesterification increased throughout exercise (2).

Another approach is to combine indirect calorimetry with measurements of glycerol and FFA turnover using stable isotopes. With this technique, a whole-body fractional reesterification of 50% to 70%, higher in trained than in untrained subjects, has been found at rest (20, 28). Once more, fractional reesterification decreased below resting levels in response to running at 40% $\dot{V}O_2max$. However, during 4 h of exercise, fractional reesterification increased again from 25% to 35% (28). Furthermore, total reesterification increased continuously from rest to end of exercise (28). Attempts to distinguish between intra- and intercellular recycling of FFA with these methods are based on the unsound assumption that fatty acids derived from muscle triglyceride are not directly oxidized but either reesterified or released to plasma. In consequence, intracellular recycling is overestimated. Accordingly, the conclusion that most of the change in fractional reesterification during exercise was caused by changes in intercellular cycling of FFA is probably correct (28).

The technique does not reveal the tissues (e.g., fat, muscle, liver) that participate in the intercellular cycling of FFAs. In future studies aiming at a detailed account of the mobilized FFAs that are traveling within and between triglyceride stores, whole-body turnover and indirect calorimetry measurements should be combined with arterial and regional venous catheterizations, allowing determination of local RQ, of net release of glycerol and FFA, and of extraction of labeled FFA. In this way the contribution of various tissues to oxidation and intra- and intercellular recycling of FFA during exercise can be evaluated.

Influence of Training

The influence of physical training on fat metabolism is an important aspect of the relationship between exercise and fat metabolism. This issue will be dealt with in subsequent chapters. However, some examples of current research directions will be given here. In order to explore the regulation in vivo of lipolysis in adipose

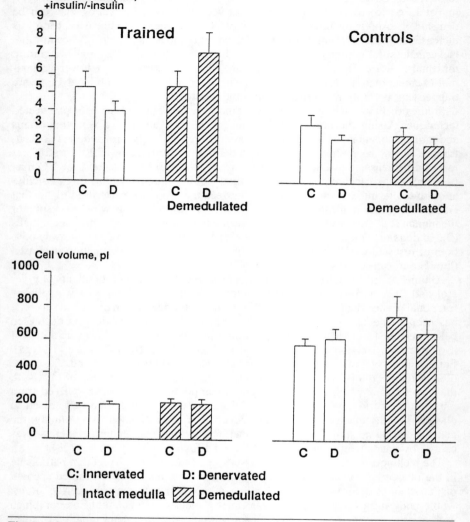

Figure 6.2   The influence of adrenodemedullation and unilateral abdominal sympathectomy on effects of training on epididymal fat cells in rats. Values are means ± *SE; n* = 6-9.

tissue from trained subjects, we infused epinephrine and measured glycerol output from the subcutaneous abdominal adipose tissue by microdialysis. We found that basal and epinephrine-induced lipolysis were identical in trained and untrained subjects (1.1 ± 0.7 vs. 1.0 ± 0.7 [*SD, n* = 6] μmol glycerol · 100 g⁻¹ · min⁻¹ during infusion of 0.3 nmol · kg⁻¹ · min⁻¹ of epinephrine) (24). This finding is compatible with the fact that a lower catecholamine response to a given work load after compared with before training is accompanied by lower turnover of plasma FFA (17). However, the finding is surprising in light of the fact that training has previously been shown to enhance both the lipolytic response to epinephrine of isolated fat cells (6) and the increases in plasma FFA and glycerol concentrations in response to a given epinephrine concentration (16). Possibly the subcutaneous abdominal adipose tissue is not representative of all fat stores.

The physiological mechanisms responsible for the development of fat cell adaptations to training are also being studied. Training enhances insulin-mediated glucose transport in fat cells, an adaptation facilitating replenishment of triglyceride stores between exercise bouts (5). We have recently studied the importance of sympathetic nervous activity for this adaptation. Rats were adrenodemedullated or sham operated and had the abdominal sympathetic chain below the first lumbar ganglion removed unilaterally. They were swim trained for 10 wk, and then fat cells were isolated from the epididymal fat pads.

It is seen from figure 6.2 that the fat cells were smaller and that the effect of a maximal insulin stimulation on glucose transport higher in trained than in untrained rats ($p < .05$). Furthermore, these effects of training were identical whether sympathetic activity had been impaired or not ($p > .05$). This indicates that neither circulating epinephrine nor local sympathetic nerve activity is crucial for development of changes in fat cell size and insulin responsiveness during training.

Finally, the molecular mechanisms underlying training-induced fat cell adaptations are also studied. Thus, it has recently been shown that the enhancement of insulin-mediated fat cell glucose transport achieved by training reflects an increase in fat cell GLUT4 mRNA and protein content (23).

Acknowledgments

The authors' research was supported by the Danish Medical Research Council, the Danish National Research Foundation, and the Novo Nordisk Foundation.

References

1. Arner, P.; Bülow, J. Assessment of adipose tissue metabolism in man: Comparison of Fick and microdialysis techniques. Clin. Sci. 85:247-256; 1993.
2. Bülow, J. Subcutaneous adipose tissue blood flow and triacylglycerol-mobilization during prolonged exercise in dogs. Pflügers Arch. 392:230-234; 1982.
3. Bülow, J.; Simonsen, L.; Madsen, J. Effects of exercise and glucose ingestion on adipose tissue metabolism. A microdialysis study. In: Sato, Y.; Poortmans, J.; Hashimoto, I.; Oshida, Y., eds. Integration of medical and sports sciences. Basel: Karger; 1992:329-335. (Med. Sport Sci.; vol. 37).
4. Coon, P.J. Effects of body composition and exercise capacity on glucose tolerance, insulin and lipoprotein lipids in healthy older men. Metabolism 38:1201-1209; 1989.
5. Galbo, H. Exercise physiology: Humoral function. Sport Sci. Rev. 1: 65-93; 1992.
6. Galbo, H. Hormonal and metabolic adaptation to exercise. New York: Thieme-Stratton Inc.; 1983.
7. Galbo, H.; Sonne, B.; Vissing, J.; Kjær, M.; Mikines, K.; Richter, E.A. Lack of accuracy of fuel mobilization in exercise. In: Benzi, G.; Packer, L.; Siliprandi,

N., eds. Biochemical aspects of physical exercise. Amsterdam: Elsevier Science Publishers B.V.; 1986:221-234.

8. Griffiths, A.J.; Humphreys, S.M.; Clark, M.L.; Frayn, K.N. Forearm substrate utilization during exercise after a meal containing both fat and carbohydrate. Clin. Sci. 86:169-175; 1994.

9. Hodgetts, V.; Coppack, S.W.; Frayn, K.N.; Hockaday, T.D.R. Factors controlling fat mobilization from human subcutaneous adipose tissue during exercise. J. Appl. Physiol. 71:445-451; 1991.

10. Hurley, B.F.; Nemeth, P.M.; Martin, W.H., III; Hagberg, J.M.; Dalsky, G.P.; Holloszy, J.O. Muscle triglyceride utilization during exercise: Effect of training. J. Appl. Physiol. 60:562-567; 1986.

11. Kiens, B.; Lithell, H.; Mikines, K.J.; Richter, E.A. Effects of insulin and exercise on muscle lipoprotein lipase activity in man and its relationship to insulin action. J. Clin. Invest. 84:1124-1129; 1989.

12. Kjær, M.; Engfred, K.; Fernandes, A.; Secher, N.H.; Galbo, H. Regulation of hepatic glucose production during exercise in humans: Role of sympathoadrenergic activity. Am. J. Physiol. 265:E275-E283; 1993.

13. Kjær, M.; Pollack, S.F.; Mohr, T.; Weiss, H.; Gleim, G.W.; Bach, F.W.; Nicolaisen, T.; Galbo, H.; Ragnarsson, K.T. Regulation of glucose turnover and hormonal responses during exercise: Electrically induced cycling in tetraplegic humans. Am. J. Physiol. (In press.)

14. Kjær, M.; Secher, N.H.; Bach, F.W.; Galbo, H. Role of motor center activity for hormonal changes and substrate mobilization in humans. Am. J. Physiol. 253:R687-R695; 1987.

15. Kjær, M.; Secher, N.H.; Bangsbo, J.; Perko, G.; Horn, A.; Mohr, T.; Galbo, H. Neural regulation of hormonal and metabolic responses to exercise studied by electrically induced cycling during epidural anesthesia. Am. J. Physiol. (In press.)

16. Martin, W.H., III; Coyle, E.F.; Joyner, M.; Santeusanio, D.; Ehsani, A.A.; Holloszy, J.O. Effects of stopping exercise training on epinephrine-induced lipolysis in humans. J. Appl. Physiol. 56:845-848; 1984.

17. Martin, W.H., III; Dalsky, G.P.; Hurley, B.F.; Matthews, D.E.; Bier, D.M.; Hagberg, J.M.; Rogers, M.A.; King, D.S.; Holloszy, J.O. Effect of endurance training on plasma free fatty acid turnover and oxidation during exercise. Am. J. Physiol. 265:E708-E714; 1993.

18. Oscai, L.B.; Essig, D.A.; Warren, K.P. Lipase regulation of muscle triglyceride hydrolysis. J. Appl. Physiol. 69:1571-1577; 1990.

19. Romijn, J.A.; Coyle, E.F.; Sidossis, L.S.; Gastaldelli, A.; Horowitz, J.F.; Endert, E.; Wolfe, R.R. Regulation of endogenous fat and carbohydrate metabolism in relation to exercise intensity and duration. Am. J. Physiol. 265:E380-E391; 1993.

20. Romijn, J.A.; Klein, S.; Coyle, E.F.; Sidossis, L.S.; Wolfe, R.R. Strenuous endurance training increases lipolysis and triglyceride–fatty acid cycling at rest. J. Appl. Physiol. 75:108-113; 1993.

21. Schlierf, G.; Dinsenbacher, A.; Kather, H.; Kohlmeier, M.; Haberbosch, W. Mitigation of alimentary lipemia by postprandial exercise-phenomena and mechanisms. Metab. Clin. Exp. 36:726-730; 1987.

22. Simonsen, L.; Bülow, J.; Madsen, J. Adipose tissue metabolism in humans determined by vein catheterization and microdialysis techniques. Am. J. Physiol. 266:E357-E365; 1994.

23. Stallknecht, B.; Andersen, P.H.; Vinten, J.; Bendtsen, L.L.; Sibbersen, J.; Pedersen, O.; Galbo, H. Effect of physical training on glucose transporter protein and mRNA levels in rat adipocytes. Am. J. Physiol. 265:E128-E134; 1993.
24. Stallknecht, B.; Simonsen, L.; Bülow, J.; Vinten, J.; Galbo, H. Effect of training on epinephrine-stimulated lipolysis determined by microdialysis in adipose tissue. Am. J. Physiol. 269:E1059-E1066; 1995.
25. Terjung, R.L.; Kaciuba-Uscilko, H. Lipid metabolism during exercise: Influence of training. Diabetes Metab. Rev. 2:35-51; 1986.
26. Turcotte, L.P.; Kiens, B.; Richter, E.A. Saturation kinetics of palmitate uptake in perfused skeletal muscle. FEBS Lett. 279:327-329; 1991.
27. Turcotte, L.P.; Richter, E.A.; Kiens, B. Increased plasma FFA uptake and oxidation during prolonged exercise in trained vs. untrained humans. Am. J. Physiol. 262:E791-E799; 1992.
28. Wolfe, R.R.; Klein, S.; Carraro, F.; Weber, J. Role of triglyceride–fatty acid cycle in controlling fat metabolism in humans during and after exercise. Am. J. Physiol. 258:E382-E389; 1990.

CHAPTER 7

Mobilization and Clearance of Fat in Exercising Humans Studied by Regional Venous Catheterization

Keith N. Frayn, Vanessa Hodgetts, A. John Griffiths
Oxford Lipid Metabolism Group, Sheikh Rashid Laboratory, Radcliffe Infirmary, Oxford, England; DRA Centre for Human Sciences, Gosport, Hampshire, England; Hammersmith Hospital, London, England

Oxidation of fatty acids is an important source of energy for physical activity. These fatty acids may be delivered to the exercising muscle in the plasma, or they may be derived from intramuscular triacylglycerol (TG) stores. If they are delivered in the plasma, they may be transported in the form of nonesterified fatty acids (NEFA) or lipoprotein TG. The transport of fatty acids in the plasma, whether in the form of NEFA or TG, may be studied by a number of techniques. The most important of these are tracer (radioactive or stable isotope) measurements of substrate turnover and measurements of arteriovenous differences across different tissues made by regional venous catheterization. While substrate turnover techniques can give important information on the relative rates of production and utilization of different substrates, and even (indirectly) on the utilization of muscle TG stores (48), they usually provide little information on processes within individual tissues. In contrast, arteriovenous difference techniques provide direct information on the (net) rates of metabolic processes in individual tissues. On the other hand, especially in the area of fat metabolism, straightforward measurement of arteriovenous differences by chemical means may give misleading results (as will be discussed), and a combination of tracer infusion and arteriovenous difference measurements can then be particularly informative. In this review, the emphasis will be on the contribution that arteriovenous difference measurements have made to our understanding of fat metabolism during exercise. As far as possible, only experiments in humans will be reviewed.

There is a common observation that oxidation of fatty acids cannot account for more than about 60% of the maximal rate of oxygen consumption. Thus, concomitant glucose oxidation is required for high-intensity endurance exercise, and power output falls when glycogen stores are exhausted. The limited contribution of fat appears paradoxical when it is considered that fat represents, even in a lean, well-trained athlete, by far the biggest potential reserve of chemical energy in the body. It is not clear whether this limited rate of oxidation of fatty acids represents a limitation in the rate at which they can be delivered to and transported in the plasma, or in the rate at which they can be taken up and oxidized by muscle. The literature on arteriovenous difference measurements will be reviewed with this question in mind.

The process of fat oxidation in exercising muscle may be divided into different stages. Those open to investigation by measurement of arteriovenous differences include the mobilization of NEFA from stored TG in adipose tissue, the uptake of NEFA by the muscle, and the uptake by muscle of fatty acids from circulating TG (figure 7.1). Circulating TG arises either from the small intestine (chylomicron TG) or the liver (very low density lipoprotein, VLDL TG). In principle, the rate of hepatic secretion of VLDL TG is open to investigation by measurement of arteriovenous differences across the splanchnic bed during exercise, but little information is available in humans, and this subject will not be reviewed here.

Fat Mobilization

The details of the process of fat mobilization from TG stored in adipose tissue have been reviewed recently by a number of authors (e.g., 5, 17). TG stored in

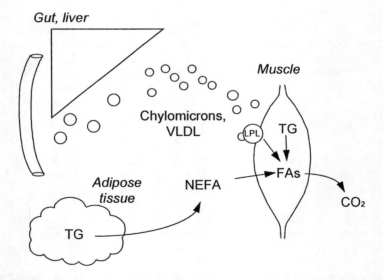

Figure 7.1 Overview of fat metabolism during exercise, showing points open to investigation by regional venous catheterization techniques: secretion of triacylglycerol (TG)-rich lipoproteins from splanchnic bed (liver and small intestine), mobilization of fatty acids from adipose tissue, muscle uptake of triacylglycerol fatty acids from plasma, and muscle uptake of nonesterified fatty acids (NEFA) from plasma. VLDL = very low density lipoprotein; LPL = lipoprotein lipase; FAs = fatty acids within muscle (substrate for oxidation).

adipocytes is hydrolyzed by the so-called hormone-sensitive lipase (HSL) and by an active monoacylglycerol lipase. Fatty acids thus released may be reesterified (to form new TG) before leaving the tissue, or they may enter the capillaries where they are bound by albumin and carried into the general circulation.

The activity of HSL is governed by a number of hormonal factors and also possibly by the sympathetic nervous system. It is activated by catecholamines and by growth hormone and cortisol (the last two being relatively slow) and suppressed by insulin. In humans, there are conflicting results about the role of glucagon (11, 32, 60), but on balance its effect on fat mobilization is probably small. The fate of fatty acids released by HSL action is governed by a number of factors. Under conditions of high glucose and insulin concentrations (as after a meal), a substantial proportion may be reesterified within the tissue (14, 15, 22), whereas in the postabsorptive state (after overnight fast), the majority (around 80-100% [16, 22]) are released into the circulation. The rate of release of fatty acids into the plasma is also governed by the perfusion of adipose tissue. Fatty acids require binding to albumin for solubility in the plasma, and under normal circumstances in the general circulation the molar ratio of NEFA to albumin is around 1:1 to 2:1, reflecting the fact that albumin has about three high-affinity binding sites for fatty acids. Thus, a restriction on the availability of albumin (e.g., when the rate of lipolysis is high relative to adipose tissue blood flow) may lead to a retention of fatty acids in the tissue in a form or location that has not been identified. This topic will be discussed further below.

One criterion for the satisfactory measurement of arteriovenous differences across a particular tissue is that the tissue must have a well-defined venous drainage, uncontaminated by the drainage from other tissues, and be accessible for sampling. In the case of adipose tissue, this presents difficulties: Most subcutaneous adipose depots have very diffuse patterns of drainage that mingle with those of the underlying muscle. For this reason, most studies in this area have been carried out in animals, particularly the dog: In this species it is possible to cannulate the pudendal vein, which drains a distinct subcutaneous adipose depot (7). More recently, a procedure has been developed for cannulation of a vein draining the subcutaneous abdominal adipose tissue in humans (20). This depot is separated from the underlying muscle by an avascular fibrous sheath, the aponeurosis of the *external oblique* muscle, and biochemical evidence suggests that the blood obtained is almost pure adipose tissue drainage (19). Studies have been made with this preparation during exercise (30).

In the postabsorptive state (after overnight fast), adipose tissue releases both NEFA and glycerol (20). The ratio between them is almost 3:1 (as would be expected for complete hydrolysis of TG and release of all the products), showing that reesterification of fatty acids is low in this state. Studies were carried out in nine recreational athletes who exercised at 50% to 70% of their $\dot{V}O_2$max for 60 min (30; figure 7.2). During exercise, as would be expected, the release of fatty acids increased as shown by an increasing arteriovenous difference for release across the tissue (30). (In these experiments, adipose tissue blood flow was not measured during exercise since this poses technical problems. The results have to be interpreted with this in mind.) Despite this increasing concentration difference, the arterial NEFA concentration rose only slightly, presumably because the rate of utilization of fatty acids by the exercising muscle also increased. (This shows the limitation of using the arterial NEFA concentration as a guide to the rate of fat mobilization.) At the end of exercise, the arterial NEFA concentration rose rapidly, as is often observed (e.g., 28, 59); presumably the rate of release remained high for a short time while the rate of utilization fell rapidly.

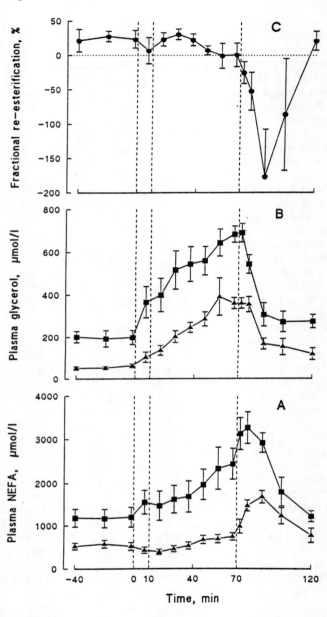

Figure 7.2   Plasma concentrations of (A) nonesterified fatty acids (NEFA) and (B) glycerol in arterialized (triangles) and adipose-venous (squares) plasma, and (C) calculated proportion of fatty acids reesterified. Values are means ± *SE* for nine subjects. Dashed vertical lines show start of warm-up (0 min); start of exercise (10 min), which consisted of bicycling at 50% to 70% of V̇O₂max; and end of exercise (70 min). The apparently negative reesterification values immediately after exercise reflect the sudden release of NEFA from adipose tissue that was not accompanied by glycerol.

Reprinted from Hodgetts, Coppack, Frayn, and Hockaday 1991.

In contrast to the slight rise in arterial NEFA concentration during exercise, the arterial plasma glycerol concentration rose markedly. Glycerol is not used to any great extent by contracting muscle, and its systemic concentration is therefore probably a better indicator of lipolysis than is the NEFA concentration. At the end of exercise, when the NEFA concentration rose sharply, the glycerol concentration did not (figure 7.2).

These studies, taken together with the animal work, show some features of the regulation of fat mobilization during exercise. The animal studies suggest that the release of fatty acids may be restricted during exercise through a lack of availability of albumin, which in turn (via high local NEFA/albumin ratios) may further decrease perfusion of the tissue (8, 9, 40). This results in a retention of fatty acids in the tissue, and it has been suggested (from animal studies) that this stimulates the reesterification of fatty acids (40). In the human studies, there was again evidence for retention of fatty acids in adipose tissue during exercise. However, there was no evidence for increased reesterification (as a proportion of fatty acids released) during exercise. The proportion of fatty acids retained in the tissue remained below about 20% and decreased to near zero toward the end of a 60-min exercise period. Immediately after exercise, however, there was a period when fatty acid release greatly exceeded that expected from glycerol release (manifested as an apparently negative reesterification rate; figure 7.2). The most likely explanation is that fatty acids were retained in the tissue in some form (not esterified) during exercise, and suddenly after exercise—with relief of a restriction of blood flow, for example—released into the plasma. It may well be that there was a restriction to their release during exercise because of lack of available albumin. However, any such limitation occurs at much greater NEFA/albumin ratios than had previously been supposed; peak NEFA/albumin molar ratios in individual subjects in the adipose tissue venous plasma ranged from 3.7:1 to 6.8:1 (30). The overall impression from these studies was that the release of fatty acids from adipose tissue might, indeed, limit their availability to the exercising muscle. There was always a marked gradient from adipose tissue venous plasma to systemic concentration, and the systemic plasma NEFA concentration remained relatively low, suggesting that fatty acids were utilized at a rate which matched their rate of release. Had the rate of utilization by muscle been the limiting step, it seems more likely that the arterial concentration would have risen and the gradient from adipose venous to systemic plasma declined. Similar conclusions were reached in an isotopic study of light (36% $\dot{V}O_2$max) and heavy (70% $\dot{V}O_2$max) exercise: During heavy exercise, systemic plasma NEFA concentrations fell and the rate of fatty acid turnover decreased, implying a limitation at the level of mobilization rather than of fatty acid utilization (34).

The factors regulating fat mobilization from adipose tissue during exercise are thus complex and conflicting. While the hormonal environment is clearly highly conducive to lipolysis (relatively low insulin concentrations, high catecholamine concentrations, and elevated growth hormone and cortisol concentrations potentially contributing during prolonged exercise), a proportion of fatty acids are nevertheless in some way entrapped in the tissue and not released until exercise ceases. This may reflect α-adrenergic vasoconstriction in adipose tissue (23), relieved at the end of exercise.

Utilization of Plasma NEFA by Exercising Muscle

The store of TG in adipose tissue, even in a lean athlete, would be sufficient to maintain high rates of energy expenditure for days or even weeks. In order for this to happen, the adipocyte TG must be hydrolyzed and NEFA released into the circulation, as previously reviewed. Once in the circulation, fatty acids must be taken up by the muscle. Fatty acid uptake into a number of tissues is now thought to occur by specific transporters in the cell membrane (27, 53). Once inside the cell, fatty acids are bound by one or more fatty acid–binding proteins to aid their transport through the cytoplasm to the mitochondria (56). After activation to their CoA esters, fatty acids enter the mitochondria for oxidation via the carnitine shuttle, which is outside the scope of this review. Early studies of fatty acid uptake and oxidation in muscle, based on the measurement of arteriovenous differences, suggested that fatty acids entering the muscle cell became esterified and entered a muscle TG pool, from which fatty acids for oxidation were derived by intramuscular lipolysis (18, 61). This view was based mainly on the delay in release of $^{14}CO_2$ from the muscle after the intraarterial infusion of ^{14}C-labeled fatty acids. It is now generally considered not to be true, although there are no good published data to refute it. While this route of fatty acid oxidation in muscle, were it to exist, would be of importance for the interpretation of tracer studies of substrate turnover, it is not really important for interpretation of arteriovenous difference studies as reviewed later.

Two preparations have been used extensively in studies of the utilization of plasma NEFA by muscle in humans: the forearm and the leg. For the former, a vein in the antecubital fossa that drains predominantly the deep (muscular) tissues can be identified and cannulated (2). Superficial blood (arising from the hand, skin, and subcutaneous adipose tissue) can be largely excluded by occlusion of the wrist with a blood pressure cuff inflated to a pressure above arterial. Exercising muscle can be studied if the subject performs intermittent isometric contraction by squeezing a handgrip dynamometer or simply a sphygmomanometer bulb (58). However, the bulk of muscle drained is not large, and arteriovenous differences are not always readily measurable, especially when blood flow is high during exercise. The exercising leg is studied by cannulation of the femoral vein in the groin. The leg can be exercised by the subject working on a bicycle ergometer (one- or two-legged exercise). The bulk of muscle drained is obviously greater than in the forearm. However, there is some limitation in interpretation because there are communicating veins that join deep and superficial venous drainage (and thus skin and adipose tissue metabolism may be included).

For either arm or leg, muscle blood flow may be measured in order to quantitate substrate uptake and release. This is done most directly using an indicator-dilution technique (3) with an indicator (thermal or dye) infused into the relevant artery: brachial for the forearm, femoral for the leg. Alternatively, ^{133}Xe may be injected into the muscle and its clearance followed (38), or whole-limb blood flow may be measured by plethysmography (24). The latter has the advantages of simplicity and noninvasiveness but the disadvantage that it is sensitive to movement and may require momentary cessation of exercise (26).

Whichever preparation is used, the direct measurement of NEFA extraction by muscle poses a problem. It was recognized more than 30 years ago that the net exchange of NEFA across a limb reflects the balance between muscle uptake and concomitant release of fatty acids from adipocytes (4; figure 7.3). Adipocytes are found interleaved within the muscle cells, and discrete intramuscular depots may also contribute. In addition, because the venous drainage is not pure (as previously discussed), there may be a contribution from subcutaneous adipose depots. For this reason, although muscle is not thought under any circumstances to release NEFA into the general circulation, it is not uncommon to measure net NEFA release from the

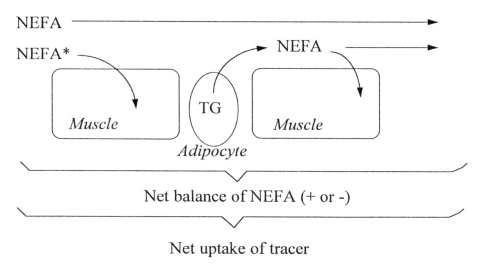

Figure 7.3 Exchange of nonesterified fatty acids (NEFA) across a muscle bed. NEFA delivered in the arterial plasma (left-hand side) may be taken up by muscle fibers. They are also produced by adipocytes within the tissue bed. Net balance of NEFA across the tissue bed may be negative or positive. Uptake may be measured separately by infusion of a tracer (labeled with a stable or radioactive isotope, shown as NEFA*). There will always be net uptake of tracer.

human forearm (4). If insulin, even at low concentrations, is infused, adipose tissue lipolysis is suppressed and the uptake of NEFA by muscle is unmasked (47). This difficulty can be overcome by simultaneous infusion of an isotopic fatty acid tracer. Fatty acid uptake can then be measured by the disappearance of the tracer across the limb, which can be observed despite a net liberation of fatty acids (figure 7.3).

In the resting state or during moderate exercise (120 min at 50% $\dot{V}O_2$max), there is a clear relationship between the rate of delivery of NEFA in the plasma and the rate of uptake by muscle, where delivery is the product of plasma flow and arterial concentration; this is true for both the leg (52; figure 7.4) and the myocardium in vivo (57). In the myocardium there is evidence for saturability, whereas in the leg the relationship was linear over the range of deliveries studied. Thus, under these conditions skeletal muscle appears able to take up and presumably oxidize fatty acids as fast as they are delivered. The ability of the muscle to extract and oxidize fatty acids is improved by training, as shown by a greater fractional uptake across the leg and greater oxidation of fatty acids in trained subjects compared with untrained, for similar plasma concentrations (55).

Studies of the uptake of NEFA by the human leg (listed in table 7.1) indicate that uptake of plasma NEFA contributes around 20% to 40% of the oxygen consumption of muscle during exercise of 1 to 2 h duration. The contribution of plasma NEFA to O_2 consumption tends to rise with time (e.g., from 37% during the first hour to 62% after 4 h), and it tends to decline with increasing intensity of exercise (e.g., 37% of leg O_2 consumption at 30% $\dot{V}O_2$max to 19% of leg O_2 consumption at 65% $\dot{V}O_2$max).

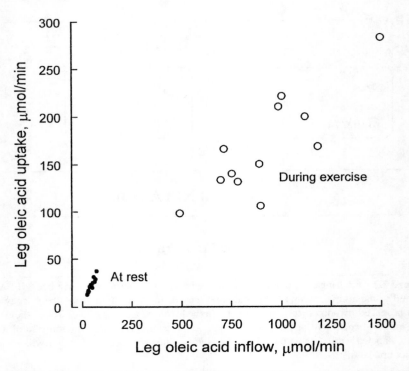

Figure 7.4   Relationship between fatty acid delivery to leg (*x* axis) and leg fatty acid uptake (*y* axis) at rest and during exercise (50% $\dot{V}O_2$max for 2 h) in seven subjects; each subject was studied on two occasions, with and without carnitine supplementation (not distinguished here; no differences were apparent). Based on data in Soop et al. 1988 (52).

The lower contribution of plasma NEFA to muscle oxygen consumption at higher exercise intensities does not seem to reflect primarily an inability of muscle to utilize plasma NEFA at high work loads: The fractional extraction of NEFA across the exercising leg falls only slightly with increasing work load (e.g., from 0.19 at 30% $\dot{V}O_2$max to 0.16 at 65% $\dot{V}O_2$max; table 7.1). Rather, it seems to reflect a failure of NEFA delivery to the muscle to increase with increasing work load (table 7.1). Again, therefore, the evidence suggests that the primary reason for the limited contribution of fatty acid oxidation to muscle oxygen consumption lies more in a limitation in the rate of fatty acid delivery to the muscle than in an inability of the muscle to utilize fatty acids. However, it should be noted that few, if any, arteriovenous difference studies have been performed at very high work intensities (> 65% $\dot{V}O_2$max), probably because of the technical difficulties involved. Other factors might, therefore, become rate limiting at higher work intensities.

Plasma Triacylglycerol Uptake by Muscle During Exercise

Plasma TG circulates mainly in two forms: chylomicron TG (derived from dietary fat) and VLDL TG (secreted by the liver). Circulating TG is utilized by a number

Table 7.1   Plasma Nonesterfied Fatty Acid (NEFA) Metabolism in the Human Leg During Exercise at Various Intensities

Reference	Subjects	Work load	% contribution of plasma NEFA to leg O_2 consumption	NEFA delivery rate to leg, mmol/min	Fractional extraction of NEFA
Ahlborg et al. 1974 (1)	Untrained	30% $\dot{V}O_2$max	40 min: 37% 240 min: 62%	40 min: 1.22 240 min: 3.06	40 min: 0.19 240 min: 0.15
Havel et al. 1967 (29)	Moderately trained	400 kg-m/min (≈40% $\dot{V}O_2$max)	1-2 h: 21%	Blood flow not measured	1-2 h: 0.17
Wahren et al. 1984 (59)	Untrained	45% $\dot{V}O_2$max	60 min: 20%	Blood flow not reported	60 min: 0.16
Soop et al. 1988 (52)	Moderately trained	50% $\dot{V}O_2$max	120 min: 32%	120 min: 2.87	120 min: 0.17
Turcotte et al. 1992 (55)	Trained	60% m.v.c.	0-2 h: 23% 2-3 h: 35%	0-2 h: 1.46* 2-3 h: 3.74*	0-2 h: 0.15 3 h: 0.15
	Untrained		0-2 h: 16% 2-3 h: 20%	0-2 h: 1.00* 2-3 h: 3.27*	0-2 h: 0.15 3 h: 0.07
Jansson & Kaijser 1987 (31)	Trained	65% $\dot{V}O_2$max	60 min: 19%	60 min: 2.20	60 min: 0.16
	Untrained		60 min: 18%	60 min: 1.90	60 min: 0.12

Percentage contribution of plasma NEFA to leg O_2 consumption refers to the proportion of leg O_2 consumption (measured by arteriovenous difference) that would be accounted for by oxidation of the NEFA uptake observed (see 21). NEFA delivery rate to leg is leg plasma flow × arterial concentration of NEFA. The data marked with an asterisk are for NEFA supply to the thigh only. Fractional extraction of NEFA refers to the fraction of the fatty acid tracer (either oleic or palmitic acid) extracted during a single passage through the leg. Some values were calculated from data contained in the papers; the percentage $\dot{V}O_2$max for the study by Havel et al. was estimated assuming a $\dot{V}O_2$max for their subjects of 3.5 L/min.

m.v.c. = maximum voluntary contraction.

of tissues, including adipose tissue and skeletal muscle. The first step in this process is hydrolysis of TG by the enzyme lipoprotein lipase (LPL) attached to the capillary endothelium. LPL releases fatty acids, which may be taken up into the tissue for oxidation or storage. Some of the fatty acids released by LPL action are also released into the plasma (22); this will be discussed again later. The fatty acids liberated by muscle LPL are taken up into the cells and metabolized following pathways that may be the same as those for plasma NEFA; it is not clear whether there are distinct pools of fatty acids arising from different sources.

A key regulatory step in this process is the activity of LPL. LPL activity is greater in oxidative than in glycolytic muscles (39) and is increased by endurance training and by prior exercise (36, 37, 43). These features suggest that uptake and oxidation of TG fatty acids will be an important source of energy for working muscle. However, the evidence from arteriovenous difference measurements does not clearly bear this out.

In early studies, Havel and co-workers examined the potential role of plasma TG during low-intensity exercise (either walking or bicycling at 40% $\dot{V}O_2$max) and concluded that plasma TG fatty acids were unlikely to contribute more than 5% to 10% of leg oxidative metabolism (28, 29). Turcotte et al. (55) could not measure TG extraction across the working thigh. This points to a technical difficulty: The fractional extraction of plasma TG across a limb may be very small (since the arterial concentration is relatively high) and difficult to measure precisely. For instance, using data from Turcotte et al. (55), it may be shown that for a contribution of 10% of thigh oxygen consumption, the fractional extraction of plasma TG would be around 1.5%; accurate quantitation is thus extremely difficult. In studies of VLDL TG extraction across the thigh (36), arteriovenous differences were easily measurable at rest (55 µmol/L in a trained thigh against 30 µmol/L in an untrained thigh). During exercise when blood flow was increased, arteriovenous differences were correspondingly decreased, representing about 8% fractional extraction (estimated from data in paper), a small difference in an inherently variable measurement. Nevertheless, this corresponds to a potential contribution of about 25% of the thigh oxygen consumption (using data for thigh O_2 consumption from ref. 55). This shows again the difficulty of measuring precisely a small contribution of plasma TG to muscle metabolism.

All the preceding studies were conducted in the overnight-fasted state, when most of plasma TG is present in the VLDL fraction. The findings may be different when chylomicron TG is present in the circulation. Chylomicrons compete with VLDL particles for hydrolysis by LPL and are its preferred substrate (6, 45). In the human (untrained) forearm at rest, extraction of VLDL TG was not measurable, while fractional extraction of chylomicron TG after a mixed meal (containing 33 g fat) was 10% to 15% (46).

In rats, chylomicrons containing labeled fatty acids are cleared more rapidly during exercise than at rest (33), and their removal by different muscles is related to muscle fiber type (more extensive in more oxidative fibers) and to muscle LPL activity (39, 54). Chylomicron TG fatty acids appear to enter a rapidly oxidizable pool (33), consistent with the idea that they may form an important substrate for muscle oxidative metabolism.

Very few studies have examined the potential for chylomicron TG to act as an energy source for contracting muscle in humans. Indirect evidence that chylomicron TG may be utilized by working muscle is provided by the observation that postprandial lipemia (the rise in plasma TG concentration after a fatty meal) is reduced if subjects exercise during the postprandial period (12, 42, 51). In addition, there is considerable evidence that postprandial lipemia is diminished in trained compared with untrained subjects (13, 41) and by a prior bout of exercise (10, 50), conditions known to elevate LPL activity in muscle. Direct measurements of chylomicron TG removal by measurement of arteriovenous differences in humans have apparently been confined to the forearm. Kaijser and Rössner (35) studied the removal of "fat particles" across the forearm at rest and during 45 min of rhythmic handgrip exercise. The fat particles were not true chylomicrons, but arose from infused lipid emulsion (Intralipid); they behave like chylomicrons in most respects. They found considerable extraction of fat particles at rest (fractional extraction around 10%), but during exercise this was no longer measurable, presumably masked by the increased blood flow. At rest, the forearm removal of TG particles was equivalent to around 2.3 times the forearm oxygen consumption (i.e., fat storage must have been occurring); this indicates the potential for replenishment of muscle TG stores by uptake of chylomicron TG during the postprandial phase. A study of HDL cholesterol production in the forearm showed some of the pitfalls of this area: No arteriovenous differences for "TG" were measured even after fat ingestion, but clearly lipolysis was occurring because HDL cholesterol was produced in the forearm (and more after fat feeding and during forearm exercise; 49). (Cholesterol is transferred to the HDL fraction during the action of LPL on the TG-rich lipoproteins [36, 44].) However, the method used for TG estimation measured total glycerol (free + esterified), and since free glycerol efflux from the forearm was probably increased during exercise, this may have masked TG uptake. Finally, in a recent study forearm uptake of substrates was studied at rest and during 60 min of intermittent handgrip exercise both after overnight fast (control) and after ingestion of a meal containing 80 g of fat and 80 g carbohydrate (26). The meal was shown both to maintain plasma NEFA concentrations (unlike pure carbohydrate loading, which will suppress the plasma NEFA concentration) and to produce a high chylomicron TG concentration. Total fatty acid flux into the forearm during exercise (NEFA plus chylomicron TG fatty acids) was increased from 300 to 980 nmol · min^{-1} · 100 ml^{-1} (control vs. fed state). Chylomicron TG uptake in the fed state during exercise potentially contributed around 40% of forearm O_2 consumption (figure 7.5). Thus, a number of studies suggest that chylomicron TG may be a good substrate for muscular metabolism during exercise.

There is a further route by which circulating TG may be utilized by muscle, which will not appear directly in studies of arteriovenous differences across muscle. It was mentioned earlier that not all the fatty acids released by LPL action enter the tissues; in adipose tissue, for instance (where this has been most closely studied), around 50% of the fatty acids generated by LPL action during the postprandial period following a high-fat meal are liberated into the plasma (22). This is a route by which plasma TG may be made available to other tissues in the form of NEFA. In a study of arteriovenous differences across muscle, this will, of course, be seen as NEFA uptake even though the fatty acids have arisen from circulating TG rather than stored (intra-adipocyte) TG. This may be one benefit of fat ingestion before exercise (25).

Conclusion

The measurement of substrate flux across tissues or limbs at rest and during exercise may provide important information about the supply and utilization of

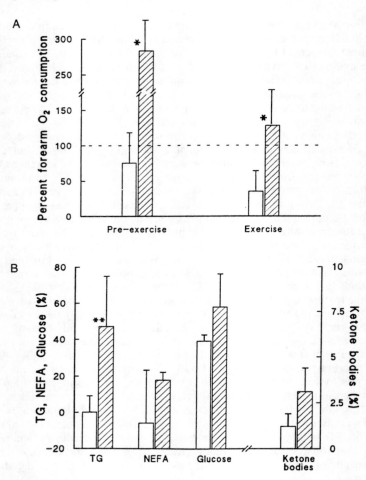

Figure 7.5 (A), potential contribution of all major substrates to forearm O_2 consumption before and during forearm exercise (algebraic sum of potential contributions of TG, NEFA, glucose, and ketone bodies); (B), potential contribution of individual blood-borne substrates to forearm O_2 consumption during exercise (the contribution of ketone bodies is plotted on a different scale). Open bars = postabsorptive state; hatched bars = exercise starting 3 h after a meal containing 80 g fat and 80 g carbohydrate; 10 normal subjects. Reprinted from Griffiths, Humphreys, Clark, and Frayn 1994.

metabolic fuels. In the area of fat metabolism, such studies suggest that the rate of supply of nonesterified fatty acids to exercising muscle may limit the rate at which fatty acids are used as an oxidative fuel during moderately intense exercise (up to 65% $\dot{V}O_2$max). There appear to be factors that limit the rate at which fatty acids can be liberated from adipose tissue and delivered to the working muscle. At such intensities of exercise, the ability of muscle to extract fatty acids from the plasma does not appear to be a major limiting factor. The contribution to muscle oxidative metabolism of plasma TG in the form of VLDL TG (i.e., after overnight fast) appears to be small, although there are severe technical difficulties in estimating it precisely. Chylomicron TG, on the other hand, may represent a more readily utilizable source of fat. Its potential for replenishment of muscle TG stores seems clear, although its role as an energy source during exercise requires further elucidation, preferably through studies involving a large muscle bulk such as the leg.

Acknowledgments

Our own studies in this area have been supported by the Oxford Diabetes Trust and Mars Inc. We thank our colleagues in the Sheikh Rashid Laboratory for their help.

References

1. Ahlborg, G.; Felig, P.; Hagenfeldt, L.; Hendler, R.; Wahren, J. Substrate turnover during prolonged exercise in man. Splanchnic and leg metabolism of glucose, free fatty acids, and amino acids. J. Clin. Invest. 53:1080-1090; 1974.

2. Andres, R.; Cader, G.; Zierler, K.L. The quantitatively minor role of carbohydrate in oxidative metabolism by skeletal muscle in intact man in the basal state. Measurements of oxygen and glucose uptake and carbon dioxide and lactate production in the forearm. J. Clin. Invest. 35:671-682; 1956.

3. Andres, R.; Zierler, K.L.; Anderson, H.M.; Stainsby, W.N.; Cader, G.; Ghrayyib, A.S.; Lilienthal, J.L.Jr. Measurement of blood flow and volume in the forearm of man; with notes on the theory of indicator-dilution and on production of turbulence, hemolysis, and vasodilatation by intra-vascular injection. J. Clin. Invest. 33:482-504; 1954.

4. Baltzan, M.A.; Andres, R.; Cader, G.; Zierler, K.L. Heterogeneity of forearm metabolism with special reference to free fatty acids. J. Clin. Invest. 41:116-125; 1962.

5. Belfrage, P. Hormonal control of lipid degradation. In: Cryer, A.; Van, R.L.R., eds. New perspectives in adipose tissue. London: Butterworths; 1985:121-144.

6. Brunzell, J.D.; Hazzard, W.R.; Porte, D.J.; Bierman, E.L. Evidence for a common, saturable, triglyceride removal mechanism for chylomicrons and very low density lipoproteins in man. J. Clin. Invest. 52:1578-1585; 1973.

7. Bülow, J. Subcutaneous adipose tissue blood flow and triacylglycerol-mobilization during prolonged exercise in dogs. Pflügers Arch. 392:230-234; 1982.

8. Bülow, J.; Madsen, J. Influence of blood flow on fatty acid mobilization from lipolytically active adipose tissue. Pflügers Arch. 390:169-174; 1981.

9. Bülow, J.; Madsen, J.; Astrup, A.; Christensen, N.J. Vasoconstrictor effect of high FFA/albumin ratios in adipose tissue in vivo. Acta Physiol. Scand. 125:661-667; 1985.

10. Burnett, R.A.; Aldred, H.E.; Hardman, A.E. Influence of the intensity of prior exercise on postprandial lipaemia in man. Proc. Nutr. Soc. 52:284A; 1993.

11. Carlson, M.G.; Snead, W.L.; Campbell, P.J. Regulation of free fatty acid metabolism by glucagon. J. Clin. Endocrinol. Metab. 77:11-15; 1993.

12. Cohen, J.; Goldberg, C. Effect of physical exercise on alimentary lipaemia. Br. Med. J. 2:509-511; 1960.

13. Cohen, J.C.; Noakes, T.D.; Spinnler Benade, A.J. Postprandial lipemia and chylomicron clearance in athletes and in sedentary men. Am. J. Clin. Nutr. 49:443-447; 1989.

14. Coppack, S.W.; Evans, R.D.; Fisher, R.M.; Frayn, K.N.; Gibbons, G.F.; Humphreys, S.M.; Kirk, M.J.; Potts, J.L.; Hockaday, T.D.R. Adipose tissue metabolism in obesity: Lipase action in vivo before and after a mixed meal. Metabolism 41:264-272; 1992.

15. Coppack, S.W.; Fisher, R.M.; Gibbons, G.F.; Humphreys, S.M.; McDonough, M.J.; Potts, J.L.; Frayn, K.N. Postprandial substrate deposition in human forearm and adipose tissues in vivo. Clin. Sci. 79:339-348; 1990.

16. Coppack, S.W.; Frayn, K.N.; Humphreys, S.M.; Whyte, P.L.; Hockaday, T.D.R. Arteriovenous differences across human adipose and forearm tissues after overnight fast. Metabolism 39:384-390; 1990.

17. Coppack, S.W.; Jensen, M.D.; Miles, J.M. In vivo regulation of lipolysis in humans. J. Lipid Res. 35:177-193; 1994.

18. Dagenais, G.R.; Tancredi, R.G.; Zierler, K.L. Free fatty acid oxidation by forearm muscle at rest, and evidence for an intramuscular lipid pool in the human forearm. J. Clin. Invest. 58:421-431; 1976.

19. Frayn, K.N.; Coppack, S.W.; Humphreys, S.M. Subcutaneous adipose tissue metabolism studied by local catheterization. Int. J. Obesity 17 (suppl. 3):S18-S21; 1993.

20. Frayn, K.N.; Coppack, S.W.; Humphreys, S.M.; Whyte, P.L. Metabolic characteristics of human adipose tissue in vivo. Clin. Sci. 76:509-516; 1989.

21. Frayn, K.N.; Lund, P.; Walker, M. Interpretation of oxygen and carbon dioxide exchange across tissue beds in vivo. Clin. Sci. 85:373-384; 1993.

22. Frayn, K.N.; Shadid, S.; Hamlani, R.; Humphreys, S.M.; Clark, M.L.; Fielding, B.A.; Boland, O.; Coppack, S.W. Regulation of fatty acid movement in human adipose tissue in the postabsorptive-to-postprandial transition. Am. J. Physiol. 266:E308-E317; 1994.

23. Galitzky, J.; Lafontan, M.; Nordenström, J.; Arner, P. Role of vascular alpha-2 adrenoceptors in regulating lipid mobilization from human adipose tissue. J. Clin. Invest. 91:1997-2003; 1993.

24. Greenfield, A.D.M.; Whitney, R.J.; Mowbray, J.F. Methods for the investigation of peripheral blood flow. Br. Med. Bull. 19:101-109; 1963.

25. Griffiths, A.J.; Humphreys, S.M.; Clark, M.L.; Fielding, B.A.; Frayn, K.N. Immediate metabolic availability of dietary fat in combination with carbohydrate. Am. J. Clin. Nutr. 59:53-59; 1994.

26. Griffiths, A.J.; Humphreys, S.M.; Clark, M.L.; Frayn, K.N. Forearm substrate utilization during exercise after a meal containing both fat and carbohydrate. Clin. Sci. 86:169-175; 1994.

27. Harmon, C.M.; Luce, P.; Abumrad, N.A. Labelling of an 88 kDa adipocyte membrane protein by sulpho-N-succinimidyl long-chain fatty acids: Inhibition of fatty acid transport. Biochem. Soc. Trans. 20:811-813; 1992.

28. Havel, R.J.; Naimark, A.; Borchgrevink, C.F. Turnover rate and oxidation of free fatty acids of blood plasma in man during exercise: Studies during continuous infusion of palmitate-1-14C. J. Clin. Invest. 42:1054-1063; 1963.

29. Havel, R.J.; Pernow, B.; Jones, N.L. Uptake and release of free fatty acids and other metabolites in the legs of exercising men. J. Appl. Physiol. 23:90-99; 1967.

30. Hodgetts, V.; Coppack, S.W.; Frayn, K.N.; Hockaday, T.D.R. Factors controlling fat mobilization from human subcutaneous adipose tissue during exercise. J. Appl. Physiol. 71:445-451; 1991.

31. Jansson, E.; Kaijser, L. Substrate utilization and enzymes in skeletal muscle of extremely endurance-trained men. J. Appl. Physiol. 62:999-1005; 1987.
32. Jensen, M.D.; Heiling, V.J.; Miles, J.M. Effects of glucagon on free fatty acid metabolism in humans. J. Clin. Endocrinol. Metab. 72:308-315; 1991.
33. Jones, N.L.; Havel, R.J. Metabolism of free fatty acids and chylomicron triglycerides during exercise in rats. Am. J. Physiol. 213:824-828; 1967.
34. Jones, N.L.; Heigenhauser, G.J.F.; Kuksis, A.; Matos, C.G.; Sutton, J.R.; Toews, C.J. Fat metabolism in heavy exercise. Clin. Sci. 59:469-478; 1980.
35. Kaijser, L.; Rössner, S. Removal of exogenous triglycerides in human forearm muscle and subcutaneous tissue. Acta Med. Scand. 197:289-294; 1975.
36. Kiens, B.; Lithell, H. Lipoprotein metabolism influenced by training-induced changes in human skeletal muscle. J. Clin. Invest. 83:558-564; 1989.
37. Kiens, B.; Lithell, H.; Mikines, K.J.; Richter, E.A. Effects of insulin and exercise on muscle lipoprotein lipase activity in man and its relationship to insulin action. J. Clin. Invest. 84:1124-1129; 1989.
38. Lassen, N.A.; Lindbjerg, J.; Munck, O. Measurement of blood-flow through skeletal muscle by intramuscular injection of xenon-133. Lancet 1:686-689; 1964.
39. Mackie, B.G.; Dudley, G.A.; Kaciuba-Uscilko, H.; Terjung, R.L. Uptake of chylomicron triglycerides by contracting skeletal muscle in rats. J. Appl. Physiol. 49:851-855; 1980.
40. Madsen, J.; Bülow, J.; Nielsen, N.E. Inhibition of fatty acid mobilization by arterial free fatty acid concentration. Acta Physiol. Scand. 127:161-166; 1986.
41. Mankowitz, K.; Seip, R.; Semenkovich, C.F.; Daugherty, A.; Schonfield, G. Short-term interruption of training affects both fasting and post-prandial lipoproteins. Atherosclerosis 95:181-189; 1992.
42. Nikkilä, E.A.; Konttinen, A. Effect of physical activity on postprandial levels of fats in serum. Lancet 1:1151-1154; 1962.
43. Nikkilä, E.A.; Taskinen, M.-R.; Rehunen, S.; Harkonen, M. Lipoprotein lipase activity in adipose tissue and skeletal muscle of runners: Relation to serum lipoproteins. Metabolism 27:1661-1671; 1978.
44. Patsch, J.R.; Gotto, A.M.; Olivecrona, T.; Eisenberg, S. Formation of high density lipoprotein$_2$-like particles during lipolysis of very low density lipoproteins in vitro. Proc. Natl. Acad. Sci. USA 75:4519-4523; 1978.
45. Potts, J.L.; Fisher, R.M.; Humphreys, S.M.; Coppack, S.W.; Gibbons, G.F.; Frayn, K.N. Chylomicrons are the preferred substrate for lipoprotein lipase in vivo. Biochem. Soc. Trans. 19:314S; 1991a.
46. Potts, J.L.; Fisher, R.M.; Humphreys, S.M.; Coppack, S.W.; Gibbons, G.F.; Frayn, K.N. Peripheral triacylglycerol extraction in the fasting and post-prandial states. Clin. Sci. 81:621-626; 1991b.
47. Rabinowitz, D.; Zierler, K.L. Role of free fatty acids in forearm metabolism in man, quantitated by use of insulin. J. Clin. Invest. 41:2191-2197; 1962.
48. Romijn, J.A.; Coyle, E.F.; Sidossis, L.S.; Gastaldelli, A.; Horowitz, J.F.; Endert, E.; Wolfe, R.R. Regulation of endogenous fat and carbohydrate metabolism in relation to exercise intensity and duration. Am. J. Physiol. 265:E380-E391; 1993.
49. Ruys, T.; Sturgess, I.; Shaikh, M.; Watts, G.F.; Nordestgaard, B.G.; Lewis, B. Effects of exercise and fat ingestion on high density lipoprotein production by peripheral tissues. Lancet ii:1119-1122; 1989.
50. Sady, S.P.; Thompson, P.D.; Cullinane, E.M.; Kantor, M.A.; Domagala, E.; Herbert, P.N. Prolonged exercise augments plasma triglyceride clearance. JAMA 256:2552-2555; 1986.

51. Schlierf, G.; Dinsenbacher, A.; Kather, H.; Kohlmeier, M.; Haberbosch, W. Mitigation of alimentary lipemia by postprandial exercise—Phenomena and mechanisms. Metabolism 36:726-730; 1987.
52. Soop, M.; Björkman, O.; Cederblad, G.; Hagenfeldt, L.; Wahren, J. Influence of carnitine supplementation on muscle substrate and carnitine metabolism during exercise. J. Appl. Physiol. 64:2394-2399; 1988.
53. Stremmel, W.; Kleinert, H.; Fitscher, B.A.; Gunawan, J.; Klaassen-Schlüter, C.; Möller, K.; Wegener, M. Mechanism of cellular fatty acid uptake. Biochem. Soc. Trans. 20:814-817; 1992.
54. Terjung, R.L.; Mackie, B.G.; Dudley, G.A.; Kaciuba-Uscilko, H. Influence of exercise on chylomicron triacylglycerol metabolism: Plasma turnover and muscle uptake. Med. Sci. Sports Exercise 15:340-347; 1983.
55. Turcotte, L.P.; Richter, E.A.; Kiens, B. Increased plasma FFA uptake and oxidation during prolonged exercise in trained vs. untrained humans. Am. J. Physiol. 262:E791-E799; 1992.
56. Veerkamp, J.H.; Maatman, R.G.H.J.; Prinsen, C.F.M. Fatty acid–binding proteins: Structural and functional diversity. Biochem. Soc. Trans. 20:801-805; 1992.
57. Vyska, K.; Meyer, W.; Stremmel, W.; Notohamiprodjo, G.; Minami, K.; Machulla, H.-J.; Gleichmann, U.; Meyer, H.; Körfer, R. Fatty acid uptake in normal human myocardium. Circ. Res. 69:857-870; 1991.
58. Wahren, J. Quantitative aspects of blood flow and oxygen uptake in the human forearm during rhythmic exercise. Acta Physiol. Scand. 67 (suppl. 269);1966.
59. Wahren, J.; Sato, Y.; Östman, J.; Hagenfeldt, L.; Felig, P. Turnover and splanchnic metabolism of free fatty acids and ketones in insulin-dependent diabetics at rest and in response to exercise. J. Clin. Invest. 73:1367-1376; 1984.
60. Wu, M.S.; Jeng, C.Y.; Hollenbeck, C.B.; Chen, Y.-D.I.; Jaspan, J.; Reaven, G.M. Does glucagon increase plasma free fatty acid concentration in humans with normal glucose tolerance? J. Clin. Endocrinol. Metab. 70:410-416; 1990.
61. Zierler, K.L. Fatty acids as substrates for heart and skeletal muscle. Circ. Res. 38:459-463; 1976.

CHAPTER 8

Regulation of Lipolysis in Exercise Studied by Microdialysis

Peter Arner
Karolinska Institute, Huddinge University Hospital, Huddinge, Sweden

Lipolysis in fat cells plays a critical role for the regulation of the energy balance during exercise. Free fatty acids, which are mobilized from adipose tissue after hydrolysis of triglycerides in adipocytes, are the most important source of energy during prolonged exercise periods.

Most of the information about lipid mobilization in vivo during exercise has so far been obtained from indirect studies based on measurements of circulating free fatty acids and glycerol (9). For a few years it has been possible to study this process directly through microdialysis, focusing on results of interest for metabolism during exercise. This review will discuss the microdialysis method and its role in exercise studies.

Principles of Microdialysis

The methodological aspects of microdialysis have been discussed in detail in several review articles (1, 2, 21, 25). In brief, the microdialysis probe consists of a hollow fiber membrane that functions as an artificial vessel. The probe is placed in the extracellular space of subcutaneous adipose tissue. Two types of probes are used (figure 8.1). One is constructed as a single dialysis tube with steel cannulas at each end. The other is a double-lumen cannula in which the microdialysis membrane is glued to the top of the cannula. A neutral dialysis solvent (usually saline or Ringer's solution) is pumped through the probe at low speed (usually 1-5 µl/min). The outgoing solvent is analyzed for molecules, which are collected from the extracellular water space.

Microdialysis is most suitable for the measurements of small water-soluble substances that easily pass through the membrane. Hydrophobic molecules, such as free fatty acids, cannot be collected by the probes with sufficient yield because of their physical properties. Usually dialysis membranes have a molecular weight (MW) cut-off point around 20,000, allowing molecules with a MW up to about 1,000 to pass rapidly in and out of the probe. It is possible to collect larger molecules, such

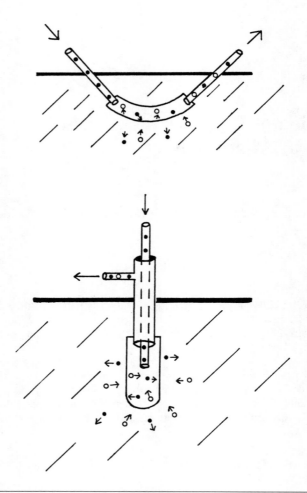

Figure 8.1   Principles of microdialysis.

as proteins, using membranes with a high MW cut-off point (around 100,000). On the other hand, the recovery (discussed later) is low, and the time to reach dialysis equilibrium is long with such membranes. Membranes with a large pore size are not suitable for kinetic experiments when there is a need for frequent sampling. A successful attempt to measure steady-state insulin levels in subcutaneous adipose tissue has recently been made with the latter type of dialysis membranes (16).

Determination of Concentration
and Turnover of Endogenous Substances

Microdialysis measures the level of a substance in the extracellular water space. This is influenced by local production and utilization by tissue cells and by delivery and removal by the tissue blood flow. Some metabolites are produced by fat cells at high rates, such as glycerol and lactate (2). The concentration of these metabolites is therefore higher in the extracellular space than in blood. Thus, local production and removal are more important determinants for the tissue level of these substances than local utilization and delivery. This is the case for glycerol. The adipose tissue level of glycerol is two to three times higher than the circulating level (6, 18), indicating that the inflow of glycerol from blood to the extracellular space is negligible because of the high concentration gradient. In addition, there is insignificant reutilization of glycerol in adipose tissue (22). This means that changes in the tissue level of glycerol are mediated above all by variations in fat cell production and removal by the bloodstream. This makes glycerol an ideal substance for studies of lipid mobilization from adipose tissue.

One problem with microdialysis is obtaining an absolute value for the subcutaneous interstitial concentration of the substance of interest. This is because microdialysis is usually performed at high speed using short probes. The length of the probe and the velocity of the dialysis solvent are the two major determinants of recovery. In addition, in vivo recovery is often much lower than in vitro recovery because of yet undefined tissue factors. It is possible to indirectly estimate the true tissue level of a certain endogenous compound by performing so-called calibration experiments (20). However, these experiments are time consuming (about 4 h) and may alter the behavior of adipose tissue. Alternatively, a long probe ($\geq$30 mm) and a slow perfusion speed ($\leq$0.5 µL/min) can be used to obtain full recovery (7). The latter technique necessitates long fraction times and is therefore less suitable in rapid kinetic experiments. However, there is no change in recovery over time during microdialysis (1, 2). Therefore, changes in the concentration of a substance in the microdialysate over time truly reflect changes in the extracellular water space, even if microdialysis is performed under conditions of incomplete recovery.

Another problem with microdialysis is evaluating the influence of blood flow on the concentration of a substance in the microdialysate. This is of particular importance in comparative studies where, for example, the true rate of lipolysis by adipose tissue is evaluated (17). It is not possible to directly measure the flow in the water space surrounding the microdialysis probe. An ethanol escape technique has been developed to study the nutritive flow in the tissue around the probe. Ethanol is added to the dialysis solvent and measured in the outgoing microdialysate. Changes in the ratio of ethanol out to in reflect changes in the nutritive blood flow around the probe (14, 15). Similar data were obtained in muscle when the ethanol escape technique was compared with the xenon washout technique (13).

In Situ Manipulation

A unique feature of microdialysis is that it allows local manipulation of adipose tissue without causing generalized effects. Therefore, detailed pharmacological experiments can be performed in situ employing very high concentrations of the agents locally. Such concentrations usually cannot be achieved through intravenous or oral administration because of toxic side effects. Pharmacological concentrations of highly active substances can be maintained locally in adipose tissue through the microdialysis probe without influencing the body as a whole, because the total given dose is very low.

For example, 10^{-6} mol/L of noradrenaline is infused to adipose tissue by microdialysis at 2.5 μl/min of flow rate for 4 h in order to reach a pharmacological local tissue concentration. It would be fatal to achieve such a high concentration of the catecholamines in the circulation. The total amount of noradrenaline infused is 2×10^{-4} mg during this period. However, recovery in vivo under the present conditions is about 10%, meaning that only 2×10^{-5} mg has entered the tissue. The recommended single injection dose of noradrenaline is 1 mg. In other words, a very high concentration of a potent agent has been maintained for several hours using a total dose which is 50,000 times lower than the recommended dose.

Regulation of Lipid Mobilization From Adipose Tissue

The microdialysis technique has so far been used to study above all the importance of catecholamines for lipid mobilization from subcutaneous adipose tissue. Among hormones, only catecholamines have an acute and pronounced effect on lipolysis in fat cells. As reviewed (19), catecholamines stimulate lipolysis through a chain of events initiated by binding to stimulatory $beta_1$- and $beta_2$-adrenoceptors or inhibitory $alpha_2$-adrenoceptors. $Beta_3$-adrenoceptors may also be of functional importance for lipolysis in vivo. Oral or local administration by microdialysis of $beta_3$-adrenoceptor agonists causes a lipolytic response in vivo in humans, which is resistant to $beta_1$/$beta_2$-adrenoceptor blockade (24, wt). The adrenergic receptors regulate adenyl cyclase activity in the plasma membrane, which catalyzes the formation of cyclic AMP. The latter nucleotide forms a complex with protein kinase, which in its turn regulates the final step in the lipolytic cascade: hormone-sensitive lipase. The latter enzyme stimulates the hydrolysis of triglycerides to diglycerides, which thereafter are broken down to free fatty acids and glycerol. Furthermore, catecholamine-induced lipolysis can be regulated by phosphodiesterase, which is a family of isozymes that stimulates breakdown of cyclic AMP.

Microdialysis studies have suggested that lipolysis in adipose tissue is very sensitive to catecholamine stimulation. A clear lipolytic response (measured as dialysate glycerol) is observed when subcutaneous adipose tissue is perfused with concentrations of noradrenaline that are lower than those in the circulation (4). This indicates, first, that local production or metabolism of noradrenaline is of major importance for the regulation of lipolysis and, second, that the catecholamine levels in adipose tissue may be very low at rest. Evidence for local production of noradrenaline in tissue has recently been presented using microdialysis (11).

Functional $beta_1$-, $beta_2$-$beta_3$-, and $alpha_2$-adrenergic receptors appear to be present in human subcutaneous adipose tissue when investigated with microdialysis. The lipolytic order of potency for classical adrenergic agonists is isoprenaline > adrenaline > noradrenaline (4). This indicates a predominance of $beta_2$-adrenoceptors. In addition, the $beta_2$ is the only beta-adrenergic subtype that stimulates blood flow in this tissue (25). However, $beta_1$-receptors may play a role in regulating the well-known catecholamine tachyphylaxia phenomenon. The lipolytic response of the classical catecholamines is only transient (4, 5). However, selective $beta_2$- and $alpha_2$-receptor stimulation causes sustained effects, whereas selective $beta_1$-receptor stimulation is transient (5). Alpha$_2$-adrenoceptors may play a unique role in the regulation of lipid mobilization (10). Selective stimulation of these receptors causes a marked retention of glycerol in adipose tissue because of inhibition of lipolysis in fat cells in combination with decreased blood flow.

The phosphodiesterase system has also been investigated with microdialysis (3). A small lipolytic- and blood flow–stimulating effect was observed after infusion with the phosphodiesterase-3 inhibitor amrinone. However, nonselective phosphodiesterase inhibition with theophylline caused marked stimulation of lipolysis and blood flow. These data are surprising and suggest that phosphodiesterase-3 only plays a minor role for lipolysis regulation in situ. In vitro data have suggested that this phosphodiesterase subclass is dominating in fat cells (23). It seems also to be the only subclass that is important for the in vivo antilipolytic effect of insulin in humans (26).

Lipid Mobilization During Exercise

During exercise for 30 min at two-thirds of maximum working capacity, there is a rapid rise in the level of glycerol in the microdialysate of adipose tissue, which gradually declines after stopping exercise (6). There is no change in blood flow, as measured by the ethanol escape technique, during the exercise and postexercise periods (12). The postexercise finding is in harmony with several earlier studies, which used the xenon washout method and showed that adipose tissue blood flow increases only during prolonged periods of exercise (8). The changes in dialysate glycerol occur in parallel with changes in venous glycerol and arterial or venous catecholamines (6, 12). Addition of the nonselective beta-adrenoceptor blocker propranolol almost completely prevented the exercise-induced increase in dialysate glycerol, whereas addition of the nonselective alpha-adrenoceptor blocker phentolamine did not influence the dialysate level of glycerol (6). There is also a correlation ($r = .60$) between changes in adipose and plasma glycerol during exercise (28). Taken together, these data strongly suggest that exercise-induced lipid mobilization is a result of increased catecholamine-induced lipolysis in fat cells, which is solely mediated by an activation of beta-adrenoceptors.

There are also gender and regional differences in the lipolytic response to exercise in subcutaneous adipose tissue. Lipolysis is activated to a much higher rate in the abdominal than in the gluteal area (6). This regional difference is most marked in women, who also have a higher rate of lipolysis during exercise in the abdominal region as compared with men (12). The rise in plasma noradrenaline is similar in either sex during exercise, whereas men have a higher rise of plasma adrenaline than women (12). The rise in plasma glycerol during exercise is also more marked in women than in men (6, 12). These data might suggest that the in vivo lipolytic sensitivity to catecholamines is higher in women than in men. In addition, alpha-adrenergic receptors seem to modulate exercise-induced lipolysis in men but not in women (12).

Acknowledgment

This study was supported in part by Medicus Bromma Ltd., Sweden.

References

1. Arner, P.; Bolinder, J. Microdialysis of adipose tissue. J. Intern. Med. 230:381-386; 1991.
2. Arner, P.; Bülow, J. Assessment of adipose tissue metabolism in man: Comparison of Fick and microdialysis technique. Clin. Sci. 85:247-256; 1993.
3. Arner, P.; Hellmér, J.; Hagström-Toft, E.; Bolinder, J. Effect of phosphodiesterase inhibition with amrinone or theophylline on lipolysis and blood flow in human adipose tissue in vivo as measured with microdialysis. J. Lipid Res. 34:1737-1743; 1993.
4. Arner, P.; Kriegholm, E.; Engfeldt, P. In situ studies of catecholamine induced lipolysis in human adipose tissue using microdialysis. J. Pharmacol. Exp. Therapeutics 254:284-288; 1990.
5. Arner, P.; Kriegholm, E.; Engfeldt, P. In vivo interactions between beta-$_1$ and beta-$_2$-adrenoceptors regulate catecholamine tachyphylaxia in human adipose tissue. J. Pharmacol. Exp. Therapeutics 259:317-322; 1991.
6. Arner, P.; Kriegholm, E.; Engfeldt, P.; Bolinder, J. Adrenergic regulation of lipolysis in situ at rest and during exercise. J. Clin. Invest. 85:893-898; 1990.
7. Bolinder, J.; Ungerstedt, U.; Arner, P. Microdialysis measurement of the absolute glucose concentration in subcutaneous adipose tissue allowing glucose monitoring in diabetic patients. Diabetologia 35:1177-1180; 1992.
8. Bülow, J. Adipose tissue blood flow during exercise. Dan. Med. Bull. 30:85-100; 1983.
9. Bülow, J. Lipid mobilization and utilization. In: Poortmans, J.R., ed. Principles of exercise biochemistry. 2nd rev. ed. Basel: Karger; 1993:158-185.
10. Galitzky, J.; Lafontan, M.; Nordenström, J.; Arner, P. Role of alpha$_2$ adrenoceptors in regulating lipid mobilization from human adipose tissue. J. Clin. Invest. 91:1997-2003; 1993.
11. Grönlund, B.; Astrup, A.; Christensen, N.J. Noradrenaline release in skeletal muscle and in adipose tissue: Studies by microdialysis. Clin. Sci. 80:595-598; 1991.
12. Hellström, L.; Blaak, E.; Hagström-Toft, E. Gender differences in adrenergic regulation of lipid mobilization during exercise. Int. J. Sports Med. (In press.)
13. Hickner, R.C.; Bone, D.; Ungerstedt, U.; Jorfeldt, L.; Henriksson, J. Muscle blood flow during intermittent exercise: Comparison of the microdialysis ethanol technique and ^{133}Xe clearance. Clin. Sci. 86:15-25; 1994.
14. Hickner, R.C.; Rosdahl, H.; Borg, I.; Ungerstedt, U.; Jorfeldt, L.; Henriksson, J. Ethanol may be used with the microdialysis technique to monitor blood flow changes in skeletal muscle: Dialysate glucose concentration is blood-flow-dependent. Acta Physiol. Scand. 143:355-356; 1991.
15. Hickner, R.C.; Rosdahl, H.; Borg, I.; Ungerstedt, U.; Jorfeldt, L.; Henriksson, J. The ethanol technique of monitoring local blood flow changes in rat skeletal muscle: Implications for microdialysis. Acta Physiol. Scand. 146:87-97; 1992.
16. Jansson, P.A.E.; Fowelin, J.P.; Von Schenck, H.P.; Smith, U.P.; Lönnroth, P.N. Measurement by microdialysis of the insulin concentration in subcutaneous interstitial fluid. Diabetes 42:1469-1473; 1993.
17. Jansson, P.A.; Larsson, A.; Smith, U.; Lönnroth, P. Glycerol production in subcutaneous adipose tissue in lean and obese humans. J. Clin. Invest. 89:1610-1617; 1992.

18. Jansson, P.A.; Smith, U.; Lönnroth, P. Interstitial glycerol concentration measured by microdialysis in two subcutaneous regions in humans. Am. J. Physiol. 258:918-922; 1990.
19. Lafontan, M.; Berlan, M. Fat cell adrenergic receptors and the control of white and brown fat cell function. J. Lipid Res. 34:1057-1092; 1993.
20. Lönnroth, P.; Jansson, P.A.; Smith, U. A microdialysis method allowing characterization of intercellular water space in humans. Am. J. Physiol. 253:228-231; 1987.
21. Lönnroth, P.; Smith, U. Microdialysis—A novel technique for clinical investigations. J. Intern. Med. 227:295-300; 1990.
22. Low, G.K.; Steinberg, D.; Vaughan, M.V.; Margolis, S. Studies of triglyceride biosynthesis in homogenates of adipose tissue. J. Biol. Chem. 236:1631-1637; 1961.
23. Manganiello, V.C. Subcellular localization and biological function of specific cyclic nucleotide phosphodiesterase. J. Mol. Cell. Cardiol. 19:1037-1040; 1987.
24. Newnham, D.M.; Ingram, C.G.; Mackie, A.; Lipworth, B.J. Beta-adrenoceptor subtypes mediating the airways response to BRL 35135 in man. Br. J. Pharmacol. 36:567-571; 1993.
25. Ungerstedt, U. Microdialysis—Principles and applications for studies in animals and man. J. Intern. Med. 230:365-373; 1991.
26. Wennlund, A.; Wahrenberg, H.; Hagström-Toft, E.; Bolinder, J.; Arner, P. Lipolytic and cardiac responses to various forms of stress in humans. Int. J. Sports Med. 15:408-413; 1994. (In press.)

CHAPTER 9

Transport and Metabolism of FFA in Muscle

Erik A. Richter, Bente Kiens, Lorraine Turcotte
Copenhagen Muscle Research Centre, August Krogh Institute, University of Copenhagen, Copenhagen, Denmark; University of Copenhagen, Copenhagen, Denmark; Department of Exercise Sciences, University of Southern California, Los Angeles, California, U.S.A.

Lipids are important energy substrates for skeletal muscle metabolism during endurance exercise, and their contribution to total oxidative metabolism is dependent on a variety of factors, including exercise intensity and duration as well as dietary and training status. Oxidizable lipid fuels include circulating plasma triacylglycerols (TGs) and free fatty acids (FFAs) as well as intramuscular triacylglycerols. Whereas circulating albumin-bound FFAs mobilized from adipose tissue contribute in significant proportions to lipid metabolism in skeletal muscle during exercise, the conditions during which FFA hydrolyzed from intramuscular TG and plasma TG–derived FFA contribute to lipid metabolism during exercise have not been clearly defined.

Metabolism of Plasma Free Fatty Acids

Within the past 15 years, experimental evidence has indicated that FFA transport across plasma membranes is not only by simple diffusion but rather is mainly carrier mediated. In hepatocytes, adipocytes, and cardiac myocytes, evidence shows that cellular uptake of long-chain FFA is not limited by the dissociation of FFA from albumin and demonstrates saturation kinetics when plotted against the unbound plasma FFA concentration (1, 26, 27). It should be noted that more than 99.9% of total FFA in vivo is bound to albumin, and consequently only a very small fraction is really "free." Furthermore, long-chain FFAs bind in a saturable fashion to freshly isolated plasma membranes (22, 27), and such binding is apparently attributable to a specific plasma-membrane fatty acid–binding protein (FABP_{PM}) of molecular mass between 40 and 43 kDa, immunologically distinct from the 12- to 14-kDa cytosolic FABP described in many tissues (22, 27). In every cell type studied to date, antibodies raised against the rat hepatic FABP_{PM} inhibit both FFA binding to and permeation of plasma membranes in a dose-dependent fashion, suggesting that FABP$_{PM}$ constitutes a functional FFA transporter (22).

Evidence is also accumulating to suggest that permeation of FFA into skeletal muscle is carrier mediated (19, 29-33). In untrained human subjects performing 2 or 3 h of one-legged dynamic knee extension exercise, FFA uptake into the exercising skeletal muscle determined either as net uptake (19; figure 9.1) or with tracer technique (32; figure 9.2) was found to saturate with an increase in plasma-unbound FFA concentration. Furthermore, FFA oxidation as determined by the liberation of radiolabeled CO_2 also displayed saturation with increasing FFA concentration (figure 9.2). Similarly, in isolated, perfused rat skeletal muscle, palmitate uptake displayed

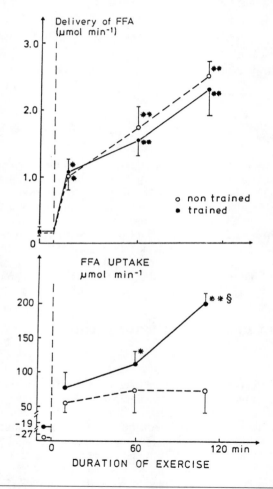

Figure 9.1 Delivery of FFA and net FFA uptake during dynamic knee extension exercise in seven subjects exercising either with the nontrained leg or with the contralateral leg that was endurance trained for 8 wk. Values are means ± *SE*. *$p < .05$ compared with rest; **$p < .05$ compared with 10-min value; §$p < .05$ compared with nontrained.
Reprinted from Kiens, Essen-Gustavsson, Christensen, and Saltin 1993.

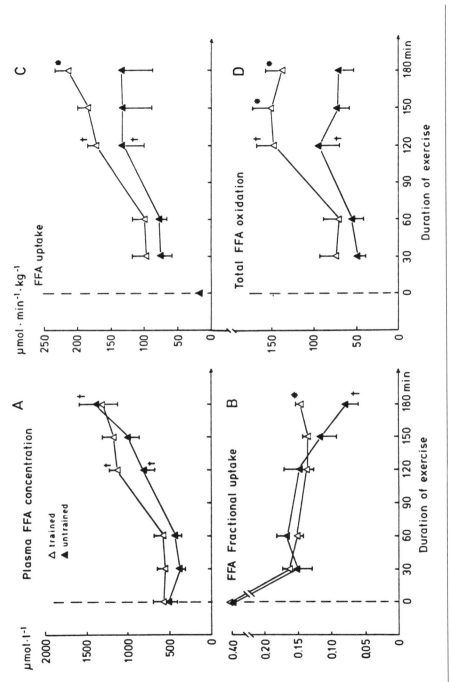

Figure 9.2 (A) Arterial plasma concentration, (B) fractional uptake, (C) uptake, and (D) total oxidation of free fatty acids (FFA) across thigh during rest and 3 h of knee extension exercise in trained and untrained subjects. Values are means ± SE of six subjects in both groups.
*p < .05 compared with untrained; †p < .05 compared with previous value.
Reprinted from Turcotte, Richter, and Kiens 1992.

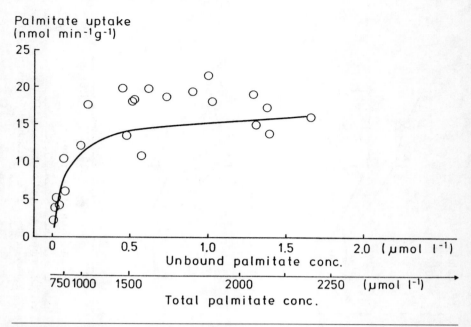

Figure 9.3   Palmitate uptake of perfused hindquarters as a function of unbound palmitate concentration. Abscissa also indicates the corresponding total palmitate concentration from which the unbound fraction was calculated. Each point represents the average uptake value of one rat ($n = 23$).
Reprinted from Turcotte, Kiens, and Richter 1991.

saturation kinetics when plotted against the unbound perfusate palmitate concentration (30; figure 9.3). Finally, immunoblotting of plasma membrane fractions of rat skeletal muscles with a polyclonal antibody against the rat hepatic $FABP_{PM}$ detected a single protein band with an apparent molecular mass of 42 kDa (33). Furthermore, $FABP_{PM}$ is more abundant in red muscle than in white and increases significantly in red muscle during fasting (34). Put together, these results suggest that, as in other cell types, FFA permeation into skeletal muscle is mediated, at least in part, by a carrier-mediated process that may play an important function in regulating the utilization of FFA by skeletal muscle.

Once inside the muscle cell, FFAs are directed either to mitochondrial oxidation or to esterification in the intramuscular TG pool. Even in conditions of increased metabolic rate, the percentage of plasma FFA taken up that is directly oxidized never reaches a value of 100%, suggesting that a certain portion of plasma FFA is available for other metabolic pathways.

Carnitine palmitoyl transferase (CPT) appears to be rate-limiting for mitochondrial long-chain fatty acid β-oxidation (4). It has been proposed that regulation of CPT activity involves inhibition by malonyl CoA, an intermediate in fatty acid synthesis. Malonyl CoA is formed by acetyl CoA carboxylase in the rate-limiting reaction of fatty acid synthesis. In vitro studies have shown that, like hepatic CPT, skeletal muscle CPT is sensitive to regulation by fluctuations in malonyl CoA concentration (20). Rat skeletal muscle malonyl CoA levels have been shown to decrease in response to fasting and to 30 min of treadmill running, suggesting that malonyl CoA levels may be a contributing factor in the regulation of FFA oxidation (20, 35).

The rate of FFA oxidation is to a large extent dependent on exercise intensity and duration. As indicated by the observed increase in respiratory exchange ratio (RER), the relative contribution of lipids to total oxidative metabolism decreases as the intensity of exercise increases (5). However, as exercise intensity increases, the decrease in the relative contribution of lipids to oxidative metabolism is minimal compared to the increase in total lipid utilization until the intensity of exercise reaches a value equal to approximately 60% to 70% of maximal oxygen uptake (11). Furthermore, as light- to moderate-intensity exercise progresses, the contribution of lipids to oxidative metabolism increases, as evidenced by a progressive decrease in RER during 4 h of light-intensity exercise (2).

The rate of FFA oxidation is in part a function of the plasma FFA concentration, and at a given FFA concentration it is also dependent on the metabolic rate (18, 21). In dogs (3) and humans (18, 13), plasma FFA turnover and oxidation have been shown to correlate with plasma FFA concentration, and during light- to moderate-intensity exercise, FFA concentration increases with exercise intensity and duration (21, 23). In humans exercising at 30% of maximal aerobic capacity, Ahlborg et al. (2) have shown that the gradual increase in plasma FFA level was accompanied by a progressive rise in the turnover rate of labeled oleate. The onset of exercise is usually accompanied by an immediate increase in the rate of FFA uptake by the active muscles. Initially, this enhanced utilization of plasma FFA is not completely matched by an increased mobilization of FFA from adipose tissue, resulting in a transient decrease in plasma FFA concentration. As exercise continues, the rate of FFA mobilization increases and eventually exceeds the rate of FFA utilization, resulting in a gradual increase in plasma FFA concentration (19, 21, 23, 32), and the higher the work intensity (as long as it remains below the level at which lactate accumulates markedly), the greater is the increase in FFA concentration. Thus, during prolonged, mild- to moderate-intensity exercise in humans and dogs, the gradual increase in plasma FFA level is associated with an increase in the rate of FFA turnover and oxidation. However, as previously indicated, at high FFA concentrations FFA uptake and oxidation plateau (19, 32). It is interesting that this relationship between FFA concentration and FFA uptake is altered by endurance training, such that leveling off is not seen in the trained state (19, 32; figures 9.1 and 9.2).

Intramuscular Triacylglycerol Metabolism

It has been suggested that intramuscular triacylglycerol (TG) functions as an important energy source for skeletal muscle metabolism, especially during prolonged exercise. This suggestion is in part based on the fact that isotopically determined plasma FFA oxidation does not match estimates of total lipid oxidation as calculated from RER measurements during prolonged exercise (14, 18). Thus, in postabsorptive exercising men and dogs, the oxidation of circulating plasma FFA can account for little more than half of the total lipid oxidation (14, 18). However, there are also some studies showing a decrease in directly measured muscle TG concentration. Thus, evidence collected from a number of studies in humans suggests that TG content in vastus lateralis muscle decreases 25% to 50% during prolonged exercise at an exercise intensity of 55% to 75% (6, 7, 8). However, high-intensity exercise of short duration has also been described to result in significant intramuscular TG depletion. Thus 5 min of intense bicycling exercise decreased intramuscular TG concentration by 29% (9).

Intramuscular TG utilization may possibly be influenced by the mode of exercise employed. Hurley et al. (17) observed no significant decrease in intramuscular TG after 2 h of bicycle exercise at 65% of $\dot{V}O_2$max in untrained subjects. After 12 wk of endurance training, the decrease was significant and numerically twice as big. Thirty minutes of intermittent, heavy-resistance exercise activating the quadriceps femoris muscle has also been reported to decrease TG content by 30% (10). Conversely, Kiens et al. (19) found no change in intramuscular TG content following 2 h of dynamic knee extension exercise at 65% of maximal kicking capacity. Although different, these results do not necessarily contradict each other but may, in fact, be a reflection of the different exercise modes employed. Bicycle and heavy-resistance exercise are associated with marked increases in plasma catecholamine levels (12, 28), whereas one-legged knee extension exercise is associated with catecholamine levels that are barely above resting concentrations (19). This lower catecholamine response could possibly affect the utilization of intramuscular TG since it has been shown in exercising humans that nonselective beta-adrenergic blockade prevented muscle lipolysis (6). In line with this finding are results that suggest that the lipase regulating intramuscular triglyceride breakdown is similar to the neutral pH optimum adipose tissue hormone-sensitive lipase (HSL; 24). Following the production of an antibody raised against the purified rat adipose tissue HSL, immunological evidence has been presented to support this hypothesis. In rat skeletal muscle extracts, immunoblotting with this antibody revealed the presence of an antigenic protein with a molecular mass similar to that of the adipose tissue HSL (15). Using a cDNA clone to perform Northern blotting, it was shown that HSL mRNA in heart and skeletal muscle was also similar in size to that found in adipose tissue (16). Furthermore, cAMP-dependent protein kinase was able to phosphorylate HSL in rat cardiac myocyte preparations (25).

On the other hand, we have repeatedly been unable to obtain decreases in muscle TG level after prolonged exhaustive bicycle exercise. Thus, in 21 subjects ranging from untrained to highly endurance trained, bicycling at 70% of $\dot{V}O_2$max to exhaustion, at which point muscle glycogen stores were very low, did not decrease muscle TG concentrations (unpublished observations).

It is thus apparent that the utilization of intramuscular TG is regulated by a number of factors that remain to be elucidated before a better understanding of the process can emerge. It is also important to keep in mind that the inability to measure an exercise-induced change in intramuscular TG content does not exclude the possibility that while FFAs are being hydrolyzed from the intramuscular TG pool, TG is also being synthesized so that no net change in concentration may be observed.

Acknowledgments

The authors were supported by grants from the Danish Medical Research Council (grant no. 12-9535), the Danish Veterinary and Agricultural Research Council (grant no. 13-4083), the Danish Natural Sciences Research Council (grant no. 11-0082), and the Danish National Research Foundation (grant no. 504-14).

References

1. Abumrad, N.A.; Perkins, R.C.; Park, J.H.; Park, C.R. Mechanism of long chain fatty acid permeation in the isolated adipocyte. J. Biol. Chem. 256(17):9183-9191; 1981.

2. Ahlborg, G.; Felig, P.; Hagenfeldt, L.; Hendler, R.; Wahren, J. Substrate turnover during prolonged exercise in man. Splanchnic and leg metabolism of glucose, free fatty acids, and amino acids. J. Clin. Invest. 53:1080-1090; 1974.

3. Armstrong, D.T.; Steele, R.; Altszuler, N.; Dunn, A.; Bishop, J.S.; DeBodo, R.C. Regulation of plasma free fatty acid turnover. Am. J. Physiol. 201:9-15; 1961.

4. Brady, P.S.; Ramsay, R.R.; Brady, L.J. Regulation of the long-chain carnitine acyltransferases. FASEB J. 7:1039-1044; 1993.

5. Christensen, E.H.; Hansen, O. Respiratorischer quotient und O_2-aufnahme. Skand. Arch. Physiol. 81:180-189; 1939.

6. Cleroux, J.; Van Nguyen, P.; Taylor, A.W.; Leenen, F.H.H. Effects of β1- vs. β1+β2-blockade on exercise endurance and muscle metabolism in humans. J. Appl. Physiol. 66(2):548-554; 1989.

7. Costill, D.L.; Gollnick, P.D.; Jansson, E.; Saltin, B.; Stein, E.M. Glycogen depletion pattern in human muscle fibres during distance running. Acta Physiol. Scand. 89:374-383; 1973.

8. Essen, B. Intramuscular substrate utilization during prolonged exercise. Ann. N.Y. Acad. Sci. 301:30-44; 1977.

9. Essen, B. Studies on the regulation of metabolism in human skeletal muscle using intermittent exercise as an experimental model. Acta Physiol. Scand. (suppl. 454):1-32; 1978.

10. Essen-Gustavsson, B.; Tesch, P. Glycogen and triglyceride utilization in relation to muscle metabolism characteristics in men performing heavy-resistance exercise. Eur. J. Appl. Physiol. 61:5-10; 1990.

11. Galbo, H. Exercise physiology: Humoral function. Sport Sci. Rev. 1:65-93; 1992.

12. Galbo, H. Hormonal and metabolic adaptation to exercise. Stuttgart, Germany: Georg Thieme Verlag; 1983:64-69.

13. Hagenfeldt, L.; Wahren, J. Human forearm muscle metabolism during exercise: II. Uptake, release and oxidation of individual FFA and glycerol. Scand. J. Clin. Lab. Invest. 21:263-276; 1968.

14. Havel, R.J.; Pernow, B.; Jones, N.L. Uptake and release of free fatty acids and other metabolites in the legs of exercising men. J. Appl. Physiol. 23:90-99; 1967.

15. Holm, C.; Belfrage, P.; Fredrikson, G. Immunological evidence for the presence of hormone-sensitive lipase in rat tissue other than adipose tissue. Biochem. Biophys. Res. Commun. 148:99-105; 1987.

16. Holm, C.; Kirchgessner, T.G.; Svenson, K.L.; Fredrikson, G.; Nilsson, G.; Miller, C.G.; Shively, J.E.; Heinzmann, C.; Sparkes, R.S.; Mohandas, T.; Lusis, A.J.; Belfrage, P.; Schotz, M.C. Hormone-sensitive lipase: Sequence, expression, and chromosomal localization to 19 cent-q 13.3. Science 241:1503-1506; 1988.

17. Hurley, B.F.; Nemeth, P.M.; Martin, W.H., III; Hagberg, J.M.; Dalsky, G.P.; Holloszy, J.O. Muscle triglyceride utilization during exercise: Effect of training. J. Appl. Physiol. 60:562-567; 1986.

18. Issekutz, B., Jr.; Bortz, W.M.; Miller, H.I.; Paul, P. Turnover rate of plasma FFA in humans and in dogs. Metabolism 16:1001-1009; 1967.
19. Kiens, B.; Essen-Gustavsson, B.; Christensen, N.J.; Saltin, B. Skeletal muscle substrate utilization during submaximal exercise in man: Effect of endurance training. J. Physiol. (London) 469:459-478; 1993.
20. McGarry, J.D.; Mills, S.E.; Long, C.S.; Foster, D.W. Observations on the affinity for carnitine, and malonyl-CoA sensitivity, of carnitine palmitoyltransferase I in animal and human tissues. Biochem. J. 214:21-28; 1983.
21. Paul, P. FFA metabolism of normal dogs during steady-state exercise at different work loads. J. Appl. Physiol. 28:127-132; 1970.
22. Potter, B.J.; Sorrentino, D.; Berk, P.D. Mechanisms of cellular uptake of free fatty acids. Annu. Rev. Nutr. 9:253-270; 1989.
23. Pruett, E.D.R. FFA mobilization during and after prolonged severe muscular work in men. J. Appl. Physiol. 29:809-815; 1970.
24. Severson, D.L. Regulation of lipid metabolism in adipose tissue and heart. Can. J. Physiol. Pharmacol. 57:923-937; 1979.
25. Small, C.A.; Garton, A.J.; Yeaman, S.J. The presence and role of hormone-sensitive lipase in heart muscle. Biochem. J. 258:67-72; 1989.
26. Sorrentino, D.; Robinson, R.B.; Kiang, C.-L.; Berk, P.D. At physiologic albumin/oleate concentrations oleate uptake by isolated hepatocytes, cardiac myocytes, and adipocytes is a saturable function of the unbound oleate concentration. Uptake kinetics are consistent with the conventional theory. J. Clin. Invest. 84:1325-1333; 1989.
27. Stremmel, W.; Strohmeyer, G.; Berk, P.D. Hepatocellular uptake of oleate is energy dependent, sodium linked, and inhibited by an antibody to a hepatocyte plasma membrane fatty acid binding protein. Proc. Natl. Acad. Sci. USA 83:3584-3588; 1986.
28. Tesch, P.A. Acute and long-term metabolic changes consequent to heavy-resistance exercise. Med. Sport Sci. 26:67-89; 1987.
29. Turcotte, L.P.; Hespel, P.; Richter, E.A. Influence of carbohydrate availability on metabolism of free fatty acids in contracting, perfused skeletal muscle. In: Devlin, J.; Horton, E.S.; Vranic, M., eds. Diabetes mellitus and exercise. London: Smith-Gordon; 1992:252.
30. Turcotte, L.P.; Kiens, B.; Richter, E.A. Saturation kinetics of palmitate uptake in perfused skeletal muscle. FEBS Lett. 279:327-329; 1991.
31. Turcotte, L.P.; Petry, C.; Kiens, B.; Richter, E.A. Electrical stimulation increases the Vmax for the uptake and oxidation of palmitate in perfused skeletal muscle. Med. Sci. Sports Exercise 24:S178; 1992.
32. Turcotte, L.P.; Richter, E.A.; Kiens, B. Increased plasma FFA uptake and oxidation during prolonged exercise in trained vs. untrained humans. Am. J. Physiol. 262:E791-799; 1992.
33. Turcotte, L.P.; Richter, E.A.; Srivastava, A.K.; Chiasson, J.-L. First evidence for the existence of a fatty acid binding protein in the plasma membrane of skeletal muscle. Diabetes 41 (suppl. 1):172A; 1992.
34. Turcotte, L.P.; Srivastava, A.K.; Chiasson, J.-L. Fasting increases plasma membrane fatty acid–binding protein ($FABP_{PM}$) in red muscle of rats. Med. Sci. Sports Exercise 26, S93, (suppl. 93); 1994.
35. Winder, W.W.; Arogyasami, J.; Barton, R.J.; Elayan, I.M.; Vehrs, P.R. Muscle malonyl-CoA decreases during exercise. J. Appl. Physiol. 67:2230-2233; 1989.

CHAPTER 10

Regulation of Muscle Triglyceride Metabolism in Exercise

Lawrence B. Oscai, Karyn Esser
University of Illinois at Chicago, Chicago, Illinois, U.S.A.

The regulation of muscle triglyceride (TG) metabolism in exercise revolves around two major identified lipases. They are hormone-sensitive lipase (HSL) and lipoprotein lipase (LPL). Aside from the fact that the presence of HSL has been demonstrated in muscle, little is known about the factors involved in the regulation of lipolysis of muscle TG. LPL is synthesized in and secreted from a variety of tissues, including skeletal muscle. The exported LPL found in the capillary beds hydrolyzes circulating TG, providing fatty acids for the replenishment of muscle lipid stores, for TG packing above control levels in response to eating a high-fat diet, and to a lesser extent for immediate substrate for muscle energy needs. The potential role of dietary fat in endurance exercise is discussed. HSL and LPL appear to be activated simultaneously in response to the same signal and to function as a coordinated unit in meeting the energy needs of muscle. The evidence suggests that both lipases are regulated, in part, through the classical cAMP cascade in muscle. LPL activity is increased in muscle in response to endurance exercise training. Recent evidence indicates that the increase in enzyme activity in muscle of trained rats occurs in the circulating plasma LPL fraction, with very little LPL activity attached to capillary walls. These results provide evidence that exercise training has a heparinlike effect on LPL activity in muscle. The finding that serum TGs were reduced at a time when LPL activity was increased in plasma provides evidence that training increases the capacity to remove TG from circulation.

Sources of Fat

Heart and skeletal muscle contain a pool of endogenous TG, which serves as an energy source during prolonged strenuous exercise (25, 40). It has been estimated that approximately 50% of the fat oxidized during exercise comes from intramuscular TG stores (21). Much of the remaining fat oxidized during exercise comes from plasma free fatty acids (FFAs) originating from adipose tissue (21). Plasma TGs are lowered acutely with prolonged exercise (40). However, the actual contribution of TG fatty acids to actively contracting muscle fibers appears to be relatively small (25, 40).

TG concentration in red skeletal muscle fibers of rats averages about 2 μmol/g wet weight (7, 18, 46). Intramuscular TG content of rats can be decreased with exercise (7, 18, 46). In most of the studies, the decrease is in the range of 25% to 68%, leaving a residual of about 1 μmol/g wet weight. At the present time, it is not known why TG stores can be only partially depleted. It has been suggested (25) that after prolonged exercise, when plasma FFA levels are high, the rate of FFA influx into the intramuscular TG pool balances the rate of efflux (i.e., synthesis and lipolysis are in equilibrium). Intramuscular TGs are also decreased in skeletal muscle of humans with exercise (25). However, although the resting levels of TGs are four to six times greater in humans than in rats, the pattern of reduction is similar. Of interest is that even under conditions of very severe exercise, such as a 7-h ski race (19) or a marathon race (54), TG stores can be only partially depleted in humans.

HSL and LPL in Muscle

In 1987, Holm, Belfrage, and Fredrikson (26) raised an antibody to purified rat adipose tissue HSL. Using Western blotting, these investigators were able to show quantitatively the existence of an antigenic protein in muscle extract that corresponded in size (84 kDa) to the HSL in adipose tissue. The development of an anti-HSL antibody permitted quantitative enzyme measurement for the first time. In a separate set of experiments, Holm et al. (27) used the antibody to HSL to screen a cDNA expression library and to obtain a specific cDNA clone to rat adipose tissue HSL. Using the cDNA clone to perform Northern blotting experiments, they were able to provide evidence for the existence of HSL mRNA in heart and skeletal muscle and evidence that it was similar in size to that found in adipose tissue. A couple of years later, Small, Garton, and Yeaman (53) simultaneously activated and phosphorylated purified HSL from bovine heart with cAMP-dependent protein kinase. The preceding results supported earlier claims by Goldberg and Khoo (20) and Heathers, Al-Muhtaseb, and Brunt (22) that HSL can be activated in muscle with cAMP or cAMP-dependent protein kinase. Because the presence of HSL in muscle has been unequivocally demonstrated, it is thought that this lipase might be responsible for intramuscular TG lipolysis. Identification and characterization of the factors involved in the regulation of lipolysis of muscle triglycerides is a fertile area for future research.

LPL is found in at least three fractions in muscle (5, 9, 47). One fraction, which is readily released from heart and skeletal muscle by perfusion with heparin, is located on the luminal surface of endothelial cells of capillaries, where it is directly involved in the hydrolysis of plasma TG. The second fraction remains in tissue after perfusion with heparin. The function of the intracellular fraction remains unknown. The third fraction is a small one that is found in circulating plasma. In the past, the plasma LPL fraction has received little attention. This fraction represents only about 1% of that which can be released into circulation by injection with heparin (9).

About 15 years ago, we began ascribing a lipolytic role for intramuscular LPL. This lipolytic role was based on a tight inverse relationship between endogenous LPL activity and muscle TG concentration under a variety of biochemical (43), pharmacological (36), and physiological (35) conditions. However, in view of evidence demonstrating the presence of HSL in muscle and results from recent molecular studies on LPL, this stand is no longer tenable. In order for LPL to serve two functions, one inside the cell and one in circulation, two isoforms of LPL must exist. A large number of LPL cDNA clones have been isolated from a variety of species, including human, bovine, guinea pig, chicken, and mouse (12, 17, 31, 50, 56). To date there is no evidence for two isoforms of LPL. Although different sizes of mRNA have been detected, these differences can be explained by different placement of the poly A tail on mRNA. Therefore, the observation that only one isoform of LPL mRNA has been found provides strong evidence for only one LPL protein.

An NH_4-terminal sequence of 16 to 30 amino acids (signal peptide) initiates transport of secretory proteins across the endoplasmic reticulum (14). Once inside the lumen of the endoplasmic reticulum, the signal peptide is cleaved from the protein. The process of secretion proceeds with further protein modification such as glycosylation, and the mature protein is then exported to the Golgi and carried forward in the transport vesicles to exit the cell. In this context, LPL mRNA encodes an NH_4-terminal signal peptide of 27 amino acids (56). Newly synthesized proteins lacking a signal peptide are left behind, permanent residents of the cytosolic compartment. The HSL mRNA does not appear to code for a signal peptide (27). Thus, it appears that LPL with a signal peptide functions outside the cell, whereas HSL with no signal peptide functions inside the cell.

Simultaneous Activation of HSL and LPL

It appears that HSL and LPL are activated simultaneously in response to the same signal (i.e., cAMP) and function as a coordinated unit in meeting the energy demands of muscle. Figure 10.1 shows a strong negative correlation between endogenous LPL activity and triglyceride content as a result of perfusing the heart with various concentrations of epinephrine. Similar results were obtained as a result of perfusing the heart with various concentrations of cAMP (43). Direct measurement of HSL activity was not made. However, because the presence of HSL in muscle has been established (26) and because TG concentration inside muscle cells was decreased, it is assumed that HSL was responsible for intramuscular TG hydrolysis. Similar results suggesting a simultaneous activation of HSL and LPL have been obtained under a variety of biochemical (43), pharmacological (36), and physiological (35) conditions in muscle. There is evidence that both lipases are regulated posttranslationally through the cAMP cascade (43, 52, 53). The mechanism of LPL activation also includes transcriptional (8, 49) as well as posttranscriptional (16, 49) modification through one or more of the steps involved in synthesis, transport, and secretion of the enzyme.

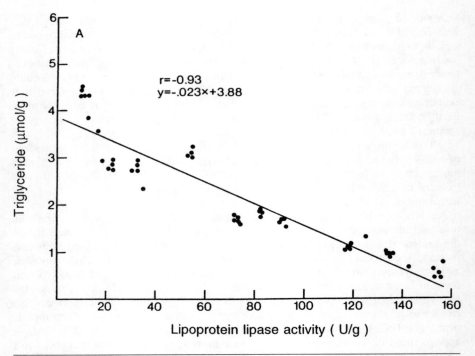

Figure 10.1   Intracellular triglyceride plotted as a function of endogenous lipoprotein lipase activity assayed on hearts perfused with various concentrations of epinephrine. Reprinted from Palmer, Caruso, and Oscai 1981 (43).

Effects of Exercise Training

An adaptation that characterizes the trained state is a greater reliance on fat oxidation as an energy substrate (23, 25). The source of these additional fatty acids oxidized in the trained state has been shown to be intramuscular TG stores (28, 33). For example, the depletion of intramuscular TG deposits during a 2-h bout of cycle ergometer work was 106% greater after than before endurance exercise training, a difference that could explain the increased whole-body oxidation of fat in the physically trained state. Moreover, endurance exercise training actually blunts the rate of adipose tissue lipolysis during submaximal exercise, resulting in a decrease in FFA turnover and oxidation (33). These results serve to emphasize the importance of intramuscular TG stores as a source of energy during exercise, especially in physically trained individuals.

The mechanisms responsible for the increased oxidation of fat in the trained state remain unclear. It is known, however, that endurance training results in an increase in the enzymes involved in the activation of fatty acids, in their transport into the mitochondria, and in β-oxidation (37). It has been speculated (25) that an increase in these enzymes responsible for fatty acid oxidation probably plays the primary role in accounting for the increased oxidation of fatty acids in the trained state.

Obviously, the partially depleted TG stores seen with exercise need to be replenished. Perhaps the strongest evidence that LPL and plasma TG play important roles in the replenishment process comes from mice born with genetic combined lipase deficiency (4, 44). LPL in tissues of these mice is very low. LPL-deficient mice develop severe hyperchylomicronemia because of an inability to clear TG from circulation. These affected mice have no intracellular lipid droplets in the heart and diaphragm, whereas the unaffected mice have numerous lipid droplets in their muscle cells. These results suggest an important role for LPL in the replenishment of muscle lipid stores.

LPL is anchored with high affinity on the luminal surface of capillary endothelial cells. Because of this binding process, hydrolysis of chylomicrons and very low density lipoproteins occurs on, or close to, the luminal surface of the vascular endothelium and not in the circulating plasma (3, 45). About 20 years ago (6), it was shown that LPL activity is markedly increased in skeletal muscle in response to endurance exercise training. However, since LPL activity was measured in whole homogenates of muscle, it was not clear whether the increase(s) occurred in circulating plasma fraction (pre-heparin-perfusate LPL activity), in the capillary-bound fraction (post-heparin-perfusate LPL activity), or in the intracellular fraction (residual LPL activity in tissue after heparin perfusion). Using heparin as a tool (48), it was possible to demonstrate that LPL activity is increased ninefold in the circulating plasma fraction (pre-heparin-perfusate LPL activity) of trained rats (42). At the same time, capillary-bound LPL activity (post-heparin-perfusate fraction) was reduced to very low levels (42). These results provide evidence that exercise training has a heparinlike effect on capillary-bound LPL. Further, the finding that the sum of the pre-heparin-perfusate LPL activity and the post-heparin-perfusate LPL activity was increased at a time when serum TGs were reduced provides evidence that training increases the capacity to remove TG from circulation. In separate experiments, it has been shown that LPL activity is also significantly increased (nearly threefold) in the intracellular fraction in soleus and fast red fibers of the quadriceps in response to endurance exercise training (39). The increase in intracellular LPL activity with training may represent an increased potential for shuttling enzyme to the circulating plasma LPL fraction.

Potential Role of Dietary Fat in Endurance Exercise

In the late 1960s and shortly thereafter, evidence appeared to show that endurance can be increased by raising, and diminished by lowering, body carbohydrate stores (2, 29). It was strongly implicated that muscle glycogen depletion is closely associated with the development of exhaustion during prolonged strenuous work (1, 23). These findings provided the basis for the common practice of glycogen loading before endurance events (11). Little attention was paid to the role of dietary fat in endurance exercise. Then in 1977, interest in the potential role of fat metabolism in exercise performance was stimulated when Hickson et al. (24) provided evidence that an increased availability of fatty acids delays the development of exhaustion in rats subjected to prolonged running. In that study (24), rats were given corn oil by stomach tube, and 3 h later an injection of heparin was given to raise their plasma free fatty acids. The rats with raised free fatty acids were able to run approximately

1 h longer than otherwise comparable control animals before becoming exhausted. Thus, an increased availability of fatty acids to working muscle fibers increases endurance. A few years later, Miller, Bryce, and Conlee (34) reported that rats exposed to a high-fat diet for as little as 1 wk or as long as 5 wk can run significantly longer than those on a high-carbohydrate diet, despite reduced glycogen storage. This report was followed by that of Simi et al. (51) in which fat feeding was shown to increase submaximal running time by 62% in highly trained rats. More recently, Muoio et al. (38) reported that run time to exhaustion was 20% greater after exposure to a high-fat diet versus a high-carbohydrate diet in highly trained collegiate distance runners. The possibility exists that an increased availability of fatty acids could have delayed the development of exhaustion in the preceding fat-feeding experiments. This possibility is of interest to us because, in the course of work on obesity in our laboratory, rats fed diets high in fat were found to have raised intramuscular TG deposits. Raised TG deposits could potentially increase the availability of fatty acids to working muscle fibers. Figure 10.2 clearly demonstrates that TG deposits were raised in heart and in the three types of skeletal muscle in rats habitually consuming fat-rich diets. Further, it shows that TG deposits increased progressively as the fat content of the diet increased. For example, TG deposits in all muscle types examined were significantly greater in rats eating a diet containing 50% energy as fat compared with those eating 30% energy as fat ($p < .05$). TG packing takes place rapidly, within a period of 24 h, provided that the fat content of the diet is sufficiently high. For example, results from a previous paper (41) show that TG deposits in heart can be significantly increased (38%; $p < .001$) after 1 d in rats eating a diet containing 60% energy as fat. TG packing also takes place in muscle of rats eating diets containing lesser amounts of fat, but the packing takes place

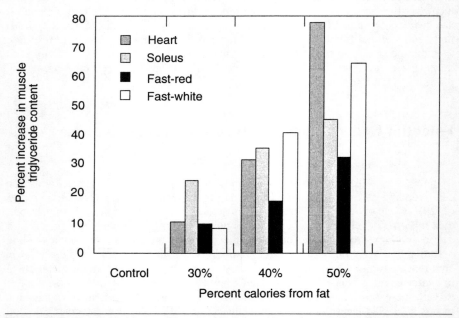

Figure 10.2 Percentage increase in muscle triglyceride content plotted as function of percentage of calories in diet from fat. Reprinted from Oscai, Miller, and Esser (41).

less rapidly. For example, the data indicate that a small but statistically significant increase (7%; $p < .02$) in the TG content of the heart occurs after 1 d in rats eating a diet containing 42% energy as fat. However, between 1 and 13 d on this diet (42% energy as fat), TG deposits in the heart increased to 43% above control ($p < .001$).

It should be pointed out that in a previous study (35), fat packing did not take place in hearts of rats eating a fat-rich diet for 1 d. In that study, rats were fasted from 12 noon until 7 A.M. to 10 A.M. the next day. Therefore, the absence of fat packing might have been due to the prolonged fast. In the experiments previously outlined, the rats were fasted overnight for a period lasting about 12 h.

In addition to playing an important role in the replenishment of muscle TG stores decreased by exercise, LPL may play a role in muscle TG packing that takes place in response to eating a fat-rich diet. For example, there is considerable evidence that LPL activity is elevated in muscle of fat-fed humans and animals (10, 13, 15, 30, 32, 55). Figure 10.3 shows that LPL activity starts to increase in heparin-perfused hearts of rats when the animals are fed a diet containing 30% energy as fat ($p < .05$), provided that there is no sugar in the diet (41). Under these conditions, LPL activity remains significantly elevated as the fat content of the diet increases. When sugar is replaced by cornstarch in the diet, LPL activity is suppressed, so that when rats are fed a diet containing 50% or 60% energy as fat, the reduction in enzyme activity is statistically significant ($p < .01$) (41). At the present time, it is not known

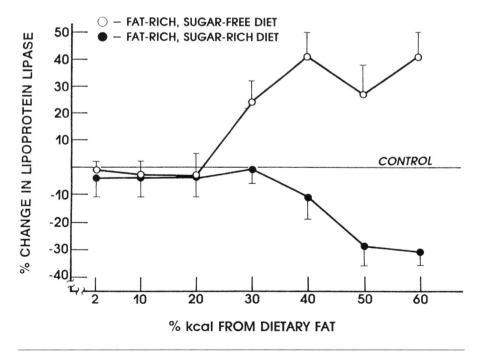

Figure 10.3 Percentage change in intracellular lipoprotein lipase activity in heart plotted as a function of percentage of calories in diet from fat. Values are means ± *SE* for six rats. Reprinted from Oscai, Miller, and Esser (41).

why dietary fat in the absence of sugar activates LPL in muscle, whereas fat in combination with sugar suppresses enzyme activity.

Acknowledgment

This research was supported by the National Institute of Diabetes and Digestive and Kidney Diseases, grant DK-42023.

References

1. Ahlborg, B.; Bergström, J.; Ekelund, L.-G.; Hultman, E. Muscle glycogen and muscle electrolytes during prolonged physical exercise. Acta Physiol. Scand. 70:129-142; 1967.
2. Bergström, J.; Hermansen, L.; Hultman, E.; Saltin, B. Diet, muscle glycogen and physical performance. Acta Physiol. Scand. 71:140-150; 1967.
3. Blanchette-Mackie, E.J.; Masuno, H.; Dwyer, N.K.; Olivecrona, T.; Scow, R.O. Lipoprotein lipase in myocytes and capillary endothelium of heart: Immunocyto-chemical study. Am. J. Physiol. 256:E818-E828; 1989.
4. Blanchette-Mackie, E.J.; Wetzel, M.G.; Chernick, S.S.; Paterniti, J.R.; Brown, W.V.; Scow, R.O. Effect of the combined lipase deficiency mutation (cld/cld) on ultrastructure of tissues in mice diaphragm, heart, brown adipose tissue, lung, and liver. Lab. Invest. 55:347-362; 1986.
5. Borensztajn, J. Heart and skeletal muscle lipoprotein lipase. Chicago: Evener Publishers, Inc.; 1987:133-148.
6. Borensztajn, J.; Rone, M.S.; Babirak, S.P.; McGarr, J.A.; Oscai, L.B. Effect of exercise on lipoprotein lipase activity in rat heart and skeletal muscle. Am. J. Physiol. 229:394-397; 1975.
7. Carlson, L.A.; Fröberg, S.O. Effect of training with exercise on plasma and tissue lipid levels of ageing rats. Gerontologia 15:14-23; 1969.
8. Carneheim, C.; Nedergaard, J.; Cannon, B. Cold-induced β-adrenergic recruitment of lipoprotein lipase in brown fat is due to increased transcription. Am. J. Physiol. 254:E155-E161; 1988.
9. Chajek-Shaul, T.; Friedman, G.; Stein, O.; Etienne, J.; Stein, Y. Endogenous plasma lipoprotein lipase activity in fed and fasting rats may reflect the functional pool of endothelial lipoprotein lipase. Biochim. Biophys. Acta 837:271-278; 1985.
10. Childs, M.T.; Tollefson, J.; Knopp, R.H.; Bowden, D.A. Lipid metabolism in pregnancy: VIII. Effects of dietary fat versus carbohydrate on lipoprotein and hepatic lipids and tissue triglyceride lipases. Metabolism 30:27-35; 1981.
11. Conlee, R.K. Muscle glycogen and exercise endurance: A twenty-year perspective. Exercise Sport Sci. Rev. 15:1-28; 1987.
12. Cooper, D.A.; Stein, J.C.; Strieleman, P.J.; Bensadoun, A. Avian adipose lipoprotein lipase: cDNA sequence and reciprocal regulation of mRNA levels in adipose and heart. Biochim. Biophys. Acta 1008:92-101; 1989.
13. Cryer, A.; Kirtland, J.; Jones, H.M.; Gurr, M.I. Lipoprotein lipase activity in the tissues of guinea pigs exposed to different dietary fats from conception to three months of age. Biochem. J. 170:169-172; 1978.

14. Darnell, J.; Lodish, H.; Baltimore, D. Molecular cell biology. New York: Scientific American Books; 1986:945.
15. DeGasquet, P.; Griglio, S.; Pequignot-Planche, E.; Malewiak, M.I. Diurnal changes in plasma and liver lipids and lipoprotein lipase activity in heart and adipose tissue in rats fed a high and low fat diet. J. Nutr. 107:199-212; 1977.
16. Doolittle, M.H.; Ben-Zeev, O.; Elovson, J.; Martin, D.; Kirchgessner, T.G. The response of lipoprotein lipase to feeding and fasting. Evidence for posttranslational regulation. J. Biol. Chem. 265:4570-4577; 1990.
17. Enerback, S.; Semb, H.; Bengtsson-Olivecrona, G.; Carlsson, P.; Hermansson, M.-L.; Olivecrona, T.; Bjursell, G. Molecular cloning and sequence analysis of cDNA encoding lipoprotein lipase of guinea pig. Gene 58:1-12; 1987.
18. Fröberg, S.O. Effects of training and of acute exercise in trained rats. Metabolism 20:1044-1051; 1971.
19. Fröberg, S.O.; Mossfeldt, F. Effect of prolonged strenuous exercise on the concentration of triglycerides, phospholipids and glycogen in muscle of man. Acta Physiol. Scand. 82:167-171; 1971.
20. Goldberg, D.I.; Khoo, J.C. Activation of myocardial neutral triglyceride lipase and neutral cholesterol esterase by cAMP-dependent protein kinase. J. Biol. Chem. 260:5879-5882; 1985.
21. Havel, R.J.; Pernow, B.; Jones, N.L. Uptake and release of free fatty acids and other metabolites in the legs of exercising men. J. Appl. Physiol. 23:90-99; 1967.
22. Heathers, G.P.; Al-Muhtaseb, N.; Brunt, R.V. The effect of adrenergic agents on the activities of glycerol 3-phosphate acyltransferase and triglyceride lipase in the isolated perfused rat heart. J. Mol. Cell. Cardiol. 17:785-796; 1985.
23. Hermansen, L.; Hultman, E.; Saltin, B. Muscle glycogen during prolonged severe exercise. Acta Physiol. Scand. 71:129-139; 1967.
24. Hickson, R.C.; Rennie, M.J.; Conlee, R.K.; Winder, W.W.; Holloszy, J.O. Effects of increased plasma fatty acids on glycogen utilization and endurance. J. Appl. Physiol. 43:829-833, 1977.
25. Holloszy, J.O. Utilization of fatty acids during exercise. In: Taylor, A.W.; Gollnick, P.D.; Green, H.J.; Ianuzzo, C.D.; Noble, E.G.; Métivier, G.; Sutton, J.R., eds. Biochemistry of exercise VII. Champaign, IL: Human Kinetics; 1990:319-327. (Int. Series Sport Sci.; vol. 21).
26. Holm, C.; Belfrage, P.; Fredrikson, G. Immunological evidence for the presence of hormone-sensitive lipase in rat tissues other than adipose tissue. Biochem. Biophys. Res. Commun. 148:99-105; 1987.
27. Holm, C.; Kirchgessner, T.G.; Svenson, K.L.; Fredrikson, G.; Nilsson, S.; Miller, C.G.; Shively, J.E.; Heinzmann, C.; Sparkes, R.S.; Mohandas, T.; Lusis, A.J.; Belfrage, P.; Schotz, M.C. Hormone-sensitive lipase: Sequence, expression, and chromosomal localization to 19 cent-q 13.3. Science 241:1503-1506; 1988.
28. Hurley, B.F.; Nemeth, P.M.; Martin, W.H.; Hagberg, J.M.; Dalsky, G.P.; Holloszy, J.O. Muscle triglyceride utilization during exercise: Effect of training. J. Appl. Physiol. 60:562-567; 1986.
29. Karlsson, J.; Saltin, B. Diet, muscle glycogen, and endurance performance. J. Appl. Physiol. 31:203-206; 1971.
30. Kiens, B.; Essen-Gustavsson, B.; Gad, P.; Lithell, H. Lipoprotein lipase activity and intramuscular triglyceride stores after long-term high-fat and high-carbohydrate diets in physically trained men. Clin. Physiol. 7:1-9; 1987.
31. Kirchgessner, T.G.; Svenson, K.L.; Lusis, A.J.; Schotz, M.C. The sequence of cDNA encoding lipoprotein lipase. J. Biol. Chem. 262:8463-8466; 1987.

32. Lawson, N.; Pollard, A.D.; Jennings, R.J.; Gurr, M.I.; Brindley, D.N. The activities of lipoprotein lipase and of enzymes involved in triacylglycerol synthesis in rat adipose tissue. Effects of starvation, dietary modification and of corticotropin injection. Biochem. J. 200:285-294; 1981.

33. Martin, W.H.; Dalsky, G.P.; Hurley, B.F.; Matthews, D.E.; Bier, D.M.; Hagberg, J.M.; Rogers, M.A.; King, D.S.; Holloszy, J.O. Effect of endurance training on plasma free fatty acid turnover and oxidation during exercise. Am. J. Physiol. 265:E708-E714; 1993.

34. Miller, W.C.; Bryce, G.R.; Conlee, R.K. Adaptations to a high-fat diet that increase exercise endurance in male rats. J. Appl. Physiol. 56:78-83; 1984.

35. Miller, W.C.; Oscai, L.B. Relationship between type L hormone-sensitive lipase and endogenous triacylglycerol in rat heart. Am. J. Physiol. 247:R621-R625; 1984.

36. Miller, W.C.; Palmer, W.K.; Oscai, L.B. Relationship between type L hormone-sensitive lipase activity and endogenous triacylglycerol in the hearts of colchicine-treated rats. Biochem. J. 224:793-798; 1984.

37. Molé, P.A.; Oscai, L.B.; Holloszy, J.O. Adaptation of muscle to exercise. Increase in levels of palmityl CoA synthetase, carnitine palmityltransferase, and palmityl CoA dehydrogenase, and in the capacity to oxidize fatty acids. J. Clin. Invest. 50:2323-2330; 1971.

38. Muoio, D.M.; Leddy, J.J.; Horvath, P.J.; Awad, A.B.; Pendergast, D.R. Effect of dietary fat on metabolic adjustments to maximal VO_2 and endurance in runners. Med. Sci. Sports Exercise 26:81-88; 1994.

39. Oscai, L.B.; Caruso, R.A.; Wergeles, A.C. Lipoprotein lipase hydrolyzes endogenous triacylglycerols in muscle of exercised rats. J. Appl. Physiol. 52:1059-1063; 1982.

40. Oscai, L.B.; Essig, D.A.; Palmer, W.K. Lipase regulation of muscle triglyceride hydrolysis J. Appl. Physiol. 69:1571-1577; 1990.

41. Oscai, L.B.; Miller, W.C.; Esser, K. Effects of fat rich diets on triglyceride deposits and lipoprotein lipase activity in muscle. (Submitted.)

42. Oscai, L.B.; Tsika, R.W.; Essig, D.A. Exercise training has a heparin-like effect on lipoprotein lipase activity in muscle. Can. J. Physiol. Pharmacol. 70:905-909; 1992.

43. Palmer, W.K.; Caruso, R.A.; Oscai, L.B. Possible role of lipoprotein lipase in the regulation of endogenous triacylglycerols in the rat heart. Biochem. J. 198:159-166; 1981.

44. Paterniti, J.R.; Brown, W.V.; Ginsberg, H.N. Combined lipase deficiency (cld): A lethal mutation on chromosome 17 of the mouse. Science 221:167-169; 1983.

45. Pedersen, M.E.; Cohen, M.; Schotz, M.C. Immunocytochemical localization of the functional fraction of lipoprotein lipase in the perfused heart. J. Lipid Res. 24:512-521; 1983.

46. Reitman, J.; Baldwin, K.M.; Holloszy, J.O. Intramuscular triglyceride utilization by red, white, and intermediate skeletal muscle and heart during exhausting exercise. Proc. Soc. Exp. Biol. Med. 142:628-631; 1973.

47. Robinson, D.S. The function of the plasma triglycerides in fatty acid transport. Comp. Biochem. 18:51-116; 1970.

48. Robinson, D.S.; Harris, P.M. The production of lipolytic activity in the circulation of the hind limb in response to heparin. Q. J. Exp. Physiol. 44:80-90; 1959.

49. Robinson, D.S.; Speake, B.K. Role of insulin and other hormones in the control of lipoprotein lipase activity. Biochem. Soc. Trans. 17:40-42; 1989.

50. Senda, M.; Oka, K.; Brown, W.V.; Oasba, P.K.; Furuichi, Y. Molecular cloning and sequence of a cDNA coding for bovine lipoprotein lipase. Proc. Natl. Acad. Sci. USA 84:4369-4373; 1987.

51. Simi, B.; Sempore, B.; Mayet, M.-H.; Favier, R.J. Additive effects of training and high-fat diet on energy metabolism during exercise. J. Appl. Physiol. 71:197-203; 1991.

52. Simsolo, R.B.; Ong, J.M.; Kern, P.A. The regulation of adipose tissue and muscle lipoprotein lipase in runners by detraining. J. Clin. Invest. 92:2124-2130; 1993.

53. Small, C.A.; Garton, A.J.; Yeaman, S.J. The presence and role of hormone-sensitive lipase in heart muscle. Biochem. J. 258:67-72; 1989.

54. Staron, R.S.; Hikida, R.S.; Murray, T.F.; Hagerman, F.C.; Hagerman, M.T. Lipid depletion and repletion in skeletal muscle following a marathon. J. Neurol. Sci. 94:29-40; 1989.

55. Weisenburg-Delorme, C.L.; Harris, K.L. Effects of diet on lipoprotein lipase activity in the rat. J. Nutr. 105:447-451; 1975.

56. Wion, K.L.; Kirchgessner, T.G.; Lusis, A.J.; Schotz, M.C.; Lawn, R.M. Human lipoprotein lipase complementary DNA sequence. Science 235:1638-1641; 1987.

PART III

Integration of Fat
and Carbohydrate Metabolism

CHAPTER 11

An Introduction to the Roles of the Glucose–Fatty Acid Cycle in Sustained Exercise

Eric A. Newsholme

University of Oxford, Oxford, England

Liver contains the only store of glycogen that can be broken down into glucose and released into the bloodstream for use by muscle. However, the quantity of this stored carbohydrate is very small in relation to the glucose requirement of the tissues. At rest, the total glucose requirement of the major carbohydrate-utilizing tissues of the body (brain, kidney, heart, and muscle) is more than 300 g/d, which is normally met by the dietary intake of carbohydrate: The liver store in the adult is about 100 g. However, the amount of carbohydrate stored in the liver of a child is very small in relation to the child's brain requirement for glucose. Since liver glycogen is broken down during starvation to provide glucose for the tissues, it can last for at most 24 h in the adult and for much shorter periods in children. Hence, the important question arises, How is it possible to survive prolonged starvation?

The lipid reserves in the average human subject are much greater than carbohydrate reserves. The reason for this marked preference for lipid as a reserve fuel, which is not unique to humans but is found in most animals, is that it is approximately nine times more efficient than carbohydrate, on the basis of weight, as a storage fuel. However, some key organs and tissues (e.g., brain, immune cells) have an obligatory requirement for glucose, so that the blood glucose level cannot fall to very low levels even when carbohydrate stress is severe (8). Hence, protection for the blood glucose level is necessary and is provided in part by the regulatory effect of fatty acid on the rate of glucose utilization by muscle and perhaps some other tissues.

The mobilization of fatty acids from the very large adipose tissue store of triacylglycerol and the increased rate of fatty acid oxidation probably begin during the overnight fast and are increased if starvation continues. However, of relevance to this publication, fatty acid oxidation not only provides energy for tissues but results in a decreased rate of glucose utilization; this regulatory effect of fatty acids is known as the glucose–fatty acid cycle.

The Glucose–Fatty Acid Cycle

For large amounts of fat to be oxidized by muscle and other tissues, it has to be mobilized from adipose tissue as free fatty acids. These are transported and bound to albumin in the plasma, and their plasma concentration in part plays a role in control of the rate of oxidation of fatty acids by muscle. However, fatty acids not only play a role as a fuel, but also, when they are oxidized, can lead under some conditions to regulation of the rate of glucose utilization and oxidation.

The concept of the glucose–fatty acid cycle was put forward in 1963 to explain the reciprocal relationship between the rates of oxidation of glucose and fatty acids by muscle (11). Although some features of the model have been modified since that time, there is now considerable evidence to support the important proposal that under conditions of carbohydrate stress (defined as when the glycogen store in the liver is depleted) fatty acid mobilization from adipose tissue is increased so that its rate of oxidation by muscle can be increased, and this in turn may decrease the rate of glucose utilization. Conversely, when the carbohydrate stress is removed (e.g., by refeeding a starved subject), the plasma level of fatty acid decreases, due to a decreased rate of release from adipose tissue plus an increased rate of uptake by liver, which leads to a decrease in the rate of fatty acid oxidation by muscle. This results in an increased rate of glucose utilization by the muscle. These responses serve to stabilize the blood glucose concentration.

Although changes in the plasma level of fatty acids undoubtedly influence their rate of oxidation, recent work by Winder (see chapter 14) has shown that conditions that favor fatty acid mobilization from adipose tissue (e.g., a low level of insulin) will also increase the rate of fatty acid oxidation in muscle by a specific activation of a key enzyme in the fatty acid oxidation pathway: carnitine palmitoyl transferase (CPT). This is achieved by changes in the intracellular level of malonyl CoA, a well-established inhibitor of CPT. Hence the muscle level of malonyl CoA may also play a role in encouraging the oxidation of fat by muscle and therefore in the glucose–fatty acid cycle.

Sustained Exercise and the Glucose–Fatty Acid Cycle

Because the liver glycogen reserves are partially depleted by the overnight fast, even moderate exercise (e.g., walking or jogging) before breakfast causes mobilization of fatty acids (5), as indicated by an increased plasma level of glycerol. It is generally accepted that after 30 min of exercise at 60% to 70% of $\dot{V}O_2$max, mobilization of fatty acids from adipose tissue increases. However, despite increased rates of mobilization, the plasma concentration of fatty acids may be only slightly increased (1); this is because the rate of uptake of the fatty acids by the active muscle is increased (encouraged by increased flow of blood to muscle). In addition, the rate of oxidation will be increased by a decrease in the malonyl CoA concentration (see chapter 14).

It is possible that the plasma fatty acid concentration increases markedly in exercise only in some conditions:

- When the muscle (and liver) glycogen store are totally depleted
- In very unfit subjects when control of fatty acid mobilization may not be very precise
- When the rate of fatty acid oxidation by muscle is somewhat restricted by the intermittent nature of the exercise that occurs in games such as soccer, rugby, tennis, or squash

Not only may large increases in the plasma fatty acid level lead to increased fatty acid oxidation and therefore play a part in the glucose–fatty acid cycle, but they may also lead to central fatigue, as discussed later. Since the importance of the plasma fatty acid level is considerable in understanding such interactions in muscle and possible fatigue, the author would wish to see more studies on the plasma level during various exercise activities.

The theoretical importance of the glucose–fatty acid cycle in exercise is probably most simply explained by reference to the marathon event as follows. The rate of energy expenditure in the marathon run appears to be considerably greater than can be supplied by the oxidation of fatty acids alone. The author suggests that, for the major period of the marathon run, the energy requirement of the runner is provided by oxidation of both glycogen and fatty acids (perhaps in the ratio 70:30, as previously discussed; 9). The importance of fatty acid oxidation is not only the provision of ATP for the muscle, but also that it may restrict the rate of utilization of glycogen to that required to supplement the energy not provided by fatty acid oxidation. If fatty acid oxidation did not restrict glycogen utilization, the glycogen reserves of the muscle would be utilized more rapidly, so that they would become depleted before completion of the race (9). However, studies on the actual effect of fatty acid oxidation on glucose and glycogen metabolism in exercise do not always confirm the validity of the theory (see chapter 12). One of the problems, however, is that even though fatty acid oxidation can inhibit the rate of utilization of glucose and glycogen, this is not an immutable effect of fatty acids. Thus this inhibitory effect is removed if the energy demand by the muscle exceeds that which can be provided by glycogen and fatty acid oxidation. The regulation of glucose utilization by fatty acid oxidation is considered to be achieved in part by the inhibitory effect of citrate on the enzyme phosphofructokinase: Citrate enhances the inhibition of the enzyme by ATP. However, it is well established that an increase in the concentration of any (or all) of the deinhibitors of phosphofructokinase (e.g., AMP, NH_4^+, inorganic phosphate [Pi], fructose diphosphate) will reduce ATP and therefore citrate inhibition of the enzyme and hence increase the rate of glycolysis and glycogen utilization. The important point from this discussion is that it will only be possible to detect an effect of fatty acid oxidation on glucose or glycogen utilization by muscle provided that the normal ATP, AMP, NH_4^+, and Pi levels are maintained. Thus, if the rate of fatty acid and glycogen oxidation provides just sufficient energy for the requirements of the working muscle, a further increase in work by that muscle might decrease the ATP/ADP concentration ratio, increase the concentrations of AMP, inorganic phosphate, and NH_4^+ (and possibly fructose diphosphate), and hence increase the flux through glycolysis. This would occur despite the inhibitory effects of fatty acid oxidation, since citrate inhibition of phosphofructokinase is relieved by increases in the concentration of AMP, Pi, and so on. Thus, if an increased energy demand by muscle could not be met by increased fat mobilization, an increase in the rate of glycogen utilization would have to occur. This will be a particularly important effect if oxygen supply to muscle is limiting performance, since to maintain the rate of ATP generation some glycogen must be converted to lactate and the activity of phosphofructokinase must be increased. Experiments to test the glucose–fatty acid cycle on exercising muscle must take this into account.

The Glucose–Fatty Acid Cycle and Pyruvate Oxidation at Rest and in Exercise

In 1964 it was shown that pyruvate oxidation by heart muscle could be inhibited by fatty acid oxidation, and it was considered that this was caused by raised concentration of NADH and acetyl CoA, which inhibited the enzyme pyruvate dehydrogenase (PDH; 4). However, when it was discovered that the enzyme could also be regulated by covalent modification (phosphorylation and dephosphorylation), the PDH kinase, which converts the enzyme to the inactive form, was found to be activated by NADH, acetyl CoA, and ATP, suggesting that this was the effect by which fatty acid oxidation would change the activity of the key enzyme PDH. Much of the basic work on the regulation of the enzyme has been done on heart rather than skeletal muscle. The interesting question is whether fatty acid oxidation in skeletal muscle will inhibit pyruvate oxidation via a decrease in PDH in the active form as it does in the heart. However, an important question is the effect of oxidation on PDH activity and on the flux of pyruvate through the reaction since the rate should change by up to 100-fold from rest to intense aerobic activity. Several detailed studies on this topic have now been carried out and are discussed by Hultman (see chapter 13).

The Triglyceride–Fatty Acid Cycle and the Glucose–Fatty Acid Cycle

The triglyceride–fatty acid cycle consists of the simultaneous activity of the processes of lipolysis of triglyceride and esterification of fatty acids. This cycle comprises several reactions such that one turn of the cycle results in the hydrolysis of at least eight molecules of ATP to adenosine diphosphate (ADP) and phosphate. Evidence for the existence of this cycle in adipose tissue has been available for many years and has recently been demonstrated in adipose tissue in vivo both in the rat and in humans (see 10 for references).

It is suggested that increases in cycling rates in general improve the sensitivity of the control of key processes in metabolism (6). Some evidence to support the view that the triglyceride–fatty acid cycle increases the sensitivity of the process of lipolysis to regulation has recently been established in human white adipose tissue in vivo. Using [1-^{13}C]palmitate and deuterated glycerol, Wolfe and Peters (14) demonstrated a 2.7-fold increase in the rate of triglyceride–fatty acid cycling in response to glucose infusion. The rate of this cycle has also been shown to be higher in burn patients and in subjects after exercise (12). Furthermore the cycle can occur within individual cells in one tissue (intracellular cycling) or it can occur between tissues, for example, between adipose tissue (lipolysis) and liver (esterification). Wolfe has obtained evidence that the rates of both these cycles are increased in some conditions, including exercise (13).

If the activity of triglyceride lipase activity is high, then the rate of release of fatty acids from stored triglyceride is high. If these fatty acids are not required for oxidation, as could be the case at rest, then the extracellular concentration of fatty acids and the intracellular concentrations of fatty acid plus fatty acyl CoA may increase to levels that could cause damage. However, if triacylglycerol–fatty acid cycling occurs, the rate of esterification will be increased by raised concentrations of fatty acyl CoA, and adipose tissue triglyceride lipase activity will be decreased by the inhibitory effect of fatty acids: In this case the operation of the cycle would help to maintain relatively constant extracellular and intracellular concentrations of fatty acid (and fatty acyl CoA), thereby providing a buffering system. This important point was first explained by Newsholme and Crabtree in 1976 (6). Evidence for this role of the extracellular triglyceride–fatty acid cycle has been obtained by Wolfe et al. (15).

This discussion can now be used to extend the concept of the triglyceride–fatty acid cycle to include the important regulatory mechanism of branched point sensitivity. The triglyceride–fatty acid substrate cycle can be considered as a branch point that occurs between the processes of esterification (cycling) and β-oxidation. Such a branch point might enable the process of β-oxidation to retain maximal possible sensitivity to its regulator(s) in tissues that can oxidize fatty acids. The high sensitivity will be achieved if the rates of lipolysis and esterification are high (i.e., the cycling rate is high) and greater than the rate of β-oxidation. Under these conditions, an increased rate of fatty acid oxidation to provide energy for the tissue will result in only a small decrease in the fatty acid concentrations both within the cell and within the plasma; these concentrations are "protected" by the lipolytic process. The triglyceride–fatty acid branch point can therefore be seen as a dynamic buffer system, since a large change in the rate of oxidation will lead only to a small change in the concentration of fatty acid, which will not cause any marked opposition to the change in the rate of oxidation. Recent results provided by Wolfe and co-workers are consistent with this concept of branch point sensitivity, particularly for the extracellular triglyceride–fatty acid cycle (15).

Plasma Fatty Acid, Free Tryptophan, Branched-Chain Amino Acid Concentrations, and Fatigue

Fatigue is defined physiologically as the inability to maintain power output. In some cases it can be explained by the excessive accumulation of end products of fuel metabolism (e.g., protons) or by too low a concentration of fuel (e.g., glycogen; 9). It is possible that too high a concentration of a fuel—that is, the plasma concentration of fatty acids—may also result in fatigue; this is the interesting conclusion based on a new hypothesis for central fatigue.

There is some evidence to support the view that a decrease in the concentration of a neurotransmitter in the brain may limit the rate of neuronal firing in some parts of the brain, especially if the rate of neuronal firing is high. This inability of one part of the brain to function satisfactorily because of a decrease in neurotransmitter concentration can result in changes in behavior. For example, in some parts of the brain a decrease in the concentration of the monoamine neurotransmitters (noradrenaline, dopamine, or 5-hydroxytryptamine) can result in depression. In addition, there is evidence to support the view that an increase in the level of 5-hydroxytryptamine (5-HT) in the brain can result in tiredness and sleep. It has therefore been suggested as a working hypothesis that an increase in the concentration of this neurotransmitter in certain areas of the brain might ensure a high rate of neuronal firing in a specific part of the brain, which then increases the sensitivity to fatigue in physical activity. This would be called central fatigue. Fatty acid could play a role in this system as follows. Since tryptophan is the precursor of 5-HT in the brain and it is unique among amino acids in that it is bound to plasma albumin, it exists in a bound form and a free form, which are in equilibrium: This equilibrium is changed in favor of free tryptophan when the plasma concentration of fatty acids increases above normal.

This change is probably caused by the binding of fatty acids to albumin. An increase in the plasma level of free tryptophan is predicted to lead to an increase in the level of 5-HT in some parts of the brain, leading to central fatigue. Preliminary evidence to support this hypothesis is described by Blomstrand and Newsholme (see chapter 15).

If there is imprecise control between the rate of mobilization of fatty acids and that of utilization in muscle and other tissues, the plasma concentration of fatty acids could increase markedly. Hence, the free tryptophan concentration may increase. It is suggested therefore that if the branch point sensitivity system is not very effective (see previous discussion), the blood fatty acid concentration could be increased to sufficiently high concentrations to markedly increase the plasma concentration of free tryptophan and lead to an increase in 5-HT levels in some parts of the brain. Furthermore, in intermittent exercise, in which there is usually a greater dependence on anaerobic exercise and, therefore, less opportunity to oxidize these fatty acids, the plasma concentrations of fatty acid and therefore free tryptophan could also reach high levels during the exercise. In addition, if a decrease in the malonyl CoA concentration plays a role in increasing fatty acid oxidation by muscle, it may minimize the increase in the plasma fatty acid level necessary to achieve satisfactory rates of oxidation. Hence, failure to lower the malonyl CoA concentration in muscle during exercise could lead to a greater increase in the plasma fatty acid level and hence contribute to central fatigue.

However, the system is more complex and certainly more interesting than this. Branched-chain amino acids (leucine, isoleucine, and valine) are not taken up by liver but by muscle, and their rate of uptake is increased during exercise. Both branched-chain amino acids and tryptophan enter the brain on the same amino acid carrier, so competition between the two types of amino acids for entry into brain can occur. In prolonged exercise it seems likely that muscle will use branched-chain amino acids for energy when the muscle glycogen is depleted, and at the same time the plasma level of free tryptophan will increase, as previously explained, so that the concentration ratio of free tryptophan to branched-chain amino acids will increase, resulting in fatigue (2, 3, 7).

Consequently, it is possible to test this hypothesis by investigating the effects of ingestion of a solution containing branched-chain amino acids sufficient to increase the plasma level of branched-chain amino acids so that the resting value of the ratio of the concentrations of free tryptophan to branched-chain amino acids is maintained during exercise. The results of a number of experiments of this nature are presented and discussed by Blomstrand and Newsholme (see chapter 15).

References

1. Bahr, R.; Hostmark, A.T.; Gronnerod, O.; Newsholme E.A.; Sejersted, O.M. Effect of exercise on recovery changes in plasma levels of FFA, glycerol, glucose and catecholamines. Acta Physiol. Scand. 143:105-115; 1991.
2. Blomstrand, E.; Hassmén, P.; Ekblom, B.; Newsholme, E.A. Administration of branched-chain amino acids during sustained exercise—Effects on physical and mental performance. Eur. J. Appl. Physiol. 63:83-88; 1991.
3. Blomstrand, E.; Hassmén, P.; Newsholme, E.A. Effect of branched-chain amino acid supplementation on mental performance. Acta Physiol. Scand. 143:225-226; 1991.

4. Garland, P.B.; Newsholme, E.A.; Randle, P.J. Regulation of glucose uptake. Biochem. J. 93:665-678; 1964.

5. Maughan, R.J.; Greenhaff, P.L.; Gleeson, M.; Fenn, C.E.; Leiper, J.B. The effect of dietary carbohydrate intake on the metabolic response to prolonged walking on consecutive days. Eur. J. Appl. Physiol. 56:583-591; 1987.

6. Newsholme, E.A., Crabtree, B. Substrate cycles in metabolic regulation and heat generation. Biochem. Soc. Symp. 41:61-110; 1976.

7. Newsholme, E.A.; Blomstrand, E.; Hassmén, P.; Ekblom, B. Physical and mental fatigue: Do changes in amino acids play a role? Biochem. Soc. Trans. 19:358-362; 1991.

8. Newsholme, E.A.; Leech, A.R. Biochemistry for the medical sciences. Chichester, England: John Wiley & Sons; 1983.

9. Newsholme, E.A.; Leech, A.R.; Duester, G. Keep on running: The science of training and performance. Chichester, England: John Wiley & Sons; 1994.

10. Newsholme, E.A.; Parry-Billings, M. Some evidence for the existence of substrate cycles and their utility in vivo. Biochem. J. 285:340-341; 1992.

11. Randle, P.J.; Garland, P.B.; Hales, C.N.; Newsholme, E.A. The glucose–fatty acid cycle: Its role in insulin sensitivity and metabolic disturbances of diabetes mellitus. Lancet 1:785-789; 1963.

12. Wolfe, R.R.; Herndon, D.; Jahoor, F.; Miyoshi, H.; Wolfe, M. Effect of severe burn injury on substrate cycling by glucose and fatty acids. N. Engl. J. Med. 317:403-408; 1987.

13. Wolfe, R.R.; Klein, S.; Carraro, F.; Weber, J.M. Role of triglyceride–fatty acid cycle in controlling fat metabolism in humans during and after exercise. Am. J. Physiol. 258:E382-E389; 1990.

14. Wolfe, R.R.; Peters, E.J. Lipolytic response to glucose infusion in human subjects. Am. J. Physiol. 252:E218-E223; 1987.

15. Wolfe, R.R.; Peters, E.J.; Klein, S.; Holland, O.B.; Rosenblott, J.I.; Gary, H. Effect of short-term fasting on lipolytic responsiveness in normal and obese subjects. Am. J. Physiol. 252:E189-E196; 1987.

CHAPTER 12

The Glucose–Fatty Acid Cycle in Skeletal Muscle at Rest and During Exercise

Lawrence L. Spriet, David J. Dyck

University of Guelph, Guelph, Ontario, Canada

Randle and co-workers originally introduced the concept of the glucose–fatty acid (G-FA) cycle to explain the interactions between carbohydrate (CHO) and fatty acid metabolism in muscle, adipose, and liver tissues. These tissue interactions were important for understanding the control of blood free fatty acid (FFA) and glucose concentrations (24, 49, 50). Their initial observations resulted from an interest in several abnormalities of CHO metabolism that were associated with high levels of FFA. The G-FA cycle spanned several tissues and described (1) the impairment of muscle glucose metabolism when the release of FFA from adipose tissue was increased and (2) the impairment of adipose tissue FFA release when blood glucose was elevated and muscle glucose uptake was increased.

The G-FA cycle described a hormone-independent mechanism whereby plasma glucose could be regulated at a constant level in animals that feed intermittently (49). The presence of insulin altered control of the cycle by enhancing muscle glucose uptake and inhibiting adipose tissue FFA release by increasing FFA reesterification to triglyceride (TG). Epinephrine, growth hormone, and the stress hormones accelerated adipose tissue FFA release, leading to a reduced muscle glucose uptake. Much of the support for the G-FA cycle was obtained by perfusing contracting heart muscle or bathing resting diaphragm muscle with high [FFA] and measuring alterations in glucose uptake; lactate and pyruvate efflux; and muscle glucose-6-phosphate (G6P), glucose, and glycogen contents.

The tissues involved in the cycle, other than blood, included adipose tissue, muscle, and to some extent the liver (FFA conversion to ketone bodies). The finding that increased exogenous FFA availability could limit muscle glucose metabolism suggested that metabolic regulators sensitive to increased fat oxidation were responsible for decreasing glucose metabolism. The theory proposed by Randle et al. (24, 49, 50) to explain the reciprocal relationship between fat and CHO metabolism in muscle is presented in schematic form in figure 12.1. Increases in the delivery of FFA to muscle enhanced FFA delivery to the mitochondria and β-oxidation, leading to an increase in muscle acetyl CoA and citrate contents. The increase in acetyl CoA was believed to inhibit the activity of pyruvate dehydrogenase (PDH) by activating PDH kinase, the enzyme responsible for phosphorylating PDH to its less

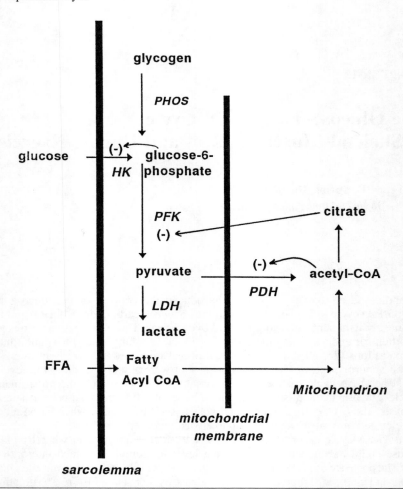

Figure 12.1   Schematic representation of the regulation of the classic glucose–fatty acid cycle in muscle. LDH = lactate dehydrogenase; PHOS = glycogen phosphorylase.

active state. The increase in mitochondrial citrate was believed to increase citrate transport into the cytoplasm, where it exerted an inhibitory effect on the regulatory glycolytic enzyme phosphofructokinase (PFK). The combined effect of decreased PDH and PFK activities increased the content of G6P, which in turn inhibited hexokinase (HK) activity and ultimately glucose uptake. This theory was supported by in vitro data demonstrating that acetyl CoA, citrate, and G6P were potent inhibitors of PDH, PFK, and HK, respectively (12, 25, 45, 46, 60).

The presence of a system in muscle that reduces the use of CHO when fat is available is very logical from a substrate storage point of view. The amount of CHO stored in the body is finite compared to fat stores. Without dietary replenishment, the CHO stores in the body are quickly depleted, and tissues that rely almost entirely on CHO for fuel are compromised. Therefore, many tissues of the body preferentially metabolize fat whenever it is available.

Over the past 30 years there has been controversy regarding the existence and regulation of the G-FA cycle in resting and exercising skeletal muscle. The questions that have been raised are as follows:

- Does the cycle exist at rest and at varying exercise intensities in skeletal muscle?
- If the cycle does exist, is the regulation between fat and CHO metabolism in skeletal muscles the same as classically proposed in heart muscle?

Certainly, one aspect that must not be overlooked when extrapolating from contracting heart muscle and resting diaphragm to skeletal muscle is that the former muscles have a duty cycle. Therefore, the majority of the substrate oxidized by these muscles must come from exogenous sources. In skeletal muscle other than diaphragm, the high demand for energy during many exercise situations dictates that a large proportion of the consumed fuel come from the endogenous glycogen store. During exercise, an increase in fat oxidation would need to be communicated not only to the PFK and PDH enzymes in the glycolytic pathway, but also to glycogen phosphorylase (PHOS), the enzyme responsible for glycogen degradation. The purpose of this chapter is to briefly review the existing information regarding the existence and regulation of the G-FA cycle in skeletal muscle. The review is not exhaustive but highlights recent work that examines the regulation of fat-CHO interaction in resting and exercising human skeletal muscle.

In Vitro Experiments

In vitro experiments with purified enzymes and muscle extracts have contributed greatly to understanding the communication between fat and CHO metabolism in resting and contracting muscle. Classic experiments demonstrated that the putative regulators of the G-FA cycle were capable of down-regulating the key glycolytic enzymes. Increases in acetyl CoA and in the acetyl CoA/CoA ratio activate PDH kinase, which phosphorylates PDH to its less active form (12, 45). High levels of citrate exert a powerful inhibition on PFK activity in heart (25) and skeletal muscle (39, 60), and HK is inhibited by high [G6P] (46).

Most of the classic in vitro studies were performed with some combination of nonphysiological concentrations of enzyme, substrates, and regulators. More recent studies have recognized the importance of enzyme concentration with respect to PFK regulation (8, 64). When PFK regulatory properties were examined at a physiological concentration of PFK in the test tube, ATP inhibition was relieved, and the potent stimulatory effect of fructose 2,6-bisphosphate was removed (8). Similar results were obtained when the enzyme was "crowded" with a 10% polyethylene glycol (PEG) solution (8). Increasing the enzyme concentration or crowding the enzyme enhances the formation of higher aggregates of the enzyme subunits, which more closely matches the in vivo state (2, 8). Even studies using dilute enzyme preparations but more physiological concentrations of substrates and effectors have demonstrated less potent effects of inhibitors such as H^+, citrate, and the bisphosphorylated hexoses (1, 14).

The regulatory properties of additional glycolytic enzymes such as PHOS, HK, and PDH appear less affected when assayed in dilute enzyme concentrations. Given the importance of examining PFK in conditions simulating the enzyme aggregation state in the cell and the important role that citrate inhibition of PFK is reported to play in the communication between fat and CHO oxidation, the in vitro potency of citrate on PFK was recently reexamined.

The regulatory properties of PFK were examined in vitro using the crowding agent PEG as described by Bosca, Aragon, and Sols (8). Physiological concentrations of effectors and substrates were added to approximate the conditions of rest, moderate aerobic exercise (40-65% maximal O_2 uptake [$\dot{V}O_2$max]), and intense aerobic exercise (75-85% $\dot{V}O_2$max), based upon measurements appearing in the literature. The potency of citrate inhibition on rabbit skeletal muscle PFK activity was examined over the physiological range of rest and exercise muscle citrate concentrations (0-0.5 mM).

Absolute PFK activities in the simulated conditions increased from rest to moderate exercise to intense exercise as expected from the higher concentrations of positive effectors (44). When the results were expressed as a percentage of maximal activity in each condition, the most powerful citrate inhibition occurred at rest (figure 12.2). At normal resting citrate concentrations (0.10-0.15 mM), PFK activity was already decreased to 50% of maximum. Increasing the citrate concentration further to 0.5 mM had little additional inhibitory effect, as 43% of maximal activity remained (figure 12.2). The two simulated exercise conditions were less affected by citrate (44). At normal exercise citrate concentrations (0.20-0.30 mM), 65% to 70% of maximal PFK activity remained, and further increases to 0.5 mM only decreased activity to 55% of maximum (figure 12.2). Therefore, at rest the most powerful inhibition of PFK by citrate is already present at normal resting citrate concentrations in the muscle cell. During exercise, less citrate

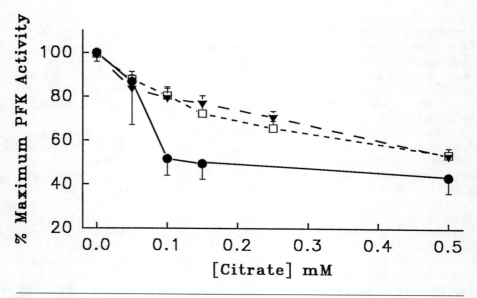

Figure 12.2   Citrate inhibition of phosphofructokinase activity with enhanced enzyme aggregation in rest (circles), moderate aerobic exercise (triangles), and intense aerobic exercise conditions (squares).

inhibition of PFK is present at normal exercise citrate concentrations compared with rest. Additional increases that may occur through experimental increases in fat availability are not expected to significantly increase citrate inhibition of PFK at rest or exercise. In conclusion, these in vitro data suggest that earlier in vitro work overestimated the potency of citrate to inhibit PFK activity during exercise. Presumably, the presence of positive regulators in significant concentrations overrides the inhibitory effect of citrate during exercise.

The Glucose–Fatty Acid Cycle in Intact Preparations

In vitro experiments are valuable for demonstrating which regulators may be important in the communication between fat and CHO oxidation in the muscle cell. However, experiments with in situ or in vivo preparations are required to confirm whether the G-FA cycle exists in skeletal muscle and to identify which regulators are important in the regulation of fat-CHO interaction. The majority of the work examining the G-FA cycle has attempted to increase the delivery of FFA to the muscle and to determine whether fat oxidation is increased and whether muscle glycogenolysis or muscle glucose uptake and oxidation are decreased. Measurements of the putative regulators of fat-CHO interaction would also determine whether communication is as classically proposed.

Animal Models: Rest Studies

Since the original studies by Randle et al. (24, 25, 49, 50), there has been controversy regarding the existence of the G-FA cycle in skeletal muscle other than diaphragm. The majority of the studies that have examined the G-FA cycle in resting and exercising skeletal muscle have employed either acute and chronic fat diets, fasting, or perfusion-incubation with elevated FFA in an attempt to enhance the uptake and subsequent oxidation of FFA. The opposite approach has also been used where nicotinic acid (NA) or acipimox ingestion inhibits FFA release from adipose tissue and decreases FFA delivery to skeletal muscle.

Hickson et al. (29) and Rennie, Winder, and Holloszy (53) fed rats corn oil via a stomach tube prior to exercise followed by heparin infusion to release lipoprotein lipase (LPL), to hydrolyze circulating TG, and to acutely elevate plasma [FFA]. Sampling of resting muscle prior to exercise demonstrated a significant elevation of citrate in red gastrocnemius (RG) muscles in both studies and in soleus (SOL) in one study (16) following elevation of plasma FFA. No measurements of glucose and FFA uptake or lactate release were made in these studies. Jenkins et al. (36) acutely raised plasma FFA in anaesthetized rats to 2 mM by Intralipid-heparin infusion, resulting in a 36% suppression in glucose utilization under basal insulin conditions. No muscle metabolite measurements were made in this study. A 24% suppression of glucose oxidation (3) and a 30% reduction in peripheral glucose utilization (57) were also reported in resting dogs following Intralipid-heparin administration.

Relatively few fasting studies have used animal models, and the results are more controversial. Zorzano et al. (66) found no evidence of classic regulation of the

G-FA cycle because rat SOL citrate content was not elevated following a 48-h fast. Paul, Issekutz, and Miller (43) elevated plasma FFA from approximately 0.3 to 1.8 mM in dogs by varying the length of fast from 18 to 72 h. Elevations in FFA increased the oxidation of [^{14}C]palmitate and decreased the respiratory exchange ratio (RER), supporting the existence of the G-FA cycle. However, administration of NA to pancreatectomized dogs depressed FFA release and oxidation but failed to elevate glucose oxidation in the absence of insulin (43). A recent study also examined the G-FA cycle from the perspective of reducing FFA availability. Jenkins et al. (37) treated conscious rats with the β-oxidation blocker methyl palmoxirate and reported no stimulation of 2-deoxy-[^{3}H]glucose uptake or PDH activation in skeletal muscle, regardless of the state of insulinemia.

Several studies have used the perfused rat hindlimb to examine fat-CHO interaction in resting skeletal muscle. PDH activity in unspecified hindlimb muscle was reduced following perfusion with approximately 2 mM acetoacetate (5, 27). Berger et al. (5) also reported a threefold elevation of muscle acetyl CoA content. However, the same authors were unable to demonstrate a reduction in hindlimb glucose uptake or lactate release when perfused with palmitate, octanoate, or acetoacetate. Additional studies have demonstrated increased muscle citrate (18, 54) and acetyl CoA (58) contents in oxidative fibers when perfused with elevated FFA at rest but no changes in hindlimb glucose uptake and lactate release (18). Only Rennie and Holloszy (52) were able to demonstrate an increase in the G6P content in oxidative fibers and reductions in resting hindlimb glucose uptake and lactate release with high-fat perfusion. In addition to the intact animal models, several studies have used isolated muscle preparations to study the G-FA cycle. Although the normal blood and nervous supply to these muscles has been disturbed, valuable information has been obtained from these in vitro studies using viable muscle preparations with intact metabolism.

Grundleger and Thenen (26) observed a reduced rate of glucose oxidation, estimated by incorporation of ^{14}C from [^{14}C]glucose into CO_2, in isolated SOL muscles from rats on a high-fat diet for 10 d. However, two additional studies using isolated muscle preparations have added controversy to the existence of the G-FA cycle in skeletal muscle. Beatty and Bocek (4) incubated isolated sartorius fibers from the rhesus monkey with 1.45 mM palmitate, and Jefferson, Koehler, and Morgan (35) perfused rat diaphragm with the same FFA concentration; both studies found no reduction in muscle glucose uptake.

It is clear from the preceding studies that the existence of the G-FA cycle in resting skeletal muscle remains controversial in animal models. However, this research has been dominated by extensive use of the rat, and it is possible that other species may provide more consistent results. In addition, manipulations such as prolonged fasting and chronic high-fat diets have the disadvantage of altering circulating hormone and tissue substrate levels, such as liver and muscle glycogen. Finally, more extensive assessments of the mechanisms of intramuscular selection of oxidizable fuels are needed. The measurements required include muscle citrate, G6P, acetyl CoA, lactate, and pyruvate contents and PDH activity, coupled with accurate metabolic tracer assessments of muscle lipid and CHO oxidation.

Animal Models: Exercise Studies

Holloszy and colleagues examined the existence and regulation of the G-FA cycle in skeletal muscle of exercising rats. Animals were fed corn oil followed by infusions of heparin to increase preexercise [FFA] to approximately 1 mM vs. 0.2 mM in a control group (29, 53). Fat-fed rats ran longer (181 vs. 118 min); used less glycogen in the SOL, red vastus lateralis (RVL), RG, and liver; and experienced a smaller decrease in blood glucose during exercise than the control animals. In all cases, citrate contents were elevated during exercise in the muscles exposed to high fat. Other studies reported decreased muscle glycogen use during exercise following 24 to 48 h of fasting in rats (41, 66). Fasting increased the FFA and ketone concentrations, leading the authors to conclude that increased fat-ketone oxidation during exercise caused the decrease in CHO use. However, there were few measurements to substantiate the conclusions, because only Zorzano et al. (66) reported an increase in SOL citrate content following exercise in fasted compared with fed groups.

Fasting studies and, to a lesser extent, acute fat feeding studies (3-4 h) cause alterations in hormonal status prior to exercise, and fasting also decreases muscle glycogen content prior to exercise. Both in vivo models also suffer from a limited ability to sample arterial and venous blood and an inability to quickly sample muscle tissue following exercise. For these reasons, investigators have employed in situ perfusion models to study the existence and regulation of the G-FA cycle. The isolated, perfused rat hindlimb model provides tight control of inflowing substrate and hormone concentrations and facilitates the sampling of arterial and venous blood and muscle tissue during exercise.

The exercise perfusion studies in this area have been dominated by the work of Rennie and Holloszy (52), which provided the strongest evidence for the existence of the G-FA cycle in red skeletal muscle. They perfused rat hindlimbs with a mixture of rejuvenated human red blood cells (RBCs) and Krebs-Henseleit solution containing either 1.8 mM oleate or no fat. Hindlimb glucose uptake and lactate release were decreased with high-fat perfusion during 10 min of electrical stimulation. Muscle glycogen utilization was reduced by 33% to 50% and lactate accumulation by 50% in the SOL and RG muscles perfused with high fat. The reduction in muscle CHO use coincided with elevations in G6P (30%) and citrate (33-57%) contents in SOL and RG muscles. Their results suggested that the G-FA cycle did operate in contracting red skeletal muscle and that the cycle was regulated as originally proposed for contracting heart and resting diaphragm muscles.

Additional perfusion studies have not been able to demonstrate the existence of the G-FA cycle in contracting red skeletal muscle (5, 16, 18, 30, 54). Perfusions with 1.3 mM palmitate, 1 mM octanoate, and 1.8 mM acetoacetate during stimulation did not significantly alter hindlimb glucose uptake, lactate release, or citrate content in samples of unidentified hindlimb muscle (5, 30). Rennie and Holloszy (52) suggested that the findings of these earlier studies were due to inadequate oxygenation of the perfused, contracting muscles. They demonstrated that perfusion of the contracting hindlimb with aged human RBCs resulted in low O_2 uptakes and did not reduce hindlimb glucose uptake or lactate release in the presence of 1.8 mM oleate. Their findings of CHO sparing with high fat were dependent on perfusions that maintained well-oxygenated muscle during stimulation.

However, more recent studies using well-oxygenated, perfused hindlimb preparations have failed to confirm the findings of Rennie and Holloszy (52). Richter et al. (54) reported no effect of perfusion with 1.6 mM palmitate on hindlimb glucose uptake or glycogen breakdown in SOL, RG, and white gastrocnemius (WG) muscles during 20 min of stimulation (180 twin pulses/min). Muscle citrate contents were also unaffected by high-fat perfusion during stimulation. Dyck and Spriet (18) were also unable to demonstrate decreased hindlimb glucose uptake or lactate release during perfusions with 1 mM oleate during 5 min of tetanic stimulation. Muscle glycogen was also not spared in the contracting SOL, RG, or WG muscles during the high-fat compared with fat-free perfusions. During exercise, muscle citrate decreased in all muscles in both conditions (except SOL with high fat) but remained higher in the SOL and RG muscles at 1 and 5 min of stimulation with high fat (figures 12.3 and 12.4). Acetyl CoA contents were not different in the high-fat and fat-free groups in either muscle after 1 and 5 min of stimulation (58; figures 12.3 and 12.4).

A more recent attempt has been made to identify a stimulation paradigm in which perfusion with high fat would produce a sparing of glycogen in muscles containing aerobic fibers (16). A series of stimulation intensities (0.4-4 Hz) that produced a wide range of hindlimb O_2 uptakes and glycogenolytic rates in the SOL, RG, and plantaris (PL) muscles were examined. The results for the RG muscle demonstrate that high-fat (1.5-1.9 mM FFA) perfusions did not produce glycogen sparing across most stimulation intensities (figure 12.5). Muscle glycogen use was significantly reduced only at a stimulation frequency of 0.7 Hz. In the SOL, high-fat perfusion had no effect on glycogen, except at one stimulation intensity (0.4 Hz), and in the PL, a significant reduction was found only at 1 Hz.

In conclusion, it seems clear that the perfused rat hindlimb model is not well suited for demonstrating the existence of the G-FA cycle during exercise. This makes it a poor model to study the regulation of fat and CHO interaction during exercise. However, it appears that the cycle does exist at certain stimulation intensities in the oxidative muscles, and these could be used to examine the regulation. It must also be noted that no investigators have attempted to exactly mimic the experimental conditions used by Rennie and Holloszy (52). The most important aspect of repeating their work may be to mimic the stimulation paradigm they employed, in which muscles were stimulated with 100-ms trains of stimuli (100 Hz) delivered at a rate of 0.5 Hz every 2 s. The voltage delivered with each stimulus was approximately 0.5 V and was varied to produce approximately 1,000 g of tension by the gastrocnemius-PL-SOL muscle group in each preparation.

Human Models: Rest Studies

Does the G-FA Cycle Exist in Resting Human Skeletal Muscle?

The existing literature strongly suggests that the G-FA cycle exists in resting human skeletal muscle. Several models have been employed to examine the cycle from the perspective of elevating circulating FFA levels, including Intralipid-heparin infusion, fasting, and high-fat diets. Acetate infusion has also recently been employed to acutely elevate muscle acetyl CoA content. The consequences of impaired fat mobilization (acipimox) on CHO metabolism and the effects of enhancing CHO availability on FFA metabolism have also been examined.

Infusion of Intralipid and low-dose heparin is an effective means of acutely elevating circulating FFA without disturbing plasma hormone and blood glucose levels or liver and muscle glycogen stores. In one study (23), Intralipid infusion caused a significant inhibition of whole-body glucose uptake determined by constant

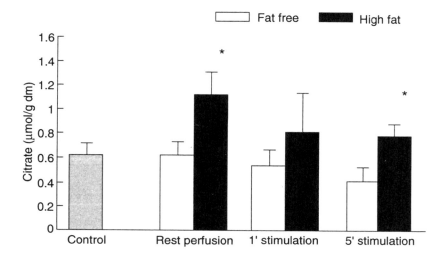

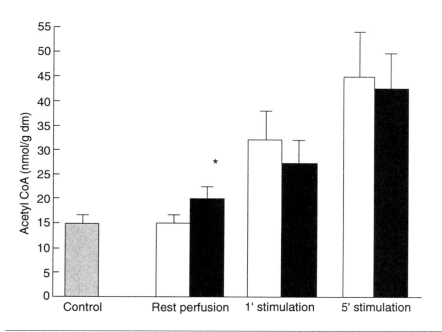

Figure 12.3   Red gastrocnemius citrate and acetyl CoA dry muscle contents during fat-free and high-fat perfusions at rest and during electrical stimulation. * = significantly different from fat free.

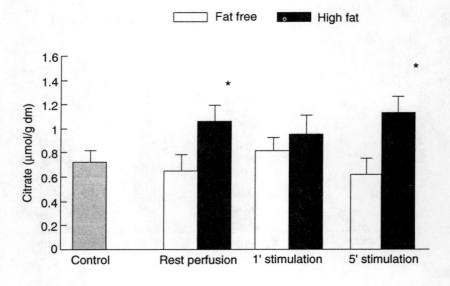

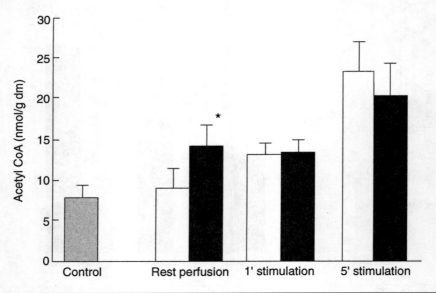

Figure 12.4 Soleus citrate and acetyl CoA dry muscle contents during fat-free and high-fat perfusions at rest and during electrical stimulation. * = significantly different from fat free.

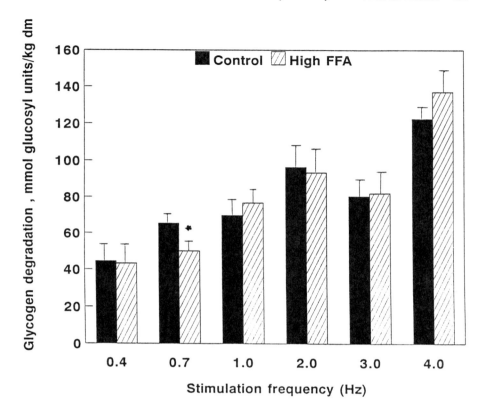

Figure 12.5   Glycogen degradation in the gastrocnemius muscles during varying twitch-stimulation frequencies for 20 min while perfused with control (fat-free) and high-fat blood. * = significantly different from control.

infusion of [3-^{2}H]glucose in the presence of either eu- or hyperglycemia and hyperinsulinemia, but not under conditions simulating the diabetic state (high glucose and glucagon and low insulin levels). Additional studies have reported 20% to 60% reductions in glucose oxidation following Intralipid infusion (7, 56). It should be stressed that these studies assessed whole-body glucose oxidation or disposal and therefore may not reflect changes in skeletal muscle. However, two studies measured glucose uptake and oxidation across specific muscle groups using arterial and venous catheterization. Intralipid infusion at rest produced decreases in leg muscle glucose uptake (38) and glucose oxidation by the forearm (62). Therefore, although there is a paucity of information regarding muscle glucose uptake and oxidation changes following manipulation of plasma FFA, that which does exist provides strong support for the existence of the G-FA cycle in resting human muscle.

Fasting has also been used to examine the G-FA cycle in resting human muscle. Subjects fasting for 3.5 d exhibited elevated FFA and decreased whole-body glucose flux ([6,6-^{2}H]glucose infusion) and CHO oxidation (RER) compared with an overnight-fast control (40).

Two recent studies examined the G-FA cycle from the perspective of enhancing the availability of CHO. The lipolytic or FFA turnover rates were measured during either a eu- or hyperglycemic clamp. Hyperglycemia failed to decrease the lipolytic rate in one study (10) but decreased lipolysis and FFA turnover by 30% in the other (9). Demonstration of a reduction in FFA oxidation subsequent to enhanced CHO availability had also been demonstrated earlier (63). However, it is difficult based on these studies to assess whether the reduction in lipolysis is actually due to hyperglycemia or to the hormonal alterations attendant with the simulated diabetes state. Using the opposite perspective, Faneill et al. (22) tested the hypothesis that FFA may mediate some of the changes in glucose metabolism that occur during counterregulation of hypoglycemia. Subjects were infused with insulin for 8 h to produce a modest state of hypoglycemia ($\approx$ 3 mM) either with or without acipimox. FFA levels decreased from 0.7 to less than 0.1 mM with acipimox, resulting in enhanced overall glucose production (40%), gluconeogenesis from alanine (70%), and glucose utilization (15%).

In summary, the evidence for the existence of the G-FA cycle in resting humans is very strong. However, most of the measurements of glucose oxidation or disposal following FFA manipulation are whole body. It is clear that additional studies need to assess actual muscle uptake and oxidation of glucose with increased or decreased fat availability to confirm the existence of the G-FA cycle at rest.

Is the G-FA Cycle in Resting Human Skeletal Muscle Regulated as Classically Proposed?

Despite the strong overall support for the existence of the G-FA cycle in resting human muscle, there is conflicting information regarding the mechanisms by which the regulation of fat-CHO interaction occurs in muscle. During infusion of Intralipid at rest, Boden et al. (7) measured an increased muscle acetyl CoA/CoA ratio. This is consistent with an inhibition of PDH activity, although it was not measured. However, other studies have reported no change in muscle acetyl CoA content (17) and either no change (17, 56) or a decreased PDH activity (38) during Intralipid infusion at rest. To add to the confusion, muscle G6P and citrate were either unchanged (7) or increased (15, 17) with Intralipid infusion at rest.

A recent study by Putman et al. (47) infused subjects with sodium acetate in an attempt to produce acute increases in muscle acetyl CoA and citrate independent of FFA metabolism. Muscle acetyl CoA content was increased twofold at rest, producing a 55% decrease in the maximal activity of the active form of PDH (PDHa). Muscle citrate was also increased twofold at rest, but G6P was unaffected.

Intralipid and acetate infusion are models in which plasma FFA and muscle acetyl CoA can be acutely increased with minimal disturbances of substrate or hormone levels. However, other models have also examined regulation of the G-FA cycle in resting muscle. Maughan and Williams (42) were unable to detect any changes in vastus lateralis citrate or G6P contents in subjects fasted for 24 h. In contrast, resting muscle citrate and G6P were elevated following 5 d on a high-fat diet, compared to a high-CHO diet (33). Following 3 d on a high-fat diet, Putman et al. (48) measured an elevated muscle acetyl CoA/CoA ratio and a 71% decrease in PDH activation at rest compared with a high-CHO diet. Muscle citrate was increased by 40% following the high-fat diet, but not significantly. Increases in resting muscle citrate and acetyl CoA have also been demonstrated within 1 h following the ingestion of caffeine (59). Last, endurance training has also been used as a model to study the regulation of fat-CHO interaction, and the results are contradictory. In one study, muscle citrate was twofold higher and G6P was significantly lower in a group of well-trained cyclists compared with a group of untrained controls (34). In a second study, resting muscle citrate and G6P contents were unaffected by 12 wk of aerobic training (11).

In conclusion, the literature generally supports the classical proposal that enhanced FFA delivery increases muscle acetyl CoA at rest and inhibits PDH activity. However, the measurements of muscle citrate and G6P are inconsistent and often do not increase when FFA availability is increased at rest. This leaves the significance of citrate-PFK and G6P-HK regulatory mechanisms unresolved in resting human skeletal muscle.

Human Models: Exercise Studies

Does the G-FA Cycle Exist in Human Skeletal Muscle During Exercise?

Numerous approaches have been employed to study the existence of the G-FA cycle in human skeletal muscle during exercise. Most have attempted to elevate plasma FFA and delivery to the working muscles during exercise and to examine whether muscle glucose uptake or glycogen utilization is reduced. The majority of studies that have examined the effects of increasing the availability of exogenous FFA to exercising skeletal muscle in humans have concluded that muscle CHO use is reduced (table 12.1). The strongest evidence comes from the studies in which Intralipid (20% TG solution) is infused or a high-fat meal is ingested, coupled with low-dose injections of heparin. All studies using the acute fat-feeding or infusion approach during moderate to intense whole-body aerobic exercise have reported significant decreases in muscle glycogen use (table 12.1). In these studies, subjects exercised (cycling and running) at 70% to 90% $\dot{V}O_2$max for 15 to 60 min and reported 15% to 44% reductions in muscle glycogen utilization as compared with a low-fat control trial (13, 17, 55, 61).

However, one study with low-intensity exercise and another with one-leg knee extension exercise reported no decrease in CHO or muscle glycogenolysis following Intralipid-heparin infusion (table 12.1). Ravussin et al. (51) reported only indirect information (RER), which was unchanged during 150 min of cycling at 44% $\dot{V}O_2$max during Intralipid infusion. Hargreaves, Kiens, and Richter (28) reported no difference in muscle glycogen use during 60 min of one-leg knee extension exercise but did find a significant reduction in muscle glucose uptake. It is interesting to note that these studies had higher [FFA] in the control trial (0.54-0.78 mM) than the studies using more intense whole-body exercise (0.20-0.30 mM; table 12.1). It is possible that FFA delivery to the working muscles was already high in the control trials of these two studies and that further increases in plasma [FFA] could not enhance muscle FFA uptake. This is supported by similar leg FFA uptake rates in the control and Intralipid conditions of the Hargreaves, Kiens, and Richter study (28).

Other models have also provided support for a reciprocal relationship between fat and CHO use in exercising human skeletal muscle (table 12.1). Acute NA

Table 12.1   Summary of Studies Examining the Existence of the G-FA Cycle in Human Skeletal Muscle During Exercise

Authors	[FFA], mM	Subjects, Training status	Intensity (%VO₂max), Duration	Modality	RER	Glycogen use	Glucose uptake	FAT use
Intralipid-heparin infusion								
Ravussin et al. 1986 (51)	1.12 vs 0.78	10 M RA	44% 150 min	Cycling	NC	—	—	—
Hargreaves et al. 1991 (28)	1.12 vs. 0.54	11 M varied	80% leg 60 min	Knee extension	NC	NC	↓33%	NC
Vukovich et al. 1993 (61)	1.25 vs. 0.30	5 M ?	70% 60 min	Cycling	→	↓28%	—	—
Dyck et al. 1993 (17)	1.00 vs. 0.20	6 M varied	85-90% 15 min	Cycling	—	↓44%	—	—
Romijn et al. 1995 (55)	1-2 vs. 0.30	6 M WT	85% 30 min	Cycling	→	↓15% (calc)	NC	↓27% (20-30 min)
Acute fat feeding/heparin infusion								
Costill et al. 1977 (13)	1.0 vs. 0.20	7 M 6 WT, 1 UT	70% 30 min	Running	→	↓40%	—	—
Vukovich et al. 1993 (61)	1.5-2.0 vs. 0.30	5 M ?	70% 60 min	Cycling	→	↓28%	—	—

Chronic fat feeding (3-5 d)

Study		Subjects	Intensity/Duration	Mode		Change		FFA
Jansson & Kaijser 1982b (32)	0.8-1.0 vs. 0.4-0.6	11 F, 9 M	65% 25 min	Cycling	→	↓22% NS, $n = 15$	NC	↑leg FFA extract.
Jansson & Kaijser 1982a (31)	0.70 vs. 0.30	3 F, 4 M ?	65% 6 min	Cycling	→	↓57% NS, $n = 6$	NC	—
Putman et al. 1993 (48)	0.5-1.25 vs. 0.35	5 M T	75% 50 min	Cycling	→	↓30%, 0-15 min ↓84%, 15-50 min	NC, a-v diff.	—

Nicotinic acid feeding

Bergström et al. 1969 (6)	0.30 vs. 0.81	15 M RA	approx. 35% 90 min	Cycling	—	↓20-34%	—	—

Starvation

Knapik et al. 1988 (40)	0.5-1.0 vs. 0.3-0.9	8M	45%	Cycling	→	↓43%	—	—

Caffeine ingestion

Essig et al. 1980 (21)	0.70 vs. 0.43	7 M RA	70% 30 min	Cycling	→	↓42%	—	↑150%
Erickson et al. 1987 (19)	0.45 vs. 0.45	1 F, 4 M WT	68% 90 min	Cycling	NC	↓31%	—	—
Spriet et al. 1992 (59)	0.46 vs. 0.24	1 F, 7 M RA	80% 75-90 min	Cycling	—	↓55%, 0-15 min	—	—

All measurements represent experimental values compared with control values (e.g., Intralipid infusion vs. control). FFA, free fatty acid. RER, respiratory exchange ratio. Subjects: M, male; F, female. Training status: UT, untrained; T, trained; WT, well trained; RA, recreationally active; varied, varied training status; ?, training status not reported. NC, no significant difference between high fat and control data. NS, not significant. —, no determination. a-v, arteriovenous.

administration decreased plasma [FFA] and increased muscle glycogen utilization by 20% to 34% during 60 to 90 min of cycling at approximately 35% $\dot{V}O_2$max (6). Chronic ingestion of high-fat, low-CHO diets for 3 to 5 d prior to exercise results in higher plasma [FFA] and less muscle glycogen use during 25 to 50 min of cycling at 65% to 75% $\dot{V}O_2$max (31, 32, 48), although muscle glucose uptake was unchanged. Fasting for 3.5 d as compared with an overnight fast (14 h) produced higher plasma [FFA], decreased RER, reduced muscle glycogen use, and decreased glucose uptake during 120 min of cycling at 45% $\dot{V}O_2$max (40). Several studies have also reported muscle glycogen sparing during exercise following caffeine ingestion (19, 21, 59). The prevailing theory to explain the glycogen-sparing effect of caffeine involves increased fat mobilization from adipose tissue. Caffeine ingestion produces a twofold increase in exercise epinephrine concentration, which is believed to increase adipose tissue FFA release, plasma [FFA], and FFA delivery to working muscle. Increased muscle fat oxidation would then decrease flux in the glycolytic pathway via the classic citrate-PFK, acetyl CoA–PDH explanation.

Aerobic training and chronic high-altitude exposure could be added to the list of models that examine the interaction of fat and CHO use. Exercise at the same absolute power output following training uses less muscle glycogen and exogenous glucose than before training, in spite of unchanged or lower FFA delivery to the muscles (11, 34). Therefore the turnover of exogenous FFA or the use of intramuscular TG must be higher during exercise in the trained state. Muscle glycogenolysis is also decreased during intense aerobic exercise (80-85% $\dot{V}O_2$max) following 18 d at 4,300 m as compared with acute altitude exposure (65). The explanation for the reduced muscle CHO use was increased mobilization of fat from adipose tissue and increased muscle FFA oxidation following altitude exposure.

In summary, there is strong evidence that the G-FA cycle exists in human skeletal muscle during exercise. The best evidence comes from studies that acutely increase FFA delivery to the working muscle and that demonstrate reductions in muscle glycogen use during whole-body exercise at 65% to 90% $\dot{V}O_2$max. There have not been enough studies to accurately conclude whether increased fat availability during exercise reduces muscle glucose uptake.

Is the G-FA Cycle in Exercising Human Skeletal Muscle Regulated as Classically Proposed?

Few attempts have been made to study the regulation of fat and CHO interaction in contracting human skeletal muscle in situations where the G-FA cycle has been demonstrated. It is often stated that increases in fat oxidation and decreases in CHO oxidation are mediated through increases in muscle citrate and decreased PFK activity, but supporting evidence is lacking. Ideally, it would be desirable to measure muscle citrate, acetyl CoA, and G6P contents and the maximal activities of the active forms of PHOS and PDH enzymes during exercise situations with increased fat availability and decreased CHO use. An increase in these muscle metabolites and a decrease in the active form of the enzymes during exercise with elevated fat availability would provide support for the classical explanation of the regulation of fat-CHO interaction.

The first work on the regulation of the G-FA cycle in human skeletal muscle was published by Jansson and Kaijser (31-33). They examined subjects who exercised for

25 min at 65% $\dot{V}O_2$max following 5 d on a high-CHO diet and again after 5 d on a high-fat diet. Less glycogen was used after the high-fat diet, although the changes were not significant (table 12.2). At 6 min into the exercise following the high-fat diet, muscle citrate was significantly elevated above the high-CHO diet content, while G6P was unaffected. Estimated leg citrate release was higher after the high-fat diet but not significantly different. The authors concluded that inhibition of glycolysis may have been due to citrate inhibition of PFK after 6 min of exercise, but not after 25 min. Putman et al. (48) reported a more complete series of regulatory measurements during cycling at 75% $\dot{V}O_2$max following 3 d of a high-CHO or high-fat diet. Subjects exhausted at 47 min following the high-fat diet and were biopsied at the same time in the high-CHO trial. After 15 and 47 min of exercise, muscle G6P, acetyl CoA, and PDHa were lower in the high-fat trial, while citrate was unaffected. Muscle glycogen use was considerably lower in the 0- to 15-min and the 15- to 47-min time periods in the high-fat trial (table 12.2). The results suggest that muscle fat oxidation and flux through the glycolytic pathway are unrelated to citrate content during exercise following diet manipulations. In addition, muscle acetyl CoA appeared to have no regulatory effect on PDH during exercise. If acetyl CoA is an inhibitor of PDH activation, then the lower acetyl CoA in the high-fat trial should have permitted greater activation of PDH, contrary to what was found. These studies suggest that the G-FA cycle does not appear to be regulated as classically proposed at all time points during exercise. However, chronic fat feeding has been criticized as a model for studying regulation of the G-FA cycle, because changes in substrate and hormone levels accompany the increases in [FFA] and FFA delivery to exercising muscle. The hormonal and substrate alterations with fat feeding may confound the conclusions of these studies. For example, the most critical change with the 3- to 5-d high-fat diet may be the decrease in muscle glycogen content prior to the onset of exercise. Therefore, reductions in glycolytic flux during moderate to intense aerobic exercise following the high-fat diet are more likely due to decreased substrate supply than down-regulation due to increases in fat oxidation and subsequent increases in muscle citrate and acetyl CoA.

Spriet et al. (59) measured muscle citrate, acetyl CoA, and free CoASH during exercise to exhaustion at 80% $\dot{V}O_2$max following placebo and caffeine ingestion. Muscle glycogen use was reduced by 55% from 0 to 15 min of exercise, but muscle citrate and acetyl CoA contents and the acetyl CoA/CoASH ratio at 15 min were unaffected by caffeine ingestion (table 12.2). The findings suggested that acetyl CoA and citrate were not involved in the decreased glycogen utilization with caffeine and that additional signals between fat and CHO utilization exist. However, it is difficult to prove that exogenous FFA utilization by muscle is augmented following caffeine ingestion and is the actual cause of the reduced muscle glycogen utilization. Direct measurements of increased exogenous FFA oxidation following caffeine ingestion have not been made. Caffeine may exert additional effects on the muscle that account for the glycogen sparing.

Jansson and Kaijser (34) compared the metabolic response of well-trained cyclists to untrained subjects during 60 min of cycling at approximately 65% to 70% $\dot{V}O_2$max. Muscle citrate was higher and G6P was lower in the trained cyclists at 15 and 60 min of exercise (table 12.2). Muscle glycogen use was considerably lower in the trained group (157 vs. 284 mmol/kg dry muscle [d.m.]). Coggan et al. (11) performed a similar study in which a group of untrained subjects exercised for 2 h at approximately 60% $\dot{V}O_2$max before and after 12 wk of endurance training. They found no effect on muscle citrate and lower G6P

Table 12.2   Summary of Studies Examining the Regulation of the G-FA Cycle in Human Skeletal Muscle During Exercise

Authors	Sampling time (min)	[G6P]	[Citrate]	[Acetyl CoA]	Leg citrate release	PDHa	PHOSa
Chronic high-fat diet (3-5 d)							
Jansson & Kaijser 1984 (33)	6	NC	↑	—	↑, NS	—	—
	25	↑	NC	—	NC	—	—
Putman et al. 1993 (48)	15	→	NC	→	—	→	—
	47	→	NC	→	—	→	—
Caffeine							
Spriet et al. 1992 (59)	15	—	NC	NC	—	—	—
	75	—	NC	NC	—	—	—
Aerobic training							
Jansson & Kaijser 1984 (34)	15	→	↑	—	—	—	—
	60	NC	↑	—	—	—	—
Coggan et al. 1993 (11)	120	→	NC	—	—	—	—
Intralipid-heparin infusion							
Dyck et al. 1993 (17)	3	—	NC	NC	—	NC	—
	15	—	NC	NC	—	NC	—
Dyck et al. 1995 (15)	1	NC	NC	NC	—	NC	NC
	5	NC	NC	NC	—	NC	NC
	15	NC	NC	NC	—	NC	NC

All measurements represent high-fat values compared with control values (e.g., Intralipid infusion vs. control). PDHa and PHOSa, maximal activities of the active form of the enzyme. NC, no significant difference between high-fat and control data. NS, not statistically significant.

contents following training when muscle was sampled after 2 h of cycling. Therefore, both studies suggest that G6P levels are unrelated to shifts in substrate use, but the conclusions are conflicting regarding the importance of citrate for lower CHO use following training. The much higher resting and exercise citrate levels in the trained cyclists may have been due to a higher proportion of type I fibers (70% vs. 40% in untrained subjects), because Essen (20) reported higher citrate contents in type I vs. type II fibers. In addition, the usefulness of the training model to study regulation of the G-FA cycle is limited by differing muscle glycogen and hormonal levels following training. Preexercise muscle glycogen levels in the untrained and trained groups were approximately 330 and 570 mmol/kg d.m. (34) and 360 and 440 mmol/kg d.m. (11) in the previous two studies. It is therefore difficult to conclude that reductions in muscle CHO use following training were strictly a function of elevated fat provision to the working muscle and of communication between increasing fat and decreasing CHO oxidation.

Dyck et al. (17) recently examined the regulation of the G-FA cycle in human skeletal muscle during 15 min of intense aerobic exercise in control and high–plasma FFA conditions. The authors used an acute Intralipid-heparin infusion to increase exercise plasma [FFA] to between 1.0 and 1.4 mM versus 0.2 and 0.3 mM in the control trial (figure 12.6). This model provides a cleaner approach to the study of G-FA cycle regulation because it avoids alterations in blood and muscle substrate levels and does not alter exercise insulin and catecholamine concentrations (17, 28). Muscle glycogen breakdown was reduced by approximately 45% in the high-fat trial (figure 12.7). Muscle citrate and acetyl CoA

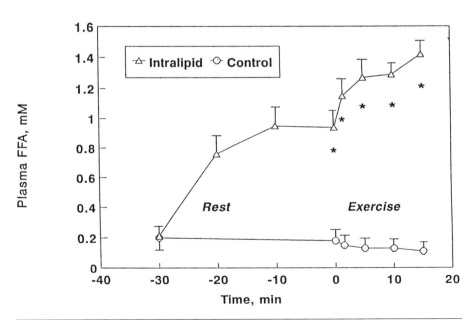

Figure 12.6 Plasma FFA concentrations at rest and during cycling at 85% $\dot{V}O_2$max with saline (control) or Intralipid-heparin infusion. * = significantly different from control. Circles = Intralipid; triangles = control.

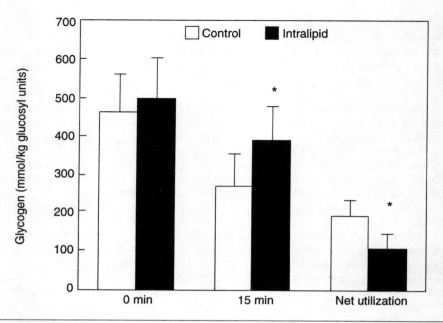

Figure 12.7   Muscle glycogen contents before and after 15 min of intense aerobic cycling and net glycogen utilization with control and Intralipid-heparin infusions. * = significantly different from control.

contents were increased at 3 and 15 min of exercise in both trials, but the increases were unaffected by fat availability (figures 12.8 and 12.9). Muscle PDHa was also unaffected by the high-fat trial (figure 12.10, p. 149). The authors concluded that the G-FA cycle was not regulated as classically proposed when exercising at approximately 85% V̇O₂max. The results suggested that the primary site of control for decreasing CHO metabolism was at glycogen PHOS. However, it was not clear what modulators were responsible for down-regulating PHOS activity when fat availability and oxidation were increased.

A subsequent study by Dyck et al. (15) extended the initial findings with biopsies at 1, 5, and 15 min of exercise at 85% V̇O₂max. The occurrence of muscle glycogen sparing with Intralipid infusion was variable, because only 7 out of 11 subjects demonstrated greater than a 20% reduction in muscle glycogenolysis. Muscle citrate, acetyl CoA, and PDH in the subjects who spared glycogen were again unaffected by high fat availability at all time points during exercise. Muscle PDHa was already maximally activated at 1 min of exercise. Muscle G6P content was also unchanged in the high-fat trial at all exercise time points (figure 12.11, p. 150). The fraction of PHOS in the active form was similar in the fat and control trials (figure 12.12, p. 151), suggesting that the decrease in PHOS activity during exercise was mediated by posttransformational, allosteric factors. Measurements of total muscle ADP and AMP and calculations of the free ADP, AMP, and inorganic phosphate (Pi) concentrations in the cell revealed no differences between the high-fat and control trials during exercise, although the free metabolite contents tended to be lower during

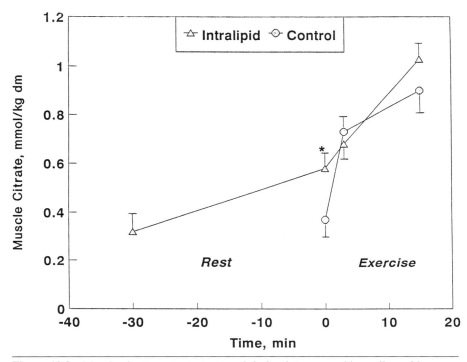

Figure 12.8 Muscle citrate content at rest and during intense aerobic cycling with control and Intralipid infusion. * = significantly different from control.

the high fat trials. Total ADP levels were significantly lower in the Intralipid trial at 15 min. When the present results were pooled with the data from the previous study (17), the free ADP, AMP, and Pi contents of all subjects who spared glycogen ($n = 13$) were significantly lower at 15 min in the Intralipid trial. The data suggest that blunted increases in free ADP, AMP, and Pi levels are involved in the decreased muscle glycogenolysis in the presence of increased fat availability at this exercise intensity.

In summary, the regulation of fat-CHO interaction in human skeletal muscle during exercise at 65% to 85% $\dot{V}O_2$max does not appear to be regulated as classically proposed for contracting heart muscle. It is likely that the major site of down-regulation of muscle glycogenolysis in the presence of increased fat availability is at glycogen PHOS. Regulation at PFK and PDH appears to be secondary at moderate to intense exercise power outputs when the majority of the CHO substrate and total substrate metabolized is muscle glycogen. The regulatory signals or modulators responsible for coupling increased muscle fat oxidation to decreased CHO use are presently unknown. However, it appears that PHOS regulation is posttransformational and that changes in muscle free ADP, AMP, and Pi contents are involved in the decreased glycogenolysis with high fat provision during high intensity exercise.

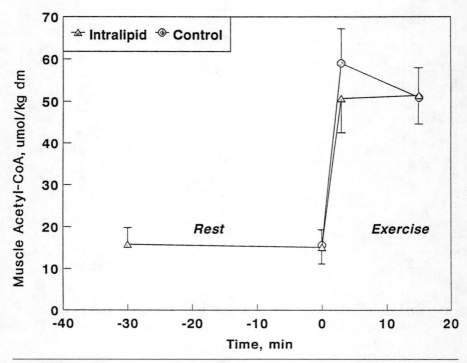

Figure 12.9   Muscle acetyl CoA content at rest and during intense aerobic cycling with control and Intralipid infusion.

Summary

In conclusion, there is considerable evidence to suggest that the G-FA cycle or fat-CHO interaction does occur in resting and exercising rat and human skeletal muscle. However, support for the cycle is not found in all resting situations or at all exercise intensities. The information examining the regulation of fat-CHO interaction in skeletal muscle is lacking and is less conclusive. At rest, the classic acetyl CoA–PDH aspect of fat-CHO regulation appears to function in skeletal muscle, where the citrate-PFK and G6P-HK aspects are less likely to be important. During exercise, the data strongly suggest that the G-FA cycle is not regulated as classically proposed.

Recent in vitro experiments reveal that previous in vitro work overestimated the potency of citrate to inhibit PFK activity during exercise because increases in positive regulators override its inhibitory effect. Work with animal models has been dominated by studies with the rat model and perfused hindlimb preparations. The majority of the evidence suggests that the G-FA cycle does not exist in most resting and exercising situations, making the perfused rat hindlimb preparation a poor model for studying the regulation of fat-CHO interaction. However, the cycle does exist

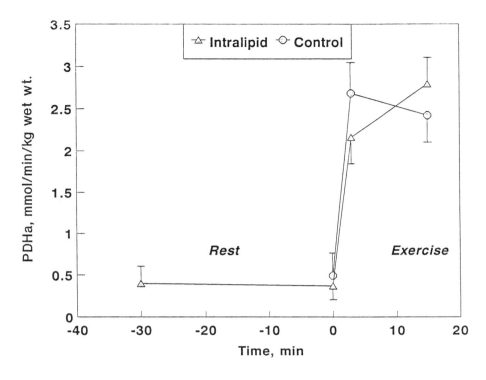

Figure 12.10   Maximal activity of the active form of pyruvate dehydrogenase (PDHa) at rest and during intense aerobic cycling with control and Intralipid infusion.

at certain stimulation intensities in selected muscles, and these could be used to examine the regulation.

The evidence for the existence of the G-FA cycle in resting humans is very strong. However, most of the measurements of glucose oxidation or disposal following FFA manipulation are whole body. Additional studies are needed to measure actual muscle uptake and oxidation of glucose with increased or decreased fat availability to confirm the existence of the G-FA cycle at rest. The literature generally supports the classical proposal that enhanced FFA delivery increases resting muscle acetyl CoA and inhibits PDH activity. However, muscle citrate and G6P are inconsistent and often do not increase when FFA availability is increased, leaving the significance of the citrate-PFK and G6P-HK regulatory mechanisms unresolved in resting human skeletal muscle.

The G-FA cycle does exist in human skeletal muscle during exercise. Acute increases in FFA delivery to the working muscle decrease muscle glycogenolysis during whole-body exercise at 65% to 90% $\dot{V}O_2$max. There have not been enough studies to accurately conclude whether increased fat availability reduces muscle glucose uptake during exercise. The regulation of fat-CHO interaction in human skeletal muscle during exercise at 65% to 85% $\dot{V}O_2$max does not appear to be regulated as classically proposed. The major site of down-regulation of muscle glycogenolysis in the presence of increased fat is at glycogen PHOS. The modulators

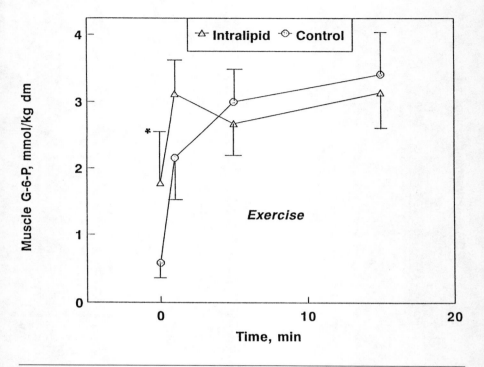

Figure 12.11   Muscle glucose-6-phosphate (G6P) content at rest and during intense aerobic cycling with control and Intralipid infusion. * = significantly different from control.

responsible for coupling increased muscle fat oxidation to decreased CHO use are presently unknown. However, it appears that PHOS regulation is posttransformational, and that a dampened increase in muscle free ADP, AMP, and Pi are involved in decreased glycogenolysis with enhanced fat provision.

Acknowledgments

The authors wish to thank all their co-workers for excellent collaboration in the investigations from their laboratories. The work from the authors' laboratories was supported with grants from the Natural Science and Engineering Research Council of Canada.

References

1. Andres, V.; Carreras, J.; Cussó, R. Regulation of muscle phosphofructokinase by physiological concentrations of bisphosphorylated hexoses: Effect of alkalinization. Biochem. Biophys. Res. Commun. 172:328-334; 1990.

Phosphorylase activation (% active)

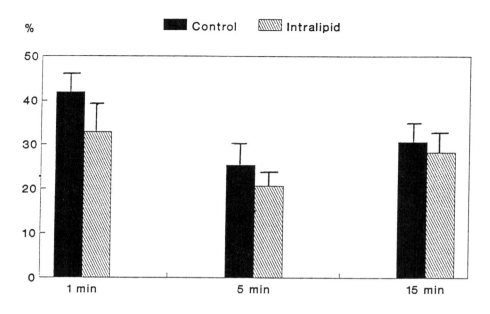

Figure 12.12   Maximal activity of the active form of phosphorylase (PHOSa) during intense aerobic cycling with control and Intralipid infusion.

2. Aragon, J.J.; Sols, A. Regulation of enzyme activity in the cell: Effect of enzyme concentration. FASEB J. 5:2945-2950; 1991.
3. Balasse, E.O. Effect of free fatty acids and ketone bodies on glucose uptake and oxidation in the dog. Horm. Metab. Res. 3:403-409; 1971.
4. Beatty, C.H.; Bocek, R.M. Interrelation of carbohydrate and palmitate metabolism in skeletal muscle. Am. J. Physiol. 220:1928-1934; 1971.
5. Berger, M.; Hagg, S.A.; Goodman, M.N.; Ruderman, N.B. Glucose metabolism in perfused skeletal muscle: Effects of starvation, diabetes, fatty acids, acetoacetate, insulin and exercise on glucose uptake and disposition. Biochem. J. 158:191-202; 1976.
6. Bergström, J.; Hultman, E.; Jorfeldt, L.; Pernow, B.; Wahren, J. Effect of nicotinic acid on physical working capacity and on metabolism of muscle glycogen in man. J. Appl. Physiol. 26:170-176; 1969.
7. Boden, G.; Jadali, F.; White, J.; Liang, Y.; Mozzoli, M.; Chen, X.; Coleman, E.; Smith, C. Effects of fat on insulin-stimulated carbohydrate metabolism in normal men. J. Clin. Invest. 88:960-966; 1991.
8. Bosca, L.; Aragon, J.J.; Sols, A. Modulation of muscle phosphofructokinase at physiological concentration of enzyme. 260:2100-2107; 1985.
9. Carlson, M.G.; Snead, W.L.; Hill, J.O.; Nurjhan, N.; Campbell, P.J. Glucose regulation of lipid metabolism in humans. Am. J. Physiol. 261:E815-E820; 1991.
10. Caruso, M.; Divertie, G.D.; Jensen, M.D.; Miles, J.M. Lack of effect of hyperglycemia on lipolysis in humans. Am. J. Physiol. 259:E542-E547; 1990.

11. Coggan, A.R.; Spina, R.J.; Kohrt, W.M.; Holloszy, J.O. Effect of prolonged exercise on muscle citrate concentration before and after endurance training in men. Am. J. Physiol. 264:E215-E220; 1993.

12. Cooper, R.H.; Randle, P.J.; Denton, R.M. Stimulation of phosphorylation and inactivation of pyruvate dehydrogenase by physiological inhibitors of the pyruvate dehydrogenase reaction. Nature 257:808-809; 1975.

13. Costill, D.L.; Coyle, E.; Dalsky, G.; Evans, W.; Fink, W.; Hoopes, D. Effects of elevated plasma FFA and insulin on muscle glycogen usage during exercise. J. Appl. Physiol. 43:695-699; 1977.

14. Dobson, G.P.; Yamamoto, E.; Hochachka, P.W. Phosphofructokinase control in muscle: Nature and reversal of pH-dependent ATP inhibition. Am. J. Physiol. 250:R71-R76; 1986.

15. Dyck, D.J.; Peters, S.J.; Wendling, P.; Chesley, A.; Hultman, E.; Spriet, L.L. Regulation of muscle glycogen phosphorylase activity during intense aerobic cycling with elevated FFA. Am. J. Physiol. 270; 1996 (In press.)

16. Dyck, D.J.; Peters, S.J.; Wendling, P.S.; Spriet, L.L. Effect of high FFA on glycogenolysis in oxidative rat hindlimb muscles during twitch stimulation. Am. J. Physiol. 270:E116-E125; 1996.

17. Dyck, D.J.; Putman, C.T.; Heigenhauser, G.J.F.; Hultman, E.; Spriet, L.L. Regulation of fat-carbohydrate interaction in skeletal muscle during intense aerobic cycling. Am. J. Physiol. 265:E852-E859; 1993.

18. Dyck, D.J.; Spriet, L.L. Elevated muscle citrate does not reduce carbohydrate utilization during tetanic stimulation. Can. J. Physiol. Pharmacol. 72:117-125; 1994.

19. Erickson, M.A.; Schwarzkopf, R.J.; McKenzie, R.D. Effects of caffeine, fructose and glucose ingestion on muscle glycogen utilization during exercise. Med. Sci. Sports Exercise 19:579-583; 1987.

20. Essen, B. Studies on the regulation of metabolism in human skeletal muscle using intermittent exercise as an experimental model. Acta Physiol. Scand. (suppl. 454):1-32; 1978.

21. Essig, D.; Costill, D.L.; Van Handel, P.J. Effects of caffeine ingestion on utilization of muscle glycogen and lipid during leg ergometer cycling. Int. J. Sports Med. 1:86-90; 1980.

22. Faneill, C.; Calderone, S.; Epifano, L.; De Vincenzo, A.; Modarelli, F.; Pampanelli, S.; Perriello, G.; De Feo, P.; Brunetti, P.; Gerich, J.E.; Bolli, G.B. Demonstration of a critical role for free fatty acids in mediating counterregulatory stimulation of gluconeogenesis and suppression of glucose utilization in humans. J. Clin. Invest. 92:1617-1622; 1993.

23. Ferrannini, E.; Barrett, S.; Bevilacqua, S.; DeFronzo, R.A. Effect of fatty acids on glucose production and utilization in man. J. Clin. Invest. 72:1737-1747; 1983.

24. Garland, P.B.; Randle, P.J. Regulation of glucose uptake by muscle: 10. Effects of alloxan-diabetes, starvation, hypophysectomy and adrenalectomy, and of fatty acids, ketone bodies and pyruvate on the glycerol output and concentrations of free fatty acids, long-chain fatty acyl-coenzyme A, glycerol phosphate and citrate-cycle intermediates in rat heart and diaphragm muscles. Biochem. J. 93:678-687; 1964.

25. Garland, P.B.; Randle, P.J.; Newsholme, E.A. Citrate as an intermediary in the inhibition of phosphofructokinase in rat heart muscle by fatty acids, ketone bodies, pyruvate, diabetes and starvation. Nature 200:169-170; 1963.

26. Grundleger, M.; Thenen, S.W. Decreased insulin binding, glucose transport, and glucose metabolism in soleus muscle of rats fed a high fat diet. Diabetes 31:232-237; 1982.

27. Hagg, S.A.; Taylor, S.I.; Ruderman, N.B. Glucose metabolism in perfused skeletal muscle: Pyruvate dehydrogenase activity in starvation, diabetes and exercise. Biochem. J. 158:203-210; 1976.

28. Hargreaves, M.; Kiens, B.; Richter, E.A. Effect of plasma free fatty acid concentration on muscle metabolism in exercising men. J. Appl. Physiol. 70:194-210; 1991.

29. Hickson, R.C.; Rennie, M.J.; Conlee, R.K.; Winder, W.W.; Holloszy, J.O. Effects of increased plasma fatty acids on glycogen utilization and endurance. J. Appl. Physiol. 43:829-833; 1977.

30. Houghton, C.R.S.; Ruderman, N.B. Acetoacetate as a fuel for perfused rat skeletal muscle. Biochem. J. 121:15-16; 1971.

31. Jansson, E.; Kaijser, L. Effect of diet on muscle glycogen and blood glucose utilization during a short term exercise in man. Acta Physiol. Scand. 115:341-347; 1982a.

32. Jansson, E.; Kaijser, L. Effect of diet on the utilization of blood-borne and intramuscular substrates during exercise in man. Acta Physiol. Scand. 115:19-30; 1982b.

33. Jansson, E.; Kaijser, L. Leg citrate metabolism at rest and during exercise in relation to diet and substrate utilization in man. Acta Physiol. Scand. 122:145-153; 1984.

34. Jansson, E.; Kaijser, L. Substrate utilization and enzymes in skeletal muscle of extremely endurance-trained men. J. Appl. Physiol. 62:999-1005; 1987.

35. Jefferson, L.S.; Koehler, J.O.; Morgan, H.E. Effect of insulin on protein synthesis in skeletal muscle of an isolated perfused preparation of rat hemicorpus. Proc. Natl. Acad. Sci. USA 69:816-820; 1972.

36. Jenkins, A.B.; Storlein, L.H.; Chisholm, D.J.; Kraegen, E.W. Effects of nonesterified fatty acid availability on tissue-specific glucose utilization in rats in vivo. J. Clin. Invest. 82:293-299; 1988.

37. Jenkins, A.B.; Storlein, L.H.; Cooney, G.J.; Denyer, G.S.; Caterson, I.D.; Kraegen, E.W. Effects of blockade of fatty acid oxidation on whole body and tissue-specific glucose metabolism in rats. Am. J. Physiol. 265:E592-E600; 1993.

38. Kelley, D.E.; Mokan, M.; Simoneau, J.-A.; Mandarino, L.L. Interaction between glucose and free fatty acid metabolism in human skeletal muscle. J. Clin. Invest. 92:91-98; 1993.

39. Kemp, R.G.; Foe, L.G. Allosteric regulatory properties of muscle phosphofructokinase. Mol. Cell. Biochem. 57:147-154; 1983.

40. Knapik, J.J.; Meredith, C.N.; Jones, B.H.; Suek, L.; Young, V.R.; Evans, W.J. Influence of fasting on carbohydrate and fat metabolism during rest and exercise in men. J. Appl. Physiol. 64:1923-1929; 1988.

41. Koubi, H.E.; Desplanches, D.; Gabrielle, C.; Cottet-Emard, J.M.; Sempore, B.; Favier, R.J. Exercise endurance and fuel utilization: A reevaluation of the effects of fasting. J. Appl. Physiol. 70:1337-1343; 1991.

42. Maughan, R.J.; Williams, C. Muscle citrate content and the regulation of metabolism in fed and fasted human skeletal muscle. Clin. Physiol. 2:21-27; 1982.

43. Paul, P.; Issekutz, B.; Miller, H. Interrelationship of free fatty acids and glucose metabolism in the dog. Am. J. Physiol. 211:1313-1320; 1966.

44. Peters, S.J.; Spriet, L.L. Skeletal muscle phosphofructokinase activity examined under physiological conditions in vitro. J. Appl. Physiol. 78:1853-1858; 1995.
45. Pettit, F.H.; Pelley, J.W.; Reed, L.J. Regulation of pyruvate dehydrogenase kinase and phosphatase by acetyl-CoA/CoA and NADH/NAD ratios. Biochem. Biophys. Res. Commun. 65:575-582; 1975.
46. Purich, D.L.; Fromm, H.J.; Rudolph, F.B. The hexokinases: Kinetic, physical, and regulatory properties. Adv. Enzymol. 39:249-326; 1973.
47. Putman, C.T.; Spriet, L.L.; Hultman, E.; Dyck, D.J.; Heigenhauser, G.J.F. Skeletal muscle pyruvate dehydrogenase activity during acetate infusion in humans. Am. J. Physiol. 268:E1007-E1017; 1995.
48. Putman, C.T.; Spriet, L.L.; Hultman, E.; Lindinger, M.I.; Lands, L.C.; McKelvie, R.S.; Cederblad, G.; Jones, N.L.; Heigenhauser, G.J.F. Pyruvate dehydrogenase activity and acetyl group accumulation during exercise after different diets. Am. J. Physiol. 265:E752-E760; 1993.
49. Randle, P.J.; Garland, P.B.; Hales, C.N.; Newsholme, E.A. The glucose fatty-acid cycle. Its role in insulin sensitivity and the metabolic disturbances of diabetes mellitus. Lancet 1:785-789; 1963.
50. Randle, P.J.; Newsholme, E.A.; Garland, P.B. Regulation of glucose uptake by muscle: 8. Effects of fatty acids, ketone bodies and pyruvate, and of alloxan-diabetes and starvation, on the uptake and metabolic fate of glucose in rat heart and diaphragm muscles. Biochem. J. 93:652-665; 1964.
51. Ravussin, E.; Bogardus, C.; Scheidegger, K.; LaGrange, B.; Horton, E.D.; Horton, E.S. Effect of elevated FFA on carbohydrate and lipid oxidation during prolonged exercise in humans. J. Appl. Physiol. 60:893-900; 1986.
52. Rennie, M.J.; Holloszy, J.O. Inhibition of glucose uptake and glycogenolysis by availability of oleate in well-oxygenated perfused skeletal muscle. Biochem. J. 168:161-170; 1977.
53. Rennie, M.J.; Winder, W.W.; Holloszy, J.O. A sparing effect of increased plasma fatty acids on muscle and liver glycogen content in the exercising rat. Biochem. J. 156:647-655; 1976.
54. Richter, E.A.; Ruderman, N.B.; Gavras, H.; Belur, E.R.; Galbo, H. Muscle glycogenolysis during exercise: Dual control by epinephrine and contractions. Am. J. Physiol. 242:E25-E32; 1982.
55. Romijn, J.A.; Coyle, E.F.; Zhang, X.-J.; Sidossis, L.S.; Wolfe, R.R. Relationship between fatty acid delivery and fatty acid oxidation during strenuous exercise. J. Appl. Physiol. 79:1939-1945; 1995.
56. Saloranta, C.; Koivisto, V.; Widen, E.; Falholot, K.; DeFronzo, R.A.; Karkonen, M.; Groop, L. Contribution of muscle and liver to glucose–fatty acid cycle in humans. Am. J. Physiol. 264:E599-E605; 1993.
57. Segffert, W.A.; Madison, L.L. Physiological effects of metabolic fuels on carbo-hydrate metabolism: I. Acute effect of elevation of plasma free fatty acids on hepatic glucose output, peripheral glucose utilization, serum insulin, and plasma glucagon levels. Diabetes 16:765-767; 1967.
58. Spriet, L.L.; Dyck, D.J.; Cederblad, G.; Hultman, E. Effects of fat availability on acetyl-CoA and acetylcarnitine metabolism in rat skeletal muscle. Am. J. Physiol. 263:C653-C659; 1992.
59. Spriet, L.L.; MacLean, D.A.; Dyck, D.J.; Hultman, E.; Cederblad, G.; Graham, T.E. Caffeine ingestion and muscle metabolism during prolonged exercise in humans. Am. J. Physiol. 262:E891-E898; 1992.

60. Tornheim, K.; Lowenstein, J.M. Control of phosphofructokinase from rat skeletal muscle. Effects of fructose diphosphate, AMP, ATP, and citrate. J. Biol. Chem. 251:7322-7328; 1976.

61. Vukovich, M.D.; Costill, D.L.; Hickey, M.S.; Trappe, S.W.; Cole, K.J.; Fink, W.J. Effect of fat emulsion and fat feeding on muscle glycogen utilization during cycle exercise. J. Appl. Physiol. 75:1513-1518; 1993.

62. Walker, M.; Fulcher, G.R.; Catalano, C.; Petranyi, G.; Orskov, H.; Albero, K.G.M.M. Physiological levels of plasma non-esterified fatty acids impair forearm glucose uptake in normal man. Clin. Sci. 99:167-174; 1990.

63. Waterhouse, C.; Baker, N.; Rostami, H. Effect of glucose ingestion on the metabolism of free fatty acids in human subjects. J. Lipid Res. 10:487-494; 1969.

64. Wu, T.-F.L.; Davis, E.J. Regulation of glycolytic flux in an energetically controlled cell-free system: The effects of adenine nucleotide ratios, inorganic phosphate, pH, and citrate. Arch. Biochem. Biophys. 209:85-99; 1981.

65. Young, A.J.; Evans, W.J.; Cymerman, A.; Pandolf, K.B.; Knapik, J.J.; Maher, J.T. Sparing effect of chronic high-altitude exposure on muscle glycogen utilization. J. Appl. Physiol. 52:857-862; 1982.

66. Zorzano, A.; Balon, T.W.; Brady, L.J.; Rivera, P.; Garetto, L.P.; Young, J.C.; Goodman, M.N.; Ruderman, N.B. Effects of starvation and exercise on concentrations of citrate, hexose phosphates and glycogen in skeletal muscle and heart. Biochem. J. 232:585-591; 1985.

CHAPTER 13

Pyruvate Dehydrogenase as a Regulator of Substrate Utilization in Skeletal Muscle

Eric Hultman

Karolinska Institute, Huddinge, Sweden

The pyruvate dehydrogenase (PDH) enzyme is one in a group of three enzymes oxidizing keto acid substrates: pyruvate, branched-chain keto acids, and α-ketoglutarate. They all have important regulatory functions in cell metabolism. The branched-chain keto acids are formed from the corresponding amino acids via specific aminotransferases distributed widely throughout the body, and the subsequent oxidation of the keto acids may, if not regulated, create the potential for depletion of the carbon skeleton, which cannot be synthesized by the body. A precise regulation of the activity of this enzyme is therefore necessary to act as a conservation mechanism to prevent depletion of these essential amino acids. The enzyme is also a key regulatory enzyme in nitrogen metabolism in the body, acting via the reversible aminotransferase reaction.

The PDH complex catalyzes the pyruvate oxidation in the mitochondrion, and it has been calculated that 50% to 80% of the energy sources in the diet are channeled through the pyruvate dehydrogenase system. This represents 200 to 400 g of glucose each day with a normal dietary intake, but during low food intake or starvation, glucose must be conserved. The glucose transfer through the PDH system, which commits pyruvate to oxidation or channeling into lipids or steroid, is essentially irreversible. A continued high flux through PDH during starvation can lead to depletion of the carbohydrate stores in the body, since the rate of de novo synthesis of glucose from amino acids and intermediates from the glycolytic pathway is limited. Another role of the PDH complex is the regulation of substrate utilization during exercise when the demand on oxidative energy release can increase by 10 to 100 times, depending on the intensity of the exercise.

The last of the three enzymes is α-ketoglutarate dehydrogenase, which has a regulatory role in the tricarboxylic acid (TCA) cycle. It determines the maximum flux through the cycle, and thus, together with PDH, it regulates both the maximum substrate utilization and the relative roles of carbohydrate and fat in the oxidative energy release.

The enzymes are multienzyme complexes that catalyze the oxidative decarboxylation of keto acids, releasing CO_2 and generating the relevant acyl CoA. The reaction

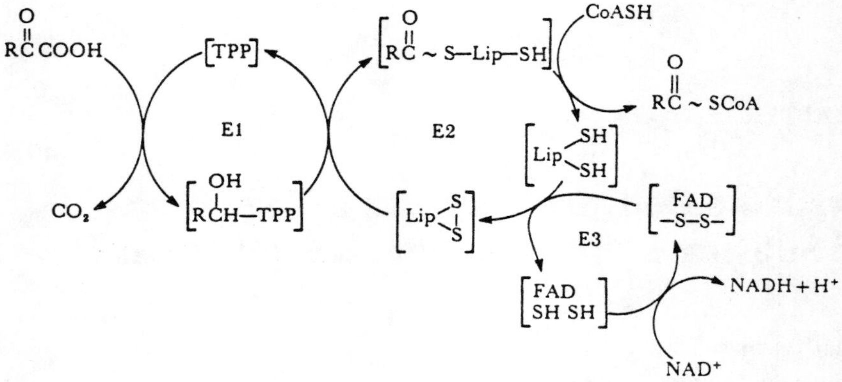

Figure 13.1   The reaction mechanism for the pyruvate and α-ketoglutarate dehydrogenase multienzyme complexes. R = CH_3 for pyruvate and R = $COOH$-CH_2 for α-ketoglutarate. TPP = thiamin pyrophosphate; Lip = lipoic acid; CoA = coenzyme A.

catalyzed is shown in schematic form in figure 13.1. The constituent enzymes for the pyruvate dehydrogenase (PDH) complex are pyruvate dehydrogenase (E1), dihydrolipoamide acetyltransferase (E2), and dihydrolipoamide dehydrogenase (E3) (see recent reviews 1, 24). Two other proteins, a kinase and a phosphatase, are associated with the pyruvate dehydrogenase complex.

Regulation of PDH Activity

The irreversible decarboxylation of pyruvate by pyruvate dehydrogenase (E1) is the rate-limiting step in the reaction catalyzed by the PDH complex. The reaction requires Mg^{2+} and the cofactor thiamine pyrophosphate. The activity of PDH is regulated by two types of mechanisms. The first is an end-product inhibition of the catalytic activity of the enzyme by acetyl CoA and NADH. The second is a conformational modification of the enzyme complex by a phosphorylation-dephosphorylation mechanism mediated via a specific protein kinase and a phospho-protein phosphatase.

At the beginning of the 1960s, it was shown that the carbohydrate utilization in a heart preparation decreased in the presence of alternative substrates, such as fatty acids or ketone bodies (9, 11, 30). This carbohydrate-sparing effect was attributed to inhibition of the catalytic activity of PDH by the end products NADH and acetyl CoA (10, 14).

In 1969, Linn, Pettit, and Reed (16) demonstrated the phosphorylation-dephosphorylation mechanism as a regulator of the PDH complex (figure 13.2). The complex is inactivated by a specific cAMP-independent protein kinase, with

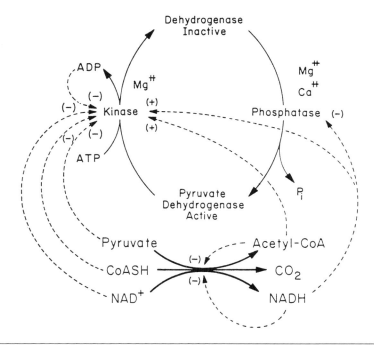

Figure 13.2   The regulation of the pyruvate dehydrogenase multienzyme complex.

Mg ATP as substrate, and reactivated by dephosphorylation via a Mg^{2+}-dependent protein phosphatase. The kinase is inhibited with respect to ATP by ADP and by the substrates to the PDH reaction, pyruvate, NAD^+, and CoASH, while the products, NADH and acetyl CoA, are stimulators. Inhibition also occurs when Ca^{2+} increases and when the coenzyme thiamine pyrophosphate is bound to the catalytic site of E1. The phosphatase is dependent on Mg^{2+} and is stimulated by Ca^{2+}, which facilitates binding of the phosphatase to the complex; NADH, the only inhibitor, is reversed by NAD^+. Thus, the main inhibitors of the complex are increased concentration ratios of acetyl CoA/CoASH and NADH/NAD^+, and the activators are pyruvate and Ca^{2+} (6, 21). Most of these studies of PDH regulation have been carried out by in vitro experiments.

Regulatory Mechanisms for PDH in Contracting Muscle

Muscle contraction is initiated by Ca^{2+} release from the sarcoplasmic reticulum, activating actomyosin ATPase, glycogen phosphorylase kinase, PDH phosphatase, and α-ketoglutarate dehydrogenase (figure 13.3).

The result of the Ca^{2+}-induced muscle contraction is an increased formation of pyruvate in the glycolytic sequence, but also an increased activation of pyruvate oxidation via PDHa and of acetyl CoA transfer in the TCA cycle via α-ketoglutarate dehydrogenase. Pyruvate accumulation further activates the fraction of PDH in

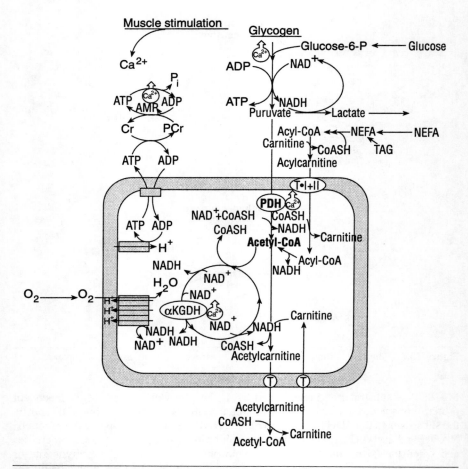

Figure 13.3   Metabolic processes in contracting muscle.

active form (PDHa), but the catalytic activity of the enzyme reaction also needs a continuous supply of NAD$^+$ and CoASH. NAD$^+$ is formed by oxidation of NADH in the electron transport chain at a rate determined by the availability of O_2 and ADP. CoASH is released when acetyl CoA is condensed with oxaloacetate in the TCA cycle.

NAD$^+$ and CoASH are also needed for simultaneous β-oxidation of fatty acyl CoA. This means that the concentration ratios NADH/NAD$^+$ and acetyl CoA/CoASH regulate the total oxidative metabolism in muscle and possibly also the relative contributions of carbohydrate and fat as substrates for metabolism. The NADH/NAD$^+$ quotient is dependent on the activity of the electron transport chain and the O_2 availability, while the acetyl CoA/CoASH ratio is regulated by the turnover rate in the TCA cycle but also by a buffer mechanism, the carnitine acetyltransferase system, by which acetyl groups are transferred to carnitine.

The total store of CoASH in muscle is small, about 50 µmol · kg^{-1} of dry muscle (d.m.) or 10 to 15 µmol · kg^{-1} of wet muscle (w.m.; 3). Ninety-five percent of this store is confined to the intramitochondrial space and 5% to the sarcoplasm (13). The maximum rate of acetyl CoA formation via PDH is 40 to 50 μmol $\cdot$ s^{-1} $\cdot$ kg^{-1} w.m., which means that the whole CoASH store can be acetylated within less than 1 s, with complete inhibition of the catalytic activity of PDH. The size of the carnitine store in muscle is about 21 mmol $\cdot$ kg^{-1} d.m. (3), that is, about 400 times larger than the CoA store. Only 10% of the carnitine store is confined to the mitochondrial space (13) but the intra- and extramitochondrial carnitine pools are linked by a carnitine-acetylcarnitine translocase (17, 20). This enzyme, which has a high activity, enables the free carnitine in the whole cell to act as a buffer for excess intramitochondrial acetyl CoA accumulation (17). An increase in extramitochondrial acetylcarnitine concentration will also acetylate part of the small extramitochondrial CoASH pool and thus reduce the availability of CoASH extramitochondrially. In this way, the acetylation of the CoASH pool both intra- and extramitochondrially can potentially regulate carbohydrate oxidation by acetyl CoA–induced inhibition of PDH or lipid oxidation by reducing the concentration of CoASH that is necessary for acyl CoA formation and transport (18).

PDH Activity During Various Types of Exercise

Isometric Exercise

The time course of PDH transformation was studied during electrical stimulation of the intact quadriceps muscle of humans (4). The stimulation was intermittent, and the frequency 20 Hz. Stimulation periods were 1.6 s with 1.6-s rest intervals. PDHa increased from 25% at rest to 64% after 10 contractions and to 80% after 20 contractions. After 46 contractions, the PDH was almost completely transformed to the active form. In the muscle tissue obtained after electrical stimulation, there was a high concentration of lactate and NADH but a very low content of acetyl CoA. To further examine the effect of NADH accumulation on the PDH activity, the study was repeated with occluded blood flow to the muscle. The stimulation was started immediately after blood flow occlusion or after 20 min of occlusion. In both situations, the transformation to PDHa was complete despite the high accumulation of NADH, but the flux through the activated enzyme, as measured by acetyl CoA formation, was, as expected, completely inhibited.

The absence of NADH oxidation during anoxia had apparently no effect on the contraction-induced transformation of PDH to its active form, but the flux through the enzyme reaction is inhibited.

Dynamic Exercise

Pyruvate dehydrogenase activity was analyzed during short periods of exercise at three different intensities corresponding to 30%, 60%, and 90% $\dot{V}O_2$max (3). It increased from 0.4 mmol $\cdot$ min^{-1} $\cdot$ kg^{-1} in resting muscle to 0.8 at 30% $\dot{V}O_2$max and to 1.2 at 60%; no further increase was observed at 95% $\dot{V}O_2$max. At the end of the exercise at the lowest work load, the lactate concentration showed only a marginal increase, while acetyl CoA and acetylcarnitine concentrations were unchanged in the exercising muscle. This suggests a close relationship between the rates of glycolysis, of pyruvate oxidation to acetyl CoA, and of acetyl CoA utilization in the TCA cycle. With increasing work intensity, both the lactate and acetyl groups accumulated in muscle tissue, showing the imbalance between pyruvate formation and oxidation during short periods of exercise at these intensities. The relationship between accumulated acetyl CoA and acetylcarnitine in muscle was 1/400, showing the rapid equilibration of acetyl groups between the CoA and carnitine pools.

In a further study by the same group (5), the exercise period was prolonged to 60 min, the work intensity corresponded to 75% $\dot{V}O_2$max, and tissue samples were obtained before the exercise, after 3, 10, 40, and 60 min of exercise, and after 20 min of rest. The PDH was transformed to the active state almost completely (approximately 92%) within the first 3 min of exercise and remained thereafter unchanged during the whole exercise period. The glycogen degradation rate was highest during the first 3 min, during which period the lactate accumulation also reached the highest value. The accumulation of acetyl groups bound to CoA and carnitine increased with the greatest rate during the first 3 min but also continued to increase during the 3- to 10-min period. After 10 min of exercise, the acetyl group accumulation ceased and remained practically unchanged until the end of the exercise period (figure 13.4).

These results indicate that the initial glycolytic rate is much higher than the flux through the PDH pathway during the first 3 min of exercise with increasing lactate accumulation. At the same time, the rate of acetyl CoA formation is higher than the condensation of the acetyl group with oxaloacetate. This imbalance also persisted in the 3- to 10-min period, but thereafter a balance was reached with a constant PDHa fraction and unchanged concentrations of acetyl CoA and acetylcarnitine. The formation of pyruvate could be estimated from the decrease in muscle glycogen and the uptake of blood glucose during exercise. The amount of pyruvate formed was 2.46 mmol $\cdot$ min^{-1} $\cdot$ kg^{-1} w.m., and after subtraction of the pyruvate used for the formation of lactate and anaplerotic substrates, the pyruvate flux through PDH was calculated as 2.1 mmol $\cdot$ min^{-1} $\cdot$ kg^{-1} w.m. The estimated in vitro activity of PDHa was 1.7 to 1.9 mmol $\cdot$ acetyl CoA $\cdot$ min^{-1} $\cdot$ kg^{-1}, corresponding to 90% of the total PDH activity.

Thus, both the transformation of PDH to its active form and the catalytic activity of PDHa were near 100%, despite the high accumulation of acetyl CoA in the muscle. The concentration ratio of acetyl CoA/CoASH increased from 0.19 in resting muscle to 1.29 at 10 min of exercise and to 1.33 at 60 min, a concentration ratio that would completely inhibit PDHa formation in isolated muscle tissue according to Cooper, Randle, and Denton (6) and Pettit, Pelley, and Reed (21).

Dietary Changes and PDH Activity

Studies by Randle and co-workers in the early 1960s (10, 11, 23) showed that enhanced fat oxidation elevates muscle citrate and acetyl CoA concentrations, resulting in a down-regulation of carbohydrate utilization due to inhibition of phosphofructokinase (PFK) and PDH. A decrease in the PDHa fraction and in the catalytic activity of PDH has also been shown in rat skeletal muscle by prolonged starvation

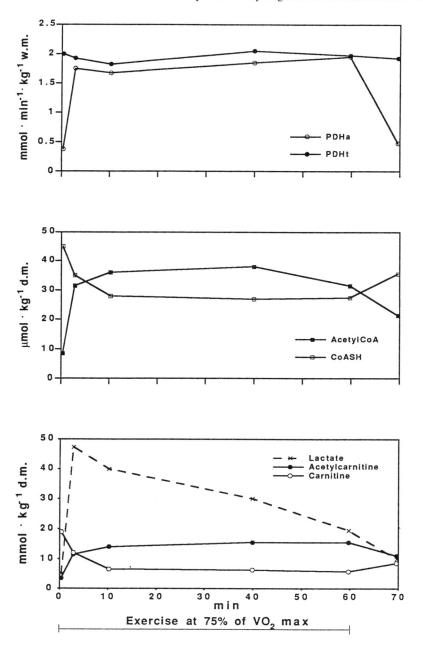

Figure 13.4 *Upper panel,* PDH activities at rest, during 58 ± 7 min of exercise at an intensity of 75% VO_2max, and after 10-min recovery. PDHa and PDHt denote active form and total PDH, respectively. *Middle panel,* muscle contents of CoASH and acetyl CoA before and during the exercise. *Lower panel,* muscle content of lactate, carnitine, and acetyl-carnitine before and during the exercise.

(8, 12, 29). In a recent investigation by Putman et al. (22), the PDH activity and the acetyl group accumulation in the quadriceps muscle was analyzed in five male subjects after two different diets. The studies commenced with glycogen-depleting exercise, followed by 3 d on a diet with a low carbohydrate content (LCD) or with a high carbohydrate content (HCD). The subjects exercised on two occasions on a bicycle ergometer at 75% $\dot{V}O_2$max for the same length of time. The first work was performed to exhaustion after the LCD. The second exercise of the same duration was performed 1 to 2 wk later after the HCD. Tissue samples for analyses of PDH and metabolites were obtained before the exercise, after 15 min of exercise, and at exhaustion (end of exercise).

After the LCD, the exercise capacity ceased after 47.7 ± 5.5 min due to a decrease in blood glucose concentration (2.38 ± 0.21 mmol $\cdot$ L^{-1}), causing symptoms in the central nervous system. This decrease can be attributed to a low glycogen content in the liver caused by the low carbohydrate intake (19). No fall in blood glucose concentration was observed during the exercise after the HCD. The plasma concentrations of FFA and glycerol were higher before and during exercise after the LCD compared with the HCD.

The muscle samples obtained at rest showed a significantly lower fraction of PDH in active form after the LCD, a large accumulation of acetyl CoA and acetyl-carnitine, a higher concentration of citrate, and a low glycogen content compared with the sample after the high carbohydrate intake (figure 13.5). The results were thus in agreement with previous findings of increased acetyl group accumulation as a result of augmented availability of fat, a resultant inhibition of PDH transformation and an accumulation of citrate.

During exercise, the PDH was rapidly transformed to its active form in both situations, but the fraction of active form was approximately 50% lower after LCD. The acetyl CoA concentration showed completely different patterns during exercise, decreasing rapidly during the first 15 min after LCD, but increasing during the same time period after HCD. Acetylcarnitine showed the same pattern. The CoASH concentration fell during the first 15 min in the LCD series, despite a decreasing acetyl CoA accumulation. This is probably due to the binding of CoASH to various other acyl groups during lipid oxidation. There was no increase in carnitine, despite a fall in acetylcarnitine in the same period. Contrary to this, the CoASH and carnitine concentrations fell after the HCD at the same rate as the acetyl group accumulated. At the end of the exercise after HCD, the CoASH concentration had decreased by about 50%.

The citrate content in muscle increased in both series, but the difference between the diets was eliminated. The glycogen utilization rate calculated over the whole work period was three times higher after the HCD than after the LCD; the difference was most pronounced during the final 16 min of exercise, when the glycogen degradation rate was about six times higher after the HCD.

The flux through the PDH enzyme during exercise after LCD was calculated to be 0.9 mmol pyruvate $\cdot$ min^{-1} $\cdot$ kg^{-1} w.m., corresponding to 50% of the maximal flux through the PDHa measured in vitro (1.88 mmol $\cdot$ min^{-1} $\cdot$ kg^{-1}), whereas after HCD the flux was 3.1 mmol $\cdot$ min^{-1} $\cdot$ kg^{-1}, corresponding to 100% of the activity of PDHa (figure 13.6, p. 167).

The maximum flux of acetyl groups in the TCA cycle has been estimated by Blomstrand, Ekblom, and Newsholme (2) as the activity of the α-ketoglutarate dehydrogenase enzyme in the quadriceps femoris muscle of well-trained athletes. The activity was 3.1 ± 0.26 mmol $\cdot$ min^{-1} $\cdot$ kg^{-1}, thus closely corresponding to the

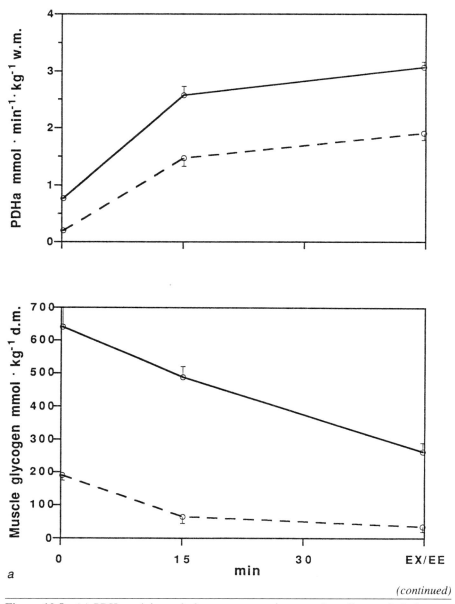

a

(continued)

Figure 13.5   (*a*) PDHa activity and glycogen content in vastus lateralis muscle before and during two bicycle exercise periods of 47-min duration at an intensity of 75% V̇O₂max. The first exercise was performed after a 3-d period on a diet with low carbohydrate content (LCD), indicated by a dashed line, and the second exercise after 3 d on a diet with high carbohydrate content (HCD), indicated by a solid line. Note the very low glycogen utilization during the period 16 to 47 min after the LCD. (*b*) The muscle content of CoASH and carnitine and their acetylated forms before and during the exercise after HCD (solid line) and after LCD (dashed line).

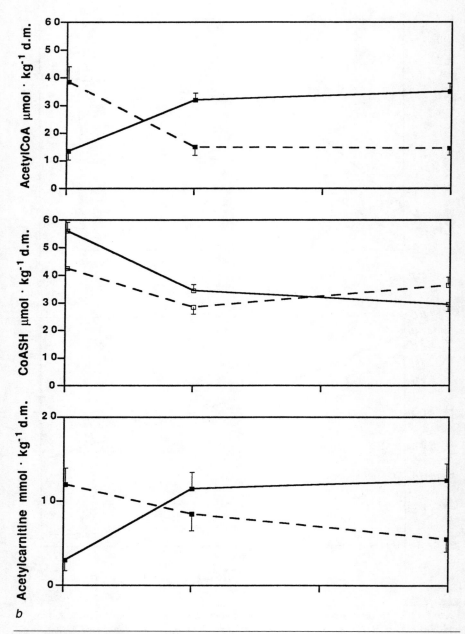

b

Figure 13.5   *(continued)*

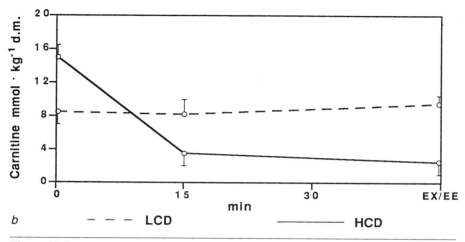

Figure 13.5   *(continued)*

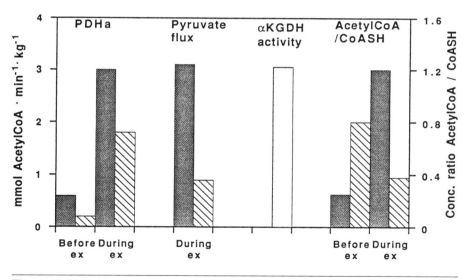

Figure 13.6   PDH activity and regulation during the two exercise periods described in figure 13.5a. Results after HCD are indicated by filled bars and after LCD by striped bars. PDHa activity in muscle samples obtained before and at the end of the exercise periods is determined in vitro. The pyruvate flux through PDH is calculated from glycogen degradation and glucose uptake, with deduction of pyruvate used for formation of lactate and anaplerotic substrates during the exercise period from 16 min to end of exercise (≈ 47 min). The activity of α-ketoglutarate dehydrogenase (αKGDH) is a measure of the maximum flux through the TCA cycle. The concentration ratios of acetyl CoA to CoASH are measured in muscle samples obtained before and at the end of the exercise periods. The activity of αKGDH is from Blomstrand, Ekblom, and Newsholme (2).

catalytic activity of PDH during exercise after the high carbohydrate diet. The conclusion would be that the oxidative energy release was completely covered by pyruvate oxidation in the quadriceps muscle during the exercise after HCD.

On the other hand, after LCD pyruvate oxidation could cover only approximately 30% of the oxidative metabolism, while about 70% was derived from fat metabolism. Substrate differences after the two diets are high fat availability and low muscle glycogen after LCD and high muscle glycogen content after HCD.

The concentration ratio of acetyl CoA to CoASH at end of exercise was 1.2 after the HCD compared with 0.4 after the LCD, and the free carnitine concentrations were 3 and 9 mmol · kg^{-1} d.m. after the HCD and the LCD, respectively. These differences could, as discussed before, possibly inhibit fat utilization after the HCD and facilitate fat utilization after the LCD. The suggested regulator is CoASH, the concentration of which regulates the activity of fatty acyl CoA synthetases extramitochondrially and also the activity of carnitine palmitoyl transferase II, necessary for acyl CoA transport into the mitochondrion (18).

This mechanism could, at least partly, explain why the fat contribution to energy metabolism decreases when exercise intensity increases from 60% to 100% $\dot{V}O_2$max. The energy release from oxidation of FFA could be determined not only by the inflow of FFA to the muscle, but also by the catalytic activity of PDHa controlling the acetyl CoA accumulation and subsequently the concentration of CoASH.

Earlier studies of starvation have shown a reduced PDHa activity in rat skeletal muscle. The decrease was attributed to an adaptive increase in PDH-kinase activity during the starvation (8, 15, 27). Prolonged exposure to high kinase activity was also shown to phosphorylate additional sites of the E1 component of PDH and to reduce the rate of PDH transformation to PDHa after stimulation of the PDH phosphatase and inhibition of the kinase (25, 28). This mechanism could probably explain the incomplete transformation of PDH to its active form during the exercise after the LCD.

Availability and Choice of Substrate

Another important factor for the substrate choice during exercise after the two diets is the availability of muscle glycogen, which could limit pyruvate formation rate after the LCD and thus limit both PDHa formation and the catalytic activity of PDHa.

Significantly lower concentrations of pyruvate were observed after 16 min of exercise after the LCD compared to the concentration after the HCD. Over the same time period, the concentrations of acetyl CoA and acetylcarnitine fell in the LCD series, whereas the concentrations increased after the HCD (see figure 13.5b). This indicates differences in the initial rates of acetyl CoA formation in the HCD series with high glycogen availability compared with the LCD series with low glycogen availability combined with increased availability of fat. During the period from 16 to 47 min, the acetyl group concentrations were practically unchanged in both exercise series but remained on different concentration levels.

In two other studies in which subjects took a normal mixed diet, the substrates to the muscle were changed by infusion of a sodium acetate solution (26) or a triacylglycerol emulsion (7). In the first series, approximately 400 mmol of sodium acetate was given during a 20-min period of rest, followed by 5 min of exercise at 40% $\dot{V}O_2$max and 15 min at 80%. A control group was given sodium bicarbonate during the same rest and exercise protocol. As expected, during the rest period acetyl CoA and acetylcarnitine concentrations in muscle tissue increased (by 100% and 150%, respectively) when acetate was infused, and the PDHa fraction decreased by 50%. During exercise, however, both the acetyl CoA concentration and the PDHa fraction increased in the same way, regardless of the acetate or bicarbonate infusions. Only the acetylcarnitine concentration remained higher when acetate was given. No difference in glycogen utilization was observed in the two exercise series.

In the other study (7), a triacylglycerol emulsion and heparin were infused 20 min before and during 15 min of exercise at an intensity of 85% $\dot{V}O_2$max. The increased availability of lipid substrates resulted in a 40% reduction in glycogen utilization, as compared with a control experiment without fat infusion. The PDHa fraction and the concentrations of acetyl CoA and of acetylcarnitine were unchanged in the rest period and showed the same increase during the exercise without and with fat infusion. The citrate concentration was increased in resting muscle during the fat infusion, signifying mitochondrial uptake and utilization of fat, but during exercise the citrate concentrations did not differ between the control and fat-infusion series. Apparently, the glycogen sparing during the exercise with fat infusion cannot be explained by acetyl CoA inhibition of PDHa formation or by citrate inhibition of PFK activity.

Summary

PDH is the flux-generating step for pyruvate oxidation in muscle. In resting muscle, the transformation of PDH to its active form is inhibited by acetyl CoA accumulation derived from oxidation of fat substrates when the availability of these are increased. The result is decreased pyruvate oxidation.

In contracting muscle, the PDH transformation to active form is stimulated by the Ca^{2+} release from the sarcoplasmic reticulum, and the inhibition of transformation by acetyl CoA and NADH is at least partially overridden. The degree of PDH transformation is directly related to the intensity of the exercise. At the start of exercise, when the rate of acetyl CoA formation is higher than the turnover rate in the TCA cycle, acetyl groups are accumulated in the form of acetyl CoA and acetylcarnitine. At an exercise intensity of 75% of $\dot{V}O_2$max, 90% to 100% of the PDH complex is in active form.

If the glycogen content in exercising muscle is sufficient, the pyruvate flux through PDH may be high enough to cover the maximal catalytic activity of the α-ketoglutarate dehydrogenase enzyme and thus the maximal flux rate of the TCA cycle. The acetyl CoA derived from pyruvate is in this situation the sole energy substrate used for the oxidative phosphorylation in contracting muscle.

If the glycogen availability is low, as after a carbohydrate-poor diet, the pyruvate formation rate during the exercise will fall, resulting in a decreased catalytic activity of PDH, and a corresponding increase in acetyl CoA formation from fat. The lower accumulation of acetyl groups in muscle during exercise after intake of a carbohydrate-poor diet may stimulate fat utilization by increasing the availability of CoASH necessary for acyl CoA formation and transport.

Acknowledgments

These studies of the pyruvate dehydrogenase complex in muscle are done in collaboration with J.I. Carlin, G. Cederblad, D. Constantin-Teodosiu, D.J. Dyck, G.J.F. Heigenhauser, N.L. Jones, L.C. Lands, M.I. Lindinger, R.S. McKelvie, C.T. Putman, and L.L. Spriet.

The work has been supported by grants from the Karolinska Institute, the Swedish Medical Research Council, the Medical Research Council of Canada, and the Natural Science and Engineering Research Council of Canada.

References

1. Behal, R.H.; Buxton, D.B.; Robertson, J.G.; Olson, M.S. Regulation of the pyruvate dehydrogenase multienzyme complex. Annu. Rev. Nutr. 13:497-520; 1993.

2. Blomstrand, E.; Ekblom, B.; Newsholme, E.A. Maximum activities of key glycolytic and oxidative enzymes in human muscle from differently trained individuals. J. Physiol. 381:111-118; 1986.

3. Constantin-Teodosiu, D.; Carlin, J.I.; Cederblad, G.; Harris, R.C.; Hultman, E. Acetyl group accumulation and pyruvate dehydrogenase activity in human muscle during incremental exercise. Acta Physiol. Scand. 143:367-372; 1991.

4. Constantin-Teodosiu, D.; Cederblad, G.; Hultman, E. PDC activity and acetyl group accumulation in skeletal muscle during isometric contraction. J. Physiol. 74(4):1712-1718; 1993.

5. Constantin-Teodosiu, D.; Cederblad, G.; Hultman, E. PDC activity and acetyl group accumulation in skeletal muscle during prolonged exercise. J. Physiol. 73(6):2403-2407; 1992.

6. Cooper, R.H.; Randle, P.J.; Denton, R.M. Stimulation of phosphorylation and inactivation of pyruvate dehydrogenase by physiological inhibitors of the pyruvate dehydrogenase reaction. Nature 257:808-809; 1975.

7. Dyck, D.J.; Putman, C.T.; Heigenhauser, G.J.F.; Hultman, E.; Spriet, L.L. Regulation of fat-carbohydrate interaction in skeletal muscle during intense aerobic cycling. Am. J. Physiol. 265 (Endocrinol. Metab. 28):852-859; 1993.

8. Fuller, S.J.; Randle, P.J. Reversible phosphorylation of pyruvate dehydrogenase in rat skeletal-muscle mitochondria: Effects of starvation and diabetes. Biochem. J. 219:635-646; 1984.

9. Garland, P.B.; Newsholme, E.A.; Randle, P.J. Effects of fatty acids and ketone bodies and of alloxan diabetes and starvation on pyruvate metabolism. Biochem. J. 93:665-678; 1964.

10. Garland, P.B.; Randle, P.J. Control of pyruvate dehydrogenase in the perfused rat heart by the intracellular concentration of acetyl CoA. Biochem. J. 91:6C-7C; 1964.

11. Garland, P.B.; Randle, P.J.; Newsholme, E.A. Citrate as an intermediary in the inhibition of phosphofructokinase in rat heart muscle by fatty acids, ketone bodies, pyruvate, diabetes and starvation. Nature 200:169-170; 1963.

12. Holness, M.J.; Sugden, M.C. Glucose utilization in heart, diaphragm and skeletal muscle during the fed-to-starved transition. Biochem. J. 270:245-249; 1990.

13. Idell-Wenger, J.A.; Grotyohann, L.W.; Neely, J.R. Coenzyme A and carnitine distribution in normal and ischemic hearts. J. Biol. Chem. 253:4310-4318; 1978.

14. Kanzaki, T.; Hayakawa, T.; Hamada, M.; Fukuyoski, Y.; Koike, M. Mammalian α-keto acid dehydrogenase complexes: Substrate specificities of the pig heart pyruvate dehydrogenase and α-ketoglutarate dehydrogenase complexes. J. Biol. Chem. 244:1183-1187; 1969.

15. Kerbey, A.L.; Radcliffe, P.M.; Randle, P.J. Diabetes and the control of pyruvate dehydrogenase in rat heart mitochondria by concentration ratios of adenosine triphosphate/adenosine diphosphate, of reduced/oxidized nicotinamide adenine dinucleotide and acetylCoA/coenzyme A. Biochem. J. 164:509-519; 1977.

16. Linn, T.C.; Pettit, F.H.; Reed, L.J. Regulation of the activity of the pyruvate dehydrogenase complex from beef kidney mitochondria by phosphorylation and dephosphorylation. Proc. Natl. Acad. Sci. USA 62:234-241; 1969.

17. Lysiak, W.; Toth, P.P.; Suelter, C.H.; Bieber, L.L. Quantitation of the efflux of acylcarnitines from rat heart, brain and liver mitochondria. J. Biol. Chem. 261: 13698-13703; 1986.

18. Newsholme, E.A.; Leech, A.R. The integration of metabolism during starvation, refeeding, and injury. In: Biochemistry for the medical sciences. Toronto: Wiley; 1988:330-331.

19. Nilsson, H.; Hson, L.; Hultman, E. Liver glycogen in man—The effect of total starvation or a carbohydrate-poor diet followed by carbohydrate refeeding. Scand. J. Clin. Lab. Invest. 32:325-330; 1973.

20. Pande, S.V.; Parvin, R. Characterization of carnitine acylcarnitine translocase system of heart mitochondria. J. Biol. Chem. 251: 6683-6691; 1976.

21. Pettit, F.H.; Pelley, J.W.; Reed, L.J. Regulation of pyruvate dehydrogenase kinase and phosphatase by acetyl-CoA/CoA and NADH/NAD$^+$ ratios. Biochem. Biophys. Res. Commun. 65:575-582; 1975.

22. Putman, C.T.; Spriet, L.L.; Hultman, E.; Lindinger, M.I.; Lands, L.C.; Cederblad, G.; Jones, N.L.; Heigenhauser, G.J.F. Pyruvate dehydrogenase activity and acetyl group accumulation during exercise after different diets. Am. J. Physiol. 265 (Endocrinol. Metab. 28):752-760; 1993.

23. Randle, P.J.; Garland, P.B.; Hales, C.N.; Newsholme, E.A. The glucose-fatty acid cycle: Its role in insulin sensitivity and the metabolic disturbances of diabetes mellitus. Lancet i:3785-3789; 1963.

24. Roche, T.E.; Patel, M.S. α-Keto acid dehydrogenase complexes: Organization, regulation and biomedical ramifications. Ann. N.Y. Acad. Sci. 573:1-473; 1989.

25. Sale, G.J.; Randle, P.J. Occupancy of phosphorylation sites in pyruvate dehydrogenase phosphate complex in rat heart in vivo. Biochem. J. 206:221-229; 1982.

26. Spriet, L.L.; Putman, C.T.; Dyck, D.J.; Heigenhauser, G.J.F.; Hultman, E. Effects of acetate infusion on muscle pyruvate dehydrogenase activity and acetyl group accumulation. Med. Sci. Sports Exercise 26 (suppl.):203; 1994.

27. Sugden, M.C.; Holness, M.J. Effects of re-feeding after prolonged starvation on pyruvate dehydrogenase activities in heart, diaphragm and selected skeletal muscles of the rat. Biochem. J. 262:669-672; 1989.

28. Sugden, P.H.; Hutson, N.J.; Kerbey, A.L.; Randle, P.J. Phosphorylation of additional sites on pyruvate dehydrogenase inhibits its re-activation by pyruvate dehydrogenase phosphate dehydrogenase. Biochem. J. 169:433-435; 1978.

29. Wieland, O.H. The mammalian pyruvate dehydrogenase complex: Structure and regulation. Rev. Physiol. Biochem. 96:123-170; 1983.

30. Williamson, J.R.; Krebs, H.A. Acetate as a fuel of respiration in the perfused rat heart. Biochem. J. 80:540-547; 1961.

CHAPTER 14

Malonyl CoA as a Metabolic Regulator

William W. Winder
Brigham Young University, Provo, Utah, U.S.A.

Malonyl CoA in Lipogenic Tissues

In the lipogenic tissues (liver, adipose tissue), malonyl CoA is an intermediate in the metabolic pathway that converts carbohydrate to fatty acids (12). It is formed by carboxylation of acetyl CoA by the cytosolic enzyme acetyl CoA carboxylase (ACC; figure 14.1; 9). Malonyl CoA then serves as the principal source of two-carbon units for synthesis of the long-chain fatty acids by fatty acid synthase (EC 6.2.1.3). In the liver, malonyl CoA also is an inhibitor of fatty acid oxidation (12, 18). When carbohydrate is present in abundance, glucose may be converted to fatty acids and triglycerides. The consequent rise in malonyl CoA inhibits fatty acid oxidation at the same time as fatty acids are being synthesized.

The transfer of long-chain fatty acids into the mitochondria where the β-oxidation enzymes are located is mediated by the carnitine palmitoyl transferase (CPT) system (figure 14.2; 12, 18, 20). CPT I (EC 1.3.99.1) is located on the inner surface of the outer mitochondrial membrane (18). This enzyme forms the carnitine derivative of the fatty acid from the CoA derivative. After traversing the inner mitochondrial membrane, the CoA derivative of the fatty acid is regenerated due to the action of CPT II. Only CPT I is specifically inhibited by malonyl CoA. The malonyl CoA–binding component of CPT I has a domain exposed to the exterior of the mitochondrion. High levels of malonyl CoA present in the cytosol can therefore prevent oxidation of fatty acids by inhibition of CPT I. In the liver, the Vmax of CPT I is increased, and the sensitivity of CPT I to malonyl CoA inhibition is decreased in response to prolonged fasting (18).

Acetyl–CoA Carboxylase

$$Acetyl-CoA + ATP + CO_2 \longrightarrow Malonyl-CoA + ADP + Pi$$

Figure 14.1 The acetyl CoA carboxylase reaction.

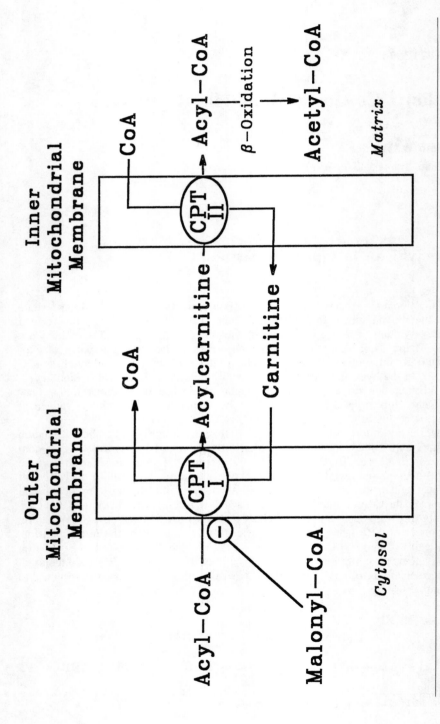

Figure 14.2   The carnitine palmitoyl transferase system.

The liver ACC that synthesizes malonyl CoA is a very large protein, consisting of a single polypeptide chain with a molecular mass of 265 kDa (2, 8). A minor 280-kDa isozyme is also present. This enzyme is subject to both long-term and rapidly acting mechanisms of regulation. Fasting results in a marked decrease in both measurable enzyme activity and in amount of protein quantitated by immunological techniques, as well as a decrease in the liver content of the product malonyl CoA (2, 8, 14, 16). Refeeding with a fat-free, high-carbohydrate diet causes a marked increase in total activity and amount of enzyme protein. The enzyme is subject to regulation by phosphorylation (3, 10). Both cAMP-dependent protein kinase and AMP-activated protein kinase phosphorylate and inactivate the liver ACC (3, 7, 10). The action of specific phosphatases activates the enzyme (10). Insulin activates ACC, apparently by phosphorylation-induced inactivation of the AMP-activated protein kinase (27). The enzyme is subject to allosteric activation by citrate and to inhibition by malonyl CoA and by long-chain fatty acyl CoA (9). In summary, when carbohydrate is present in abundance, plasma insulin concentration is elevated, resulting in activation of ACC, elevation of malonyl CoA, and consequent inhibition of fatty acid oxidation and ketogenesis. Carbons originating in carbohydrate are incorporated into fatty acids, malonyl CoA being the intermediate. When carbohydrate supply is limited (as is the case during fasting or prolonged exercise), glucagon and catecholamines are elevated, ACC is phosphorylated and inactivated, malonyl CoA is decreased, and fatty acid oxidation and ketogenesis proceeds.

Malonyl CoA in Heart and Skeletal Muscle

Heart and skeletal muscle are generally thought of as being nonlipogenic tissues; that is, they do not have a high capacity to convert carbohydrate carbon to fatty acids. It therefore came as somewhat of a surprise to find malonyl CoA, an intermediate in the pathway from glucose to fatty acids, present in these tissues (13). The CPT I of skeletal muscle and heart appears to be more sensitive to inhibition by malonyl CoA than is the CPT I of liver (13, 15, 18). The concentration of malonyl CoA that gives 50% inhibition (I_{50}) of CPT I is in the range of 1.7 μM for liver and 0.04 μM for skeletal muscle. The role of malonyl CoA in these nonlipogenic tissues has been postulated to be principally that of regulation of fatty acid oxidation (13, 18, 25).

Recent studies in perfused hearts and in cardiac myocytes have yielded important information concerning the role of malonyl CoA in this tissue. Saddik and co-workers (17) demonstrated an inverse correlation between the rate of fatty acid oxidation and malonyl CoA content in isolated, perfused, contracting rat hearts. Saggerson's laboratory (1) demonstrated in cardiac myocytes that malonyl CoA content could be increased with insulin and decreased with epinephrine treatments.

Skeletal Muscle Malonyl CoA During Exercise

Initial studies by McGarry demonstrated that skeletal muscle malonyl CoA decreased in response to fasting (13). We reasoned that if malonyl CoA is an important regulator of fatty acid metabolism in muscle, we would expect to see a decrease in malonyl CoA during exercise. In an initial experiment (23), rats were run on a treadmill for 30 min up a 15% grade. Rats were anesthetized rapidly by intravenous infusion of pentobarbital, and gastrocnemius muscles were frozen for malonyl CoA analysis. During the course of the 30-min run, malonyl CoA decreased to 38% of the resting value.

In a subsequent study (25), the time course of the change in malonyl CoA was examined during a prolonged bout of exercise (figure 14.3). Rats were initially taught to run on the treadmill for 2 wk for 5 to 10 min/d. Jugular catheters were installed 3 d prior to the final exercise test to allow rapid induction of anesthesia and rapid removal of the muscles. Rats ran at 21 m/min up a 15% grade for intervals ranging from 5 min to 120 min. Samples of the superficial quadriceps (having a high concentration of type IIb fibers), of the region of the quadriceps near the femur (having a high concentration of type IIa fibers), and of the soleus (composed of type I fibers) were quick-frozen in liquid nitrogen and later analyzed for malonyl CoA. In resting rats, the concentration of malonyl CoA was higher in the muscles having a higher capacity to oxidize fatty acids. A significant decrease in the red region of the quadriceps was observed after 5 min of exercise (figure 14.3). Malonyl CoA continued to decrease to a plateau at 30 min of exercise. The decline was more gradual in the white quadriceps. The time course of the decline in malonyl CoA appeared to follow the general time course of decline in muscle glycogen in these two muscle types. This may be related to the recruitment pattern. The white fibers of the superficial quadriceps would be expected to be recruited later during the course of the exercise than would the red fibers at this work rate. The slower rate in decline of glycogen in the white quadriceps provides some evidence for this supposition.

The decline in malonyl CoA in the red quadriceps appeared to precede the rise in plasma free fatty acids, implying that the muscle becomes metabolically set for an increase in fatty acid oxidation even prior to the time when fatty acids become available for oxidation in large quantities. Increase in fatty acid availability by intramuscular lipolysis may not be reflected by plasma FFA, however. Previous studies have implied that intramuscular triglyceride stores can be a significant source of fatty acids for oxidation during exercise, particularly in endurance-trained individuals (11, 19). The time course of utilization of this source of fatty acids is not obvious at this time, however.

Synthesis of Malonyl CoA in Muscle by Acetyl CoA Carboxylase

It seems clear, then, that the concentration of malonyl CoA in muscle can change markedly in response to different physiological perturbations. The next question of how malonyl CoA is controlled in the muscle is of particular importance if the concentration of malonyl CoA is critical for governing the rate of fatty acid oxidation. The synthesis of malonyl CoA appears to be catalyzed by an ACC, as in liver (22). High-speed (50,000 × g) supernatants were prepared from hindlimb muscles and were assayed for capacity to catalyze malonyl CoA formation from acetyl CoA. Elimination of any one of the substrates for ACC (ATP, bicarbonate, or acetyl CoA) markedly decreased the rate of malonyl CoA appearance in the reaction mixture.

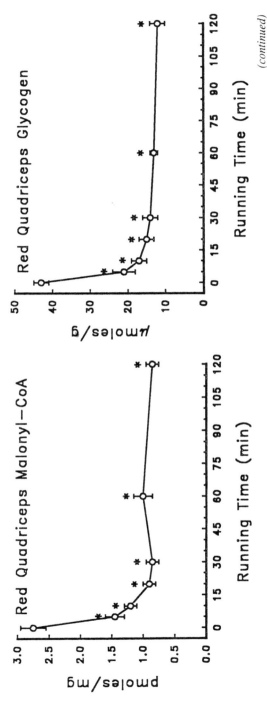

Figure 14.3 Effect of treadmill exercise (21 m/min, 15% grade) on malonyl CoA and glycogen in red and white quadriceps muscle of rats. Values are means ± *SE*.
Adapted from Winder, Arogyasami, Elayan, and Cartmill 1990.

(continued)

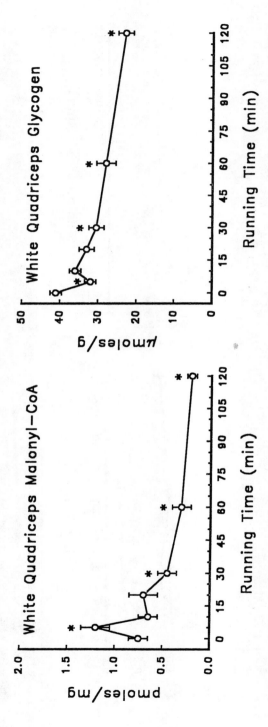

Figure 14.3 *(continued)*

The synthesis of malonyl CoA was found to be almost entirely dependent on the presence of citrate in the medium. Inclusion of avidin, which inhibits biotin-containing enzymes, completely prevented synthesis of malonyl CoA by the high-speed supernatant. These data clearly point to ACC as the enzyme in muscle responsible for synthesis of malonyl CoA. The enzyme has now been isolated and purified using ammonium sulfate precipitation followed by avidin-sepharose affinity chromatography (23). The enzyme is inhibited by palmitoyl CoA and malonyl CoA and is stimulated by citrate. The molecular weight appears to be in the range of 272 kDa, near that reported for the principal isoform in heart (2, 8, 21).

Muscle Malonyl CoA Decreases During Electrical Stimulation

In the initial observation of the decline in malonyl CoA during exercise, an increase in plasma catecholamines and muscle cAMP accompanied the change in muscle malonyl CoA. The liver ACC is subject to regulation by cAMP-dependent protein kinase (10). Phosphorylation by this kinase causes a decrease in Vmax for the enzyme. The liver enzyme is also inactivated by phosphorylation induced by an AMP-activated (cAMP-independent) protein kinase (3, 10). We hypothesized that the muscle form of the enzyme may also be sensitive to regulation by a process initiated by the rise in free calcium or some other intracellular change (e.g., increase in AMP) associated with muscle contraction. We therefore investigated the effects of in situ electrical stimulation of the sciatic nerve on malonyl CoA in the gastrocnemius-plantaris group in anesthetized rats (5). Electrical stimulation of one sciatic nerve would be expected to increase sarcoplasmic free calcium in the muscles innervated by that nerve but not in the contralateral muscles. Measurement of malonyl CoA and other metabolites in the resting contralateral muscles controls for possible humoral changes. By trial and error, a stimulation pattern was selected that had no effect on muscle ATP, citrate, or cAMP that could influence ACC activity. Muscles were stimulated at a frequency of 5/s (10-ms duration) at a voltage that produced maximal twitch tension. A 45% decrease in malonyl CoA was observed after 5 min of stimulation. No change was noted in ATP, citrate, or cAMP. The significance of this finding is that it clearly demonstrates that the decrease in malonyl CoA can occur in the absence of a change in cAMP. This indirectly implicates a calcium-mediated system of control or another cAMP-independent means of control of malonyl CoA synthesis in muscle.

Epinephrine Unessential for the Decrease in Malonyl CoA During Exercise

The idea of a cAMP-independent control of muscle malonyl CoA synthesis receives additional support from an in vivo study (26). The purpose of this study was to determine if the usual exercise-induced increase in epinephrine (with consequent rise in muscle cAMP) is responsible for the decrease in muscle malonyl CoA.

Rats were either adrenodemedullated or sham operated and allowed to recover for at least 3 wk. They were then subjected to a run of 60 min in the fed state or a 15- or 30-min run after fasting 24 h. Plasma epinephrine increased in sham-operated rats during exercise, but not in adrenodemedullated rats. Malonyl CoA decreased to the same extent in adrenodemedullated rats as in sham-operated rats. These studies clearly establish the fact that a rise in plasma epinephrine is not essential for inducing the exercise-induced decline in muscle malonyl CoA. It is conceivable, however, that the ACC activity can be decreased by more than one mechanism. The enzyme may in fact be sensitive to control by epinephrine, but a second cAMP-independent mechanism may induce the decline in malonyl CoA during exercise. Although the possibility of epinephrine being involved in the regulation of skeletal muscle ACC cannot be ruled out by this experiment, the data clearly indicate that a rise in plasma epinephrine is not essential for causing the decline in malonyl CoA during exercise.

Insulin and Glucose Are Necessary for Maintaining Malonyl CoA

Additional information concerning the regulation of malonyl CoA in muscle comes from hindlimb perfusion studies (4). We hypothesized that if malonyl CoA is important in controlling the fat-carbohydrate oxidation mix in muscle, then the muscle concentration of malonyl CoA should be elevated when glucose and insulin are present in abundance and should be decreased when the supply of glucose is decreased. Isolated rat hindlimbs were perfused with Krebs-Henseleit bicarbonate buffer containing fresh erythrocytes (hematocrit = 41), a complete amino acid mixture, and albumin for 60 min. Two experiments were performed. In the first, hindlimbs were perfused with medium containing 10 mM glucose and 100 μU/ml of insulin (regular bovine/porcine, Eli Lilly) or with medium containing no glucose and no insulin. Without glucose and insulin, the malonyl CoA content of the gastrocnemius-plantaris decreased to 31% of the level in the contralateral control muscle. Inclusion of 10 mM glucose and 100 μU/ml of insulin in the perfusion medium markedly attenuated this decline in muscle malonyl CoA. In the second perfusion experiment, hindlimbs were perfused with medium containing a combination of 10 mM glucose and 200 μU/ml insulin or with glucose or insulin alone. Malonyl CoA was decreased in gastrocnemius-plantaris perfused with glucose alone and with insulin alone compared with hindlimbs perfused with a combination of glucose and insulin (figure 14.4). Muscles perfused with different media had no change in citrate or cAMP. ATP was slightly lower in muscles perfused without glucose and insulin but was not influenced in muscles perfused with only glucose or only insulin. Thus, the decrease in malonyl CoA was not dependent on changes in citrate, cAMP, or ATP. The liver ACC is activated by insulin. It appears that muscle ACC is also subject to regulation by insulin.

Glucose Infusion Into Exercising Rats Attenuates Decrease in Malonyl CoA

An in vivo study has been performed to determine the effect of provision of excess carbohydrate on these muscle changes in malonyl CoA (figure 14.5; 6).

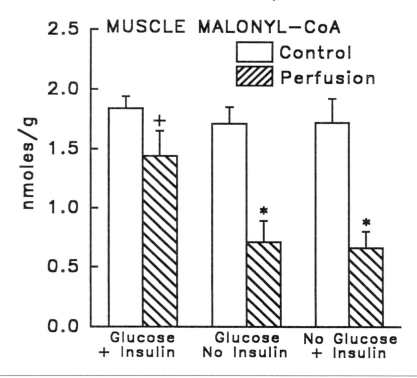

Figure 14.4   Muscle malonyl CoA concentration in gastrocnemius-plantaris taken before perfusion (control) and after 50-min perfusion with medium containing 10 mM glucose and 200 µU/ml insulin, 10 mM glucose alone, or 200 µU/ml insulin alone. Medium contained washed bovine erythrocytes and albumin in Krebs-Henseleit bicarbonate buffer. * = significantly different from control. + = significantly different from muscles perfused with glucose alone and insulin alone; $p < .05$.
Reprinted from Duan and Winder 1993.

During 30 or 60 min of treadmill exercise, rats were infused with either glucose (0.625 g/ml) or saline at a rate of 1.5 ml/h. This rate of glucose infusion increased blood glucose concentration to 10 mM, prevented liver glycogen utilization, and reduced the rate of muscle glycogenolysis. Glucose infusion also prevented the normal exercise-induced rise in plasma FFA. Gastrocnemius muscle malonyl CoA decreased from 1.2 to 0.7 nmol/g with glucose infusion and to 0.4 nmol/g with saline infusion. In the liver, glucose infusion prevented the exercise-induced drop in malonyl CoA. Plasma insulin was also significantly elevated in glucose-infused rats compared with saline-infused rats. Thus, the normal exercise-induced decrease in malonyl CoA in muscle is attenuated when the supply of glucose is supplemented by infusion.

Summary

In summary, malonyl CoA is present in skeletal muscle, a nonlipogenic tissue. Malonyl CoA inhibits skeletal muscle CPT I. Malonyl CoA is synthesized in skeletal

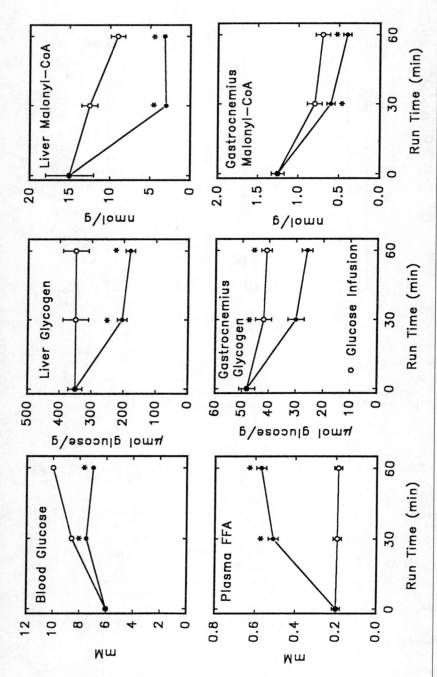

Figure 14.5 Effect of glucose infusion (1.5 ml/h; 0.625 g/ml) on blood glucose, plasma FFA, liver and muscle glycogen, and malonyl CoA in exercising rats (21 m/min, 15% grade). * = significantly different from glucose-infused rats (open circles); *p* < .05. Closed circles = data from saline-infused rats.

muscle by an ACC. It decreases in response to fasting and exercise. Both glucose and insulin are required for maintenance of malonyl CoA in perfused hindlimb muscle. Epinephrine is not required for the exercise-induced decrease in malonyl CoA. Infusion of glucose attenuates the decrease in muscle malonyl CoA during exercise. These observations are consistent with the hypothesis that malonyl CoA plays a role in regulation of fatty acid oxidation in working skeletal muscle during exercise.

Acknowledgment

This work was supported by a grant from the National Institute of Arthritis and Musculoskeletal and Skin Diseases, grant AR-41438.

References

1. Awan, M.M.; Saggerson, E.D. Malonyl-CoA metabolism in cardiac myocytes and its relevance to the control of fatty acid oxidation. Biochem. J. 295:61-66; 1993.
2. Bianchi, A.; Evans, J.L.; Iverson, A.J.; Nordlund, A.; Watts, T.D.; Witters, L.A. Identification of an isozymic form of acetyl-CoA carboxylase. J. Biol. Chem. 265:1502-1509; 1990.
3. Carling, D.; Clarke, P.R.; Zammit, V.A.; Hardie, D.G. Purification and characterization of the AMP-activated protein kinase. Eur. J. Biochem. 186:129-136; 1989.
4. Duan, C.; Winder, W.W. Control of malonyl-CoA by glucose and insulin in perfused skeletal muscle. J. Appl. Physiol. 74:2543-2547; 1993.
5. Duan, C.; Winder, W.W. Nerve stimulation decreases malonyl-CoA in skeletal muscle. J. Appl. Physiol. 72:901-904; 1992.
6. Elayan, I.M.; Winder, W.W. Effect of glucose infusion on muscle malonyl-CoA during exercise. J. Appl. Physiol. 70:1495-1499; 1991.
7. Hardie, D.G. Regulation of fatty acid synthesis via phosphorylation of acetyl-CoA carboxylase. Prog. Lipid Res. 28:117-146; 1989.
8. Iverson, A.J.; Bianchi, A.; Nordlund, A.; Witters, L.A. Immunological analysis of acetyl-CoA carboxylase mass, tissue distribution and subunit composition. Biochem. J. 269:365-371; 1990.
9. Kim, K.H. Regulation of acetyl-CoA carboxylase. Curr. Top. Cell. Regul. 22:143-176; 1983.
10. Kim, K.H.; Lopez-Casillas, F.; Bai, D.H.; Luo, X.; Pape, M.E. Role of reversible phosphorylation of acetyl-CoA carboxylase in long-chain fatty acid synthesis. FASEB J. 3:2250-2256; 1989.
11. Martin, W.H.; Dalsky, G.P.; Hurley, B.F.; Matthews, D.E.; Bier, D.M.; Hagberg, J.M.; Rogers, M.A.; King, D.S.; Holloszy, J.O. Effect of endurance training on plasma free fatty acid turnover and oxidation during exercise. Am. J. Physiol. 265:E708-E714; 1993.
12. McGarry, J.D.; Foster, D.W. Regulation of hepatic fatty acid oxidation and ketone body concentration. Annu. Rev. Biochem. 49:395-420; 1980.

13. McGarry, J.D.; Mills, S.E.; Long, C.S.; Foster, D.W. Observation on the affinity for carnitine, and malonyl-CoA, of carnitine palmitoyl transferase I in animal and human tissue. Biochem. J. 214:21-28; 1983.

14. McGarry, J.D.; Stark, M.J.; Foster, D.W. Hepatic malonyl-CoA levels of fed, fasted and diabetic rats as measured using a simple radioisotopic assay. J. Biol. Chem. 253:8291-8293; 1978.

15. Mills, S.E.; Foster, D.W.; McGarry, J.D. Interaction of malonyl-CoA and related compounds with mitochondria from different rat tissues. Biochem. J. 214:83-91; 1983.

16. Moir, M.B.; Zammit, V.A. Changes in the properties of cytosolic acetyl-CoA carboxylase studied in cold-clamped liver samples from fed, starved, and starved-refed rats. Biochem. J. 272:511-517; 1990.

17. Saddik, M.; Gamble, J.; Witters, L.A.; Lopaschuk, G.D. Acetyl-CoA carboxylase regulation of fatty acid oxidation in the heart. J. Biol. Chem. 268:25836-25845; 1993.

18. Saggerson, D.; Ghadiminejad, I.; Awan, M. Regulation of mitochondrial carnitine palmitoyl transferases from liver and extrahepatic tissues. Adv. Enzyme Regul. 32:285-306; 1992.

19. Saltin, B.; Astrand, P. Free fatty acids and exercise. Am. J. Clin. Nutr. 57 (suppl.):752S-758S; 1993.

20. Sugden, M.C.; Holness, M.J. Interactive regulation of the pyruvate dehydrogenase complex and the carnitine palmitoyltransferase system. FASEB J. 8:54-61; 1994.

21. Thampy, K.G. Formation of malonyl-coenzyme A in rat heart. J. Biol. Chem. 264:17631-17634; 1989.

22. Trumble, G.E.; Smith, M.A.; Winder, W.W. Evidence of a biotin dependent acetyl-coenzyme A carboxylase in rat muscle. Life Sci. 49:39-43; 1991.

23. Trumble, G.E.; Smith, M.A.; Winder, W.W. Purification and characterization of rat skeletal muscle acetyl-CoA carboxylase. Eur. J. Biochem. 231:192-198; 1995.

24. Winder, W.W.; Arogyasami, J.; Barton, R.J.; Elayan, I.M.; Vehrs, P.R. Muscle malonyl-CoA decreases during exercise. J. Appl. Physiol. 67:2230-2233; 1989.

25. Winder, W.W.; Arogyasami, J.; Elayan, I.M.; Cartmill, D. Time course of exercise-induced decline in malonyl-CoA in different muscle types. Am. J. Physiol. 259:E266-E271; 1990.

26. Winder, W.W.; Braiden, R.W.; Cartmill, D.C.; Hutber, C.A.; Jones, J.P. Effect of adrenodemedullation on decline in muscle malonyl-CoA during exercise. J. Appl. Physiol. 74:2548-2551; 1993.

27. Witters, L.A.; Kemp, B.E. Insulin activation of acetyl-CoA carboxylase accompanied by inhibition of the 5'-AMP-activated protein kinase. J. Biol. Chem. 267:2864-2867; 1992.

CHAPTER 15

Glucose–Fatty Acid Cycle and Fatigue Involving 5-Hydroxytryptamine

Eva E. Blomstrand, Eric A. Newsholme

Pripps Bryggerier, Research Laboratories, Stockholm, Sweden;
University of Oxford, Oxford, England

The mechanisms that underlie fatigue during physical exercise have attracted the attention of physiologists and biochemists for many years. A large number of studies have been published concerning muscle (peripheral) fatigue, and several causative factors have been identified, for example, accumulation of protons, depletion of glycogen, and failure of neuromuscular transmission. However, very little is known about the mechanisms of central fatigue (i.e., fatigue resulting from failure or limitations within the central nervous system). A few mechanisms have been suggested to cause central fatigue, including changes in brain monoamine concentrations (25) and accumulation of ammonia in the brain during exercise (27). In 1986 it was suggested (25) that changes in plasma amino acid concentrations could play a role in central fatigue by influencing the synthesis and release of neurotransmitters, particularly 5-hydroxytryptamine (5-HT), in the brain. Because 5-HT is known to be involved in the regulation of, for example, sleep and changes in mood, it was suggested that this neurotransmitter might also be involved in the type of fatigue that occurs during and after vigorous and sustained physical exercise. Furthermore, the synthesis and metabolism of 5-HT in the brain has been shown to increase in response to exercise.

The rate of 5-HT synthesis is known to be sensitive to the supply of its precursor, tryptophan (Trp). The first reaction in the synthesis of 5-HT is catalyzed by the enzyme tryptophan mono-oxygenase, which is considered to be the rate-limiting step in the synthesis of 5-HT (26). Since this enzyme may not be saturated with substrate, an increased supply of Trp could increase the rate of 5-HT synthesis. This implies that the uptake of Trp by the brain is an important factor in the regulation of 5-HT synthesis. The transport of Trp into the brain is known to be regulated by both the availability of Trp in the bloodstream and the concentration of other large neutral amino acids (LNAA), including tyrosine, phenylalanine, methionine, and the branched-chain amino acids (BCAA) that compete with Trp for transport into the brain (28).

Exercise and Brain Monoamine Metabolism

The first report on the effect of strenuous exercise on brain monoamine metabolism was presented in a study by Barchas and Freedman in 1963 (4), who found an increase in the concentration of 5-HT in the brain after rats had swum to exhaustion. These results were supported by the findings of Romanowski and Grabiec (31), who also reported that exhausting exercise, in this case running, caused the brain 5-HT level to rise in the rat. In fact, the latter authors suggested that the observed increase in 5-HT during exercise could cause central fatigue. However, the mechanism behind the increase in 5-HT was not known. Further support for an effect of exercise on brain 5-HT metabolism can be found in studies by Chaouloff and co-workers (see 11). In these studies, 1 h of treadmill exercise was reported to increase the brain level of Trp and the 5-HT metabolite, 5-hydroxyindoleacetic acid (5-HIAA), but no effect of exercise on the 5-HT concentration was found. However, the 5-HIAA level was increased in the ventricular cerebrospinal fluid after exercise, indicating that the rate of release of 5-HT had been increased during exercise.

When rats were exercised on a treadmill to exhaustion, an increased level of both 5-HT and 5-HIAA was found in the brain stem and hypothalamus. An increased level of 5-HIAA was also found in the striatum and hippocampus, but no changes were found in the cortex and cerebellum (10). One possible explanation of the variable response to exercise in different areas of the brain might be that an enzyme in the biochemical pathway from Trp to 5-HT approaches saturation with substrate in some parts of the brain. Since the Trp level was elevated in all parts of the brain that were measured, the increased rate of synthesis of 5-HT would only occur in those parts in which the enzyme is not saturated with substrate, namely the brain stem and hypothalamus. It should also be noted that the variation in the results of different studies might be explained by different types of exercise, different work intensities, or different durations of exercise.

Further supporting evidence for the involvement of 5-HT in fatigue has recently been presented in three studies: Administration of a 5-HT agonist to rats was reported to impair running performance in a dose-related manner (2); administration of a 5-HT antagonist improved running performance (3); and administration of a 5-HT reuptake blocker to human subjects lowered the physical performance in terms of exercise time to exhaustion during standardized exercise as compared with a control condition (36). No signs of circulatory effects of the drug were discovered during exercise. However, it cannot be ruled out that these drugs, especially at high doses, might have effects on the peripheral metabolism or central circulation that may influence performance.

Exercise has also been reported to increase the synthesis and metabolism of dopamine (DA) and noradrenaline (NA) in the whole brain or in specific parts of the brain (6, 12, 17, 20). Chaouloff et al. (12) suggested that an increased concentration of DA in some parts of the brain could inhibit the synthesis of 5-HT during exercise and thereby delay fatigue. An increase in the central DA activity has also been suggested to improve physical performance (19). This was based on the observation that rats treated with apomorphine, a DA-receptor agonist, increased their exercise capacity. Treatment with clonidine, a NA-receptor agonist, had no effect on exercise performance. However, there are a few studies in which exercise is reported to cause no change in the synthesis of brain catecholamines (17, 33). It is also possible in this case that the variability of the results can be explained by different types of exercise, different intensities, and different durations of the exercise period.

Changes in the Plasma Concentration Ratio of Free Trp to Other LNAA During and After Exercise

Several studies have shown that during physical exercise there is a change in the rates of uptake or release of amino acids from various tissues in the body, particularly the liver and the working muscles (1, 16, 32). The changes that occur in plasma levels of amino acids are largely dependent on the type of exercise and its intensity and duration. Mild, short-term exercise caused no change in the arterial concentration of aromatic and branched-chain amino acids, whereas at heavier work loads their concentrations increased by 8% to 35% during exercise, most likely caused by an altered splanchnic exchange rather than increased peripheral release (16). On the other hand, Bergström, Fürst, and Hultman (5) found a decrease in BCAA after 10 and 20 min of exercise at 70% of maximal oxygen uptake ($\dot{V}O_2$max).

With 4 h of exercise at 30% of $\dot{V}O_2$max, there is an uptake of BCAA by the working muscle, but there is also a release of BCAA from the splanchnic bed, causing the arterial concentration of these amino acids to increase. Also, the level of the aromatic amino acids was increased after 4 h of exercise (1). When subjects exercised at 50% of $\dot{V}O_2$max for 3.5 h, the concentration of the aromatic and branched-chain amino acids increased during the first 90 min of exercise, but as exercise progressed, the levels of amino acids fell progressively, and at the end of exercise, the BCAA concentration was slightly lower than at rest (30). During exercise at 75% of $\dot{V}O_2$max, the level of BCAA remained approximately unchanged or increased slightly, while the level of the aromatic amino acids increased by 40% to 50% during exercise (23, 32). However, when exercise starts with reduced muscle glycogen stores, a decrease in the plasma concentration of BCAA has been reported during exercise (35). Some time after the end of exercise (100-km race, 70-km cross-country ski race, marathon race), the plasma concentration of BCAA is markedly decreased (20-85%) and that of the aromatic amino acids had returned to the preexercise level (7, 15, 29).

Tryptophan is the only amino acid that is transported bound to albumin in the plasma (24). In the resting condition, approximately 10% is in the free form, and therefore approximately 90% is bound to albumin. There has been controversy in the literature as to whether the albumin-bound Trp is taken up by the brain from the plasma or whether only the free Trp pool is available for uptake. We consider that the free concentration of Trp rather than the total governs the rate of entry of Trp into the neurons and that the free Trp therefore competes with other LNAA for transport into the brain. The plasma concentration of free Trp has been found to increase during, and especially after, prolonged exercise (7, 14). This change in free Trp can be related to an increased rate of release of free fatty acids (FFA) from adipose tissue during exercise and to an increased plasma level of FFA. Thus, like Trp, the FFA are transported bound to albumin in the plasma, and an increase in their concentration decreases the binding of Trp to albumin (13) and thereby increases the plasma free-Trp level.

Consequently, the type of exercise during which the plasma concentration ratio of free Trp to other LNAA increases is mainly sustained heavy exercise. Based on experience, the type of exercise that causes mental fatigue is sustained heavy exercise or intermittent activity, which leads to a faster depletion of the muscle glycogen stores. Unfortunately, no data on changes in the plasma concentration of amino acids during intermittent exercise are available in the literature.

According to the theory presented earlier, an increase in the free Trp/other LNAA plasma concentration ratio will favor the transport of Trp into the brain and also the synthesis and the level of 5-HT in the brain; this may maintain or allow higher rates of neuronal firing in some 5-HT neurons, which might cause fatigue at the end of or after such exercise. An important prediction of the theory is that, to maintain the concentration ratio of free Trp to other LNAA, an increase in the plasma concentration of the other LNAA (e.g., the BCAA) should maintain the normal rate of transport of Trp into the brain. This would prevent an increase in the rate of synthesis of 5-HT and therefore prevent an increase in the level of 5-HT, which may delay fatigue and improve mental alertness during such exercise.

Effect of Supplementing Branched-Chain Amino Acids Alone or in Combination With Carbohydrates During Exercise

When BCAA were taken during exercise, their plasma concentration increased (figure 15.1), which was to be expected from earlier studies in which BCAA were given either orally or intravenously to healthy subjects. Also, the plasma concentration of free Trp increased 35% during exercise and 140% 5 min after exercise, causing a similar increase in the plasma concentration ratio of free Trp to other LNAA (figure 15.1). Intake of BCAA prevented an increase in this ratio during and after exercise, which in previous studies has been found to maintain or increase mental alertness evaluated as performance on different psychological tests after exercise (9, 18). However, these studies were carried out during competitive exercise, and no evaluation of mental fatigue was made during the exercise. In a recent study, supplying BCAA (90-100 mg/kg body weight; 40% valine, 35% leucine, 25% isoleucine) to subjects with reduced body glycogen stores was shown to decrease the feeling of both mental and overall fatigue during standardized exercise at 70% of $\dot{V}O_2$max as compared with supplying flavored water (table 15.1). Since the available data in the literature suggest an increased rate of metabolism of BCAA during exercise with reduced levels of muscle glycogen (35), the subjects performed 75 min of heavy exercise (exercise at 70% $\dot{V}O_2$max interrupted by 2-min intervals of exercise at 85% $\dot{V}O_2$max) the evening before the supplementation exercise and remained fasted until the experiment the next morning. The muscle glycogen at the start of the morning exercise averaged 80 mmol/kg wet weight. During the morning exercise, the subjects exercised for 60 min at a standardized work rate corresponding to 70% of their $\dot{V}O_2$max, after which they were encouraged to perform at their maximum for another 20 min, which would be expected to result in similar ratings of perceived exertion at the end of exercise in both conditions (table 15.1). Immediately before exercise and after every 15 min of exercise, the subjects were given either a mixture of BCAA in an aqueous solution flavored to mask the bitter taste of amino acids or flavored water. The drinks were given in random order, and the

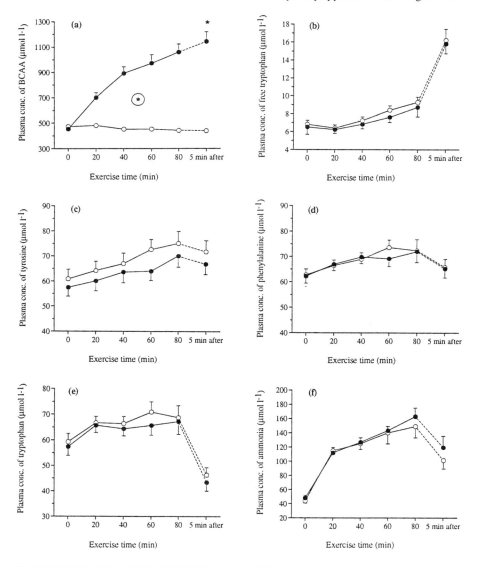

Figure 15.1. The plasma concentrations of the aromatic and branched-chain amino acids (BCAA), free tryptophan, and ammonia, during and 5 min after cycle ergometer exercise. The subjects exercised at a standardized work rate for 60 min, after which they were encouraged to perform at their maximum for another 20 min. Immediately before and during exercise the subjects were given a mixture of the three BCAA in an aqueous solution (closed circles) or flavored water (open circles). Values are means ± *SE* of means for seven subjects. ⊛ and * indicate a difference ($p < 0.05$) between the trials over the whole exercise period and 5 min after exercise, respectively.

Table 15.1 Effects of BCAA on Ratings of Perceived Exertion (RPE) and Mental Fatigue (CR-10) During Ergometer Cycle Exercise With Reduced Muscle Glycogen Stores

Borg scale	Intake	Rest	Exercise								
			10 min	20 min	30 min	40 min	50 min	60 min	70 min	80 min
RPE	BCAA	7.6 ± 0.5	11.1 ± 1.0	12.7 ± 1.0	13.6 ± 1.0	14.5 ± 0.9	15.1 ± 0.7*	15.6 ± 0.7*	16.4 ± 0.9	17.3 ± 1.0
	Placebo	7.9 ± 0.4	11.4 ± 1.2	12.7 ± 1.0	14.2 ± 0.9	15.1 ± 0.8	16.2 ± 0.7	16.8 ± 0.5	16.8 ± 0.9	18.1 ± 0.5
CR-10	BCAA	1.3 ± 0.4	2.3 ± 0.6	2.9 ± 0.5	3.4 ± 0.6*	4.1 ± 0.7*	4.9 ± 0.7*	5.4 ± 0.9*	6.1 ± 0.9	6.6 ± 1.1
	Placebo	1.3 ± 0.4	2.4 ± 0.5	3.4 ± 0.6	4.1 ± 0.6	5.1 ± 0.7	5.6 ± 0.9	6.1 ± 0.7	6.8 ± 0.7	7.9 ± 1.0

The subjects exercised for 60 min at a standardized work rate, after which they were encouraged to perform at their maximum for another 20 min. Immediately before and during exercise the subjects were supplied with a mixture of the three BCAA in an aqueous solution or a placebo that consisted of flavored water. Values are means ± *SE* of means for seven subjects. *Indicates $p < .05$ for BCAA vs. placebo using a two-way ANOVA for repeated measures.

experiment was carried out using a double-blind design. The subjects were carefully instructed to rate their overall degree of perceived exertion on the 15-degree (6-20) category scale devised by Borg. Ratings of mental fatigue were made on the CR-10 category-ratio scale with an absolute 0. The physical performance, evaluated as the amount of work performed during the last 20 min, improved in three of the subjects when BCAA were taken during exercise, while the remaining four subjects performed equally well whether BCAA or flavored water was supplied. It has been suggested that an intake of BCAA might be detrimental to physical performance due to an increased production of ammonia originating from the metabolism of BCAA during exercise (34). However, when healthy subjects in a glycogen-depleted state were supplied with a mixture of BCAA or leucine alone in large doses (350 mg/kg body weight) 1.5 h before an exhausting bout of exercise lasting approximately 30 min, no effect on the physical performance of the subjects was actually found despite high plasma levels of ammonia (34). When smaller amounts of BCAA are supplied, as in our study previously described in which a total of 6 to 8 g of BCAA were supplied, no further increase in the plasma concentration of ammonia was found as a consequence of BCAA supplementation; that is, exercise caused the same increase in plasma ammonia concentration whether BCAA or water was supplied (see figure 15.1).

When BCAA were supplied together with carbohydrates (CHO) during exercise, no difference in perceived mental and overall fatigue could be detected during 80 min of exercise at 75% of $\dot{V}O_2$max when compared with a supply of CHO alone. As expected, no difference in physical performance, evaluated as the amount of work performed during the exercise, was found between the two conditions (unpublished observations). A supply of CHO before or during exercise has been reported to depress the increase in plasma FFA concentration during exercise, which is probably caused by a stimulation of insulin secretion, which is known to inhibit lipolysis (37). Thus, on the basis of the relationship between the concentration of FFA and free Trp in plasma (previously discussed), CHO intake during exercise is also expected to depress or prevent the increase in free Trp concentration. In a recent study, Davis et al. (14) report that supplementation of CHO attenuates, in a concentration-related manner, the increase in the plasma free-Trp concentration during sustained exercise to fatigue (2-4 h duration) at approximately 70% of $\dot{V}O_2$max. Therefore, when CHO was supplied during 80 min of exercise, the increase in the plasma concentration of free Trp and also the increase in the plasma concentration ratio of free Trp to other LNAA might be too small to influence the brain level of 5-HT, so that administration of BCAA would not be expected to have an effect. It should also be kept in mind that an intake of CHO will prevent a fall in the blood glucose concentration, which could also have a direct effect on the brain to prevent or delay mental fatigue. However, when the exercise continues for longer than 2 to 3 h, there is an increase in the plasma concentration of FFA and free Trp even when CHO is consumed in amounts of 150 to 200 g (14, 37). This might explain why it was possible to detect an effect of BCAA supplementation on the marathon performance even when CHO drinks were consumed during the race (8). It should be pointed out, however, that a competitive marathon is an extremely heavy exercise situation. Furthermore, a large number of subjects participated in the study, which made it possible to detect a difference of less than 3% in performance between the subjects who were supplied with BCAA and the subjects who were supplied with the placebo in a subgroup of ''slower'' runners.

Supplementation of BCAA has also been suggested to have anabolic effects on skeletal muscle, either through a direct effect on the rate of protein synthesis or degradation in muscle or as a result of altered hormonal response to exercise (see 22). This aspect of BCAA supplementation could be of importance, especially in relation to physical performance.

Exercise Training and the 5-Hydroxytryptamine System

The effects of endurance training on cardiovascular parameters and skeletal muscle enzyme activities are well documented. It is also well known that exercise training enhances physical performance and delays fatigue. In contrast to our knowledge of how training affects physical fatigue, very little is known about the effects of training on mental fatigue. Can exercise training also delay mental fatigue through an effect on the 5-HT system in the brain?

Results from animal studies have shown that acute exercise to fatigue caused more pronounced changes in the plasma concentrations of free Trp and BCAA in trained than in sedentary rats (10). This is most likely an effect of the longer exercise time for the trained rats; the average running time to fatigue was 72 min for the sedentary rats and 180 min for the trained ones. Also, the increase in the Trp level in the six brain areas studied was larger in the trained animals, while there were no significant differences between trained and sedentary rats concerning the changes in the levels of 5-HT and 5-HIAA in the brain (10). However, there was a limited number of animals in each group, which may limit the possibility to detect small differences. Furthermore, 11 wk of endurance training did not influence the maximal activity of the enzyme monoamine oxidase, which catalyzes the conversion of 5-HT to 5-HIAA, in the brain areas that were studied.

No comparisons between trained and untrained subjects have been made to study the effects of training on the change in the plasma ratio of free Trp to other LNAA during exercise. Recently, however, some evidence was presented that endurance training alters the sensitivity of the serotonergic system. The release of prolactin after a challenge with a 5-HT agonist, which should provide an index of 5-HT sensitivity, was lower in endurance-trained athletes than in untrained individuals (21). This further supports the theory that the 5-HT system is involved in central fatigue during endurance exercise and furthermore that central fatigue, like peripheral fatigue, is affected by physical training. Thus, effects of BCAA supplementation on physical and mental fatigue may depend not only on the changes in the plasma free-Trp concentrations, but also on the sensitivity of the 5-HT system to changes in the level of 5-HT in neurons in specific parts of the brain.

Conclusion

During and after sustained heavy exercise, there is an increased plasma concentration ratio of free Trp to other LNAA (including the BCAA). This would favor the transport of Trp into the brain and also the synthesis and release of 5-HT, which is suggested to cause central and mental fatigue during or after sustained exercise. Supplementing BCAA has been shown to decrease the mental and overall fatigue that occurs during standardized exercise and also to maintain or enhance mental alertness after different types of competitive exercise. Furthermore, a supply of CHO before or during exercise attenuates the increase in the plasma free-Trp concentration and also the plasma ratio of free Trp to other LNAA. Therefore, in addition to maintaining the blood glucose level, intake of CHO is also likely to decrease the synthesis and release of 5-HT and thereby delay fatigue. When CHO are taken, an effect of BCAA supplementation on fatigue can be noted only when the exercise continues for longer periods or possibly during sustained intermittent exercise.

References

1. Ahlborg, G.; Felig, P.; Hagenfeldt, L.; Hendler, R.; Wahren, J. Substrate turnover during prolonged exercise in man. J. Clin. Invest. 53:1080-1090; 1974.
2. Bailey, S.P.; Davis, J.M.; Ahlborn, E.N. Effect of increased brain serotonergic activity on endurance performance in the rat. Acta Physiol. Scand. 145:75-76; 1992.
3. Bailey, S.P.; Davis, J.M.; Ahlborn, E.N. Neuroendocrine and substrate responses to altered brain 5-HT activity during prolonged exercise to fatigue. J. Appl. Physiol. 74:3006-3012; 1993.
4. Barchas, J.D.; Freedman, D.X. Brain amines: Response to physiological stress. Biochem. Pharmacol. 12:1232-1235; 1963.
5. Bergström, J.; Fürst, P.; Hultman, E. Free amino acids in muscle tissue and plasma during exercise in man. Clin. Physiol. 5:155-160; 1985.
6. Bliss, E.L.; Ailion, J. Relationship of stress and activity to brain dopamine and homovanillic acid. Life Sci. 10:1161-1169; 1971.
7. Blomstrand, E.; Celsing, F.; Newsholme, E.A. Changes in plasma concentrations of aromatic and branched-chain amino acids during sustained exercise in man and their possible role in fatigue. Acta Physiol. Scand. 133:115-121; 1988.
8. Blomstrand, E.; Hassmén, P.; Ekblom, B.; Newsholme, E.A. Administration of branched-chain amino acids during sustained exercise—Effects on performance and on plasma concentration of some amino acids. Eur. J. Appl. Physiol. 63:83-88; 1991.
9. Blomstrand, E.; Hassmén, P.; Newsholme, E.A. Effect of branched-chain amino acid supplementation on mental performance. Acta Physiol. Scand. 143:225-226; 1991.
10. Blomstrand, E.; Perrett, D.; Parry-Billings, M.; Newsholme, E.A. Effect of sustained exercise on plasma amino acid concentrations and on 5-hydroxytryptamine metabolism in six different brain regions of the rat. Acta Physiol. Scand. 136:473-481; 1989.
11. Chaouloff, F. Physical exercise and brain monoamines: A review. Acta Physiol. Scand. 137:1-13; 1989.
12. Chaouloff, F.; Laude, D.; Merino, D.; Serrurrier, B.; Guezennec, Y.; Elghozi, J.L. Amphetamine and α-methyl-p-tyrosine affect the exercise-induced imbalance between the availability of tryptophan and synthesis of serotonin in the brain of the rat. Neuropharmacology 26:1099-1106; 1987.
13. Curzon, G.; Friedel, J.; Knott, P.J. The effect of fatty acids on the binding of tryptophan to plasma protein. Nature 242:198-200; 1973.

14. Davis, J.M.; Bailey, S.P.; Woods, J.A.; Galiano, F.J.; Hamilton, M.T.; Bartoli, W.P. Effects of carbohydrate feedings on plasma free tryptophan and branched-chain amino acids during prolonged cycling. Eur. J. Appl. Physiol. 65:513-519; 1992.

15. Décombaz, J.; Reinhardt, P.; Anantharaman, K.; von Glutz, G.; Poortmans, J.R. Biochemical changes in a 100 km run: Free amino acids, urea, and creatinine. Eur. J. Appl. Physiol. 41:61-72; 1979.

16. Felig, P.; Wahren, J. Amino acid metabolism in exercising man. J. Clin. Invest. 50:2703-2714; 1971.

17. Gordon, R.; Spector, S.; Sjoerdsma, A.; Udenfriend, S. Increased synthesis of norepinephrine and epinephrine in the intact rat during exercise and exposure to cold. J. Pharmac. Exp. Ther. 153:440-447; 1966.

18. Hassmén, P.; Blomstrand, E.; Ekblom, B.; Newsholme, E.A. Branched-chain amino acid supplementation during 30-km competitive run: Mood and cognitive performance. Nutrition 10:405-410; 1994.

19. Heyes, M.P.; Garnett, E.S.; Coates, G. Central dopaminergic activity influences rats ability to exercise. Life Sci. 36:671-677; 1985.

20. Heyes, M.P.; Garnett, E.S.; Coates, G. Nigrostriatal dopaminergic activity is increased during exhaustive exercise stress in rats. Life Sci. 42:1537-1542; 1988.

21. Jakeman, P.M.; Hawthorne, J.E.; Maxwell, S.R.J.; Kendall, M.J.; Holder, G. Evidence for downregulation of hypothalamic 5-hydroxytryptamine receptor function in endurance-trained athletes. Exp. Physiol. 79:461-464; 1994.

22. Kreider, R.B.; Miriel, V.; Bertun, E. Amino acid supplementation and exercise performance. Sports Med. 16:190-209; 1993.

23. MacLean, D.A.; Spriet, L.L.; Hultman, E.; Graham, T.E. Plasma and muscle amino acid and ammonia responses during prolonged exercise in humans. J. Appl. Physiol. 70:2095-2103; 1991.

24. McMenamy, R.H.; Oncley, J.L. The specific binding of L-tryptophan to serum albumin. J. Biol. Chem. 233:1436-1447; 1958.

25. Newsholme, E.A. Application of knowledge of metabolic integration to the problem of metabolic limitations in middle distance and marathon running. Acta Physiol. Scand. 128 (suppl. 556):93-97; 1986.

26. Newsholme, E.A.; Leech, A.R. Biochemistry for the medical sciences. Chichester, England: John Wiley & Sons; 1983:784-787.

27. Okamura, K.; Matsubara, F.; Yoshioka, Y.; Kikuchi, N.; Kikuchi, Y.; Kohri, H. Exercise-induced changes in branched chain amino acid/aromatic amino acid ratio in the rat brain and plasma. Japan. J. Pharmacol. 45:243-248; 1987.

28. Pardridge, W.M. Kinetics of competitive inhibition of neutral amino acid transport across the blood-brain barrier. J. Neurochem. 28:103-108; 1977.

29. Refsum, H.E.; Gjessing, L.R.; Strömme, S.B. Changes in plasma amino acid distribution and urine amino acids excretion during prolonged heavy exercise. Scand. J. Clin. Lab. Invest. 39:407-413; 1979.

30. Rennie, M.J.; Edwards, R.H.T.; Krywawych, S.; Davies, C.T.M.; Halliday, D.; Waterlow, J.C.; Millward, D.J. Effects of exercise on protein turnover in man. Clin. Sci. 61:627-639; 1981.

31. Romanowski, W.; Grabiec, S. The role of serotonin in the mechanism of central fatigue. Acta Physiol. Pol. 25:127-134; 1974.

32. Sahlin, K.; Katz, A.; Broberg, S. Tricarboxylic acid cycle intermediates in human muscle during prolonged exercise. Am. J. Physiol. 259 (Cell Physiol. 28):C834-C841; 1990.

33. Sheldon, M.I.; Sorscher, S.; Smith, C.B. A comparison of the effects of morphine and forced running upon the incorporation of ^{14}C-tyrosine into ^{14}C-catecholamines in mouse brain, heart and spleen. J. Pharmac. Exp. Ther. 193:564-575; 1975.

34. Wagenmakers, A.J.M. Role of amino acids and ammonia in mechanisms of fatigue. In: Marconnet, P.; Komi, P.V.; Saltin, B.; Sejersted, O.M., eds. Muscle fatigue mechanisms in exercise and training. Basel: Karger; 1992:69-86. (Med. Sport Sci.).

35. Wagenmakers, A.J.M.; Beckers, E.J.; Brouns, F.; Kuipers, H.; Soeters, P.B.; van der Vusse, G.J.; Saris, W.H.M. Carbohydrate supplementation, glycogen depletion, and amino acid metabolism during exercise. Am. J. Physiol. 260 (Endocrinol. Metab. 23):E883-E890; 1991.

36. Wilson, W.M.; Maughan, R.J. Evidence for a possible role of 5-hydroxytryptamine in the genesis of fatigue in man: Administration of paroxetine, a 5-HT re-uptake inhibitor, reduces the capacity to perform prolonged exercise. Exp. Physiol. 77:921-924; 1992.

37. Wright, D.A.; Sherman, W.M.; Dernbach, A.R. Carbohydrate feedings before, during, or in combination improve cycling endurance performance. J. Appl. Physiol. 71:1082-1088; 1991.

PART IV

Molecular Biology: A Tool to Study Muscle

CHAPTER 16

Translational Control in Skeletal and Cardiac Muscle in Response to Energy Status

Donald B. Thomason, Jiwei Yang, Zhu Ku, Vandana Menon
University of Tennessee Health Science Center, Memphis, Tennessee, U.S.A.

Both skeletal and cardiac muscle rapidly regulate protein synthesis (time scale of hours) in response to a change in functional demand (1). The ability of muscle to rapidly modulate translation is among the first changes in gene expression; modulation of transcription and protein degradation, both potent factors controlling gene expression, generally change on a much slower time scale. It is therefore tempting to hypothesize that the intracellular signals that convey a change in functional demand to the translation machinery may, if they become chronic, also modulate transcriptional and posttranslational control of gene expression.

We have begun to examine the mechanisms for the rapid down-regulation of skeletal and cardiac muscle protein synthesis that occurs with the tail-traction model of hindlimb non–weight bearing (6). At the onset of the inactivity, both the soleus and cardiac muscles exhibit a nearly identical decrease in protein synthesis rate ($t_{1/2} = 0.3$ d). Recently, we have shown that the decrease in soleus muscle protein synthesis is a decrease in nascent polypeptide elongation rate (2). As we will show here, our hypothesis that cardiac muscle similarly regulates its protein synthesis is incorrect; the heart apparently uses a mechanism involving decreased initiation of protein synthesis. We will further show that both the soleus muscle and the heart exhibit a strong relationship between their high-energy phosphate status and the mechanism for down-regulation of protein synthesis. We present a hypothesis whereby functional demand may control protein synthesis in part by a mechanism that senses high-energy phosphate levels.

Materials and Methods

Animal Care and Tissue and Cell Collection

Female Sprague-Dawley rats (200-250 g) were used for all experiments. Animals were housed in light- and temperature-controlled quarters where they received food and water ad libitum. Animals were randomly assigned to control or experimental groups, and all of the procedures began at approximately 1600 h. Control animals were handled and housed identically to the experimental animals. Animals in the hindlimb non-weight-bearing group received a tail-traction bandage as previously described (7). The non-weight-bearing animals were placed in a suspension cage where they had free access to food and water but were prevented from bearing weight with their hindlimbs. All procedures were approved by the Animal Care and Use Committee of the University of Tennessee, Memphis, Tennessee, United States.

L8 cell lines were maintained at low density in DMEM, 10% calf serum. Prior to ATP treatment, cells were replicate plated. While the cultures were still in a rapid phase of growth (approximately 50-80% confluent), the experimental cells were treated for 10 min with 20 µg/ml digitonin in the medium. Cells were washed twice with PBS and incubated for 30 min in PBS containing different concentrations of ATP. Polysomes were then immediately isolated from control and experimental cultures.

Polysome Isolation

The homogenization buffer was prepared by autoclaving a solution of 50 mM tris-HCl, 250 mM KCl, 25 mM $MgCl_2$, 0.2% Triton X-100, 200 mM sucrose, 0.25 mM dithiothreitol, 1.0 mM EGTA, pH 7.4, to which the following were added prior to use: 0.5% nonidet-P40, 0.5% sodium deoxycholate, 200 µg/ml sodium heparin, 1 µg/ml cycloheximide, and 4 U/ml RNasin (Promega Corporation, Madison, Wisconsin, United States). Tissue collection began at the 18 h non-weight-bearing time point (approximately 1000 h the next day). The soleus muscles from anesthetized experimental and control animals were quickly excised, blotted to remove blood, and finely minced in ice-cold homogenization buffer. The tissue was then gently homogenized briefly to suspend the intact polysomes. Cell debris was removed by brief centrifugation at 4k × g for 5 min at 4° C. The polysome-containing supernatant was further centrifuged at 12k × g for 15 min at 4° C to obtain the postmitochondrial supernatant.

Polysomes were isolated from cells in culture by first washing the cells with phosphate-buffered saline and then lysing the cells on ice with the homogenization buffer previously detailed. The plates were scraped and washed to collect the lysate and cell debris. The postmitochondrial supernatant was obtained by differential centrifugation as with the tissue (previously described).

Analysis of Polysome Blots

Eight percent SDS-PAGE of the polysomes isolated from tissue or cells allowed immunoblotting for heat-shock protein 70 (hsc70). The anti-hsc70 monoclonal antibody was obtained from Stressgen (Victoria, British Columbia, Canada). The secondary antibody was an HRP-conjugate that was detected using the Renaissance kit (New England Nuclear). A permanent record for analysis was formed on Xomat-AR film (Kodak). Digital densitometric scanning of the film was done using the NIH Image package.

Statistical Analysis

A one-way ANOVA tested for differences between groups. A difference occurring with a $p < .05$ is considered significant.

Results and Discussion

Molecular chaperone levels change with changes in muscle protein synthesis. The rapid decrease of protein synthesis rate in both soleus and cardiac muscle with non–weight-bearing activity suggests a similar translational control mechanism for both tissues. However, such is not the case. Previous data indicate that the soleus muscle modulates nascent polypeptide elongation rate: Polysome size increases (more ribosomes per mRNA) as protein synthesis decreases (2). Recent data indicate that the opposite is true for cardiac muscle: Polysome size decreases as protein synthesis decreases (summarized in table 16.1). The only explanation of fewer ribosomes per mRNA is a decreased rate of initiation of protein synthesis (2).

As shown in table 16.1, the level of the constitutive (or cognate) hsc70 associated with the polysomes from soleus muscle and cardiac muscle change in opposite directions. Within the first 8 h of non–weight bearing, the soleus muscle shows a $29 \pm 14\%$ decrease in the hsc70 levels associated with the polysomes ($p < .05$) despite the mobilization of RNA into the polysome pool (2). Because the hsc70 binds to the nascent polypeptide and may help guide the protein through the ribosome channel (5), the observed decrease in polysomal hsc70 may explain the slowing of elongation rate in the soleus muscle. Can the increase in polysomal hsc70 in the cardiac muscle explain the decreased initiation observed in the polysome profiles? Hsc70, in addition to having the chaperone role of guiding the nascent polypeptide through the ribosome channel, also binds to the heme-regulated inhibitor (HRI) of protein synthesis initiation (3, 4). HRI is a kinase for initiation factor 2-α (IF2-α) and in the absence of hsc70 becomes active and inhibits protein synthesis initiation. Thus, the heart data presented in table 16.1 are consistent with the mechanism of action: A shift of hsc70 onto the polysomal nascent polypeptides activates HRI and decreases protein synthesis through decreased initiation (discussed later).

Table 16.1   Comparison of Soleus and Cardiac Muscle Translational Control Mechanisms During 8 h Non–Weight Bearing by Tail Traction

Muscle	$t_{1/2}$ for decrease in protein synthesis rate (d)	Change in polysome size	Mechanism	Polysomal hsc70
Soleus	0.3	Increase	Elongation	↓$29 \pm 14\%$
Left ventricle	0.3	Decrease	Initiation	↑$55 \pm 8\%$

Molecular chaperone association with the polysomes is sensitive to ATP levels. Hsc70 is an ATPase, and its dissociation from unfolded protein is accelerated by ATP hydrolysis. We hypothesized that if hsc70 regulates protein synthesis through either initiation or elongation, then these mechanisms should be sensitive to the cellular ATP levels. To test this hypothesis, we modulated intracellular levels of ATP of L8 myoblasts in culture by permeabilizing them with a low dose of digitonin (20 µg/ml) for 10 min prior to replacing the media with PBS containing various levels of ATP. As shown in figure 16.1, for ATP levels greater than 1 mM, there is a linear relationship between the amount of hsc70 associated with the polysomes and the rate of incorporation of radiolabeled leucine into cellular protein. At ATP levels between 1 mM and 0 mM, there is no change (or even a decrease) in protein synthesis, while hsc70 associated with the polysomes increases.

By the proposed mechanism of hsc70 action, a decrease of hsc70 associated with the polysomes will decrease protein synthesis by decreasing elongation rate; an increase in ATP level would promote dissociation of the hsc70 from the nascent polypeptide and facilitate the decrease in protein synthesis rate (figure 16.2). The data of figure 16.1 are consistent with this hypothesis. On the other hand, an increase of hsc70 association with the polysomes will also decrease protein synthesis through a mass action shift of hsc70 from HRI, causing phosphorylation of IF2-α. The data of figure 16.1 are not inconsistent with this hypothesis because the decreased ATP

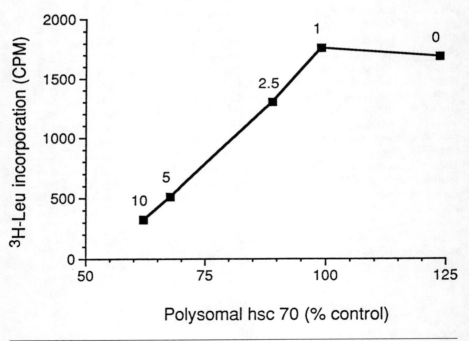

Figure 16.1   The relationship between the hsc70 associated with the polysomes and the incorporation of [³H]leucine depends upon ATP concentration. Digitonin-permeabilized L8 cells were treated for 30 min with media containing different concentrations of ATP (in mM, shown next to each point).

Increased ATP: elongation inhibition

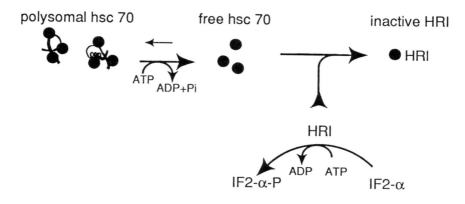

Decreased ATP: initiation inhibition

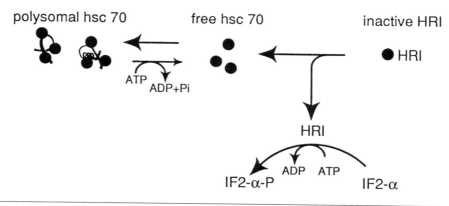

Figure 16.2   Proposed mechanism whereby protein synthesis is modulated by intracellular ATP levels affecting the distribution of hsc70. Increased intracellular ATP will dissociate hsc70 from the nascent polypeptide, slowing elongation rate. Decreased ATP will slow dissociation of hsc70, shifting it away from HRI and slowing initiation rate.

levels in the experimental manipulation would also decrease the substrate available as a phosphate donor.

ATP levels change in the non-weight-bearing muscle. Based upon these data for the mechanism of hsc70 action, we predicted that the soleus muscle would exhibit an increase in ATP levels following 8 h of non–weight bearing, whereas the cardiac muscle would exhibit a decrease in ATP levels. Flash-frozen tissue was extracted, and the ATP levels analyzed by HPLC. As predicted, soleus muscle ATP levels increased 17% following 8 h of non–weight bearing, and cardiac muscle ATP levels were decreased 45%. Thus, the protein synthesis machinery may sense these changes in ATP level through a mechanism involving hsc70 (figure 16.2).

Summary

The rapid decrease in protein synthesis rate for both cardiac and skeletal muscle during non–weight bearing is an important phenomenon to understand, not only because of its rapidity but also because of its functional consequences in long-term adaptation. We propose separate mechanisms for each tissue that have the same net effect. Each mechanism is sensitive to intracellular ATP levels: increased in the skeletal muscle and decreased in the cardiac muscle. Furthermore, the transduction of ATP levels in each mechanism is through the hsc70 molecular chaperones. Thus, the mechanism proposed in figure 16.2 provides a means whereby the muscle's protein synthesis machinery is acutely sensitive to functional demand through an ATP-sensitive signal transduction mechanism.

Acknowledgments

This work was supported by USPHS AR40901 and American Heart Association 92-013800.

References

1. Booth, F.W.; Thomason, D.B. Molecular and cellular adaptation of muscle in response to exercise: Perspectives of various models. Physiol. Rev. 71:541-585; 1991.
2. Ku, Z.; Thomason, D.B. Soleus muscle nascent polypeptide chain elongation slows protein synthesis rate during non-weightbearing. Am. J. Physiol. 267: C115-C126; 1994.
3. Matts, R.L.; Hurst, R. The relationship between protein synthesis and heat shock proteins levels in rabbit reticulocyte lysates. J. Biol. Chem. 267:18168-18174; 1992.
4. Matts, R.L.; Xu, Z.; Pal, J.K.; Chen, J.J. Interactions of the heme-regulated eIF-2 alpha kinase with heat shock proteins in rabbit reticulocyte lysates. J. Biol. Chem. 267:18160-18167; 1992.
5. Nelson, R.J.; Ziegelhoffer, T.; Nicolet, C.; Werner-Washburne, M.; Craig, E.A. The translation machinery and 70 kd heat shock protein cooperate in protein synthesis. Cell 71:97-105; 1992.
6. Thomason, D.B.; Biggs, R.B.; Booth, F.W. Protein metabolism and β-myosin heavy-chain mRNA in unweighted soleus muscle. Am. J. Physiol. 257:R300-R305; 1989.
7. Thomason, D.B.; Herrick, R.E.; Surdyka, D.; Baldwin. K.M. Time course of soleus muscle myosin expression during hindlimb suspension and recovery. J. Appl. Physiol. 63:130-137; 1987.

CHAPTER 17

Metabolic and Contractile Protein Adaptations in Response to Increased Mechanical Loading

Richard W. Tsika, Liying Gao

University of Illinois at Urbana-Champaign, Urbana, Illinois, U.S.A.

The phenotype of adult skeletal muscle fibers is not static but is remarkably malleable as demonstrated by its ability to adapt to a broad range of physiological and pathophysiological stimuli. In particular, the imposition of a sustained increase in mechanical load (work overload) results in the hypertrophic growth of postmitotic skeletal muscle fibers and is associated with a quantitative and qualitative change in metabolic and contractile protein gene expression. Both fast and slow fiber types respond to work overload with functional and biochemical adaptations that are consistent with a transition of fast- to slow-twitch properties. These adaptations have been documented using a variety of experimental models that result in a sustained increase in muscle mechanical load. These paradigms include (1) an in vitro stretch model in which either cardiac or skeletal myocytes are cultured on a deformable substrate that when perturbed places an increased mechanical load (stretch) on the myocytes, (2) stretch overload induced by attaching a weight to the wing of a chicken, (3) interventions that are designed to mimic a cardiovascular pathology (pressure or volume overload) and result in either atrial or ventricular hypertrophy (such as aortic coarctation), and (4) compensatory overload, which involves the surgical removal or ablation of a muscle's synergists. Although striated muscle hypertrophy has been characterized morphologically, functionally, and biochemically, the genetic basis that underlies these adaptations remains obscure. Until recently, a major limitation into the molecular genetics of striated muscle hypertrophy has been the lack of a suitable in vivo genetic model system. However, the recent evolution of transgenic mouse technology and its implementation in biology have overcome this limitation, providing us with an intact animal system with which to study adaptational biology and genetics (28). In order to better understand the molecular mechanism(s) and biochemical pathway(s) that underlie striated muscle plasticity in response to an increased mechanical load, we have undertaken an in vivo (transgenic mice) analysis of both metabolic and contractile protein genes using the compensatory overload model. The following will briefly review some of our ongoing studies, which are designed to characterize work overload–induced adaptations in mouse fast- and slow-twitch muscle.

Gene Expression in Overloaded Mouse Skeletal Muscle: Early Response

The development of striated muscle hypertrophy by work overload is associated with the induction of a battery of immediate early response genes. In particular, the induction of the proto-oncogenes c-*myc* and c-*fos* has been documented in the work-overloaded rat and mouse heart (8, 10, 21) and in rat skeletal muscle (34). However, the significance of the rapid and transient induction of these c-oncogenes in striated muscle by the physiological stimulus of mechanical loading is not well understood at present; the induction of these genes has been shown to occur in response to many stimuli, including growth factors. The observation that both of these c-oncogenes are rapidly induced in cells exposed to growth factors has led to the hypothesis that they are involved in the control of some aspect of cell proliferation, that is, the recruitment of quiescent cells or perhaps cell cycle control. Numerous observations support this notion: (1) When quiescent 3T3 cells expressing antisense c-*fos* RNA are exposed to serum, they fail to reenter the cell cycle; (2) the inhibition of cellular proliferation has also been demonstrated in cells expressing antisense c-*myc* RNA; (3) c-*myc* is highly expressed in proliferating myoblast, but its expression decreases dramatically during differentiation; (4) the constitutive expression of c-*fos* or c-*myc* results in the inhibition of differentiation of various cell types, including myoblast (12, 16); and (5) in transgenic mice that overexpress c-*myc*, the number of heart cells were increased (9), and the magnitude of hypertrophic heart cell growth differed in a stimulus-dependent manner (20).

Of interest, the structure of the c-Myc protein shares sequence homology with two different classes of nuclear proteins; that is, it harbors both a basic helix-loop-helix (b-HLH) and a leucine zipper (L-zip) domain characteristic of members of the muscle regulatory factors family (MRF, MyoD, myogenin, Myf-5 and herculin/MRF4, Myf-6) and of both c-Fos and c-Jun proteins, respectively. Members of the MRF family of proteins form heterodimers with other tissue-specific and ubiquitously expressed HLH proteins (E12, E47; products of E2a gene) and activate transcription of a variety of muscle-specific genes by binding to an E-box core sequence (CANNTG). Based on the structural similarity between c-myc (involved in proliferation) and the MRF proteins (involved in differentiation), a number of potential mechanisms leading to alterations in muscle growth can be inferred. For example, the c-Myc protein may alter muscle growth by interfering with the action of the MRFs by associating with the ubiquitously expressed E2a proteins or with the MRFs themselves or by interacting with the same or similar DNA-binding motifs as the MRF. Regarding c-*fos*, its early induction in response to many stimuli has led to the idea that it serves the function of converting early signals into more sustained changes in gene expression (4). In support of this, c-*fos* has been shown to associate with c-Jun (c-*fos*/c-Jun) and to interact with a specific DNA recognition element called an AP-1 site (TGACTCA) located in the promoter region of many other genes (3). It is interesting that the activation of these c-oncogenes has been shown to proceed through a diversity of signal transduction pathways (4). This observation is important because the recent work of Sadoshima and Izumo (24) and Vandenburgh, Shansky, and Karlisch (32) demonstrates that an increased mechanical load (stretch) placed on cultured cardiocytes or skeletal muscle cells activates a deluge of second messenger pathways, some of which are the same as those known to induce c-*fos*. Since these c-oncogenes encode nuclear proteins and the early induction of these genes has been associated with cellular growth, it may be that their early induction in response to an increased work load acts to direct early gene expression events leading to striated muscle hypertrophic growth.

Since the mouse has not been used extensively in the study of skeletal muscle hypertrophy, we investigated the expression pattern of c-*myc* and c-*fos* in the fast-twitch plantaris muscle during the first 48 h after the imposition of a work overload. Work overload was created bilaterally by the surgical removal of the gastrocnemius and soleus muscles (31). As illustrated in figure 17.1, Northern blot analysis revealed that the levels of c-*fos*-specific mRNA transcripts were increased in the overloaded plantaris muscle at 1 h, peaked at 3 h, and returned to control levels at 12 h postoverload. In contrast, c-*myc*-specific mRNA transcripts were first observed at 3 h, peaked at 12 h, then remained elevated at a reduced level over the 48-h time course. The level of c-*fos*- and c-*myc*-specific mRNA transcripts were barely detectable in sham-operated, control plantaris muscles. After 2 d of overload, we observed that the plantaris muscle had hypertrophied by 31%. Whether the early induction of these c-oncogenes is directly or indirectly involved in the hypertrophic growth in this overload model is not known at present. However, since the initial phase of hypertrophy has been shown to be associated with an inflammatory response (1), and as we have not compared myofibrillar protein content between control and overloaded plantaris muscles as a measure of true hypertrophic growth, it is possible that the overlapping time course of c-*myc* and c-*fos* induction with that of the early hypertrophic growth phase of the overloaded plantaris muscle may be purely coincidental and not causative. In this study, we have documented an increase in

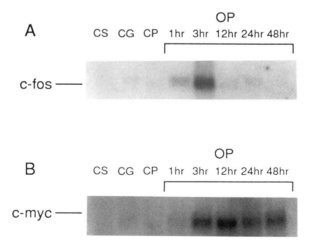

Figure 17.1   Proto-oncogene induction during the early phase of skeletal muscle hypertro-phy. Total cellular RNA (10 μg) from bilaterally overloaded (OP) or sham-operated (CP) plantaris muscles were analyzed for c-*myc*- and c-*fos*-specific transcripts at 1, 3, 12, 24, 48 h on a gel containing 1.5% agarose and 2.2 M formaldehyde. Each lane contains RNA from the muscles of three independent animals. (A) c-*fos* induction occurred as early as 1 h and peaked at 3 h. (B) c-*myc* induction peaked at 12 h and remained elevated. CG = control gastrocnemius; CS = control soleus.

c-*myc* and c-*fos* mRNA but have not formally shown the localization of the Fos or c-Myc proteins in the nucleus. Therefore at present we can only speculate as to whether these c-oncogenes are involved in the work overload–induced hypertrophic growth of the plantaris muscle. In contrast, Sadoshima, Jahn, and Takahashi (25) have shown an increase in c-*fos* mRNA and the nuclear localization of the Fos protein in cardiocytes stretched for 60 min. Although this finding would seem to support the notion that c-*fos* induction may be involved in hypertrophic growth, additional work is required before a definitive function for these c-oncogenes is identified.

Transcriptional Regulation in Overloaded Mouse Skeletal Muscle: Metabolic Adaptations

α-Glycerophosphate Dehydrogenase (GPDH)

In skeletal muscle, reducing equivalents (NADH) produced in the reaction catalyzed by glyceraldehyde-3-phosphate dehydrogenase (G3PDH) are transferred from the cytosol into the mitochondria via a shuttle system. The shuttle requires the coordinated action of the cytosolic and mitochondrial isoforms of α-glycerophosphate dehydrogenase (GPDH). The cytosolic isoform of GPDH is an NAD$^+$-linked enzyme that catalyzes the transfer of electrons from NADH to dihydroxyacetone phosphate (DAP) to produce glycerol-3-phosphate (G3P). G3P then enters the mitochondria, where electrons are transferred from G3P to FAD by the mitochondrial FAD-linked isoform of GPDH, producing FADH2 and DAP. The regenerated DAP returns to the cytosol, where this sequence of reactions can begin again. These sequential reactions constitute the glycerol phosphate shuttle, and under normal situations they ensure that the NADH produced by glycolysis is reoxidized to NAD$^+$, allowing glycolysis to proceed.

In the mouse, cytosolic GPDH is encoded by two distinct genes, termed *Gdc*-1 and *Gdc*-2 (11). *Gdc*-1 is predominantly expressed in adult tissues, whereas *Gdc*-2 is expressed in embryonic tissues. The expression pattern of the adult isoform of GPDH is regulated developmentally and hormonally (5, 11). During muscle cell differentiation, the transcriptional activation of GPDH occurs relatively late in comparison to other muscle proteins such as the myosin heavy-chain (MHC) and myosin light-chain 1/3 (MLC 1/3) genes. The developmental stage-specific expression of GPDH has recently been shown to involve both 5' promoter and 3' intragenic sequences (15). In adult mice, GPDH has been shown to be ubiquitously expressed; however, between tissue types the constitutive levels of GPDH expression can vary by several orders of magnitude. Some tissues with high mRNA expression levels and enzyme activities are adipose cells, brain, liver, and skeletal muscle.

Previous work has shown that the specific activity of GPDH varies according to fiber type; that is, slow oxidative (SO) muscle fiber demonstrates low GPDH-specific activity, while fast glycolytic (FG) fibers have high specific activities (2, 23). Furthermore, when the fast-twitch rat plantaris muscle is functionally overloaded for 9 to 12 wk, there is a significant decrease in the specific activity of GPDH, as well as a decrease in histochemical staining intensity of GPDH in these muscles (2). Based on these observations, it appears as though measured alterations in

GPDH expression levels and activity can serve as a suitable indicator of fiber type conversion. However, the mechanism of GPDH regulation in response to work overload has not been assessed as yet. Accordingly, we have assessed the expression levels of endogenous GPDH mRNA in overloaded mouse plantaris muscles. Northern analysis (figure 17.2) shows that GPDH-specific mRNA transcripts are expressed at high levels in the fast-twitch gastrocnemius muscle, while the slow-twitch soleus muscle contains low levels. The constitutive expression levels of GPDH in the control plantaris (CP) muscle are abundant but slightly less than those in the control gastrocnemius (CG) muscle and significantly higher than those of the control soleus (CS) muscle. This expression pattern is consistent with previous observations describing the specific activities of GPDH in these muscles. The imposition of a work overload to the plantaris muscle (OP) resulted in a dramatic reduction in GPDH expression levels after 2 d of overload. GPDH-specific transcripts remained at reduced levels over a 6-wk time period and resembled the expression levels observed in the soleus muscle. Collectively, these data suggest that some fiber type conversion had occurred in the OP muscle and that the regulation of GPDH expression in response to work overload most likely occurs at the level of transcription. The significance of the early changes (2 d) in GPDH mRNA expression levels is not known at present, but we have also observed similar decreases in mRNA expression levels in our studies that focus on muscle creatine kinase (MCK) and glyceraldehyde-3-phosphate dehydrogenase (G3PDH) gene expression in OP muscles (29). In addition, our analysis of transgenic mice harboring MCK transgenes revealed a 5.6-fold decrease in chloramphenicol acetyltransferase (CAT) activity in OP muscles at 2 d and 6 wk (29). It may be that the early changes in cytosolic energy metabolism act in part as a signal that leads to contractile and metabolic protein remodeling, that is, fiber type conversion.

Transcriptional Regulation in Overloaded Mouse Skeletal Muscle: Contractile Protein Adaptations

Alkali Myosin Light Chain 1 (MLC1)

The alkali MLCs are the products of a multigene family constituted by at least five different striated muscle genes. The localization of the alkali MLC to the head region of the myosin heavy chain has led to speculation that the light chain may serve a modulatory role in actomyosin interactions. This concept is supported by the following findings: (1) distinct alkali MLC isoforms are expressed throughout development and in different fiber types; (2) type IIb fibers of the rabbit psoas and tibialis anterior muscles contain MHCs that are indistinguishable but contain different ratios of MLCs and demonstrate differences in their maximum shortening velocity (Vmax; 26); (3) the normal in vivo actin-activated ATPase activity is absent in *Dictyostelium* overexpressing antisense MLC1 mRNA (19); and (4) by using a motility assay, it was shown that the interaction of the MLCs with the MHC was essential for mechanical transduction of shortening velocity but not for myosin ATPase activity, and, in addition, distinct MLC isoforms affected shortening velocity differently (13, 14).

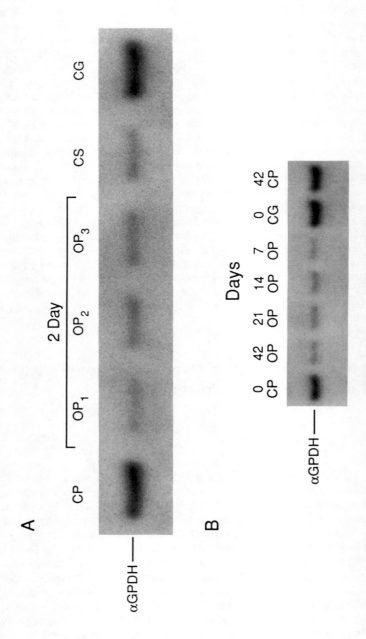

Figure 17.2 GPDH regulation in the hypertrophied mouse plantaris muscle. Endogenous GPDH mRNA transcript levels in the overloaded plantaris muscle (OP) were significantly decreased when compared with control plantaris muscle (CP) at 2 d (A) and remained depressed throughout a 42-d time course (B). CG = control gastrocnemius; CS = control soleus.

It has been well documented that the distinct alkali MLC genes are expressed in a developmental and tissue specific pattern. Alkali FMLC1 and FMLC3 proteins are the products of a single gene locus that is transcribed from two distinct promoters, and its primary transcripts are alternatively spliced (18). Of interest, the expression pattern of these two proteins differs during development and in adult muscle fibers. This gene locus also contains a strong muscle-specific enhancer element located approximately 24 kb downstream from the MLC1 promoter (6). The MLC enhancer harbors multiple cis-acting sequence motifs known to bind myogenic factors and constitutively expressed general transcriptional factors (33). While the FMLC1 and FMLC3 promoters alone can direct muscle specific expression of MLC/CAT fusion genes in primary cultures of muscle cells, the enhancer element is required for expression when permanent muscle cell lines are used. In established muscle cell lines, the expression levels of MLC/CAT reporter genes that contain the 3' enhancer are dramatically increased only in differentiated myotubes (6). The muscle specificity and developmental stage-specific action of the MLC enhancer has recently been demonstrated in transgenic mice, confirming the results obtained using muscle cells in culture (22). While this gene locus and adjacent downstream enhancer element have been extensively studied during myogenesis, understanding of its regulation in response to mechanical loading in adult skeletal muscle is incomplete.

Five native myosin isoforms have been identified in the rat and mouse plantaris muscle (30). These isoforms have been termed slow myosin (Sm), intermediate myosin (Im), and fast myosin 1, 2, and 3 (Fm1, Fm2, Fm3). Native myosin is a hexameric molecule composed of two heavy chains and two pairs of light chains. The alkali FMLC1 protein is associated with Im and Fm2 as a heterodimer and with Fm3 as a homodimer (30). Under conditions of work overload, we (31) and others (2, 7) have documented a dramatic increase in Sm and Im isoforms and a reduction in the total percentage of Fm isoform. The transition in native isomyosin profiles in the OP muscle were accompanied by alterations in light chain composition, resulting in a decrease in both FMLC1 and FMLC3 (2, 31). Although the shift in myosin light chain composition was not quantified by us, visualization of the gels (31, figure 4) and densitometric scans (2, figure 3) obtained in these studies suggests that the decrease in both FMLC proteins was significant. In contrast, Periasamy, Gregory, and Martin (17) found a nonsignificant change in the levels of FMLC1 and FMLC3 mRNA-specific transcripts and protein in the rat plantaris muscle after 11 wk of work overload when compared with CP levels. This apparent discrepancy can probably be explained by the difference in overload protocols employed in these studies. Periasamy, Gregory, and Martin (17) created an overload by removing the gastrocnemius muscle bilaterally, whereas we (31) removed the gastrocnemius and soleus muscles, resulting in a greater overload on the plantaris muscle. Nevertheless, a change in FMLC composition was observed in these studies, but the level of regulation has not yet been definitively determined. Therefore, we have initiated transgenic studies to determine if the change in FMLC1 levels in the OP muscle is transcriptionally regulated.

The FMLC1 transgene [pMLC1CAT(920)] used in this study contained 1.5 kb of FMLC1 5' promoter sequence fused to the 5' end of the CAT gene and 920 bp of downstream enhancer sequence fused to the 3' end of the CAT gene (22). Our preliminary results show that after 6 wk of work overload the FMLC1 transgene expression levels are decreased, on average, 2.5- to 3-fold as assessed by CAT activity (figure 17.3). This gene has also been shown to be expressed in a fiber type–specific manner; that is, the highest levels are seen in type IIb fibers with

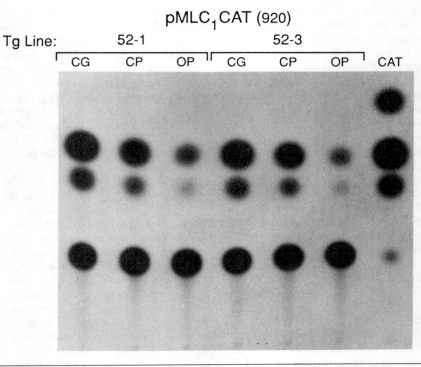

Figure 17.3 Analysis of CAT activity in control (CP) and overloaded (OP) plantaris muscle of adult transgenic mice harboring a myosin light chain 1 transgene [pMLC1CAT(920)]. CAT activity was assessed by incubation of 1 μg of extract protein for 30 min with 4 mM acetyl CoA and [^{14}C]chloramphenicol (0.1 μCi/μl) in 300 mM tris-HCl. Acetylated [^{14}C]chloramphenicol was separated from nonacetylated forms by thin layer chromatography (1 h, RT). Transgene expression levels (CAT activity) revealed an approximate threefold decrease in OP muscles when compared with CP.

progressively decreasing levels observed in type IIx, IIa, and I fibers. In good agreement with this observation, our analysis shows that the FMLC1 transgene is expressed at higher levels in the gastrocnemius muscle than in the plantaris muscle (figure 17.3) and at very low levels in the soleus muscle (unpublished observation). These preliminary studies demonstrate that the FMLC1 transgene is transcriptionally repressed in the fast-twitch plantaris muscle in response to work overload. This is not surprising, since after 6 wk of work overload we observed a significant induction of β-MHC-specific mRNA transcripts in the OP muscle, which suggests that a fiber type conversion of fast to slow had occurred (figure 17.4). Similarly, our analysis of transgenic mice harboring β-MHC transgenes revealed a 4- to 12-fold increase in chloramphenicol acetyltransferase (CAT) activity in OP muscles at 6 wk (35).

Summary

Collectively, the data reported herein and those briefly mentioned but reported elsewhere (29, 35, 36), serve to establish the transgenic mouse as an excellent

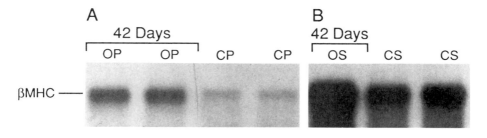

Figure 17.4   Northern blot analysis of β-MHC mRNA induction in overloaded mouse plantaris (OP) and soleus (OS) muscle. There is a significant induction of β-MHC mRNA transcripts after 6 wk of work overload (A) in the plantaris muscle and (B) in the soleus muscle.

model with which to study the molecular mechanisms that underlie transcriptional regulation in response to increased mechanical loading. In mechanically overloaded mouse skeletal muscle, we observe a rapid and transient induction of immediate early response genes, which occurs over a 48-h time course. This pattern of induction is similar to that observed during the development of cardiac hypertrophy. The significance of this event is not known at present, but in mechanically loaded striated muscle it may represent an early signal leading to enhanced cell growth and long-term changes in gene expression. In addition, increased mechanical loading resulted in changes in the expression levels of specific mRNA transcripts and transgenes representing enzymes that function in various pathways of energy metabolism. These changes occurred within 48 h postoverload and persisted for 6 wk. Finally, transcriptional regulation of sarcomeric proteins, such as FMLC1 and β-MHC, has been documented in the overloaded plantaris muscle of transgenic mice. Further work that focuses on identifying the cis-acting DNA sequence(s) that directs either repression or induction of these genes in response to work overload is currently under way. Our second line of inquiry involves investigation into the role of immediate early gene induction and signal transduction pathways activated in mechanically overloaded skeletal muscle. Information gathered from this work should lead to a better understanding of how mechanical overload leads to hypertrophic growth and altered fiber phenotypes in striated muscle.

References

1. Armstrong, R.B.; Marum, P.; Tullson, P. Acute hypertrophic response of skeletal muscle to the removal of synergists. J. Appl. Physiol. 46:835-842; 1979.
2. Baldwin, K.M.; Valdez, V.; Herrick, R.E. Biochemical properties of overloaded fast-twitch skeletal muscle. J. Appl. Physiol. 52(2):467-472; 1982.
3. Chiu, R.; Boyle, W.J.; Meek, J. The c-Fos protein interacts with c-Jun.AP-1 to stimulate transcription of AP-1 responsive genes. Cell 54:541-552; 1988.
4. Curran, T.; Franza, B.R.J. fos and jun: the AP-1 connection. Cell 55:395-397; 1988.

5. Dobson, D.E.; Groves, D.L.; Spiegelman, B.M. Nucleotide sequence and hormonal regulation of mouse glycerophosphate dehydrogenase mRNA during adipocyte and muscle cell differentiation. J. Biol. Chem. 262:1804-1809; 1987.

6. Donoghue, M.; Ernst, H.; Wentworth, B. A muscle-specific enhancer is located at the 3' end of the myosin light-chain 1/3 gene locus. Genes Dev. 2:1779-1790; 1988.

7. Gregory, P.; Low, R.B.; Stirewalt, W.S. Changes in skeletal-muscle myosin isozymes with hypertrophy and exercise. Biochem. J. 238:55-63; 1986.

8. Izumo, S.; Nadal-Ginard, B.; Mahdavi, V. Protooncogene induction and reprogramming of cardiac gene expression produced by pressure overload. Proc. Natl. Acad. Sci. USA 85:339-343; 1988.

9. Jackson, T.; Allard, M.F.; Sreenan, C.A. The c-*myc* proto-oncogene regulates cardiac development in transgenic mice. Mol. Cell. Biol. 10:3709-3716; 1990.

10. Komuro, I.; Kaida, T.; Shibazaki, Y. Stretching cardiac myocytes stimulates protooncogene expression. J. Biol. Chem. 265:3595-3598; 1990.

11. Kozak, L.P.; Burkart, D.L.; Hjorth, J.P. Unlinked structural genes for the developmentally regulated isozymes of *sn*-glycerol-3-phosphate dehydrogenase in mice. Dev. Genet. 3:1-6; 1982.

12. Lassar, A.B.; Thayer, M.J.; Overell, R.W. Transformation by activated *ras* or *fos* prevents myogenesis by inhibiting expression of MyoD. Cell 58:659-667; 1989.

13. Lowey, S.; Waller, G.S.; Trybus, K.M. Function of skeletal muscle myosin heavy and light chain isoforms by an in vitro motility assay. J. Biol. Chem. 268:20414-20418; 1993.

14. Lowey, S.; Waller, G.S.; Trybus, K.M. Skeletal muscle light chains are essential for physiological speeds of shortening. Nature 365:454-456; 1993.

15. Madden, H.M.; Perrin, S.N.; Dobson, D.E. Intragenic regulatory elements mediate the late induction of the glycerophosphate dehydrogenase gene during skeletal myogenesis. J. Cell. Biochem. (suppl. 18D):501; 1994 (abstract W236).

16. Miner, J.H.; Wold, B.J. c-*myc* inhibition of MyoD and myogenin-initiated myogenic differentiation. Mol. Cell. Biol. 11:2842-2851; 1991.

17. Periasamy, M.; Gregory, P.; Martin, B.J. Regulation of myosin heavy-chain gene expression during skeletal-muscle hypertrophy. Biochem. J. 257:691-698; 1989.

18. Periasamy, M.; Strehler, E.; Garfinkel, L. Fast skeletal muscle myosin light chain 1 and 3 are produced from a single gene by a combined process of differential RNA transcription and splicing. J. Biol. Chem. 259:13595-13604; 1984.

19. Pollenz, R.S.; Chen, T.-L.L.; Chisholm, R.L. The dictyostelium essential light chain is required for myosin function. Cell 69:951-962; 1992.

20. Robbins, R.J.; Swain, J.L. C-*myc* protooncogene modulates cardiac hypertrophic growth in transgenic mice. Am. J. Physiol. 262 (Heart Circ. Physiol. 31):H590-H597; 1992.

21. Rockman, H.A.; Ross, R.S.; Harris, A.N. Segregation of atrial-specific and inducible expression of an atrial natriuretic factor transgene in an in vivo murine model of cardiac hypertrophy. Proc. Natl. Acad. Sci. USA 88:8277-8281; 1991.

22. Rosenthal, N.; Kornhauser, J.M.; Donoghue, M. Myosin light chain enhancer activates muscle-specific, developmentally regulated gene expression in transgenic mice. Proc. Natl. Acad. Sci. USA 86:7780-7784; 1989.

23. Roy, R.R.; Baldwin, K.M.; Martin, T.P. Biochemical and physiological changes in overloaded rat fast- and slow-twitch ankle extensors. J. Appl. Physiol. 59(2):639-646; 1985.

24. Sadoshima, J.-I.; Izumo, S. Mechanical stretch rapidly activates multiple signal transduction pathways in cardiac myocytes: Potential involvement of an autocrine/paracrine mechanism. EMBO J. 12:1681-1692; 1993.

25. Sadoshima, J.-I.; Jahn, L.; Takahashi, T. Molecular characterization of the stretch-induced adaptation of cultured cardiac cells: An in vitro model of load-induced cardiac hypertrophy. J. Biol. Chem. 267:10551-10560; 1992.

26. Sweeny, L.H.; Kushmerick, M.J.; Mabuchi, K. Myosin alkali light chain and heavy chain variations correlate with altered shortening velocity of isolated skeletal muscle fibers. J. Biol. Chem. 263:9034-9039; 1988.

27. Tsika, G.L.; Wiedenman, J.L.; Gao, L.; Rivera, I.; Sheriff-Carter, K.; Tsika, R.W. βmyosin heavy chain induction in skeletal muscle is not eliminated by the simultaneous mutation of conserved regulatory elements. (Submitted.)

28. Tsika, R.W. Transgenic animal models. In: Holloszy, J.O., editor. Exercise Sport Science Review. Baltimore: Williams & Wilkins 22:361-388; 1994.

29. Tsika, R.W.; Hauschka, S.; Gao, L. M-creatine kinase gene expression in mechanically overloaded skeletal muscle of transgenic mice. Am. J. Physiol. 269(Cell Physiol. 38):C665-C674; 1995.

30. Tsika, R.W.; Herrick, R.E.; Baldwin, K.M. Subunit composition of rodent isomyosins and their distribution in hindlimb skeletal muscle. J. Appl. Physiol. 63(5):2101-2110; 1987.

31. Tsika, R.W.; Herrick, R.E.; Baldwin, K.M. Time course adaptations in rat skeletal muscle isomyosins during compensatory growth and regression. J. Appl. Physiol. 63(5):2111-2121; 1987.

32. Vandenburgh, H.H.; Shansky, J.; Karlisch, P. Mechanical stimulation of skeletal muscle generates lipid-related second messengers by phospholipase activation. J. Cell. Physiol. 155:63-71; 1993.

33. Wentworth, B.M.; Donoghue, M.; Engert, J.C. Paired MyoD-binding sites regulate myosin light chain gene expression. Proc. Natl. Acad. Sci. USA 88:1242-1246; 1991.

34. Whitelaw, P.F.; Hesketh, J.E. Expression of c-*myc* and c-*fos* in rat skeletal muscle. Biochem. J. 281:143-147; 1992.

35. Wiedenman, J.L.; Rivera-Rivera, I.; Vyas, D.; Tsika, G.L.; Gao, L.; Sheriff-Carter, K.; Xin, W.; Kwan, L.T.; Tsika, R.W. βMHC and SMLC transgene induction in overloaded skeletal muscle of transgenic mice. Am. J. Physiol. 270 (Cell Physiol. 39):C1111-C1121; 1996.

36. Wiedenman, J.L.; Tsika, G.L.; Gao, L.; McCarthy, J.J.; Rivera, I.; Vyas, D.; Sheriff-Carter, K.; Tsika, R.W. Muscle-specific and inducible expression of 293-base-pair βMyosin heavy chain promoter in transgenic mice. Am. J. Physiol. (Regulatory, Integrative and Comp. Physiol.) (In press.)

PART V

Biochemistry
of High-Intensity Exercise

CHAPTER 18

Dietary Creatine Supplementation and Fatigue During High-Intensity Exercise in Humans

Paul L. Greenhaff, Kristina Bodin, Anna Casey,
Dumitru Constantin-Teodosiu, Allison Green, Karin Söderlund,
Jamie Timmons, Eric Hultman
University Medical School, Queens Medical Centre, Nottingham, England;
Karolinska Institute, Huddinge, Sweden; University Medical School, Queens
Medical Centre, Nottingham, England; University Medical School, Queens
Medical Centre, Nottingham, England; University Medical School, Queens
Medical Centre, Nottingham, England; Karolinska Institute, Huddinge, Sweden;
University Medical School, Queens Medical Centre, Nottingham, England;
Karolinska Institute, Huddinge, Sweden

The Biosynthesis and Distribution of Creatine

Creatine (Cr), or methyl guanidine acetic acid, is a naturally occurring compound and, in a 70-kg man, the total body creatine pool amounts to approximately 120 g, of which 95% is found in muscle (41, 48). Creatine is of greatest abundance in fast-twitch skeletal muscle, its concentration being about 45% and 55% higher than in slow-twitch and cardiac muscles, respectively (figure 18.1). Creatine is also found in small quantities in brain, liver, kidney, and testes.

Creatine was first identified in 1835 in meat extract by Chevreul. Then in 1847, Liebig showed that it could be extracted from several kinds of muscle, but not from the other organs he investigated. During the following years, there was much debate as to whether the Cr concentration of muscle increased during contraction. However, not long before the discovery of phosphocreatine (PCr) by Fiske and Subbarow between the years of 1927 and 1929, Schlossmann and Tiegs showed that "diffusible" Cr increased during contraction (for further information see 49). Thus, even in the early parts of this century, there was already literature pointing to an important function for Cr in muscle contraction, the knowledge of its fairly specific distribution, and its absence from normal urine, leading to the realization that it was not merely a waste product of metabolism. This realization was confirmed

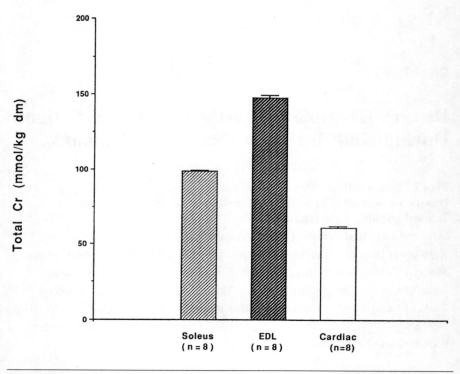

Figure 18.1   The total creatine (Cr) concentration of rat soleus, extensor digitorum longus (EDL), and cardiac muscles. Values represent mean ± *SE*.

when Chanutin (15) observed that creatine administration resulted in a major portion of the compound being retained by the body.

The precursors of Cr were first determined by labeling nitrogenous compounds with ^{15}N and isolating any creatine formed (10). Synthesis has been shown to proceed via two successive reactions involving two enzymes (figure 18.2). The first reaction is catalyzed by glycine transamidinase and results in an amidine group being reversibly transferred from arginine to glycine, forming guanidinoacetic acid. The second reaction involves irreversible transfer of a methyl group from S-adenosylmethionine (SAM) catalyzed by guanidinoacetate methyltransferase, resulting in the methylation of guanidinoacetate and the formation of Cr (20, 61). The distribution of the two enzymes differs among tissues across mammalian species. Generally however, glycine transamidinase is found in the kidney, liver, pancreas, and spleen, and guanidino-acetate methyltransferase is present in the pancreas and liver. It is generally stated that the initial reaction in Cr biosynthesis occurs in the kidneys and the second in the liver. However, in the case of humans, both the pancreas and the liver have the capability of achieving de novo Cr synthesis (61). Creatine administration in animal studies has been shown to suppress transamidinase activity without affecting methyl-transferase (61), thus suggesting that synthesis is regulated by feedback inhibition of the former. Because little creatine is found in the major sites of synthesis, it is logical to assume that transport of creatine from sites of synthesis to storage must occur, thus allowing a separation of biosynthesis from utilization.

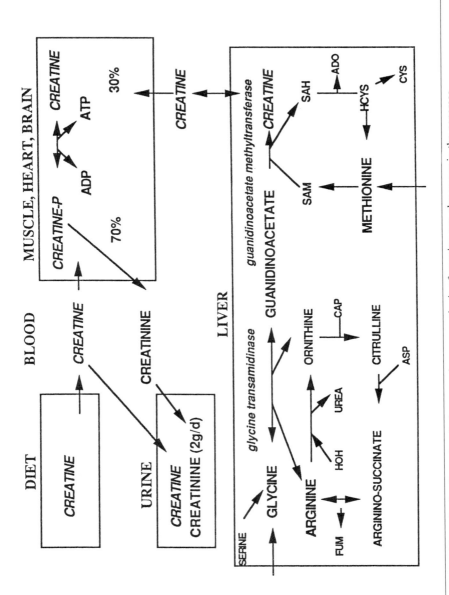

Figure 18.2   The biosynthesis of creatine. In humans, de novo synthesis of creatine can also occur in the pancreas.

The two mechanisms that have been proposed to explain the very high Cr concentration within skeletal muscle involve first, the transport of Cr into muscle by a specific saturable entry process and second, the intracellular trapping of Cr within muscle (20, 22, 23). Early studies demonstrated that creatine entry into muscle occurs actively against a concentration gradient, possibly involving Cr interacting with a specific membrane site that recognizes the amidine group (20, 22, 23). Very recently, a specific Cr transporter has been identified in rat skeletal muscle, heart, and brain (54). It has been suggested that some skeletal muscles do not demonstrate a saturable uptake process, thereby supporting the idea of intracellular entrapment of Cr (20). About 60% of muscle total Cr exists in the form of phosphocreatine and is therefore unable to pass through membranes because of its polarity; thus Cr is trapped. This entrapment will result in the generation of a concentration gradient, but phosphorylation alone cannot be the sole mechanism of cellular retention of Cr. Other mechanisms that have been proposed include binding to intracellular components and the existence of restrictive cellular membranes (20).

In normal, healthy individuals, muscle Cr is replenished at a rate of approximately $2 \text{ g} \cdot \text{d}^{-1}$ by endogenous Cr synthesis or dietary Cr intake, such as meat (61). Oral ingestion of Cr has also been demonstrated to suppress biosynthesis, an effect that has been shown to be removed upon cessation of supplementation (61).

Creatinine has been established as the sole end product of Cr degradation, formed nonenzymatically in an irreversible reaction (22, 24). Because skeletal muscle is the major store of the body Cr pool, this is the major site of creatinine production. The daily renal creatinine excretion is relatively constant in an individual, but can vary between individuals (20), being dependent on the total muscle mass in healthy individuals (35). Once generated, creatinine enters the circulation by simple diffusion and is filtered by the glomerulus and excreted in urine. Studies involving intravenous administration of labeled creatinine have shown 96% recovery in urine within 24 h, with no evidence of degradation or conversion to Cr (10, 16).

The Role of Creatine
in Muscle Energy Metabolism and Fatigue

In human skeletal muscle, Cr is present at a concentration of about 125 mmol · kg^{-1} dry muscle (d.m.), of which approximately 60% is in the form of PCr at rest. A reversible equilibrium exists between Cr and PCr (PCr + ADP + H$^+$ ↔ ATP + Cr), and together they function to maintain intracellular ATP availability, modulate metabolism, and buffer hydrogen ion accumulation during contraction. The availability of PCr has been suggested to be one of the most likely limitations to muscle performance during intense, fatiguing, short-lasting contractions. This conclusion has been drawn from studies involving short bouts of maximal electrically evoked contraction (39) and voluntary exercise (43) and from animal studies in which the muscle Cr store has been depleted prior to maximal electrical stimulation using the Cr analogue β-guanidinopropionate (β-GPA; 21, 46) or manipulated using cyclocreatine (ischemic heart, 52).

The availability of free Cr has also been ascribed a central role in the control of phosphocreatine resynthesis, its role in the regulation of mitochondrial ATP production having been subject to much debate (6, 7, 47, 55, 56, 62). While it is widely accepted that Cr is a recipient of mitochondrially derived ATP, studies demonstrating that the depletion of muscle Cr as a result of β-GPA feeding has little influence on submaximal contractile function, oxygen consumption, or energy metabolism during contraction (55, 56) directly oppose those studies suggesting a central role for Cr in the regulation of muscle metabolism during contraction, that is, the PCr-Cr shuttle (7, 62). However, it is known that, in addition to decreasing Cr availability by blocking Cr uptake, β-GPA will produce biochemical, functional, and structural abnormalities in skeletal muscle, and therefore the interpretation of these data can be misleading (62). Irrespective of this, human studies involving maximal electrically evoked and voluntary contraction (39) and animal preparation studies (53, 59), including those involving depletion of muscle Cr stores by β-GPA feeding (21, 46), generally agree that creatine-phosphocreatine availability is essential to muscle function during short-duration, fatiguing maximal exercise.

Table 18.1 shows the rates of ATP resynthesis from PCr and glycolysis (glycolysis in this situation comprises almost exclusively glycogen degradation) during 30 s of near maximal isometric contraction in humans. Notice first that the rate of PCr utilization begins to decline after only 1.3 s of contraction, while the corresponding rate from glycolysis does not peak until after approximately 3 s of contraction, suggesting that the rapid initial utilization of PCr buffers the momentary lag in energy provision from glycolysis. Second, there is a progressive decline in ATP provision from both substrates after their initial peaks. For example, the rates of ATP provision from PCr and glycolysis during the final 10 s of contraction amount to 2% and 40%, respectively, of their peak rates of production. Similar findings, involving isokinetic and dynamic exercise, have been reported by other research groups (11, 42). Of interest, in all of these studies, parallel with the decline in anaerobic ATP production was a decline in force production and power output. It is tempting to postulate therefore that the development of fatigue was attributable to the decline in ATP provision. Alternatively, however, the decline in energy provision could simply be a function of a decline in the rate of ATP utilization, which will accompany any decline in force production.

Table 18.1   Rates of Anaerobic ATP Production From Phosphocreatine (PCr) and Glycolysis During Maximal Contraction in Human Skeletal Muscle

Duration of stimulation (s)	ATP production $(\text{mmol} \cdot \text{s}^{-1} \cdot \text{kg}^{-1} \text{ d.m.})$	
	PCr	Glycolysis
0-1.3	9.0	2.0
0-2.6	7.5	4.3
0-5	5.3	4.4
0-10	4.2	4.5
10-20	2.2	4.5
20-30	0.2	2.1

Rates were calculated from metabolite changes measured in muscle biopsy samples obtained during intense, intermittent, electrically evoked isometric contraction (38, 40).

The values shown in table 18.1 were calculated from the metabolite changes measured in muscle biopsy samples obtained from the vastus lateralis muscle of normal, healthy volunteers. However, it is known that human skeletal muscle is composed of at least two functionally and metabolically different fiber types. Type I fibers are characterized as slow contracting, fatigue resistant, having a low power output, and favoring aerobic metabolism for ATP resynthesis during contraction. Conversely, type II fibers are fast contracting, fatigue rapidly, have a high power output and favor mainly anaerobic metabolism for ATP resynthesis (for comprehensive review see 27). Evidence from animal studies performed on muscles composed of predominantly type I or type II fibers (3, 13, 17, 36) and from one study performed using bundles of similar human muscle fiber types (19) suggests that the rapid, marked rise and subsequent decline in maximal power output observed during intense muscle contraction in humans may be closely related to activation and rapid fatigue of type II fibers during contraction.

More recent human studies have implicated the availability of PCr in type II muscle fibers as being of critical importance to the maintenance of performance during maximal, short-lasting exercise. Briefly, these studies involved muscle biopsy samples obtained from the quadriceps muscle group before and after intense isometric contraction, induced by percutaneous electrical stimulation (58) or following intense sprinting exercise (31). Individual muscle fiber fragments were then dissected from each biopsy sample and, after fiber type characterization, were used to determine the changes in selected energy metabolites during contraction. Figure 18.3 shows the changes in ATP and PCr concentrations in type I and II fibers after 10 and 20 s of electrical stimulation and the decline in whole-muscle force production throughout stimulation. During the first 10 s of stimulation, the rates of PCr utilization in type I and II fibers were 3.3 and 5.3 mmol $\cdot$ kg^{-1} d.m. $\cdot$ s^{-1}, respectively. During the second period of stimulation, the rate of PCr utilization in type I fibers declined by 15% to 2.8 mmol $\cdot$ kg^{-1} d.m. $\cdot$ s^{-1}, and the corresponding rate in type II fibers declined by 60% to 2.1 mmol $\cdot$ kg^{-1} d.m. $\cdot$ s^{-1}. At the end of the stimulation period, the PCr store of type II fibers was nearly exhausted. After the initial few seconds, whole-muscle force production declined throughout the stimulation period to approximately 80% of its initial value. In short, therefore, the declining rate of ATP resynthesis arising from the decreased availability of PCr principally in type II fibers will have been insufficient to maintain force production, and fatigue will have occurred.

Figure 18.4a shows the degradation of PCr and ATP in type I and II muscle fibers during 32 s of electrically evoked maximal isometric contraction (20 contractions, 1.6 s stimulation, 1.6 s rest, 50 Hz), which produced a 40% decline in power output. While it is difficult to prove that PCr availability in type II muscle fibers was a principal cause of fatigue here, the significantly higher type II fiber PCr degradation in parallel with the higher ATP loss in this fiber type implies that this may be the case. This is in agreement with the data shown in figure 18.4b, which was obtained from a study again involving 32 s of electrically evoked contraction (20 contractions, 1.6 s stimulation, 1.6 s rest, 50 Hz), but on this occasion with muscle blood flow occluded. In this extreme metabolic situation, muscle force production declined by nearly 60%, and total PCr depletion occurred in both fiber types. However, the loss of ATP was twofold greater in the type II fibers compared with type I fibers, suggesting that the depletion of PCr in this fiber type resulted in the necessary high rate of ATP turnover during contraction not being maintained.

It perhaps seems pertinent to suggest therefore that any mechanism capable of increasing muscle Cr availability may delay PCr depletion and the rate of ATP

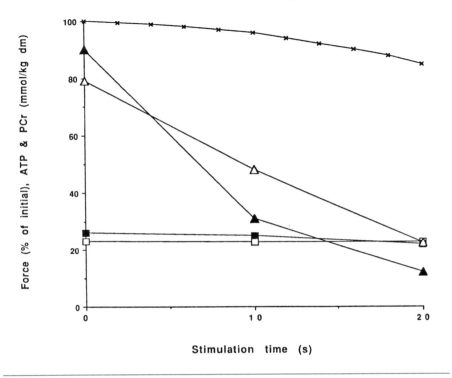

Figure 18.3 Muscle isometric force production (x) and ATP (squares) and PCr (triangles) concentrations in type I (open symbols) and type II (filled symbols) muscle fibers during 20 s of intense electrical stimulation (1.6 s stimulation, 1.6 s rest; 50 Hz) in humans.

degradation during maximal exercise or may influence PCr resynthesis during recovery. This being the case, it is rather surprising that little work appears to have been devoted to the influence of Cr ingestion on exercise performance in humans.

The Effect of Creatine Ingestion on Muscle Creatine Concentration in Humans

Early studies demonstrated that Cr administration resulted in a small increase in urinary creatinine excretion. In general, urinary creatinine excretion rose slowly during prolonged Cr administration and, upon cessation, around 5 wk elapsed before a significant fall in creatinine excretion was observed (4, 15). From these early studies, Cr retention in the body pool was thought to be much greater during the initial stages of administration. These early studies also demonstrated that there was no increase in creatinine excretion until a significant amount of the administered Cr had been retained (4, 15). In 1939, Bloch and Schoenheimer (10) demonstrated that urinary creatinine was derived from Cr by administering labeled Cr to rats.

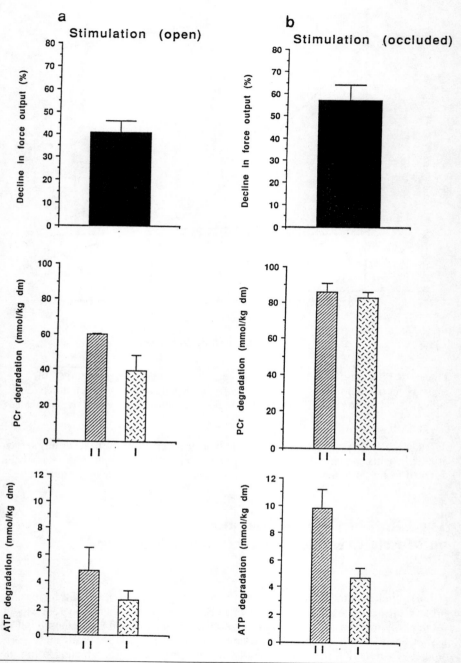

Figure 18.4   Decline in muscle isometric force production and PCr and ATP concentrations in type II and I muscle fibers during 32 s of intense electrical stimulation (1.6 s stimulation, 1.6 s rest; 50 Hz) in humans. Experiments were performed with limb blood flow open (a) and occluded (b). Values represent mean ± *SE*.

Administration resulted in urinary excretion of labeled creatinine, confirming that creatinine is derived from Cr. However, as the amount of radioactivity recovered was less than the amount administered, the authors concluded that ingested Cr must mix with the body Cr pool before degradation to creatinine. Alternatively, the inability to account for all of the labeled Cr as creatinine could have been a consequence of incomplete intestinal absorption or degradation. In 1948, Hoberman, Sims, and Peters (37) with the aid of isotopic nitrogen demonstrated that it was possible to observe Cr deposition in men.

These early studies invariably involved periods of chronic Cr ingestion. However, with the application of the muscle biopsy technique, it has recently become clear that the ingestion of 20 g of Cr each day for 5 d (4×5-g doses) by healthy volunteers can lead to, on average, more than a 20% increase in muscle total Cr concentration, of which approximately 20% is in the form of PCr (33; figure 18.5). In agreement with earlier work, the authors demonstrated that the majority of tissue Cr uptake occurred during the initial days of supplementation, with close to 30% of the administered dose being retained during the initial 2 d of supplementation, compared with 15% from days 2 to 4. Furthermore, when submaximal exercise was performed during the period of supplementation, muscle uptake appeared to be increased by a further 10%.

The mechanism by which muscle Cr uptake is achieved is presently unclear. However, muscle contraction (33) and insulin (12, 44), have both been shown to augment tissue Cr uptake, possibly by an effect on the number or activity of the membrane Cr transporter, which has recently been isolated in skeletal muscle (54). It is tantalizing to suggest that, similar to muscle glucose uptake, exercise achieves its augmentative effect on Cr uptake by increasing muscle insulin sensitivity. Furthermore, the observed sequential decrease in Cr uptake during daily feeding (33), the greater than normal retention of Cr by vegetarians (P.L. Greenhaff, personal observation) as a consequence of having a low body Cr pool (18), and the augmented loss of Cr from muscle during fasting (61) and disease (20) may be related to the up- and down-regulation of the Cr transporter. It is important, however, to point out first that human muscle appears to have an upper-limit Cr concentration of 145 to 160 mmol · kg^{-1} d.m.; therefore, once achieved by supplementation, this cannot be exceeded. Second, individuals with the lowest muscle Cr concentrations appear to achieve the most pronounced increases with ingestion. What determines whether a person has a high or low muscle Cr concentration is not yet clear. Of interest, females, for reasons as yet unknown, appear to have a slightly higher muscle Cr concentration than males (25). This may be a consequence of their muscle mass and therefore their Cr distribution space being smaller.

Based on recently obtained unpublished experimental findings, it would appear that, as might be expected, low-dose Cr supplementation (3 g · d^{-1}) over a 4-wk period is less effective, at least during the initial 2 wk of ingestion, at raising tissue Cr levels compared with the 5-d regimen of 20 g · d^{-1} (figure 18.6). Further recent work clearly demonstrates that muscle Cr stores remain elevated for several weeks when a supplementation dose of 20 g · d^{-1} for 5 d is followed by lower dose supplementation (2 g · d^{-1}), which seems to agree with the earlier suggestions of Fitch (20) that Cr is "trapped" within skeletal muscle once absorbed (figure 18.7). The natural time course of muscle Cr decline following 5 d of 20 g · d^{-1} ingestion is presently unknown, but based on earlier studies that investigated the time course of creatinine excretion following Cr ingestion (4, 15), it is likely to be over the course of several weeks rather than days.

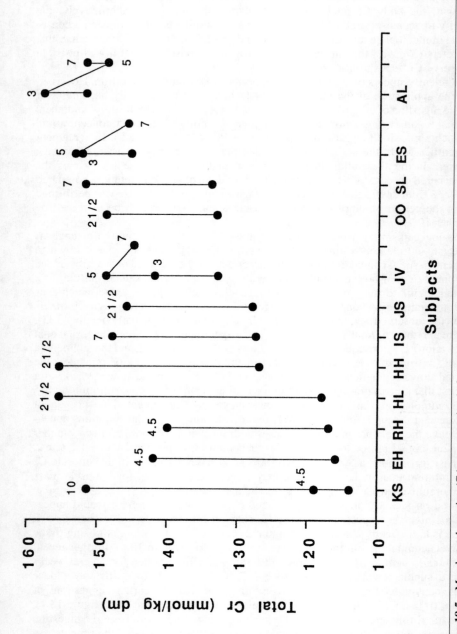

Figure 18.5 Muscle total creatine (Cr) concentration before and after different durations (3–21 d) of Cr ingestion at rates of 20 g · d^{-1} (subjects KS, EH, RH, IS, SL, and ES) and 30 g · d^{-1} (subjects HL, HH, JS, JV, OO, and AL). 21/2 indicates creatine was ingested every other day for a duration of 21 d.

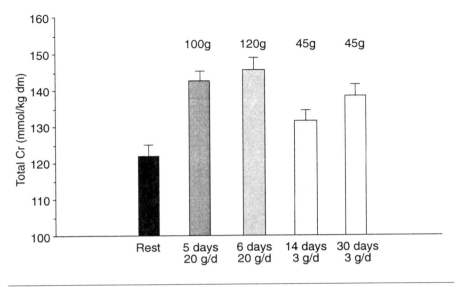

Figure 18.6   Muscle total creatine (Cr) concentrations before and after Cr ingestion. Units at the base of each bar graph indicate the duration and rate of creatine ingestion. Units above each bar graph indicate the total amount of Cr ingested over the entire experimental period. Values represent mean ± *SE*.

The Effect of Creatine Ingestion on Exercise Performance

As stated previously, a reversible equilibrium exists between Cr and PCr, and the development of fatigue during high-intensity exercise is associated with the depletion of muscle PCr. Creatine in its free and phosphorylated forms therefore occupies a pivotal role in the regulation and homeostasis of skeletal muscle energy metabolism and fatigue.

In 1934, Boothby (see 14) reported that the development of fatigue in humans could be delayed by the addition of large amounts of the Cr precursor glycine to the diet, which he attributed to an effect on muscle Cr concentration. Later, in 1939, Ray, Johnson, and Taylor (51) concluded that the ingestion of 60 g of gelatin · d^{-1} for several weeks could also postpone the development of fatigue in humans. The authors reasoned that because glycine constitutes 25% of gelatin by weight, the increased ingestion of gelatin would result in an increased muscle Cr concentration and thereby an increase in muscle function. Maison (45), however, could not reproduce these findings and concluded that gelatin, and therefore glycine, had no effect on work capacity during repeated bouts of fatiguing muscle contractions. Shortly after this, however, Chaikelis (14) reported that the ingestion of 6 g of glycine · d^{-1} in tablet form for 10 wk markedly improved performance (approximately 20%) in a number of different muscle groups and reduced creatinine excretion by 30%. In the discussion of results, the author implicated a change in the muscle Cr pool as being responsible for his observations.

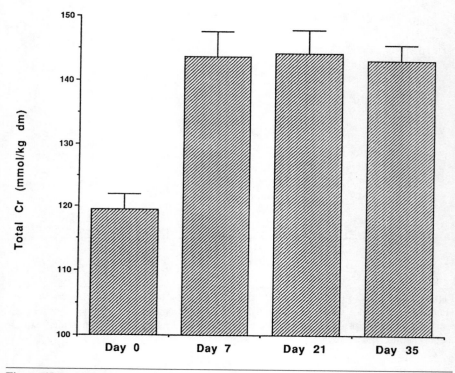

Figure 18.7   Muscle total creatine (Cr) concentration before and after 34 d of Cr inges-tion. Creatine was ingested at a rate of 20 g · d⁻¹ for the initial 6 d and at a rate of 2 g · d⁻¹ thereafter. Values represent mean ± *SE*.

Other than these initial reports, which do not relate to Cr ingestion per se, little has been published relating to Cr ingestion and exercise performance. In 1981, Sipila et al. (57) reported that, in a group of patients receiving 1 g of Cr · d⁻¹ as a treatment for gyrate atrophy, there was a comment from some of a sensation of strength gain following a 1-yr period of supplementation. Indeed, Cr ingestion was shown to reverse the type II muscle fiber atrophy associated with this disease, and one athlete in the group of patients improved his personal best record for the 100 m by 2 s. Muscle Cr availability has been implicated in the control of muscle protein synthesis (8), and muscle wasting diseases have been related to abnormalities of Cr metabolism (20, 24). In this respect, the influence of chronic Cr ingestion on skeletal muscle mass and composition is of obvious scientific interest but is beyond the scope of this review.

Based on recently published results from placebo-controlled laboratory experi-ments, it is now clear that the ingestion of 4 × 5 g of Cr · d⁻¹ for 5 d can significantly increase the amount of work that can be performed by healthy, normal volunteers during repeated bouts of maximal knee extensor exercise (29). These findings have been confirmed by additional laboratory studies involving repeated bouts of maximal dynamic (1) and isokinetic (9) cycling exercise and by controlled field experiments undertaken by athletes over 4 × 300 m and 4 × 1000 m (34). The consistent finding from these studies is that Cr ingestion can significantly increase exercise performance by sustaining force or work output during exercise. For example, in the study by Greenhaff et al. (29), two groups of subjects ($n = 6$) performed five bouts of 30 maximal, voluntary, unilateral knee extensions at a constant angular velocity of $180° \cdot s^{-1}$ before and after placebo and Cr ingestion (4×5 g of Cr $\cdot$ d^{-1} for 5 d). No difference was seen when comparing muscle torque production during exercise before and after placebo ingestion. However, following Cr ingestion, torque production was increased by 5% to 7% in all subjects during the final 10 contractions of exercise bout 1 and throughout the whole of exercise bouts 2, 3, and 4. In the study by Birch, Noble, and Greenhaff (9), two groups of seven healthy male subjects performed three bouts of maximal isokinetic cycling exercise at 80 rpm before and after Cr or placebo ingestion (4×5 g of Cr $\cdot$ d^{-1} for 5 d). Each exercise bout lasted for 30 s and was interspersed by 4 min rest. The total amount of work performed during bouts 1 to 3 were similar when comparing values obtained before and after placebo ingestion (< 2% change). After Cr ingestion, work output was increased in all seven subjects during exercise bouts 1 ($p < .05$) and 2 ($p < .05$), but no difference was observed during exercise bout 3. Figure 18.8 shows the change in work output during each exercise bout following placebo and Cr ingestion.

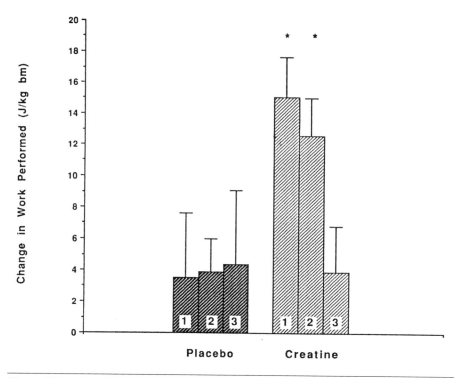

Figure 18.8   The change in work production during 3×30-s bouts of maximal isokinetic cycling (80 rpm) in men following 5 d of placebo (20 g glucose polymer $\cdot$ d^{-1}) and creatine (20 g $\cdot$ d^{-1}) ingestion. Each bout of exercise was separated by 4 min rest. Values represent mean $\pm$ *SE*. *($p < .05$) indicates significant increase from presupplementation work production.

Recent results (2, 26) suggest that Cr ingestion has no effect on performance or metabolism during submaximal exercise. The latter study demonstrated that Cr ingestion at a rate of 20 g · d^{-1} for 5 d had no effect on respiratory gas exchange or blood lactate accumulation during steady-state incremental treadmill running (figure 18.9).

Creatine's Mechanism of Action

The exact mechanism by which short-term Cr ingestion improves performance during maximal exercise is not yet clear. The available data indicate that it may be related to the stimulatory effect that Cr has on preexercise PCr availability and PCr resynthesis during recovery from exercise. Given that PCr availability is generally thought to limit exercise capacity during maximal exercise, both of these effects would increase muscle contractile capability by maintaining ATP turnover during exercise. This suggestion is supported by reports showing that the accumulation of plasma ammonia and hypoxanthine (accepted markers of skeletal muscle adenine nucleotide loss) are reduced during maximal exercise following Cr ingestion, despite a higher work output being achieved (1, 29). More convincing evidence comes from a recent study showing that creatine supplementation can reduce the extent of muscle ATP degradation during maximal isokinetic cycling exercise, while at the same time increasing work output (30). In this particular study, eight healthy male subjects familiarized with the experimental procedures undertook two bouts of maximal isokinetic cycling each lasting 30 s (80 rpm) interspersed with 4 min of recovery, before and after 5 d of Cr ingestion (4×5 g · d^{-1}). Muscle biopsy samples were obtained immediately before and after each exercise bout. Creatine ingestion resulted, on average, in a 25 mmol · kg^{-1} d.m. increase in muscle total Cr concentration, of which approximately 8.5 mmol · kg^{-1} d.m. was in the form of PCr and 16.5 mmol · kg^{-1} d.m. was in the form of Cr at rest before exercise. Following Cr ingestion, total work output was increased by 11.8 ± 3.7 J · kg^{-1} body weight (4.3%, $p < .05$) and 10.9 ± 2.9 J · kg^{-1} body weight (4.1%, $p < .05$) in exercise bouts 1 and 2, respectively. Irrespective of treatment, total work production was always greatest during the first bout of exercise.

When comparing treatments, the mean loss of ATP during exercise was 10% and 65% less during exercise bouts 1 and 2, respectively, following Cr ingestion, but this difference was not significant. However, when comparing the total ATP loss over the two bouts of exercise (i.e., Σ exercise bouts 1 and 2), the degradation was 25% less after Cr ingestion (6.2 ± 1.3 mmol · kg^{-1} d.m.) compared with before Cr ingestion (8.5 ± 1.0 mmol · kg^{-1} d.m.; $p < .05$). Figure 18.10 shows the mean total ATP degradation over the two exercise bouts and the data for individual subjects before and after Cr ingestion.

Concerning recovery, recent results from our laboratory clearly show that those individuals who experience a marked ($25 \pm 3\%$) increase in muscle total Cr following oral Cr ingestion show an accelerated rate of PCr resynthesis during recovery from intense muscle contraction (28). Figure 18.11 shows the changes in muscle free Cr and PCr during 2 min of recovery in those subjects who "responded" to Cr feeding. Both before and after Cr feeding, the muscle free Cr concentration declined during recovery, but the free Cr concentration was at all times greater following Cr ingestion.

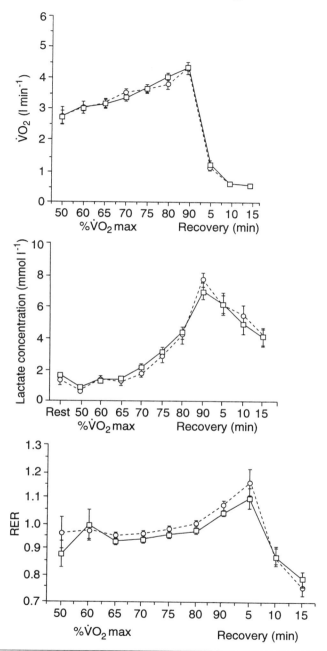

Figure 18.9   Oxygen consumption ($\dot{V}O_2$), blood lactate concentration, and respiratory exchange ratio (RER) during treadmill running and recovery before (circles) and after (squares) 5 d of Cr ingestion (20 g · d^{-1}) in humans. Exercise was performed for 6 min at intensities equivalent to 50%, 60%, 65%, 70%, 75%, 80%, and 90% of maximal oxygen consumption ($\dot{V}O_2$max). Values represent mean ± SE.

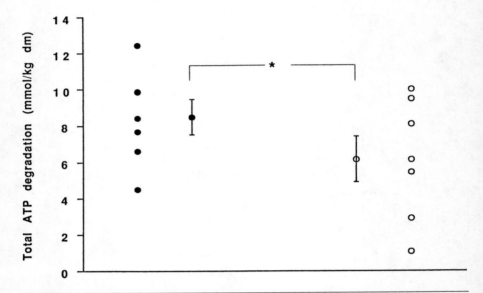

Figure 18.10 Total muscle ATP degradation during 2×30-s bouts of maximal iso-kinetic cycling (80 rpm) in men before and after 5 d of creatine ingestion ($20 \text{ g} \cdot \text{d}^{-1}$). The two exercise bouts were separated by 4 min of passive recovery. Values shown represent mean $\pm$ SE and individual values recorded for each subject. *($p < .05$) indicates significant difference in degradation pre- and postcreatine intake.

As expected, PCr resynthesis began almost immediately following the cessation of contraction. The extent of resynthesis was almost identical during the initial 40 s of recovery when comparing pre- and postfeeding concentrations. However, during the remainder of recovery, the rate of resynthesis was greater after Cr feeding, resulting in the muscle concentration being 30% higher at the end of the 2-min recovery period. In general, PCr resynthesis follows an exponential curve after intense muscle contraction (32, 50) and the half time for resynthesis in human skeletal muscle is approximately 30 to 40 s (32). It is generally accepted that the resynthesis of PCr during recovery is mediated by mitochondrial membrane–bound creatine kinase (CK), thus linking oxidative ATP production to cytoplasmic PCr resynthesis (6, 47, 62). Factors that will undoubtedly influence the rate of resynthesis include free ATP, ADP, H$^+$, and Cr concentrations, due to their role in the CK equilibrium reaction. The in vitro Michaelis constant (K_m) values of CK for ATP and ADP are relatively low, approximately $0.6 \text{ mmol} \cdot \text{l}^{-1}$ and $1 \text{ mmol} \cdot \text{l}^{-1}$, respectively (5). Conversely, the K_m of CK for Cr is comparatively high, close to 18 mmol $\cdot \text{l}^{-1}$. It is known that muscle free Cr can range in concentration from approximately 13 mmol $\cdot$ l^{-1} intracellular water at rest (33) to approximately 40 mmol $\cdot$ l^{-1} intracellular water following maximal exercise (60). Thus, during the initial stages of recovery from maximal exercise, when the rate of mitochondrial

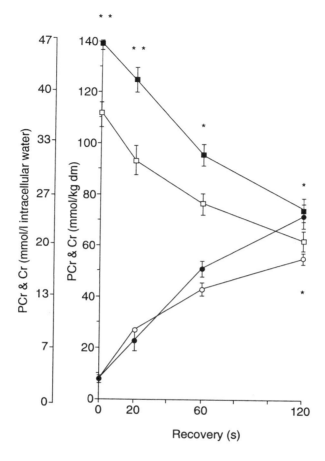

Figure 18.11   Phosphocreatine (PCr, circles) and free creatine (Cr, squares) concentrations measured in muscle biopsy samples obtained after 0, 20, 60, and 120 s of recovery from intense contraction before (open symbols) and after (filled symbols) Cr ingestion. Values represent mean $\pm$ *SE* for a group of five subjects who showed a 25 $\pm$ 3% increase in muscle total Cr concentration during 5 d of Cr ingestion (20 g $\cdot$ d^{-1}). *($p < 0.05$) and **($p < 0.01$) represent significant difference between corresponding pre- and postsupplementation concentrations.

ADP rephosphorylation to ATP will be at its highest, it is unlikely that the rate of PCr formation by mitochondrial CK will be dependent on the availability of free Cr, because its concentration will be far in excess of the K_m value. However, as PCr resynthesis continues and muscle free Cr concentration declines towards 19 mmol $\cdot$ l^{-1}, it is suggested that free Cr concentration may then begin to be a determinant of the rate of PCr resynthesis. The results of the experiment previously outlined support this suggestion. Figure 18.11 demonstrates that the rates of PCr resynthesis were almost identical during the initial 20 s of recovery when comparing values obtained before and after Cr ingestion. This, based on the preceding explanation, might be expected because the free Cr concentration was at all times in excess of 27 mmol $\cdot$ l^{-1} intracellular water. However, as recovery proceeded beyond 40 s, Cr feeding was associated with a higher rate of resynthesis. We would like to suggest that this occurred as a result of Cr ingestion maintaining the muscle free Cr concentration higher than the K_m of CK for Cr throughout the second half of recovery, thereby sustaining a high flux through the CK reaction in favor of PCr resynthesis and ADP formation. The latter will have in turn provided mitochondria with substrate to maintain a high rate of ATP formation. The role of Cr as an acceptor of mitochondrial ATP has been discussed in a series of previously published papers (6, 7, 47, 56, 62).

A series of reports have previously been published indicating that dietary Cr supplementation can have a positive effect on performance during maximal exercise (1, 9, 29, 34). However, we would now like to suggest that Cr ingestion can be of greater benefit to some individuals than others. Recent results indicate that those individuals who have a muscle Cr concentration of close to or less than 120 mmol $\cdot$ kg^{-1} d.m. prior to Cr ingestion can expect to see a 25% increase in muscle total Cr concentration following 5 d of Cr ingestion at a rate of 20 g $\cdot$ d^{-1} (28). It is important, however, that while these individuals showed an accelerated rate of PCr resynthesis during recovery from intense muscular contraction (figure 18.11), those individuals who experienced no or little muscle Cr uptake during ingestion (approximately 8% uptake) showed no measurable change in PCr resynthesis during recovery following Cr feeding. Figure 18.12a shows the individual changes in muscle total Cr concentration following 5 d of Cr ingestion (4 × 5 g $\cdot$ d^{-1}) in the group of eight subjects. The subjects have been numbered 1 to 8 based on their initial muscle total Cr concentration. As can be seen, five subjects (1, 2, 3, 4, and 7) experienced a marked 29 ± 3 mmol $\cdot$ kg^{-1} d.m. increase in total Cr concentration. In particular, the four subjects with the lowest initial total Cr concentration experienced the most dramatic increase in total Cr (25-35 mmol $\cdot$ kg^{-1} d.m.), which was equivalent to 20% to 32% of their initial total Cr concentration. The remaining three subjects (5, 6, and 8) each experienced a relatively small increase in total Cr concentration with Cr ingestion (7-9 mmol $\cdot$ kg^{-1} d.m.).

Figure 18.12b shows the increase in muscle total Cr with Cr feeding, plotted against the change in PCr resynthesis during 2 min of recovery from maximal exercise after Cr feeding. As can be seen, the same subjects who experienced a marked increase in muscle total Cr concentration with Cr ingestion also showed an increased rate of PCr resynthesis during recovery following Cr ingestion. Conversely, the three subjects who had less than a 10 mmol $\cdot$ kg^{-1} d.m. increase in muscle total Cr concentration with feeding showed very little change in PCr resynthesis during recovery after Cr feeding. Thus, these data point to the importance of maximizing tissue Cr uptake when attempting to increase exercise performance by Cr feeding. The preceding findings and the results of Harris, Söderlund, and Hultman (33) indicate that the prefeeding muscle Cr concentration will be an important determinant of the extent of tissue uptake. However, it is important to note that the average Cr concentration of human skeletal muscle is 125 mmol $\cdot$ kg^{-1} d.m. (mean of 81 biopsy samples) and follows a normal distribution ranging from 90 to 160 mmol $\cdot$ kg^{-1} d.m., and therefore a concentration of 120 mmol $\cdot$ kg^{-1} d.m. should not be viewed as appreciably low.

The importance of maximizing muscle Cr uptake when attempting to improve subsequent maximal exercise performance is clearly illustrated by our most recent

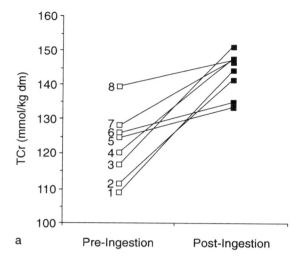

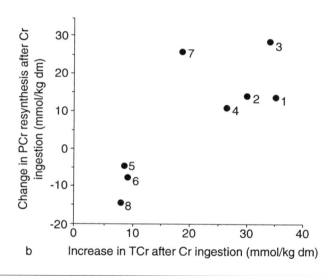

Figure 18.12.   (a) Individual values for muscle total creatine (Cr) concentration before and after 5 d of Cr ingestion (20 g · d⁻¹). Subjects have been numbered 1 to 8 based on their initial total Cr concentration. (b) Individual increases in muscle total Cr for the same group of subjects depicted in (a), plotted against the change in PCr resynthesis during re-covery from intense contraction after Cr ingestion. Values on the y axis were calculated by subtracting PCr resynthesis during 2 min of recovery before Cr ingestion from the cor-responding value after Cr ingestion.

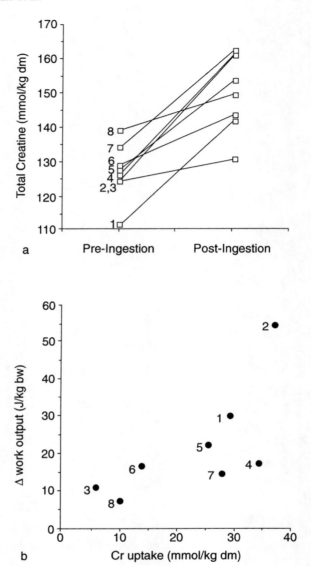

Figure 18.13. (a) Individual values for muscle total creatine (Cr) concentration before and after 5 d of Cr ingestion (20 g · d⁻¹). (b) Individual increases in muscle total Cr for the same group of subjects depicted in (a), plotted against the change in work production during 2 × 30-s bouts of maximal isokinetic cycling after Cr ingestion. Values on the *y* axis were calculated by subtracting total work output during exercise before Cr ingestion from the corresponding value after Cr ingestion.

findings. In this study, eight male subjects undertook two bouts of maximal isokinetic cycling (80 rpm) before and after 5 d of Cr ingestion (4×5 g $\cdot$ d^{-1}). Each exercise bout lasted for 30 s and was interspersed with 4 min of recovery. Figure 18.13a shows the increase in muscle total Cr concentration with Cr feeding for each individual. As in figure 18.12a, the subjects have been numbered 1 to 8 based on their initial total Cr concentration. On average, subjects 3, 6, and 8 demonstrated a 10 mmol $\cdot$ kg^{-1} d.m. increase in muscle total Cr with feeding. However, all of the remaining subjects (1, 2, 4, 5, 7) showed a greater than 30 mmol $\cdot$ kg^{-1} d.m. increase in muscle Cr with ingestion. Figure 18.13b shows the change in work output over the two bouts of exercise following Cr feeding plotted against muscle Cr uptake with feeding. This figure clearly demonstrates that those individuals who demonstrated the greatest muscle uptake of Cr during feeding also experienced the greatest improvement in exercise performance. Thus, it would appear that the extent of Cr uptake during feeding is critical to subsequent exercise performance. Future work should therefore focus on elucidating the principal factors regulating muscle Cr uptake in humans. With this in mind, figure 18.13a suggests that the initial muscle total Cr concentration was not the sole determinant of muscle Cr uptake in this particular study.

Acknowledgment

The authors would like to thank the Wellcome Trust for its support of some of the work described in this review.

References

1. Balsom, P.D.; Ekblom, B.; Söderlund, K.; Sjödin, B.; Hultman, E. Creatine supplementation and dynamic high-intensity intermittent exercise. Scand. J. Med. Sci. Sports 3:143-149; 1993.
2. Balsom, P.D.; Harridge, S.D.R.; Söderlund, K.; Sjödin, B.; Ekblom, B. Creatine supplementation *per se* does not enhance endurance exercise performance. Acta Physiol. Scand. 149:521-523; 1993.
3. Barany, M. ATPase activity of myosin correlated with speed of muscle shortening. J. Gen. Physiol. 50 (suppl. 2):197-218; 1967.
4. Benedict, S.R.; Ostergerg, E. The metabolism of creatine. J. Biol. Chem. 56:229-230; 1923.
5. Bergmeyer, H.U. Methods of enzymatic analysis. 2nd ed. London: Academic Press; 1965.
6. Bessman, S.P.; Fonyo, A. The possible role of mitochondrial bound creatine kinase in regulation of mitochondrial respiration. Biochem. Biophys. Res. Commun. 22:597-602; 1966.
7. Bessman, S.P.; Geiger, P.J. Transport of energy in muscle. The phosphoryl-creatine shuttle. Science 211:448L-452L; 1981.
8. Bessman, S.P.; Savabi, F. The role of the phosphocreatine energy shuttle in exercise and muscle hypertrophy. In: Taylor, A.W.; Gollnick, P.D.; Green, H.J.; Ianuzzo, C.D.; Noble, E.G.; Métivier, G.; Sutton, J.R., eds. Biochemistry of

exercise VII. Champaign, IL: Human Kinetics Books; 1990:167-178. (Int. Series Sports Sci.; vol. 21).

9. Birch, R.; Noble, D.; Greenhaff, P.L. The influence of dietary creatine supplementation on performance during repeated bouts of maximal isokinetic cycling in man. Eur. J. Appl. Physiol. 69:268-270; 1994.

10. Bloch, K.; Schoenheimer, R. The metabolic relation of creatine and creatinine studied with isotopic nitrogen. J. Biol. Chem. 131:111-121; 1939.

11. Boobis, L.H.; Williams, C.; Wooton, S.A. Human muscle metabolism during brief maximal exercise in man. J. Physiol. 338:21P-22P; 1982.

12. Brivio, R.H.; Chang, D.T. Insulin effect on creatine transport in skeletal muscle. Proc. Soc. Exp. Med. 148:1-4; 1975.

13. Burke, R.E.; Levine, D.N.; Zajac, F.E., III; Tsaris, P.; Engel, W.K. Mammalian motor units: Physiological-histochemical correlation in three types of cat gastrocnemius. Science 174:709-712; 1971.

14. Chaikelis, A.S. The effect of glycocoll (glycine) ingestion upon the growth, strength and creatinine-creatine excretion in man. Am. J. Physiol. 133:578-587; 1940.

15. Chanutin, A. The fate of creatine when administered to man. J. Biol. Chem. 67:29-37; 1926.

16. Clarke, J.T. Colorimetric determination and distribution of urinary creatine and creatinine. Clin. Chem. 7:217-283; 1961.

17. Close, R.I. Dynamic properties of mammalian skeletal muscles. Physiol. Rev. 52:129-197; 1972.

18. Delanghe, J.; De Slypere, J.-P.; Debuyzere, M.; Robbrecht, J.; Wieme, R.; Vermeulen, A. Normal reference values for creatine, creatinine and carnitine are lower in vegetarians. Clin. Chem. 35:1802-1803; 1989.

19. Faulkner, J.A.; Claflin, D.R.; McCully, K.K. Power output of fast and slow fibres from human skeletal muscles. In: Jones, N.L.; McCartney, N.; McComas, A.J., eds. Human muscle power. Champaign, IL: Human Kinetics Publishers; 1986:81-89.

20. Fitch, C.D. Significance of abnormalities of creatine metabolism. In: Rowland, L.P., ed. Pathogenesis of human muscular dystrophies. Amsterdam: Excerpta Medica; 1977:328-340.

21. Fitch, C.D.; Jellinek, M.; Fitts, R.H.; Baldwin, K.M.; Holloszy, J.O. Phosphorylated β-guanidinopropionate as a substitute for phosphocreatine in rat muscle. Am. J. Physiol. 288:1123-1125; 1975.

22. Fitch, C.D.; Lucy, D.D.; Bornhofen, J.H.; Dalrymple, G.V. Creatine metabolism in skeletal muscle. Neurology 18:32-39; 1968.

23. Fitch, C.D.; Shields, R.P. Creatine metabolism in skeletal muscle. I. Creatine movement across muscle membranes. J. Biol. Chem. 241:3611-3614; 1966.

24. Fitch, C.D.; Sinton, D.W. A study of creatine metabolism in diseases causing muscle wasting. J. Clin. Invest. 43:444-452; 1964.

25. Forsberg, A.M.; Nilsson, E.; Werneman, J.; Bergström, J.; Hultman, E. Muscle composition in relation to age and sex. Clin. Sci. 81:249-256; 1991.

26. Green, A.L.; Greenhaff, P.L.; Macdonald, I.A.; Bell, D.; Holliman, D.; Stroud, M.A. The influence of oral creatine supplementation on metabolism during submaximal incremental treadmill exercise. Clin. Sci. 87:707-710; 1994.

27. Green, H.J. Muscle power: Fibre type recruitment, metabolism and fatigue. In: Jones, N.L.; McCartney, N.; McComas, A.J., eds. Human muscle power. Champaign, IL: Human Kinetics Publishers; 1986:65-79.

28. Greenhaff, P.L.; Bodin, K.; Söderlund, K.; Hultman, E. The effect of oral creatine supplementation on skeletal muscle phosphocreatine resynthesis. Am. J. Physiol. 266:E725-E730; 1994.

29. Greenhaff, P.L.; Casey, A.; Short, A.H.; Harris, R.C.; Söderlund, K.; Hultman, E. Influence of oral creatine supplementation on muscle torque during repeated bouts of maximal voluntary exercise in man. Clin. Sci. 84:565-571; 1993.

30. Greenhaff, P.L.; Constantin-Teodosiu, D.; Casey, A.; Hultman, E. The effect of oral creatine supplementation on skeletal muscle ATP degradation during repeated bouts of maximal voluntary exercise in man. J. Physiol. 476:84; 1994.

31. Greenhaff, P.L.; Nevill, M.E.; Söderlund, K.; Bodin, K.; Boobis, L.H.; Williams, C.; Hultman, E. The metabolic responses of human type I and II muscle fibres during maximal treadmill sprinting. J. Physiol. 478:149-155; 1994.

32. Harris, R.C.; Edwards, R.H.T.; Hultman, E.; Nordesjö, L.-O.; Nylind, B.; Sahlin, K. The time course of phosphorylcreatine resynthesis during recovery of the quadriceps muscle in man. Pflügers Arch. 367:137-142; 1976.

33. Harris, R.C.; Söderlund, K.; Hultman, E. Elevation of creatine in resting and exercised muscle of normal subjects by creatine supplementation. Clin. Sci. 83:367-374; 1992.

34. Harris, R.C.; Viru, M.; Greenhaff, P.L.; Hultman, E. The effect of oral creatine supplementation on running performance during maximal short term exercise in man. J. Physiol. 467:74; 1993.

35. Heymsfield, S.B.; Arteaga, C.; McManus, C.; Smith, J.; Moffitt, S. Measurement of muscle mass in humans: Validity of the 24-hour urinary creatinine method. Am. J. Clin. Nutr. 36:478-494; 1983.

36. Hintz, C.S.; Chi, M.M.-Y.; Fell, R.D.; Ivy, J.L.; Kaiser, K.K.; Lowry, C.V.; Lowry, O.H. Metabolite changes in individual rat muscle fibres during stimulation. Am. J. Physiol. 242:C218-C228; 1982.

37. Hoberman, H.D.; Sims, E.A.H.; Peters, J.H. Creatine and creatinine metabolism in the normal male adult studied with the aid of isotopic nitrogen. J. Biol. Chem. 172:45-53; 1948.

38. Hultman, E.; Bergström, M.; Spriet, L.L.; Söderlund, K. Energy metabolism and fatigue. In: Taylor, A.W.; Gollnick, P.D.; Green, H.J.; Ianuzzo, D.C.; Noble, E.G.; Métivier, G., Sutton, J., eds. Biochemistry of exercise VII. Champaign, IL: Human Kinetics Books; 1990:73-79. (Int. Series Sports Sci.; vol. 21).

39. Hultman, E.; Greenhaff, P.L.; Ren, J.-M.; Söderlund, K. Energy metabolism and fatigue during intense muscle contraction. Biochem. Soc. Trans. 19:347-353; 1991.

40. Hultman, E.; Sjoholm, H. Substrate availability. In: Knuttgen, H.G.; Vogel, J.A.; Poortmans, J., eds. Biochemistry of exercise. Champaign: Human Kinetics Publishers, 1983:63-75. (Int. Series Sports Sci.).

41. Hunter, A. The physiology of creatine and creatinine. Physiol. Rev. 2:586-599; 1922.

42. Jones, N.L.; McCartney, N.; Graham, T.; Spriet, L.L.; Kowalchuk, J.M.; Haigenhauser, G.J.F.; Sutton, J.R. Muscle performance and metabolism in maximal isokinetic cycling at slow and fast speeds. J. Appl. Physiol. 59:132-136; 1985.

43. Katz, A.; Sahlin, K.; Henriksson, J. Muscle ATP turnover rate during isometric contractions in humans. J. Appl. Physiol. 60:1839-1842; 1986.

44. Koszalka, T.R.; Andrew, C.L. Effect of insulin on the uptake of creatine-1-^{14}C by skeletal muscle in normal and X-irradiated rats. Proc. Soc. Exp. Biol. Med. 139:1265-1271; 1972.

45. Maison, G.L. Failure of gelatin or amino-acetic acid to increase the work ability. JAMA 115:1439-1441; 1940.

46. Meyer, R.A.; Brown, T.R.; Krilowicz, B.L.; Kushmerick, M.J. Phosphagen and intracellular pH changes during contraction of creatine-depleted rat muscle. Am. J. Physiol. 250:C264-C274; 1986.

47. Meyer, R.A.; Sweeney, H.L.; Kushmerick, M.J. A simple analysis of the "phosphocreatine shuttle." Am. J. Physiol. 246:C365-C377; 1984.

48. Myers, V.C.; Fine, M.S. The metabolism of creatine and creatinine. VII. The fate of creatine when administered to man. J. Biol. Chem. 21:377-383; 1915.

49. Needham, D.M. Machina carnis. The biochemistry of muscular contraction in its historical development. Cambridge: Cambridge University Press; 1971.

50. Piper, J.; Spiller, P. Repayment of O_2 debt and resynthesis of high-energy phosphates in gastrocnemius muscle of the dog. J. Appl. Physiol. 28:657-662; 1970.

51. Ray, G.B.; Johnson, J.R.; Taylor, M.M. Effect of gelatin on muscular fatigue. Proc. Soc. Exp. Biol. Med. 40:157-161; 1939.

52. Roberts, J.J.; Walker, J.B. Feeding a creatine analogue delays ATP depletion and onset of rigor in ischemic heart. Am. J. Physiol. 243:H911-H916; 1982.

53. Sahlin, K.; Edström, L.; Sjöhölm, H. Force relaxation and energy metabolism of rat soleus muscle during anaerobic contraction. Acta Physiol. Scand. 129:1-7; 1987.

54. Schloss, P.; Mayser, W.; Betz, H. The putative rat choline transporter chot1 transports creatine and is highly expressed in neural and muscle-rich tissues. Biochem. Biophys. Res. Commun. 198:637-645; 1994.

55. Shoubridge, E.A.; Bland, J.L.; Radda, G.K. Regulation of creatine kinase during steady-state isometric twitch contraction in rat skeletal muscle. Biochim. Biophys. Acta 805:72-78; 1984.

56. Shoubridge, E.A.; Radda, G.K. A ^{31}P-nuclear magnetic resonance study of skeletal muscle metabolism in rats depleted of creatine with the analogue β-guanidinopropionic acid. Biochim. Biophys. Acta 805:79-88; 1984.

57. Sipila, I.; Rapola, J.; Simell, O.; Vannas, A. Supplementary creatine as a treatment for gyrate atrophy of the choroid and retina. N. Engl. J. Med. 304:867-870; 1981.

58. Söderlund, K.; Greenhaff, P.L.; Hultman, E. Energy metabolism in type I and type II human muscle fibres during short term electrical stimulation at different frequencies. Acta Physiol. Scand. 144:15-22; 1992.

59. Spande, J.I.; Schottelius, B.A. Chemical basis for fatigue in isolated mouse soleus muscle. Am. J. Physiol. 219:1490-1495; 1970.

60. Spriet, L.L.; Söderlund, K.; Bergström, M.; Hultman, E. Anaerobic energy release in skeletal muscle during electrical stimulation in man. J. Appl. Physiol. 62:611-615; 1987.

61. Walker, J.B. Creatine: Biosynthesis, regulation and function. Adv. Enzymol. Relat. Areas Mol. Med. 50:177-242; 1979.

62. Walliman, T.; Wyss, M.; Brdiczka, D.; Nicolay, K.; Eppenberger, H.M. Intracellular compartmentation, structure and function of creatine kinase isoenzymes in tissues with high and fluctuating energy demands: The "phosphocreatine circuit" for cellular energy homeostasis. Biochem. J. 281:21-40; 1992.

CHAPTER 19

Muscle Metabolism and Performance During Sprinting

Mary E. Nevill, Gregory C. Bogdanis, Leslie H. Boobis, Henryk K.A. Lakomy, Clyde Williams
Loughborough University, Loughborough, England; Loughborough University, Loughborough, England; Sunderland District Hospital, Sunderland, England; Loughborough University, Loughborough, England; Loughborough University, Loughborough, England

Over the past 15 years, there has been an explosion of interest in the biochemistry of sprinting, which may be defined as an activity in which the exercise is performed at a maximal rate from the onset of exercise. While the term *maximal exercise* has, in the past, been synonymous with an exercise intensity that elicits maximum oxygen uptake, it is now appreciated that the average power output during sprinting of 30 s duration is approximately two to three times higher than that required to elicit maximum oxygen uptake (38). The rapid expansion of the information base regarding sprinting has been facilitated by methodological developments. The needle biopsy technique was reintroduced by Bergström (6) and was used initially to examine muscle metabolism during submaximal exercise (19). The development of a maximal cycle ergometer test by Bar-Or and Cumming in the 1970s (4, 12), subsequently described as the *Wingate test,* allowed determination of power output during sprint exercise in the laboratory. Together these two techniques led to a number of abstracts and papers being produced in the early 1980s that described the metabolic responses to sprint cycling. Since that date, methodologies have been further developed to allow examination of sprint running in addition to sprint cycling, and greater sophistication in the analysis of muscle biopsy samples has allowed examination of muscle metabolism in single fibers. In dynamic exercise using small muscle groups and during electrically induced contractions, the techniques of arterial and venous cannulation, together with the muscle biopsy and studies using ^{31}P magnetic resonance spectroscopy (^{31}P-MRS), have added greatly to the knowledge base concerning muscle metabolism during high-intensity exercise. However, these latter techniques are not yet suitable for use in examining sprint performance because of the large muscle mass and body movement involved in such activity. Examination of sprinting, per se, has the dual aims of furthering understanding of, first, the limitations of performance and causes of fatigue in an activity that is crucial to performance in most sports and, second, the integration and control of metabolism in an activity in which all energy-supplying pathways appear to be taxed to their maximum. This paper examines muscle metabolism and performance during sprinting with these two questions in mind.

Exercise Models for Examining Sprint Performance

Recently, there have been a number of improvements in the methodology for determining power output during sprinting that have allowed a closer examination of the relationship between performance and muscle metabolism. Traditionally, during cycle ergometer sprinting, power output has been calculated from the product of resistive mass and flywheel velocity. However, this methodology fails to take account of the work done during acceleration and therefore underestimates peak power output. Lakomy (22) has introduced a modification that involves prior calibration of the bicycle so that changes in kinetic energy of the flywheel during acceleration can be incorporated into the power output calculations. A typical power and pedal speed profile generated from a 30-s cycle sprint is shown in figure 19.1. As

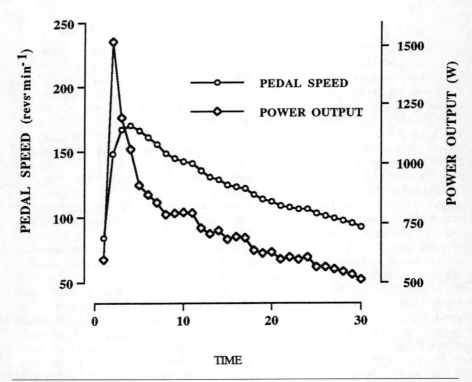

Figure 19.1   Power output (corrected for kinetic energy of the flywheel) and pedal speed during a maximal 30-s cycle ergometer sprint ($n = 1$).

one would expect theoretically for a mechanical system free to accelerate, peak power is reached before peak speed, and thereafter power declines to approximately 50% of the peak value by the end of the test. In addition, Lakomy (23) instrumented a nonmotorized treadmill for determining the horizontal component of power output during sprint running. Other than the early efforts of Best and Partridge (7), this is the first test to allow sprint running to be performed in the laboratory. The metabolic responses to such treadmill and track sprinting are very similar, with the same number of strides taken during, and the same metabolic responses in the blood to, 30 s of treadmill and 30 s of track sprinting (21). Development of such laboratory tests that allow the subjects to accelerate, sprint maximally, and slow down as fatigue occurs allow examination of the relationship between metabolism and performance.

Metabolic and Hormonal Responses to Sprinting

An example of the metabolic and hormonal responses to treadmill sprinting is shown in table 19.1. Although the sprint was of only 30-s duration, the increases in blood lactate concentration and growth hormone are some of the highest values observed after any type and duration of exercise. For the sprinters, growth hormone peaked at 30 min postexercise and remained 10 times above the basal value after 1 h of recovery (28). The magnitude of these metabolic and hormonal responses illustrates the very demanding nature of, and the large muscle mass recruited during, this type of exercise. The stress of performing sprint running is also reflected by the catecholamine and β-endorphin response to a single 30-s sprint, which is shown

Table 19.1   Blood Lactate and Serum Growth Hormone After a 30-s Treadmill Sprint in Male Sprint- and Endurance-Trained Athletes

| | Rest | Minutes postsprint | | |
		10 min post	30 min post	60 min post
Blood lactate (mmol · L^{-1})				
ST	1.1 ± 0.1	19.7 ± 0.7	12.5 ± 1.3	3.8 ± 0.3
ET	1.2 ± 0.1	13.8 ± 0.9	8.3 ± 0.9	2.9 ± 0.4[a, b, c]
Serum growth hormone (mU · L^{-1})				
ST	4.0 ± 0.8	57.7 ± 8.1	84.4 ± 21.1	44.9 ± 11.0
ET	4.8 ± 1.3	24.3 ± 8.8	25.1 ± 6.7	23.5 ± 6.8[a, b, c]

ST $n = 6$, ET $n = 6$; mean + SE. Data from Nevill et al. 1993 (28) and unpublished results by the same authors.

[a]Main effect time.

[b]Main effect group (sprint vs. endurance).

[c]Interaction (all $p < .05$).

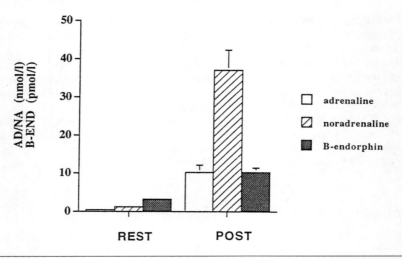

Figure 19.2   Plasma catecholamine (rest and 1 min post, *n* = 10 males) and β-endorphin (rest and 3 min post, *n* = 10 males) before and after a maximal 30-s treadmill sprint (mean ± *SE*). Catecholamine data from Allsop et al. 1990 (1); β-endorphin data from Brooks et al. 1988 (11).

in figure 19.2. Adrenaline and noradrenaline were increased from 0.4 and 1.2 nmol · L⁻¹ at rest to 10.2 ± 1.9 and 37.1 ± 5.2 nmol · L⁻¹, respectively, at 1 min postexercise (1), while β-endorphin was increased from an estimated 3.2 ± 1.5 pmol · L⁻¹ at rest to 10.2 ± 3.9 pmol · L⁻¹ after 3 min of recovery (11).

Muscle Metabolites During Sprints of Different Durations

The changes in muscle metabolites as a result of treadmill and cycle ergometer sprinting are shown in tables 19.2 and 19.3. A modified 5-mm Bergström needle with suction applied was used to provide samples of up to 100 mg wet weight. Samples were taken and frozen in the needle within 5 to 10 s of asking the subject to stop sprinting. During a single 30-s treadmill sprint (table 19.2), muscle glycogen was decreased by approximately 32%, phosphocreatine (PCr) by at least 67%, and ATP by 28% (all *p* < .01 in comparison with rest). This decrease in ATP is a consistent and common observation during maximal exercise of this duration and intensity and reflects the deamination of AMP to IMP and ammonia under conditions of high ATP turnover and low pH (36). The glycolytic intermediates were markedly increased as illustrated by the 17-fold increase in G6P. Similarly, muscle lactate was increased to 19 times the resting value. When the metabolic responses were reexamined after a period of training, there was a further increase in muscle lactate, indicating that the enhanced performance was accompanied by a greater ATP provision from anaerobic metabolism (27).

The muscle metabolic responses to 10 and 20 s of cycle ergometer sprinting are shown in table 19.3, with the most noticeable observation being that the greatest

Table 19.2   Muscle Metabolites Before and After a Maximal 30-s Treadmill Sprint

	Rest	Post
Glycogen	317.0 ± 19.3	214.5 ± 18.9
PCr	84.0 ± 4.4	28.0 ± 4.5
Total creatine	119.2 ± 4.0	116.0 ± 5.6
ATP	26.7 ± 1.4	19.2 ± 4.0
G1P	0.2 ± 0.1	2.5 ± 0.6
G6P	1.2 ± 0.2	20.7 ± 2.2
F6P	0.3 ± 0.1	5.6 ± 0.5
Pyruvate	1.0 ± 0.2	3.8 ± 0.7
Lactate	4.1 ± 0.4	86.0 ± 10.8
Posttraining lactate	5.1 ± 1.4	103.6 ± 10.0*

mmol · kg^{-1} dry muscle; $n = 6$, 3 males and 3 females; mean ± SE. Data from Nevill et al. 1989 (27).

*$p < .05$ significant difference between experimental and control group (data not shown) in response to exercise after training (group × training × exercise interaction)

Table 19.3   Muscle Metabolites at Rest and After 10 and 20 s of Cycle Ergometer Sprinting

	Rest	10 s	20 s
Glycogen	403.8 ± 20.1	357.4 ± 18.6	329.7 ± 21.4[b]
PCr	80.7 ± 3.2	36.1 ± 3.0	21.4 ± 2.2[a]
ATP	25.6 ± 0.7	20.2 ± 1.3	19.8 ± 1.4
HMP	1.5 ± 0.1	21.2 ± 2.3	29.0 ± 1.7[a]
*Pi	2.9	14.8 ± 1.8	17.4 ± 2.0
Lactate	4.5 ± 0.4	51.0 ± 4.6	81.7 ± 4.7[a]

mmol · kg^{-1} dry muscle; $n = 8$ males; mean ± SE. Data from Bogdanis et al. 1994.

[a]$p < .01$, [b]$p < .05$ different from 10 s sprint

*calculated inorganic phosphate (mmol · L^{-1} muscle water)

proportion of the metabolic changes occurs within the first 10 s (8). PCr, for example, was reduced by about 55% after 10 s and about 73% after 20 s. For ATP the disparity was even greater, with a reduction of 21% during the first 10 s and no further change after 20 s of sprinting. Similarly, the calculated inorganic phosphate increased fivefold after 10 s with no further increase after 20 s. Although 62% of the lactate accumulated over 20 s was present after 10 s, there was a further approximately 30 mmol · kg⁻¹ dry muscle (d.m.) increase in lactate from 10 to 20 s ($p < .01$, 10 vs. 20 s). From these changes in muscle metabolites, the estimated utilization of ATP derived from anaerobic metabolism (no account taken of possible losses of lactate and pyruvate to the circulation) can be calculated using the following equation (20):

$$\text{ATP utilization from anaerobic metabolism} =$$
$$-2(\Delta\text{ATP}) - \Delta\text{ADP} - \Delta\text{PCr} + 1.5(\Delta\text{pyruvate}) + 1.5(\Delta\text{lactate})$$

The ATP utilization from anaerobic metabolism during sprints of differing durations is shown in figure 19.3. During a sprint of 6-s duration, the rate of ATP utilization is extremely high with a mean value of 14.9 mmol · kg⁻¹ · s⁻¹ d.m., and approximately 50% of the ATP is supplied by the degradation of PCr (13). For a sprint of 30-s duration, the rate of ATP utilization is considerably lower at 7.5 mmol · kg⁻¹ · s⁻¹ d.m., and PCr supplies only 28% of the ATP (9, 10). Although the data in figure 19.3 is taken from different studies, it is clear that the rate of ATP utilization, the percentage contribution of PCr to ATP utilization, and the mean power output all decline as sprint duration is increased.

However, if the 10- and 20-s sprint data (which are for the same subjects) are examined more closely, there was a 49% decrease in anaerobic ATP utilization from the 10- to the 20-s sprint, but only a 28% decrease in mean power output (8). Similarly, if sprints are repeated, the decline in anaerobic ATP utilization is greater than the decline in power output. For example, during ten 6-s cycle ergometer sprints (13), the decline in power output from sprint 1 to 10 was 27%. However, the decline in ATP utilization was 64%. This decline in anaerobic ATP utilization was due largely to an almost complete inhibition of the glycolytic rate, which occurred in spite of adrenaline peaking at 5 nmol · L⁻¹ just before sprint 10.

This mismatching of the decline in power output and the decline in ATP utilization may be partly explained by an increasing efficiency as pedaling speed slows (from approximately 170 to approximately 100 rpm) during a 30-s single sprint or during repeated sprints (9). This slowing of pedal speed may increase efficiency because subjects may be cycling closer to their optimal speed according to the power-velocity relationship (32) and because the contribution of type I fibers to power generation may be higher during slower contraction velocities (5). However, it is doubtful that changes in efficiency could completely account for such large discrepancies, and a further possibility is the failure to take account of the contribution of aerobic metabolism to ATP resynthesis during sprinting.

Estimated Aerobic Contribution to Sprint Performance

During maximal sprint exercise of approximately 30-s duration, it is generally assumed that anaerobic metabolism provides a large proportion of the ATP required, and the term *anaerobic test* to describe such exercise is not uncommon. However, using the oxygen deficit method and later the oxygen deficit method in combination with muscle biopsy, Medbo and Tabata have shown that approximately 40% of the total energy requirement for cycling exercise at 90 rpm, which caused exhaustion

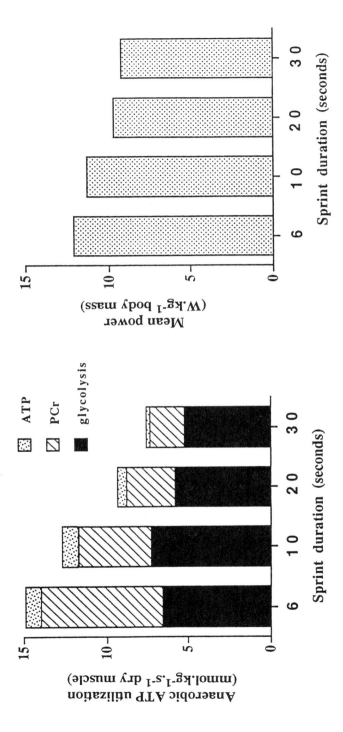

Figure 19.3 Utilization of ATP derived from anaerobic metabolism and mean power output during maximal sprint cycling of 6-, 10-, 20-, and 30-s duration (6 s: *n* = 8; 10 s and 20 s: *n* = 8; 30 s: *n* = 16; all males). Data for 6-s sprint from Gaitanos et al. 1993 (13); data for 10- and 20-s sprints from Bogdanis et al. 1994 (8); data for 30-s sprint from Bogdanis et al. (9) and Bogdanis et al. 1994 (10).

in 30 s, was supplied by aerobic metabolism (24, 25). On the basis of these findings, it is possible that aerobic metabolism could contribute significantly to sprint and repeated sprint exercise of 30-s duration. Therefore, we have recently examined both oxygen uptake and muscle metabolism during two 30-s sprints (10). Eight subjects performed two 30-s sprints separated by 4 min of passive recovery. Muscle biopsies were taken before and after each sprint, and oxygen uptake was measured during both sprints. On a separate occasion, subjects also performed a 30-s sprint followed by a 10-s sprint to allow examination of changes in performance and metabolism during the second sprint. Initially, the results for the two 30-s sprints will be presented.

Mean power output during the two sprints was reduced by 18%, from 724 ± 34 W in sprint 1 to 594 ± 17 W in sprint 2. The changes in muscle metabolites during the first and second 30-s sprints are shown in table 19.4. The total utilization of ATP derived from anaerobic metabolism was reduced from 232.5 ± 9.2 mmol · kg^{-1} d.m. in sprint 1 to 139.4 ± 8.4 mmol · kg^{-1} d.m. in sprint 2, with a 25% reduction in the contribution from PCr degradation to ATP resynthesis and a 43% reduction in the contribution from glycolysis (all $p < .01$, sprint 1 vs. sprint 2). Glycogenolysis was reduced by 55% from sprint 1 to sprint 2 ($p < .01$). Once again this overall 40% reduction in the ATP utilization derived from anaerobic metabolism was much greater than the 18% reduction in power output.

Oxygen uptake was increased by approximately 19% from 2.7 ± 0.1 to 3.2 ± 0.1 L · min^{-1} during sprint 1 and 2, respectively. If it is assumed (a) that the active muscle mass during the sprint was 20% of the body mass (38), (b) that 290 mmol of ATP were supplied per liter of oxygen consumed, and (c) that the oxygen stored in myoglobin and capillary blood was 10 mmol · kg^{-1} d.m. (18), and if the small (nonsignificant) increase in oxygen uptake before sprint 2 in comparison with before sprint 1 is subtracted, then aerobic metabolism supplied 96 ± 7 and 107 ± 9 mmol · kg^{-1} dry mass ATP during the first and second sprints, respectively ($p < .01$, sprint 1 vs. sprint 2). Thus, if the contribution of aerobic and anaerobic metabolism to the provision of ATP during the two sprints is examined (figure 19.4), there was only a 24% decrease in the utilization of ATP from sprint 1 to sprint 2, which is very

Table 19.4   Muscle Metabolites Before and After Two 30-s Sprints Separated by 4 min of Passive Recovery

	Rest	Post-sprint 1	Pre-sprint 2	Post-sprint 2
Glycogen	320.7 ± 14.9	218.4 ± 19.5[a]	240.5 ± 23.9[a]	184.0 ± 15.8[a, d]
PCr	76.5 ± 4.3	13.5 ± 1.4[a]	56.6 ± 1.4[a, b]	9.4 ± 2.4[a, c]
ATP	27.3 ± 0.8	20.7 ± 1.3[a]	22.2 ± 1.0[a]	20.8 ± 1.2[a]
G6P	1.4 ± 0.1	26.3 ± 1.7[a]	14.2 ± 0.7[a, b]	22.3 ± 1.3[a, b, c]
Lactate	5.6 ± 0.9	106.1 ± 4.5[a]	72.8 ± 5.5[a, b]	130.5 ± 4.9[a, b, c]

mmol · kg^{-1} dry muscle; $n = 8$ males, mean ± SE. Data from Bogdanis et al. (9).
[a]$p < .01$ from rest; [b]$p < .01$ from post-sprint 1; [c]$p < .01$ from pre-sprint 2; [d]$p < .05$ from pre-sprint 2.

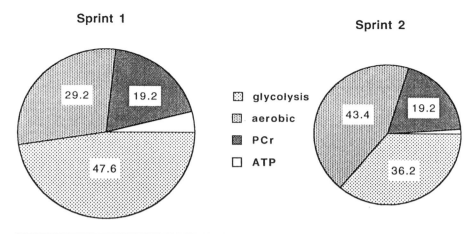

Figure 19.4   Estimated total ATP utilization from aerobic and anaerobic metabolism during two maximal 30-s sprints separated by 4 min of passive recovery ($n = 8$ males, see text for assumptions).
Data from Bogdanis et al. 1994 (10).

close to the 18% decrease in power output. The small difference remaining between the decline in ATP utilization and the decline in power output could be explained by a change in efficiency. Thus the results of this study suggest that there is a similar decline in the rate of ATP utilization and power output even during repeated bouts of exercise.

Also in this study, biopsies were taken at 10 s into the second sprint. From the first 10 s to the last 20 s of the second sprint there was an approximately 90% reduction in the contribution of PCr to ATP resynthesis and an approximately 65% reduction in the rate of anaerobic glycolysis. Thus, PCr contributes significantly to ATP provision only during the first 10 s of a second 30-s sprint, and the glycolytic rate is further reduced after only 10 s of exercise. This reduction in the glycolytic rate may be partly explained by the further reduction in muscle pH in the second sprint from 6.80 ± 0.03 at the start of the second sprint to 6.69 ± 0.03 after 10 s and 6.61 ± 0.03 after 30 s. However, reduced pH seems unlikely to be the only explanation, because unchanged glycogenolytic and glycolytic rates have been observed during electrically induced contractions when muscle pH fell from 6.70 to 6.45 (34).

Recovery of Muscle Metabolism and Sprint Performance

A further way of examining the relationship between muscle metabolism and performance is to examine the recovery of muscle metabolites together with the recovery of power output. This experimental design has the advantage that some of those variables that may be important in fatigue, such as muscle pH and PCr, may recover at different rates after maximal exercise.

In this study (9), 14 subjects, 8 of whom were biopsied, performed cycle ergometer sprints on four separate occasions. On three occasions, subjects performed two 30-s sprints separated by 90 s, 3 min, or 6 min of recovery, whereas on one occasion subjects performed only one 30-s sprint, and muscle biopsies were taken after the same recovery intervals (i.e., 90 s, 3 min, and 6 min). The muscle metabolites during recovery from a single 30-s sprint are shown in table 19.5. Glycogen and ATP were reduced by 34% and 29% respectively in the first postexercise sample taken 7.5 ± 1.6 s after the end of the sprint and did not change during the 6-min recovery period. Phosphocreatine, in contrast, was reduced to about 20% of the resting value and recovered rapidly to 64% after 90 s and 85% after 6 min of recovery. The glycolytic intermediates and lactate recovered slowly with 90%, 80%, and 69% of the peak lactate content remaining after 90 s, 3 min, and 6 min of recovery, respectively.

The PCr resynthesis data was modeled by Alan Nevill (9) using a monoexponential model with a separate power function exponent for each subject. The individual recovery curves are shown in figure 19.5. The average half time predicted from the model was 57 ± 7 s, and PCr values during recovery seem to lie between the higher values observed after dynamic exercise of lower intensity and the lower values observed after isometric contraction at 66% maximal voluntary contraction to fatigue (17). We were also able to show from the modeling process that PCr concentration at time zero (at the end of the sprint) was not significantly different from zero. The large interindividual variation in the rate of recovery of PCr among subjects may be dependent on the proportion of type I and type II fibers (35) and on the endurance fitness of the subjects. In the study previously described (10), the correlation between the percentage recovery of PCr and the $\%\dot{V}O_2$max at which blood lactate concentration reached a reference value of 4 mmol · L^{-1} was 0.94, supporting the suggestion that the adaptations associated with endurance training, such as an increase in mitochondrial volume and number, may be beneficial in the resynthesis of PCr (26).

Table 19.5   Muscle Metabolites at Rest and During Recovery After a Single 30-s Cycle Ergometer Sprint

	Rest	Post	1.5 min	3 min	6 min
Glycogen	321.5 ± 18.2	211.6 ± 18.5[a]	223.2 ± 19.5[a]	217.2 ± 21.0[a]	221.0 ± 18.3[a]
PCr	77.1 ± 2.4	15.1 ± 1.0[a]	49.7 ± 1.1[a, b]	57.2 ± 2.0[a, b, c]	65.5 ± 2.2[a, b, c, d]
Pi	2.9	18.5 ± 1.4[a]	7.7 ± 1.1[a, b]	7.4 ± 1.3[a, b]	6.4 ± 0.7[a, b]
ATP	25.6 ± 0.4	18.1 ± 1.7[a]	19.1 ± 0.9[a]	18.8 ± 1.1[a]	19.5 ± 0.9[a]
G6P	1.21 ± 0.2	22.8 ± 1.2[a]	20.9 ± 0.6[a]	16.6 ± 0.8[a, b, c]	11.0 ± 1.2[a, b, c, d]
Lactate	3.8 ± 0.3	119.0 ± 4.6[a]	107.3 ± 3.8[a]	95.4 ± 5.6[a, b]	81.9 ± 6.0[a, b, c, e]

mmol · kg^{-1} dry muscle; muscle glycogen in mmol glucosyl units · kg^{-1} dry muscle; mean ± SE, n = 8 males. Pi, calculated inorganic phosphate (mmol · L^{-1} muscle water). Data from Bogdanis et al. 1994 (10).

[a]$p < .01$ from rest; [b]$p < .01$ from post; [c]$p < .01$ from 1.5 min; [d]$p < .01$ from 3 min; [e]$p < .05$ from 3 min.

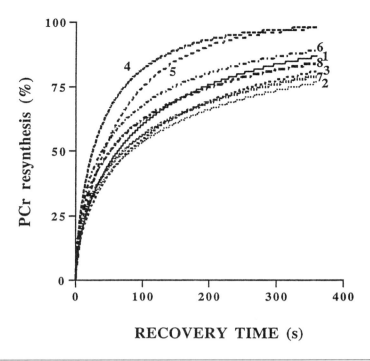

RECOVERY TIME (s)

Figure 19.5   Individual phosphocreatine (PCr) resynthesis curves, fitted using a mono-exponential model, during passive recovery after a maximal 30-s cycle ergometer sprint. Values for PCr are expressed as a percentage of the resting concentration. Numbers 1 to 8 represent individual subjects.
Reprinted from Bogdanis, Nevill, Boobis, Lakomy, and Nevill 1995.

Such an idea is supported by the observation that PCr and Pi kinetics after exercise are faster in distance runners than in untrained controls (39).

The recovery of PCr together with the recovery of peak power output are shown in figure 19.6. At the end of the 30-s sprint, power output was 36% of the peak value and recovered to 78%, 89%, and 91% of the highest value during the previous sprint after 90 s, 3 min, and 6 min of recovery. The correlation between the percentage recovery of peak power output and percentage recovery of PCr after 3 min was 0.86 ($p < .01$). This recovery of peak power output occurred in spite of a lack of change in muscle pH. Muscle pH decreased from 7.05 ± 0.01 at rest to 6.72 ± 0.04 after the 30-s sprint ($p < .01$). After 90 s of recovery, there was a further (nonsignificant) fall in muscle pH to 6.64 ± 0.02, while at the same time power output had recovered from 36% to 78% ($p < .01$, end of sprint vs. 90 s post) of the peak value achieved in sprint 1. There were no statistically significant changes in muscle pH for the first 3 min of recovery, with a small increase to 6.79 after 6 min ($p < .01$). This slower recovery of muscle pH than of PCr has been shown previously during recovery from lower intensity exercise using ^{31}P-MRS (40) and after a 2-min voluntary isometric contraction (2). It is also interesting to note that between 1.5 and 6 min, when peak power output recovered from 78% to 91% ($p < .01$, 1.5 min vs.

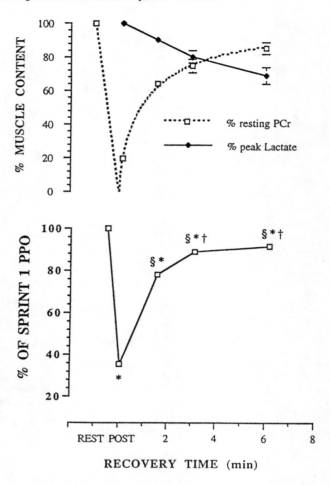

Figure 19.6   Time course of phosphocreatine (PCr) resynthesis and muscle lactate disappearance (*top*) and peak power recovery (*bottom*) after a 30-s maximal cycle ergometer sprint. Values for PCr are expressed as a percentage of the peak concentration (mean ± *SE, n* = 8). The curve fitted to the PCr data represents the mean of the curves fitted on the individual data for each subject. *$p < .01$ from sprint 1; §$p < .01$ from POST; †$p < .01$ from 1.5 min; see p. 253.

Reprinted from Bogdanis, Nevill, Boobis, Lakomy, and Nevill 1995.

6 min) of the peak values, there were no changes in the calculated inorganic phosphate or in the fraction of inorganic phosphate in the acidic form. The recovery of mean power was slower than the recovery of peak power ($p < .01$) . For example, after 3 min of recovery, peak power was recovered to 89% and mean power to 85% of the values achieved in sprint 1 ($p < .01$). This slower recovery of mean than of peak power may be the result of mean power being affected to a greater extent than peak power by the reduction in the glycolytic rate during the final 20 s of the second sprint (see earlier discussion). These data suggest that energy supply and particularly

PCr availability may be limiting performance during sprint exercise. Such suggestions are supported by the observation that creatine supplementation for 5 d at 280 mg · kg^{-1} body mass · d^{-1} improves performance during the last sprint of six 10-s treadmill sprints by as much as 10% (Bogdanis, Nevill, Lakomy, Jenkins, and Williams, unpublished observations).

Muscle Metabolism in Single Fibers During Treadmill Sprinting

Recently, the changes in muscle metabolites in single fibers during treadmill sprinting have been described for the first time (14). At rest, PCr and glycogen were respectively 11% and 26% higher in type II than in type I fibers ($p < .01$, type I vs. type II), which is in agreement with earlier findings (16, 35). However, during the 30-s sprint the rates of glycogen utilization were 4.21 ± 0.53 and 2.57 ± 0.48 mmol · kg^{-1} · s^{-1} d.m. in type II and type I fibers, respectively ($p < .01$, type I vs. type II). This type II glycogen degradation rate is higher than any previously reported value for 30 s of dynamic exercise. The type I glycogen degradation rate is also high and is in contrast to the response during electrical stimulation with the circulation to the leg intact, where the rate of glycogenolysis was 20 times higher in type II than in type I fibers (15). However, the type I response is similar to that achieved during electrical stimulation with blood flow occluded (16) and during electrical stimulation after epinephrine infusion, when the rate of glycolysis in type II fibers was only 3.5 times higher than in type I fibers (15). The rate of PCr utilization during the 30-s sprint was 2.48 and 1.97 mmol · kg^{-1}· s^{-1} d.m. in type I and type II fibers, respectively ($p < .01$, type I vs. type II). However, because most of the reduction in PCr will have occurred in the first 10 s, these values may not reflect true differences in the potential rate of PCr degradation in type I and type II fibers.

Implications for the Integration and Control of Metabolism

Two major issues arise from these studies: the more marked reduction in the rate of glycolysis than in the reduction in power output during repeated bouts of sprint exercise and the increase in oxygen uptake from the first to the second 30-s sprint when power output is reduced. The reason for the reduction in the rate of glycolysis during repeated sprints in these studies is not known. The decrease in muscle glycogen in repeated sprints or in a single 30-s sprint was no more than 27%, even in type II muscle fibers, and would seem unlikely to have affected the glycogenolytic and glycolytic rates (3). Furthermore, the reduction in the rates of glycogenolysis and glycolysis in repeated sprints occurred in spite of an increase in positive modulators of the pathway—such as adrenaline, Pi, and probably free ADP and AMP—while ATP was decreased. Such findings support earlier suggestions, based on results from ischemic voluntary contractions and recovery, that the glycogenolytic and glycolytic rates are not solely controlled by an elevated concentration of potent activators (29), but that factors intimately linked to the contractile process may dominate (30). One possibility for the inhibition of glycogenolysis and glycolysis during contraction is that the decrease in pH is not fully overcome by increases in positive modulators of the pathway. While it has been shown that the rates of glycogenolysis and glycolysis may be reduced in the absence of pH differences during repeated bouts of exercise (3), this does not preclude the possibility that an increased acidity, particularly in type II fibers, may be a contributory factor. Another possibility for the reduction in the glycogenolytic and glycolytic rates during repeated sprints is a reduction in cytosolic calcium (Ca^{2+}), due mainly to reduced Ca^{2+} release (37) during a second or in subsequent sprints. However, in the studies presented here, the reduction in the glycogenolytic and glycolytic rates was greater than the reduction in power output and greater than the number of contractions as reflected by pedal rate. Thus, it would seem that glycolysis is regulated not only by the total demand for ATP, as reflected by contractions, but also by the rate at which ATP can be supplied by the combination of PCr degradation and aerobic metabolism. Such a suggestion is supported by the maintenance of a good balance between ATP utilization and performance during two 30-s sprints, in spite of the reduction in the glycolytic rate, from the increase in aerobic metabolism from sprint 1 to sprint 2. This increased oxygen uptake probably arises from faster oxygen kinetics at the start of sprint 2. Also, it is interesting to note that preliminary findings suggest that the rate of glycolysis may be reduced when ATP resynthesis from PCr degradation is facilitated by creatine supplementation (33). Thus, although Ca^{2+} may initiate the glycolytic flux, the key to understanding the control of glycolysis may lie in this integration of the metabolic pathways, which possibly is mediated through transient changes in the products of ATP hydrolysis (31) and pH. Finally, one cannot preclude the possibility that a failure to activate the highly glycolytic type II fibers (14) during repeated sprints is the main cause of the reduction in the glycogenolytic and glycolytic rates in mixed muscle.

Implications for the Etiology of Fatigue During Sprinting

The studies presented in this paper have shown that there is a close coupling between muscle metabolism and performance during sprinting, with the relative contributions from PCr degradation, "anaerobic" glycolysis, and aerobic metabolism varying with the power output and duration of exercise. In repeated bouts of exercise, the reduction in the glycolytic rate is compensated for, to a large extent, by the increase in aerobic metabolism. During recovery from maximal exercise, power output recovers more rapidly than muscle pH, while peak power seems to recover in parallel with the recovery of PCr. In addition, creatine supplementation enhances sprint and high-intensity exercise performance (see chapter 18). These studies together would suggest that energy supply and particularly availability of PCr are important limiting factors in the maintenance of power output in sprinting and in repeated sprint performance. Furthermore, it seems that energy supply is more important than the direct effect of H^+ on the contractile mechanism. However, whether or not energy supply is the cause of fatigue in sprinting remains in question. The demand for ATP, together with PCr availability, the rate of "anaerobic" glycolysis, the rate of aerobic metabolism, and the activity of AMP deaminase, will determine the extent to which ADP (and Pi) accumulate and ATP decreases. In this way (controlling both the hydrolysis and the free energy of hydrolysis of ATP), energy supply may be seen as crucial to performance in sprinting. It is also possible, though, that the performance is inhibited by other mechanisms, such as problems with excitation-contraction coupling, thus reducing the demand for ATP. In summary, the series of studies presented here would suggest that energy supply, probably influencing the activity of all ATPases, is an important, but not the only, limitation of the ability to maintain power output during sprint exercise.

References

1. Allsop, P.; Cheetham, M.; Brooks, S.; Hall, G.M.; Williams, C. Continuous intramuscular pH measurement during the recovery from brief, maximal exercise in man. Eur. J. Appl. Physiol. 59:465-470; 1990.
2. Baker, A.J.; Carson, P.J.; Green, A.T.; Miller, R.G.; Weiner, M.W. Influence of human muscle length on energy transduction studied by 31P-NMR. J. Appl. Physiol. 73(1):160-165; 1992.
3. Bangsbo, J.; Graham, T.E.; Keins, B.; Saltin, B. Elevated muscle glycogen and anaerobic energy production during exhaustive exercise in man. J. Physiol. 451:205-227; 1992.
4. Bar-Or, O. A new anaerobic capacity test—Characteristics and applications. Proceedings of the 21st World Congress of Sports Medicine, Brasilia, Brazil. 1978:1-27.
5. Beelen, A.; Sargeant , A.J. Effect of fatigue on maximal power output at different contraction velocities in humans. J. Appl. Physiol. 71(6):2332-2337; 1991.
6. Bergström, J. Muscle electrolytes in man determined by neutron activation analysis on needle biopsy specimens: A study on normal subjects, kidney patients and patients with chronic diarrhoea. Scand. J. Clin. Lab. Invest. 14 (suppl. 68); 1962.
7. Best, C.H.; Partridge, R.C. The equation of motion of a runner exerting maximal effort. Proc. Royal Soc. London, B, 103:218-225; 1928.
8. Bogdanis G.C.; Nevill, M.E.; Boobis, L.H.; Lakomy, H.K.A. Recovery of power output and muscle metabolism after 10 s and 20 s of maximal sprint exercise in man. Clin. Sci. (suppl. 87):121-122; 1994.
9. Bogdanis, G.; Nevill, M.E.; Boobis, L.H.; Lakomy, H.K.A.; Nevill, A.M. Recovery of power output and muscle metabolites following 30 s of maximal sprint cycling in man. J. Physiol. 482(2): 467-480; 1995.
10. Bogdanis, G.; Nevill, M.E.; Lakomy, H.K.A.; Boobis, L.H. Muscle metabolism during repeated sprint exercise in man. J. Physiol. 475:25P-26P; 1994.
11. Brooks, S.; Burrin, J.; Cheetham, M.E.; Hall, G.M.; Yeo, T.; Williams, C. The responses of the catecholamines and B-endorphin to brief maximal exercise in man. Eur. J. Appl. Physiol. 57:230-234; 1988.
12. Cumming, G.R. Correlation of athletic performance and aerobic power in 12-17 year old children with bone age, calf muscle, total body potassium, heart volume and two indices of aerobic power. In: Bar- Or, O., ed. Pediatric work physiology. Netanya, Israel: Wingate Institute; 1975:109-134.

13. Gaitanos, G.C.; Williams, C.; Boobis, L.H.; Brooks, S. Human muscle metabolism during intermittent maximal exercise. J. Appl. Physiol. 75(2):712-719; 1993.

14. Greenhaff, P.L.; Nevill, M.E.; Söderlund, K.; Bodin, K.; Boobis, L.H.; Williams, C.; Hultman, E. The metabolic responses of human type I and II muscle fibres during maximal treadmill sprinting. J. Physiol. 478:149-155; 1994.

15. Greenhaff, P.L.; Ren, J.; Söderlund, K.; Hultman, E. Energy metabolism in single human muscle fibres during contraction without and with epinephrine infusion. Am. J. Physiol. 260 (Endocrinol. Metab. 23):E713-E718; 1991.

16. Greenhaff, P.L.; Söderlund, K.; Ren, J.; Hultman, E. Energy metabolism in single human muscle fibres during intermittent contraction with occluded circulation. J. Physiol. 460:443-453; 1993.

17. Harris, R.C.; Edwards, R.H.T.; Hultman, E.; Nordesjo, L.O.; Nylind, B.; Sahlin, K. The time course of phosphorylcreatine resynthesis during recovery of the quadriceps muscle in man. Pflügers Arch. 367:137-142; 1976.

18. Harris, R.C.; Hultman, E.; Kaijser, L.; Nordesjo, L.O. The effect of circulatory occlusion on isometric exercise capacity and energy metabolism of the quadriceps muscle in man. Scand. J. Clin. Lab. Invest. 35:87-95; 1975.

19. Hultman, E.; Bergström, J.; McLennan-Anderson, N. Breakdown and resynthesis of phosphorylcreatine and adenosine triphosphate in connection with muscular work in man. Scand. J. Clin. Lab. Invest. 19:56-66; 1967.

20. Katz, A.; Sahlin, K.; Henriksson, J. Muscle ATP turnover rate during isometric contraction in humans. J. Appl. Physiol. 60(6):1839-1842; 1986.

21. Lakomy, H.K.A. Measurement of external power output during high intensity exercise. Loughborough, England: Loughborough Univ.; 1988. PhD thesis.

22. Lakomy, H.K.A. Measurement of work and power output using friction-loaded cycle ergometers. Ergonomics 29(4):509-517; 1986.

23. Lakomy, H.K.A. The use of a non-motorized treadmill for analysing sprint performance. Ergonomics 30(4):627-637; 1987.

24. Medbo, J.I.; Tabata, I. Anaerobic energy release in working muscle during 30 s to 3 min of exhausting bicycling. J. Appl. Physiol. 75(4):1654-1660; 1993.

25. Medbo, J.I.; Tabata, I. Relative importance of aerobic and anaerobic energy release during short-lasting exhausting bicycle exercise. J. Appl. Physiol. 67:1881-1886; 1989.

26. Meyer, R.A. A linear model of muscle respiration explains monoexponential phosphocreatine changes. Am. J. Physiol. 254(23):C548-C553; 1988.

27. Nevill, M.E.; Boobis, L.H.; Brooks, S.; Williams, C. Effect of training on muscle metabolism during treadmill sprinting. J. Appl. Physiol. 67(6):2376-2382; 1989.

28. Nevill, M.E.; Holmyard, D.J.; Hall, G.M.; Allsop, P.; van Oosterhout, A.; Burrin, J.M. Growth hormone responses to treadmill sprinting in sprint- and endurance-trained male athletes. J. Physiol. 473:73P; 1993.

29. Quistorff, B.; Johansen, L.; Sahlin, K. Absence of phosphocreatine resynthesis in human calf muscle during ischaemic recovery. J. Biochem. 291:681-686; 1993.

30. Richter, E.A.; Ruderman, N.B.; Gavras, H.; Belur, E.R.; Galbo, H. Muscle glycogenolysis during exercise: Dual control by epinephrine and contractions. Am. J. Physiol. 242:E25-E32; 1982.

31. Sahlin, K.; Gorski, J.; Edstrom, L. Influence of ATP turnover and metabolite changes on IMP formation and glycolysis in rat skeletal muscle. Am. J. Physiol. 259(28):C409-C412; 1990.

32. Sargeant, A.J.; Hoinville, E.; Young, A. Maximum leg force and power output during short-term dynamic exercise. J. Appl. Physiol. 51(5):1175-1182; 1981.

33. Söderlund, K.; Balsom, P.D.; Ekblom, B. Creatine supplementation and high intensity exercise: Influence on performance and muscle metabolism. Clin. Sci. (suppl. 87):120-121; 1994.

34. Spriet, L.L.; Söderlund, K.; Bergström, M.; Hultman, E. Skeletal muscle glycogenolysis, glycolysis, and pH during electrical stimulation in men. J. Appl. Physiol. 62(2):616-621; 1987.

35. Tesch, P.A.; Thorsson, A.; Fujitsuka, N. Creatine phosphate in fibre types of skeletal muscle before and after exhaustive exercise. J. Appl. Physiol. 66:1756-1759; 1989.

36. Tullson, P.C.; Terjung, R.L. Adenine nucleotide metabolism in contracting skeletal muscle. Exercise Sport Sci. Rev. 19:507-537; 1991.

37. Westerblad, H.; Lee, J.A.; Lannergren, J.; Allen, D.G. Cellular mechanisms of fatigue in skeletal muscle. Am. J. Physiol. 261(30):C195-C209; 1991.

38. Wootton, S.A. The influence of diet and training on the metabolic responses to maximal exercise in man. Loughborough, England: Loughborough Univ.; 1984. PhD thesis.

39. Yoshida, T.; Watari, H. Metabolic consequences of repeated exercise in long distance runners. Eur. J. Appl. Physiol. 67:261-265; 1993.

40. Yoshida, T.; Watari, H. 31P nuclear magnetic resonance spectroscopy study of the time course of energy metabolism during exercise and recovery. Eur. J. Appl. Physiol. 66:494-499; 1993.

CHAPTER 20

Regulation of Muscle Glycogenolysis and Glycolysis During Intense Exercise: In Vivo Studies Using Repeated Intense Exercise

Jens Bangsbo

Copenhagen Muscle Research Centre, August Krogh Institute, University of Copenhagen, Copenhagen, Denmark

Muscle metabolism during intense exercise has received a considerable amount of attention for more than 100 years. Since Mosso (38) in 1891 electrically stimulated human finger flexor muscles, a variety of experimental models have been used. A substantial number of in vitro studies have focused on specific aspects of metabolism during muscle contraction, and a great deal of valuable information has been obtained. Many potential modulators and inhibitors of glycogenolysis and glycolysis have been identified (figure 20.1). However, from in vitro studies the complex interplay that occurs between the various regulators in vivo can be examined only to a limited extent. Thus, in vivo studies are needed to evaluate how potential regulators such as muscle glycogen, pH, and nucleotides are influencing the rate of glycogenolysis and glycolysis.

In a series of experiments, we have used various models in which subjects exercised an isolated muscle group. In one set of studies, the subjects contracted the calf muscles in a magnet, and nuclear magnetic resonance (NMR) measurements were obtained. In another set of experiments, the subjects kicked with one leg in a controlled fashion, keeping the exercise confined to the quadriceps muscle (figure 20.2). By collecting muscle tissue samples as well as arterial and femoral venous blood samples before and during exercise, a precise quantitative metabolic evaluation could be made of the metabolic events related to the work performed (4, 47).

Muscle Glycogenolysis and Glycolysis During Repeated Intense Exercise

Intermittent exercise can be used as an experimental model to examine muscle metabolism during intense exercise, since previous exercise may cause changes in the regulators of metabolic pathways such as glycogenolysis and glycolysis.

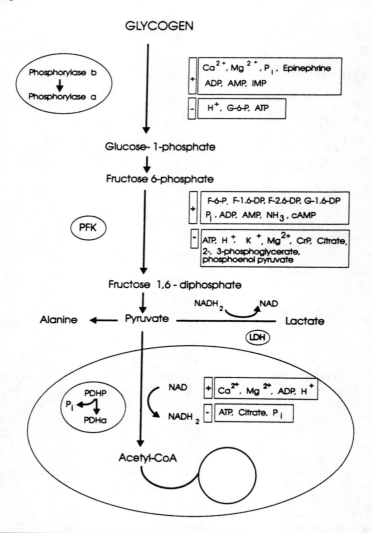

Figure 20.1 Schematic representation of the metabolic pathways related to carbohydrate utilization and a number of the potential regulators in skeletal muscle determined by in vitro experiments. *Note.* + denotes positive modulators; − denotes negative modulators.

We performed a study in which the subjects carried out two knee extensor exercise bouts to exhaustion (5). The bouts were separated by a 16-min period consisting of 10 min of rest followed by intense intermittent exercise (3.5 min) and then 2.5 min of rest. Total lactate production and rate of lactate produced during the second exercise bout were reduced by 59% and 52%, respectively (figure 20.3). The differences do not appear to be explained by the 20% shorter exercise time for the second exercise bout (2.98 vs. 3.73 min), since it is likely that the rate of lactate production during the last part of the first exercise period was lower than the average for the entire exercise period.

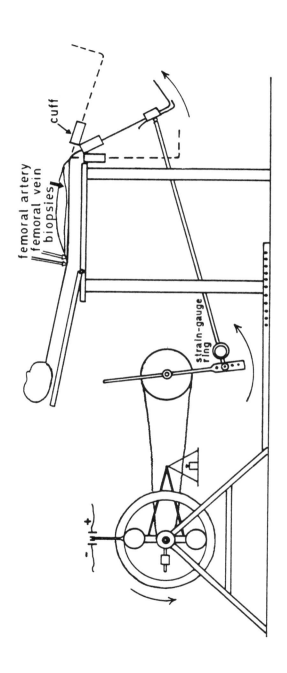

Figure 20.2   Illustration of the knee extensor exercise ergometer. The ankle is attached to the crank of a Krogh bicycle ergometer via an aluminum bar. The exercise consists of kicking the lower part of one leg forward by contracting the knee extensors. The repositioning of the leg after a kick is completely passive (i.e., by gravity and momentum of the wheel).

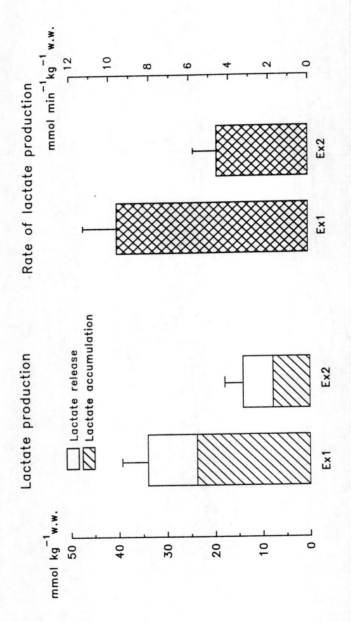

Figure 20.3 Total net lactate production (*left*) and net rate of lactate production (*right*) during the first and second exhaustive knee extensor exercise bouts. Mean ± *SE*; *n* = 6. Adapted from Bangsbo et al. 1992 (5). Adapted from Bangsbo et al. 1992.

In line with these findings were our observations from an NMR study of repeated isometric contractions with the calf muscles of one leg (3). The creatine phosphate (CP) utilization was the same during each of four 30-s maximal contractions despite a progressive reduction in the work output. No change or a slight increase in muscle pH was observed when the maximal contractions were repeated (figure 20.4). The estimated production of lactate during the second exercise bout was reduced by 65% compared with the first exercise bout, and almost no lactate was produced during the third and fourth exercise periods. Similar observations have been obtained in other studies focusing on the metabolic responses during intense intermittent exercise (19, 22, 29, 34, 37, 50).

An interesting question to be raised is the cause of the lower accumulation and release of lactate from the active muscles during the second exercise bout in the

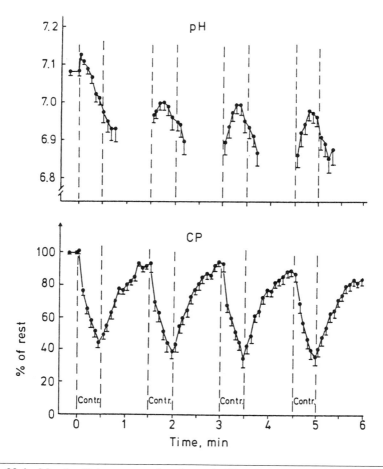

Figure 20.4   Muscle pH (*upper panel*) and muscle CP concentrations (*lower panel*) as determined by NMR during repeated 30-s maximal isometric contractions with the calf muscles. The CP concentrations are expressed in relation to the concentration at rest. Mean ± *SE; n = 18.*

knee extensor study (see figure 20.3). Lactate dehydrogenase is a near equilibrium enzyme, and therefore the direction of the flux is dictated by the concentrations of substrates and products. Thus, the formation of lactate is the net result of the rate of pyruvate and NADH production in the cytosol and of the uptake of these substances by the mitochondria, as well as of the formation of alanine from pyruvate. In the knee extensor study, the production of alanine was minor, and the uptake by the mitochondria appeared to be unaltered, since the leg oxygen uptake was the same during the two exercises (5). Thus, the lower lactate production may have been due to a reduced production of three carbon skeletons via glycolysis. Then the question to be raised is, What may be the cause of the lowered rate of glycolysis when intense exercise is repeated? There are many possibilities (see figure 20.1). Adenosine triphosphate (ATP) appears to bind to a high-affinity catalytic site of phosphofructokinase (PFK) and also to a low-affinity allosteric site at resting physiological concentrations of 5 to 7 mmol $\cdot$ L^{-1} (9, 10, 20). The binding of ATP to the allosteric site is responsible for the inhibition of the enzyme. Most modulators of PFK activity appear to function by changing the binding of ATP to the allosteric site of PFK.

Influence of Muscle Glycogen

It could be proposed that a progressive decrease in the muscle glycogen concentration caused the reduction in glycolytic activity when intense exhaustive exercise was repeated, since it has been suggested that the muscle glycogen level determines the rate of glycolysis and glycogenolysis. In studies using rats, increased muscle glycogen storage was shown to induce higher glycogenolytic and glycolytic rates (26, 44). It was observed that in fast-twitch fibers, glycogen utilization and lactate release were linearly related to the initial muscle glycogen concentration over both a 1- and a 15-min exercise period. In contrast, Spriet et al. (49) found no relationship between muscle glycogen storage and glycogenolysis during 1 min of electrical stimulation in rat red and white gastrocnemius.

In several human studies, it has been concluded that the rate of glycogenolysis is a function of muscle glycogen content when muscle carbohydrate storage is supercompensated (2, 24, 25, 31, 35). On the other hand, several other investigators have failed to verify these findings (27, 42, 47, 48, 52). There are no obvious explanations for the differences between results either in humans or in other species. The design and protocol of the various studies do, however, vary markedly. Furthermore, in many of the human studies only blood substrates and metabolites were analyzed to evaluate the metabolic responses. This limits the degree of direct comparison and may explain why no firm conclusions have been reached.

In the previously described knee extensor study (5), the muscle glycogen level prior to the second exercise bout was significantly lower than before the first exercise bout (figure 20.5). However, the rate of decline in muscle glycogen for the second exercise bout was not significantly different from the rate during the first exercise bout (figure 20.5). These findings speak against the lowered muscle glycogen content being the cause of the reduction in glycolysis. Nevertheless, due to the discrepancies in the literature, we reinvestigated the role of muscle glycogen using a model in which one leg had a normal glycogen level and the other leg had an above-normal glycogen level (6). The different muscle glycogen levels were achieved by dietary manipulation and exercise during the days before the experiment. On a separate

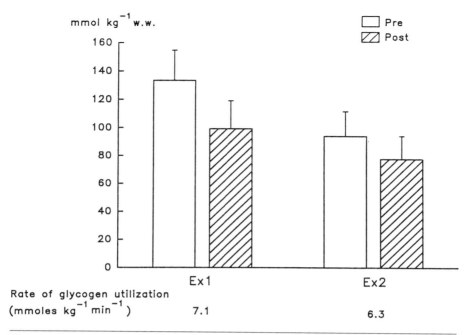

Figure 20.5   Muscle glycogen prior to and at the end of two exhaustive knee extensor exercise bouts. The mean rate of glycogen utilization is given below the bar graphs. Mean ± *SE; n* = 6. Adapted from Bangsbo et al. 1992 (5).
Adapted from Bangsbo et al. 1992.

occasion, the subjects were also tested without having exercised during the days preceding the experiment. Thus, the effect of the muscle glycogen content could be isolated as the sole factor studied. In a randomized order, each leg performed intense exhaustive exercise. The exercise time, glycogen breakdown, and lactate production were the same whether the leg had normal or elevated muscle glycogen concentrations (figure 20.6).

The study showed that the glycogenolytic and glycolytic rates during short-term intense exercise in humans were independent of initial muscle glycogen concentrations above 50 mmol · kg⁻¹ wet weight. This value is lower than that observed after the second exercise bout in the original knee extensor study (5). Thus, a progressive decline in muscle glycogen concentration is an unlikely explanation for the reduced glycolytic rate.

Influence of Muscle pH

In the original knee extensor study (5), the muscle pH was lower prior to the second exercise bout compared with the first exercise bout (6.85 vs. 7.04). This may have impaired glycolysis in the second exercise bout, since it has been demonstrated that lowered pH per se has an inhibitory effect on phosphorylase and PFK, which are considered the key regulatory enzymes of glycogenolysis and glycolysis,

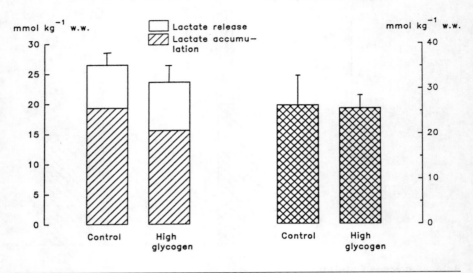

Figure 20.6   Net lactate production (*left*) and net muscle glycogen utilization (*right*) during exhaustive knee extensor exercise for one leg with normal glycogen levels (87 ± 14.4 mmol · kg^{-1} w.w.; control) and for one leg with elevated muscle glycogen level (176.8 ± 22.9 mmol · kg^{-1} w.w.; high glycogen). Mean ± *SE; n* = 6. Adapted from Bangsbo, Graham, Kiens, and Saltin 1992 (6).
Adapted from Bangsbo, Graham, Kiens, and Saltin 1992.

respectively (1, 12, 14, 30, 32). However, when a knee extensor exercise bout was repeated after 1 h of recovery, the rate of lactate production was also significantly reduced, although muscle lactate and pH were back to resting levels prior to the second exercise bout and muscle lactate was significantly lower during the second exercise bout (6). Furthermore, it is questionable whether the reduction in pH during intense exercise is large enough to inhibit these enzymes in vivo. Recent studies on the allosteric regulation of muscle PFK within the physiological range have shown that the effect of pH is negligible at levels above 6.6 (17, 51). This is lower than what was observed in muscle for any of the subjects at the end of the second exercise. Thus, it appears that an elevated muscle H^+ concentration is not the only explanation for the reduction in the glycolytic rate when exercise is repeated. This proposition is supported by findings in a study in which exhaustive leg exercise was performed with and without previous intense arm exercise (Bangsbo et al., unpublished). The rate of muscle lactate production was the same for the two exercises, although muscle pH was significantly lower during the exercise performed after the arm exercise.

Influence of Muscle Nucleotides

In addition to muscle pH, there are several other regulatory mechanisms that may contribute to the control of PFK activity (see figure 20.1). Adenosine diphosphate

(ADP), adenosine monophosphate (AMP), and ammonia/ammonium (NH_3) are positive modulators of PFK, while ATP is a negative regulator (11, 56). In the knee extensor study, the ATP concentration was lower, and the AMP and NH_3 concentrations were higher prior to the second exercise bout compared with the first exercise bout (5). These factors may have stimulated glycolysis at the onset of the second exercise, but because the glycolytic rate was lowered, strong counteracting reactions must have occurred. At the end of the second exercise period, the ATP concentration was still lower and the AMP concentration remained higher, while the NH_3 concentration was similar for the two exercise bouts. This appears to have caused a higher degree of PFK activation during the exercise. However, it cannot be excluded that the ratio between bound and unbound nucleotides was changed when the intense exercise was repeated. A higher binding of the nucleotides during the second exercise would lower the stimulating effect on PFK and thus the rate of glycolysis. On the other hand, the observation of a progressively elevated free ADP concentration when maximal isometric contractions were repeated, as estimated from NMR measurements, does not support this assumption (3).

The apparently limited role of nucleotides in the regulation of glycolysis is supported by findings in other in vivo studies. When intense knee extensor exercise was repeated after 1 h, the lactate production was markedly reduced, although the reduction in ATP and accumulation of ADP and AMP were similar for the two exercise bouts (6). Similarly, elevated concentrations of nucleotides and NH_3 do not appear by themselves to be sufficient to activate glycogenolysis and glycolysis. It has been observed that muscle CP, G6P, and lactate concentrations were unaltered when blood flow was occluded to the muscle during the first 3 min of recovery from exhaustive cycle exercise (figure 20.7), although muscle ADP, AMP, and NH_3 (figure 20.8) were markedly elevated, and muscle ATP lowered (Bangsbo et al., unpublished). Thus, it appears that a contraction related factor is required for activation of the creatine kinase reaction, glycogenolysis, and glycolysis. In accordance with these observations were findings in other studies that the muscle CP concentration remained almost constant when blood flow to previously exercising muscle was occluded during recovery (8, 41, 43, 45).

Other Factors

The question remains as to what causes the impairment of glycolysis when exercise is repeated. An accumulation of cytosolic citrate could play a role, because it has been demonstrated in vitro that citrate inhibits PFK activity by potentiating the inhibitory effect of ATP on PFK and that citrate stimulates fructose-1,6-diphosphatase activity (11, 21, 39, 40, 53, 56). Essén (18) observed that muscle citrate concentration was increased after 5, 10, and 30 min of intermittent cycling alternating between 15 s of exercise (at a work rate eliciting $\dot{V}O_2max$) and 15 s of rest. Furthermore, muscle citrate concentrations were higher at the end of the rest period than immediately after exercise. It was believed that this was caused by continuous acetyl CoA production from fatty acid oxidation, together with a decreased citric acid cycle activity during the rest periods. Essén (18) found that less glycogen was used and that lactate accumulation per unit of time was smaller when intense exercise was performed intermittently as compared with continuously. It was suggested that the citrate accumulated during the intermittent exercise penetrated the mitochondrial

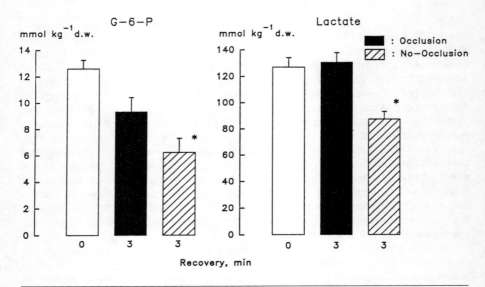

Figure 20.7 Muscle G6P (*left*) and muscle lactate (*right*) concentrations immediately after exhaustive cycling exercise (0 min) and 3 min into recovery with either intact muscle blood flow (striped bar) or occluded blood flow (filled bar). Mean ± *SE; n* = 8.

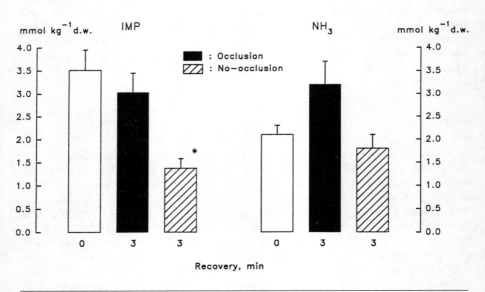

Figure 20.8 Muscle IMP (*left*) and muscle NH_3 (*right*) immediately after exhaustive cycling exercise (0 min) and 3 min into recovery with either intact muscle blood flow (striped bar) or occluded blood flow (filled bar). Mean ± *SE; n* = 8.

membrane and retarded glycolysis and that citrate was the primary cause of the metabolic changes.

It is possible that the citrate concentration at the onset of the second exercise bout in the original knee extensor study (5) was elevated and that this inhibited glycolysis, particularly during the initial phase of exercise. This is supported by a lower efflux of lactate after 45 s, despite a higher muscle lactate concentration prior to the second exercise bout, thus indicating retardation of glycolysis from the start of exercise (5). On the other hand, the same reduction in the glycolytic rate was observed whether the leg was resting (passive) or performing low intensity exercise (active) prior to the second exercise bout (7). A similar reduction occurred for the two conditions in spite of a higher oxygen uptake prior to the second exercise for the active leg as compared with the passive leg. This might have led to a difference in muscle citrate concentration. In addition, since citrate also inhibits the activity of pyruvate dehydrogenase (PDH), it would have been expected that the ratio between lactate production and pyruvate oxidation was higher during the second exercise period (39). However, this ratio was lower during the second exercise. Alternatively, the inhibitory effect on the PDH reaction may have been counteracted by the lowered muscle pH during the initial phase of the second exercise, because it has been suggested that an elevated H^+ concentration inhibits the inactivating kinase that stimulates the phosphorylation of active PDH to inactive PDH (28). Furthermore, an elevated H^+ concentration has also been suggested to raise the intramitochondrial Ca^{2+} levels, which in turn increase PDH activation (15). Nevertheless, it is questionable whether an elevated cytosolic citrate concentration prior to contraction was the main cause of the lowered glycolytic activity when intense exercise was repeated. Similarly, it seems that this difference cannot be explained by a higher citrate accumulation during the second exercise, because the rate of oxidation was similar for the first and second exercise bouts. This suggests that the supply of acetyl CoA from β-oxidation or the decarboxylation of pyruvate was not enhanced during the second exercise bout.

It can be speculated that the reduction in glycolytic activity was linked to the cytosolic Ca^{2+} concentration, because the release and reuptake of Ca^{2+} in the sarcoplasmic reticulum can be affected by intense exercise (23). However, the Ca^{2+} concentration per se does not appear to influence PFK activity (54). On the other hand, it has been proposed that activation of PFK during muscle contraction involves the formation of Ca^{2+}-calmodulin complexes, which accelerate the production of fructose-1,6-diphosphate (36). Thus, it is possible that alterations in the Ca^{2+}-calmodulin complexes play a role in changing the rate of glycolysis during intense intermittent exercise. However, the effects of Ca^{2+}-calmodulin on PFK are minimal at physiological concentrations of ATP and fructose-6-phosphate (36).

It is clear that further studies, both in vitro and in vivo, are needed before the cause of the reduction in glycolysis in relation to repeated exercise can be identified.

Energy Turnover During Repeated Intense Exercise

During the second exercise bout in the original knee extensor exercise study (5), the anaerobic energy turnover, determined from changes in metabolites, could account for only 64% of the estimated oxygen deficit, which may represent the total anaerobic energy production (4). In contrast, the same value was 90% for the first exercise bout (5). A corresponding difference, although less pronounced, was also observed when an exhaustive exercise bout was repeated after 1 h of recovery (6). Similarly, Spriet et al. (49) found that the total work performed during a 30-s all-out exercise bout, repeated a third time, was only slightly reduced in spite of a large decline in the glycogenolytic and glycolytic rate. Furthermore, it was demonstrated that the energy cost per unit force was reduced by 30% when an intense exhaustive isometric contraction was repeated after 2 min of recovery (46). These studies indicate that the energy demand is lowered when intense exercise is repeated. It is unclear what causes such a reduction in ATP utilization. It has been demonstrated that the efficiency of a muscle contraction is increased if contraction time is prolonged (16, 33). However, this does not appear to explain the lower use of energy during the second exercise bout, because there was no indication of a change in the contraction pattern from the first to the second exercise bout (5, 6). Another possibility is that the fiber type recruitment pattern changed when the exercise was repeated. Certain muscle fibers, particularly fast-twitch fibers, might not have recovered completely from the first exercise even after 1 h of rest. Consequently, more slow-twitch fibers might have been involved during the second exercise bout. This may explain the diminished rate of energy utilization, because it is known that slow-twitch fibers have a lower energy cost per unit force (13). An additional factor could be an elevation in the efficiency of the fast-twitch fibers during the second exercise bout, because it has been demonstrated that ATP turnover in mouse fast-twitch muscles decreased as an isometric contraction continued (13). However, further studies are needed to clarify the cause of an apparent reduction in the energy turnover when an intense muscle contraction is repeated. It should be noted that Vøllestad, Wesche, and Sejersted (55) have suggested that the energy turnover increases when intermittent static contractions are repeated.

Summary

We have studied the in vivo regulation of glycogenolysis and glycolysis during intense exercise by using models in which isolated muscles were contracted. It was observed that the rate of lactate production was markedly lowered when intense exercise was repeated, which could not be explained by a reduction in muscle glycogen or in muscle pH or by alterations in muscle nucleotides. It is apparent that further studies are required of how glycolysis is regulated and coupled to ATP turnover.

Acknowledgments

The experiments reported in this article were performed in collaboration with B. Saltin, T. Graham, L. Johansen, B. Kiens, S. Strange, and B. Quistorff. The studies were supported by grants from Team Danmark, the Danish Natural Science Foundation (11-0082), the Danish National Research Foundation (504-14), and Brandts Legat.

References

1. Amorena, C.F.; Wilding, T.J.; Manchester, J.K.; Roos, A. Changes in intracellular pH caused by high K in normal and acidified frog muscle. J. Gen. Physiol. 96:959-972; 1990.
2. Asmussen, E.; Klausen, K.; Nielsen, L.; Egelund, L.; Techow, O.S.A.; Tonder, P.J. Lactate production and anaerobic work capacity after prolonged exercise. Acta Physiol. Scand. 90:731-742; 1974.
3. Bangsbo, J. The physiology of soccer—With special reference to intense intermittent exercise. Acta Physiol. Scand. 151 (suppl. 619); 1994.
4. Bangsbo, J.; Gollnick, P.D.; Graham, T.E.; Juel, C.; Kiens, B.; Mizuno, M.; Saltin, B. Anaerobic energy production and O_2 deficit-debt relationship during exhaustive exercise in humans. J. Physiol. 422:539-559; 1990.
5. Bangsbo, J.; Graham, T.E.; Johansen, L.; Strange, S.; Christensen, C.; Saltin, B. Elevated muscle acidity and energy production during exhaustive exercise in man. Am. J. Physiol. 263:R891-R899; 1992.
6. Bangsbo, J.; Graham, T.E.; Kiens, B.; Saltin, B. Elevated muscle glycogen and anaerobic energy production during exhaustive exercise in man. J. Physiol. 451:205-222; 1992.
7. Bangsbo, J.; Saltin, B. Recovery of muscle from exercise, its importance for subsequent performance. In: Macleod, D.A.D.; Maughan, R.J.; Williams, C.; Madeley, C.R.; Sharp, J.C.M.; Nutton, R.W., eds. Intermittent high intensity exercise. Preparation, stresses and damage limitation. London and New York: E. & F.N. Spon; 1992:49-69.
8. Blei, M.L.; Conley, K.E.; Kushmerick, M.J. Separate measures of ATP utilization and recovery in human skeletal muscle. J. Physiol. 465:203-222; 1993.
9. Bock, P.E.; Frieden, C. Phosphofructokinase I. Mechanism of the pH-dependent inactivation and reactivation of the rabbit muscle enzyme. J. Biol. Chem. 251:5630-5636; 1976.
10. Bock, P.E.; Frieden, C. Phosphofructokinase II. Role of ligands in pH-dependent structural changes of the rabbit muscle enzyme. J. Biol. Chem. 251:5637-5643; 1976.
11. Bosca, L.; Aragon, J.J.; Sols, A. Modulation of muscle phosphofructokinase at physiological concentration of enzyme. J. Biol. Chem. 260:2100-2107; 1985.
12. Chasiotis, D. The regulation of glycogen phosphorylase and glycogen breakdown in human skeletal muscle. Acta Physiol. Scand. (suppl. 518):1-68; 1983.
13. Crow, M.T.; Kushmerick, M.J. Chemical energetics of slow- and fast-twitch muscles of the mouse. J. Gen. Physiol. 79:147-166; 1982.
14. Danforth, W.H. Activation of glycolytic pathway in muscle. In: Chance, B.; Estrabrook, B.W.; Williamson, J.R., eds. Control of energy metabolism. New York: Academic Press; 1965:287-297.
15. Denton, R.M.; McCormick, J.G.; Edgell, N.J. Role of calcium ions in the regulation of intramitochondrial metabolism. Biochem. J. 190:107-117; 1980.
16. di Prampero, P.E.; Boutellier, U.; Marguerat, A. Efficiency of work performance and contraction velocity in isotonic tetani of frog sartorius. Pflügers Arch. 412:455-461; 1988.
17. Dobson, G.P.; Yamamoto, E.; Hochachka, P.W. Phosphofructokinase control in muscle: Nature and reversal of pH-dependent ATP inhibition. Am. J. Physiol. 250:R71-R76; 1986.

18. Essén, B. Studies on the regulation of metabolism in human skeletal muscle using intermittent exercise as an experimental model. Acta Physiol. Scand. (suppl. 454):1-32; 1978.

19. Fox, E.L.; Robinson, D.; Wiegman, D.L. Metabolic energy sources during continuous and interval running. J. Appl. Physiol. 27:174-178; 1969.

20. Frieden, C.; Gilbert, H.R.; Bock, P.E. Phosphofructokinase III. Correlation of the regulatory kinetic and molecular properties of the rabbit muscle enzyme. J. Biol. Chem. 251:5644-5647; 1976.

21. Fu, J.Y.; Kemp, R.G. Activation of muscle fructose 1,6-diphosphatase by creatine phosphate and citrate. J. Biol. Chem. 248:1124-1125; 1973.

22. Gaitanos, G.C. Human muscle metabolism during intermittent maximal exercise. J. Appl. Physiol. 75:712-719; 1993.

23. Gollnick, P.D.; Körge, P.; Karpakka, J.; Saltin, B. Elongation of skeletal muscle relaxation during exercise is linked to reduced calcium uptake by the sarcoplasmic reticulum in man. Acta Physiol. Scand. 142:135-136; 1991.

24. Greenhaff, P.L.; Gleeson, M.; Maughan, R.J. The effects of dietary manipulation on blood acid-base status and the performance of high intensity exercise. Eur. J. Appl. Physiol. 56:331-337; 1987.

25. Greenhaff, P.L.; Gleeson, M.; Maughan, R.J. The effects of a glycogen loading regimen on acid-base status and blood lactate concentration before and after a fixed period of high intensity exercise in man. Eur. J. Appl. Physiol. 57:254-259; 1988.

26. Hespel, P.; Richter, E.A. Mechanism linking glycogen concentration and glycogenolytic rate in perfused contracting rat skeletal muscle. Biochem. J. 284:777-780; 1992.

27. Jacobs, I. Lactate concentrations after short, maximal exercise at various glycogen levels. Acta Physiol. Scand. 111:465-469; 1981.

28. Jones, N.L.; Heigenhauser, G.J.F. Effects of hydrogen ions on metabolism during exercise. In: Lamb, D.R.; Gisolfi, C.V., eds. Energy metabolism in exercise and sport. Perspectives in exercise science and sports medicine. Vol. 5. Dubuque, IA: Brown & Benchmark; 1992:107-147.

29. Karlsson, J.; Saltin, B. Diet, muscle glycogen and endurance performance. J. Appl. Physiol. 31:203-206; 1971.

30. Kavinsky, P.J.; Meyer, W.L. The effect of pH and temperature on the kinetics of native and altered glycogen phosphorylase. Arch. Biochem. Biophys. 181:616-631; 1977.

31. Klausen, K.; Sjøgaard, G. Glycogen stores and lactate accumulation in skeletal muscle of man during intense bicycle exercise. Scand. J. Sports Sci. 2:7-12; 1980.

32. Krebs, H.A. Glyconeogenesis. Croonian Lecture, 1963. Proc. Royal Soc. London, B. Biol., 159:545-560; 1964.

33. Kushmerick, M.J. Patterns in mammalian muscle energetics. J. Exp. Biol. 115:165-177; 1985.

34. Margaria, R.; Oliva, R.D.; di Prampero, P.E.; Ceretelli, P. Energy utilization in intermittent exercise of supramaximal intensity. J. Appl. Physiol. 26:752-756; 1969.

35. Maughan, R.J.; Poole, D.C. The effects of a glycogen loading regimen on the capacity to perform anaerobic exercise. Eur. J. Appl. Physiol. 46:211-219; 1981.

36. Mayr, G.W. Interaction of calmodulin with muscle phosphofructokinase. Eur. J. Biochem. 143:521-529; 1984.

37. McCartney, N.; Spriet, L.L.; Heigenhauser, J.F.; Kowalchuk, J.M.; Sutton, J.R.; Jones, N.L. Muscle power and metabolism in maximal intermittent exercise. J. Appl. Physiol. 60:1164-1169; 1986.
38. Mosso, U. Die Ermüdung. Leipzig, Germany: Hirzel; 1892.
39. Parmeggiani, A.; Bowman, R.H. Regulation of phosphofructokinase activity by citrate in normal and diabetic muscle. Biochem. Biophys. Res. Commun. 12:268-273; 1963.
40. Passonneau, J.V.; Lowry, O.H. P-fructokinase and the control of the citric acid cycle. Biochem. Biophys. Res. Commun. 13:372-379; 1963.
41. Quistorff, B.; Johansen, L.; Sahlin, K. Absence of phosphocreatine resynthesis in human calf muscle during ischaemic recovery. Biochem. J. 291:681-686; 1992.
42. Ren, J.M.; Broberg, G.; Sahlin, K.; Hultman, E. Influence of reduced glycogen level on glycogenolysis during short-term stimulation in man. Acta Physiol. Scand. 139:467-474; 1990.
43. Ren, J.M.; Chasiotis, D.; Bergström, M.; Hultman, E. Skeletal muscle glycolysis, glycogenolysis and glycogen phosphorylase during electrical stimulation in man. Acta Physiol. Scand. 133:101-107; 1988.
44. Richter, E.A.; Galbo, H. High glycogen levels enhance glycogen breakdown in isolated contracting skeletal muscle. J. Appl. Physiol. 61:827-831; 1986.
45. Sahlin, K.; Harris, R.C.; Hultman, E. Resynthesis of creatine phosphate in human muscle after exercise in relation to intramuscular pH and availability of oxygen. Scand. J. Clin. Lab. Invest. 39:551-558; 1979.
46. Sahlin, K.; Ren, J.M. Relationship of contraction capacity changes during recovery from a fatiguing contraction. J. Appl. Physiol. 67:648-654; 1989.
47. Saltin, B.; Hermansen, L. Glycogen stores and prolonged severe exercise. In: Blix, G., ed. Symposium of Swedish Nutrition Foundation. Uppsala, Sweden: Almquist and Wiksell; 1967.
48. Spencer, M.K.; Katz, A. Role of glycogen in control of glycolysis and IMP formation in human muscle during exercise. Am. J. Physiol. 260:E859-E864; 1991.
49. Spriet, L.L.; Berardinucci, L.; Marsh, D.R.; Campell, C.B.; Graham, T. Glycogen content has no effect on skeletal muscle glycogenolysis during short-term tetanic stimulation. J. Appl. Physiol. 68(5):1883-1888; 1990.
50. Spriet, L.L.; Lindinger, M.I.; McKelvie, S.; Heigenhauser, G.J.F.; Jones, N.L. Muscle glycogenolysis and H^+ concentration during maximal intermittent cycling. J. Appl. Physiol. 66:8-13; 1989.
51. Spriet, L.L.; Söderlund, K.; Bergström, M.; Hultman, E. Skeletal muscle glycogenolysis, glycolysis and pH during electrical stimulation in men. J. Appl. Physiol. 62:616-621; 1987.
52. Symons, J.D.; Jacobs, I. High-intensity exercise performance is not impaired by low intramuscular glycogen. Med. Sci. Sports Exercise 21:550-557; 1989.
53. Taylor, W.M.; Halperin, M.L. Regulation of pyruvate dehydrogenase in muscle. J. Biol. Chem. 248:6080-6083; 1973.
54. Vaughan, H.; Thornton, S.D.; Newsholme, E.A. The effects of calcium ions on the activities of trehalase, hexokinase, phosphofructokinase, fructose diphosphatase and pyruvate kinase from various muscles. Biochem. J. 132:527-535; 1973.
55. Vøllestad, N.K.; Wesche, J.; Sejersted, O.M. Gradual increase in leg oxygen uptake during repeated submaximal contractions in humans. J. Appl. Physiol. 68(3):1150-1156; 1990.
56. Wu, T.L.; Davis, E.J. Regulation of glycolytic flux in an energetically controlled cell-free system: The effects of adenine nucleotide ratios, inorganic phosphate, pH and citrate. Arch. Biochem. Biophys. 209:85-99; 1981.

PART VI

Exercise and Aging

CHAPTER 21

Overview of Exercise and Aging

Albert W. Taylor, Earl G. Noble
University of Western Ontario, London, Ontario, Canada

It has been recognized for a long time that the mammalian body begins to deteriorate near middle age (2, 31, 32). Signs of this deterioration include a decrease in sensory perception, reduced reaction and movement time, and altered neuromuscular transmission. Perhaps even more obvious is a progressive loss of muscular strength and an inability to successfully carry out protracted exercise or work (2). The loss of muscular strength is accompanied by a loss of muscle mass, which results from a decrease in the number and size of muscle cells. This decline approaches 10% per decade after about 30 yr of age until about 60 yr of age. Thereafter the rate of decline per decade increases to a greater magnitude (32, 33). The ability of muscle to carry out protracted work also declines with age. Several laboratories have observed distinct reductions in the activity of a number of metabolic enzymes with age, enzymes which may be important for energy provision adequate to prevent fatigue and maintain cell viability. The exact cause(s) of these age-related changes in muscle are unknown but could result from cell death due to a variety of factors that lead to genetic mutation (13, 14). The extent to which exercise and exercise training have the potential to retard the aging process are important research questions addressed in the present symposium and introduced in the following overview.

Aging and Muscle Strength

The primary role of skeletal muscle is to generate force, and this occurs when motor units are activated (33). It has been suggested that muscle mass is the major determinant of the age- and sex-related differences in strength (15). The decline in muscle mass and strength that accompanies aging results from a number of factors (2), which include the loss of motor unit and muscle fiber numbers (4, 5, 33). Recently, Doherty et al. (5) have observed an age-associated loss in the contractile function of arm musculature and demonstrated that the motor unit estimate in older adults decreased by 45% in relation to young subjects. Using multiple point stimulation, they also noted that the estimate of the number of motor units in the thenar muscle decreased with age (4). In addition to a loss of motor units and a reduced muscle fiber size (22, 29, 33), aging is accompanied by a gradual reorganization of the motor unit pool and the appearance of transitional or intermediate fiber types (21, 27). This reorganization is probably secondary to the loss of muscle mass and a result of altered recruitment patterns.

Aging is accompanied by a change in the rate of muscle protein turnover (table 21.1; 28) and by a change in the effect of exercise on this protein turnover. For example, Fielding et al. (12), who demonstrated that eccentric exercise produces an increase in whole-body protein breakdown as compared with concentric exercise, noted that myofibrillar proteolysis contributes a greater proportion of the total protein breakdown in older individuals. The aging process may also cause muscle to be more susceptible to exercise-induced injury and the subsequent metabolic consequences (9, 12). The greater muscle damage observed with aging may be related to the smaller muscle mass and lower $\dot{V}O_2$max seen in older subjects (9, 23). Despite these aging-associated effects on muscle mass and susceptibility to injury, skeletal muscle of the aged can adapt (tables 21.2 and 21.3). For example, weight training decreases the rate of loss of muscle strength (15) and age-associated changes in muscle myosin phenotype (20). Readers are referred to reviews by Bill Evans and co-investigators to further study exercise and protein metabolism (8) and the effects of aging and exercise training on skeletal muscle (29).

Table 21.1   Protein Turnover With Exercise and Aging

Parameter measured	Pre	Post	Age of subjects (yr)	Effects of age	Sex	Exercise or type of contraction	Reference
3-methyl histidine (μmol/gm creatine)	34	66	58+	↑	M	Single bout eccentric 45°	7
Leucine turnover (μmol · kg^{-1} · h^{-1})	176	192	59-63	?	M	3 × 15 eccentric	12
Leucine oxidation (μmol · kg^{-1} · h^{-1})	34	40	59-63	?	M	3 × 15 eccentric	12
Cross-sectional area (cm^2)	10	14	60-72	↓	M	Weight lifting plus protein supplement	8
Cross-sectional area (cm^2)		+11%	66 ± 2	↓	M	Concentric/ eccentric 3 sets/ 8 reps	15
Cross-sectional area (cm^2)		+15%	90 ± 1	↑	M3 F6	Progressive re- sistance training	11

Table 21.2   Effects of Exercise on Fiber Area in Older Human Subjects

Exercise or condition	Type I fiber area (μm^2)		Type II fiber area (μm^2)		Sex	Reference
	Pre	Post	Pre	Post		
Strength trained	3,967	4,205	2,532	2,988	F	3
Strength trained	45-8,200	40-7,800	32-5,100	59-6,200	M	33
Endurance trained	45-8,200	36-1,010	32-5,100	47-11,300	M	33
Strength trained	27-7,200	33-7,100	25-5,000	48-6,900	F	33
Endurance trained	27-7,200	31-10,000	25-5,000	40-7,500	F	33

Table 21.3   Effects of Exercise and Aging on Enzyme Activities in Selected Skeletal Muscle of Human Subjects

Enzyme	Age effects on activity (IU)	Age of subjects (yr)	Sex	Muscle	Training effect	Reference
Ca^{2+}-ATPase	↓	60-79	M	Pectoralis major	↓→	32
Phosphofructokinase (PFK)	↑→	55+	M	Vastus lateralis	↑→	32
Phosphofructokinase (PFK)	↓	63-76	M	Gastrocnemius	↑→	18
Citrate synthase	↓	55+	M	Vastus lateralis	→	32
Succinic dehydrogenase	↓	63-76	M	Gastrocnemius	↑	18
Lactate dehydrogenase	↓	55+	M	Vastus lateralis	→↑	32

Aging and Muscle Fiber Characteristics

Muscle fibers in different motor units may possess different physiological, biochemical, and morphological characteristics (33). A heterogeneous mixture of motor unit types is found in virtually all human muscles and most muscles of other mammals. The different characteristics of the muscle fibers representative of a motor unit have been extensively studied and categorized over the past several decades. Within most quadrupeds, there is a relative consistency in architectural and fiber type distribution properties of individual hindlimb muscles. Human skeletal muscle, on the other hand, is characterized by a wide range of distribution variability among individuals for a given muscle. However, certain muscles or muscle groups possess a large population of a particular fiber type, and this distribution pattern has a functional basis (30).

In the past two decades, a great deal of study has been carried out on the plasticity of muscle (26), that is, the capability of muscle to adapt to extensive stimuli by changing either the fiber type or the internal milieu of specific fibers or motor units (e.g., enzyme activities, organelles, transport mechanism and rate, calcium sequestration and release), thus affecting the contractile properties or capabilities of the muscle. The relationship between histochemical, biochemical, and contractile properties with aging has recently been reviewed in our laboratories (18, 32), and there is clearly an aging effect. A high correlation was noted among fiber distribution, enzyme activities, and contractile properties when various types of exercise, in particular endurance and sprint, were used as modulators of muscle response. Although previous literature has been equivocal as to whether aging is associated with a decrease or with little change in the activities of certain enzymes, the more recent literature presents a more homogeneous picture of the effects of aging and exercise on fiber adaptability and enzyme activity changes (table 21.3). In general, aging is accompanied by a decline in the activity of the enzymes of intermediary metabolism (18, 29, 32). Regular endurance exercise appears to retard the age-related changes in activity of succinate dehydrogenase, citrate synthase, and other aerobic enzymes (18). Exercise may therefore retard the age-associated decline in the capacity of muscle to carry out protracted work.

Changes in the aforementioned indices of muscle function may start at an early age. In rats, a remodeling of the motor unit profile appears to occur throughout the life-span (27). In humans, Glenmark, Hedberg, and Jansson have recently investigated changes in skeletal muscle fiber type from adolescence to adulthood (16). Age-related changes (16-27 yr) were noted for the vastus lateralis muscle. Muscle in women tended to increase in type I fiber percentage, whereas muscle in men tended to decrease in type I fiber proportion, and fiber areas remained unchanged in both sexes. When differences in anaerobic exercise performance between sexes were evaluated, the relative differences in the anaerobic metabolic properties of muscle were directly related to performance (6). If a sex-related, age-associated fiber adaptation does occur, it would be most interesting to investigate potential hormonal causes, possibly in postmenopausal women.

Aging and Cell Death

In addition to a loss of muscle mass and strength and a reduction in metabolic enzyme activity and hence reduced resistance to fatigue, aging is associated with an increased incidence of cell death. Work from the laboratory of Franceschi (13, 14) suggests that longevity is regulated through a complex network influencing the genetic control of cellular maintenance. The results do not support the idea that cell death is regulated by a central clock or that aging evolved as an active process of self-destruction. Interestingly, induction of several nuclear oncogenes occurs in cells undergoing both proliferation and apoptosis (17).

Many factors, including changes in metabolic capacity and alterations in cellular defense mechanisms, may contribute to the age-associated shift in the rate of cell death (19; table 21.4). Franceschi's group has studied programmed cell death (apoptosis) from the viewpoints of exposure to genotoxic agents, such as oxygen free radicals (25), and found that an age-related failure of the efficiency of such a system can affect cell proliferation and death. These two phenomena appear to be tightly linked and regulated as demonstrated with models of precocious aging (Down syndrome) and longevity (centenarians; 13, 14). Most Down syndrome patients show phenotypical signs of aging several decades in advance, and both precocious aging and longevity are characterized by modifications to the immune system. Premature aging and longevity are also characterized by a differential susceptibility to oxidants (14). In fact, Franceschi et al. (14) have hypothesized that peripheral blood lymphocyte sensitivity to oxidative stress is a biomarker of aging and longevity. Antioxidant agents such as nicotinamide and L-carnitine (13) and vitamin E (24) protect human cells from oxygen free radical–induced damage and are possible candidates as antiaging substances.

As mentioned previously, muscle from older mammals appears to have a reduced rate of recovery from muscle injury, including that accompanying exercise (2). Using eccentric exercise, which may result in oxidative damage to muscle, elevated myofibrillar proteolysis (12) and delayed recovery of contractile parameters (1) are observed in the aged. However, supplementation with vitamin E has been found to suppress exercise-induced oxidative damage to skeletal muscle in both young and elderly subjects (24).

What role exercise may play in retarding the loss of muscle mass, the decline in metabolic capacity, and incidence of cell death associated with aging is still unclear. However, research on these questions is certain to reveal information critical to understanding the causes of aging and the interaction between exercise and senescence.

Table 21.4   Potential Factors Associated With Age-Related Cell Death

Parameter measured	Aging effects	Reference
Sensitivity to oxygen free radicals (Down syndrome)	↑	14
Sensitivity to oxygen free radicals (centenarians)	↓	14
Sensitivity to DNA-damaging agents	↑	13
Spontaneous increase in sister chromatid exchanges	↑	13
Stimulated cytokine production	↑	10

References

1. Brooks, S.V.; Faulkner, J.A. Contraction-induced injury: Recovery of skeletal muscle in young and old mice. Am. J. Physiol. 258:C436-C442; 1988.
2. Buckwalter, J.A.; Woo, S.L.-Y.; Goldberg, V.M.; Hadley, E.C.; Booth, F.; Oegema, T.R; Eyre, D.R. Soft-tissue aging and musculoskeletal function. J. Bone Joint Surg. 75:1533-1548; 1993.
3. Charette, S.L.; McEvoy, L.; Pyka, G.; Snow-Harter, C.; Guido, D.; Wiswell, R.A.; Marcus, R. Muscle hypertrophy response to resistance training in older women. J. Appl. Physiol. 70:1912-1916; 1991.
4. Doherty, T.J.; Brown, W.F. The estimated numbers and relative sizes of thenar motor units as selected by multiple point stimulation in young and older adults. Muscle Nerve 16:355-366; 1993.
5. Doherty, T.J.; Vandervoort, A.A.; Taylor, A.W.; Brown, W.F. Effects of motor unit losses on strength in older men and women. J. Appl. Physiol. 74:868-874; 1993.
6. Esbjörnsson, M.; Sylvén, C.; Holm, I.; Jansson, E. Fast twitch fibres may predict anaerobic performance in both females and males. Int. J. Sports Med. 14:257-263; 1993.
7. Evans, W.J. Exercise, nutrition and ageing. J. Nutr. 122:796-801; 1992.
8. Evans, W.J. Exercise and protein metabolism. In: Simopoulos, A.P.; Pavlou, K.N., eds. Nutrition and fitness for athletes. Basel: Karger; 1993:23-33. (World Rev. Nutr. Diet).
9. Evans, W.J.; Meredith, C.N.; Cannon, J.G.; Dinarello, C.A.; Frontera, W.R.; Hughes, V.A; Jones, B.H.; Knuttgen, H.G. Metabolic changes following eccentric exercise in trained and untrained men. J. Appl. Physiol. 61:1864-1868; 1986.
10. Fagiolo, U.; Cossarizza, A.; Scala, E.; Fanales-Belasio, E.; Ortolani, C.; Cozzi, E.; Monti, D.; Franceschi, C.; Paganelli, R. Increased cytokine production in mononuclear cells of healthy elderly people. Eur. J. Immunol. 23:2375-2378; 1993.
11. Fiatarone, M.A.; O'Neill, E.F.; Doyle, N.; Clements, K.M.; Roberts, S.B.; Kehayias, J.J.; Lipsitz, L.A.; Evans, W.J. The Boston FICSIT study: The effects of resistance training and nutritional supplementation on physical frailty in the oldest old. J. Am. Geriatr. Soc. 41:333-337; 1993.
12. Fielding, R.A.; Meredith, C.N.; O'Reilly, K.P.; Frontera, W.R.; Cannon, J.G.; Evans, W.J. Enhanced protein breakdown after eccentric exercise in young and older men. J. Appl. Physiol. 71:674-679; 1991.
13. Franceschi, C.; Monti, D.; Cossarizza, A.; Fagnoni, F.; Passeri, G.; Sansoni, P. Aging, longevity, and cancer: Studies in Down's syndrome and centenarians. Ann. N.Y. Acad. Sci. 621:428-441; 1991.
14. Franceschi, C.; Monti, D.; Scarfi, M.R.; Zeni, O.; Temperani, P.; Emilia, G.; Sansoni, P.; Lioi, M.B.; Troiano, L.; Agnesini, C.; Salvioli, S.; Cossarizza, A. Genomic instability and aging. Studies in centenarians (successful aging) and in patients with Down's syndrome (accelerated aging). Ann. N.Y. Acad. Sci. 663:4-16; 1992.
15. Frontera, W.R.; Hughes, V.A.; Lutz, K.J.; Evans, W.J. A cross-sectional study of muscle strength and mass in 45- to 78-yr-old men and women. J. Appl. Physiol. 71:644-650; 1991.

16. Glenmark, B.; Hedberg, G.; Jansson, E. Changes in muscle fibre type from adolescence to adulthood in women and men. Acta Physiol. Scand. 146:251-259; 1992.

17. Grassilli, E.; Carcereri de Prati, A.; Monti, D.; Troiano, L.; Menegazzi, M.; Barbieri, D.; Franceschi, C.; Suzuki, H. Studies of the relationship between cell proliferation and cell death. II. Early gene expression during oncanavalin A–induced proliferation or dexamethasone-induced apoptosis of rat thymocytes. Biochem. Biophys. Res. Commun. 188:1261-1266; 1992.

18. Keh-Evans, L.; Rice, C.L.; Noble, E.G.; Paterson, D.H.; Cunningham, D.A.; Taylor, A.W. Comparison of histochemical, biochemical and contractile properties of triceps surae of trained aged subjects. Can. J. Aging 11:412-425; 1992.

19. Kirkwood, T.B.L.; Franceschi, C. Is aging as complex as it would appear? New perspectives in aging research. Ann. N.Y. Acad. Sci. 663:412-417; 1992.

20. Klitgaard, H.; Mantoni, N.; Sciaffino, S.; Ausoni, S.; Gorza, L.; Laurent-Winter, C.; Schnokr, P.; Saltin, B. Function, morphology and protein expression of ageing skeletal muscle: A cross-sectional study of elderly men with different training backgrounds. Acta Physiol. Scand. 140:41-54; 1990.

21. Klitgaard, H.; Zhou, M.; Sciaffino, S.; Betto, R.; Salviati, E. Ageing alters the myosin heavy chain composition of single fibres from human skeletal muscle. Acta Physiol. Scand. 140:55-62; 1990.

22. Lexell, J. Ageing and human muscle: Observations from Sweden. Can. J. Appl. Physiol. 18:2-18; 1993.

23. Manfredi, T.G.; Fielding, R.A.; O'Reilly, K.P.; Meredith, C.N.; Lee, H.Y.; Evans, W.J. Plasma creatine kinase activity and exercise-induced muscle damage in older men. Med. Sci. Sports Exercise 23:1028-1034; 1991.

24. Meydani, M.; Evans, W.J.; Handelman, G.; Biddle, L.; Fielding, R.A.; Meydani, S.N.; Burrill, J.; Fiatarone, M.A.; Blumberg, J.B.; Cannon, J.G. Protective effect of vitamin E on exercise-induced oxidative damage in young and older adults. Am J. Physiol. 264:R992-R998; 1993.

25. Monti, D.; Troiano, L.; Tropea, F.; Grassilli, E.; Cossarizza, A.; Barozzi, D.; Pelloni, M.C.; Tamassia, M.G.; Bellomo, G.; Franceschi, C. Apoptosis—programmed cell death: A role in the aging process? Am J. Clin. Nutr. 55:1208S-1214S; 1992.

26. Pette, D., ed. Plasticity of muscle. Berlin: Walter de Gruyter; 1980.

27. Pettigrew, F.P.; Noble, E.G. Shifts in rat plantaris motor unit characteristics with aging and compensatory overload. J. Appl. Physiol. 71:2365-2368; 1991.

28. Rattan, S.I.S.; Derventzi, A.; Clark, B.F.C. Protein synthesis, posttranslational modifications and aging. Ann. N.Y. Acad. Sci. 663:48-62; 1992.

29. Rogers, M.A.; Evans, W.J. Changes in skeletal muscle with aging: Effects of exercise training. In: Holloszy, J.O., ed. Exercise and sport sciences reviews. Baltimore: Williams and Wilkins; 1993:65-102.

30. Saltin, B.; Gollnick, P.D. Skeletal muscle adaptability: Significance for metabolism and performance. In: Peachey, L.E., ed. Skeletal muscle. Bethesda, MD: American Physiological Society; 1983:555-631.

31. Taylor, A.W. Muscle metabolism and exercise: The effects of aging. In: Lawson, D., ed. Physical activity: A universal and unifying factor. Melbourne: FIT Press; 1993:136-143.

32. Taylor, A.W.; Noble, E.G.; Cunningham, D.A.; Paterson, D.H.; Rechnitzer, P. Ageing, skeletal muscle contractile properties and enzyme activities with exercise. In: Sato, Y.; Poortmans, J.; Hashimoto, I.; Oshida, Y., eds. Integration of medical and sports sciences. Basel: Karger; 1992:109-125. (Med. Sport Sci.).

33. Thayer, R.E.; Rice, C.L.; Pettigrew, F.P.; Noble, E.G.; Taylor, A.W. The fibre composition of skeletal muscle. In: Poortmans, J., ed. Principles of exercise biochemistry. Basel: Karger; 1993:25-50. (Med. Sport Sci.).

CHAPTER 22

Aging, Exercise, and Protein Metabolism

William J. Evans
Pennsylvania State University, University Park, Pennsylvania, U.S.A.

Body Composition

Advancing age is associated with profound changes in body composition. Using total body potassium as an index of fat-free mass, Novak (34) assessed the body composition of more than 500 men and women between the ages of 18 and 85. He determined that body fat increased from 18% to 36% and from 33% to 44% in men and women, respectively. In an 18-yr longitudinal study, Flynn and co-workers found that the most rapid rate of total body potassium loss occurred between the ages of 41 and 60 yr for men, whereas the rapid loss in women did not take place until after the age of 60 yr (14). Cohn and co-workers (10), using total body neutron activation procedures, determined that the principal component of the decline in fat-free mass was a decrease in muscle mass, with minimal change in nonmuscle mass. They also observed that total body nitrogen declined in very close association with total body calcium, suggesting a link between sarcopenia and osteopenia. Skeletal muscle is the largest reservoir of protein in the body. Age-related reductions in muscle are a direct cause of the age-related decrease in muscle strength (7, 15, 27, 36, 44).

Loss of muscle mass with age in humans has been demonstrated both indirectly and directly. The excretion of urinary creatinine, reflecting muscle creatine content and total muscle mass, decreases by nearly 50% between the ages of 20 and 90 (41). Computed tomography (CT) of individual muscles shows that after age 30 there is a decrease in cross-sectional areas of the thigh, together with decreased muscle density associated with increased intramuscular fat. These changes are most pronounced in women (21). Muscle atrophy may result from a gradual and selective loss of muscle fibers. The number of muscle fibers in the midsection of the vastus lateralis of autopsy specimens is lower by about 110,000 in elderly men (age 70-73) than in young men (age 19-37), a 23% difference (28). The decline is more marked in type II muscle fibers, which fall from an average 60% in sedentary young men to below 30% after the age of 80 (24), and is significantly related to age-related decreases in strength ($r = .54$, $p < .001$).

A reduction in muscle strength is a major component of normal aging. Data from the Framingham study (22) indicate that 40% of the female population aged 55 to

64, almost 45% of women aged 65 to 74, and 65% of women aged 75 to 84 yr were unable to lift 4.5 kg. In addition, a similarly high percentage of women in this population reported that they were unable to perform some aspects of normal household work. Larsson et al. (27) studied 114 men between the ages of 11 and 70 yr and found that isometric and dynamic strength of the quadriceps increased up to the age of 30 yr and decreased after the age of 50. They saw reductions in strength between the ages of 50 and 70 from 24% to 36%. They concluded that much of the reduction in strength was due to a selective atrophy of type II muscle fibers, which were 36% smaller in diameter when compared with 40-yr-olds. It appears that muscle strength losses are most dramatic after the age of 70 yr. Knee extensor strength of a group of healthy 80-yr-olds studied in the Copenhagen City Heart Study (11) was found to be 30% lower than a previous population study (1) of 70-yr-old men and women. Thus, cross-sectional as well as longitudinal data indicate that muscle strength declines by approximately 15% per decade in the sixth and seventh decade and about 30% thereafter (11, 19, 25, 33). While there is some indication that muscle function is reduced with advancing age, the overwhelming majority of the loss in strength results from an age-related decrease in muscle mass. We (15) examined more than 200 men and women between the ages of 45 and 78 yr old. Isokinetic and isometric strength of the upper and lower body were significantly different between men and women and decreased with advancing age. However, when corrected for fat-free mass (estimated from hydrostatic weighing) and total body muscle mass (estimated from 24-h urinary creatinine), age-related differences disappear (table 22.1).

Strength and Functional Capacity

Bassey, Bendall, and Pearson (3) measured muscle strength and the amount and speed of customary walking in a large sample of men and women older than 65 yr. They found an age-related decline in muscle strength and a significant negative correlation between strength and chosen normal walking speed for both sexes ($r = .041$, $p < .001$ for men; $r = .36$, $p < .01$ for women). Bassey and co-workers (5) measured flexibility and found that the mean value for the elderly was 30° less than that accepted for younger men and women. Nearly one-half of the distribution fell

Table 22.1   Strength Corrected for Body Composition in Older Women

Age (yr)	Strength (N · m)	N · m/fat-free mass	N · m/muscle mass
45-54	108 ± 22	2.7 ± 0.4	6.1 ± 0.9
55-64	98 ± 20	2.6 ± 0.4	5.9 ± 1.2
65-78	89 ± 15*	2.5 ± 0.4	5.8 ± 1.1

*Different from age 45-54 group ($p < .05$)
Reprinted from Frontera, Hughes, and Evans 1991.

below the accepted threshold level of 120° for adequate function. Fiatarone and colleagues (12) observed a closer relationship between quadriceps strength and habitual gait speed ($r = -.745$, $p < .01$) in a group of frail, institutionalized men and women above the age of 86 yr. In these subjects, fat-free mass ($r = .732$) and regional muscle mass ($r = .752$) estimated by CT were correlated with muscle strength. In the same population, we (4) recently demonstrated that leg power is closely associated with functional performance. In older, frail women, leg power was highly correlated with walking speed ($r = .93$, $p < .001$), accounting for up to 86% of the variance in walking speed. Leg power, which represents a more dynamic measurement of muscle function, may be a useful predictor of functional capacity in the very old. These data suggest that with advancing age and very low activity levels seen in institutionalized patients, muscle strength is a critical component of walking ability.

Energy Metabolism

Daily energy expenditure declines progressively throughout adult life (30). In sedentary individuals, the main determinant of energy expenditure is fat-free mass (35), which declines by about 15% between the third and eighth decades of life, contributing to a lower basal metabolic rate in the elderly (10). Tzankoff and Norris (41) saw that 24-h creatinine excretion (an index of muscle mass) was closely related to basal metabolic rate at all ages. Nutrition surveys of those over the age of 65 yr show a very low energy intake for men (1,400 kcal $\cdot$ d^{-1}; 23 kcal $\cdot$ kg^{-1} $\cdot$ d^{-1}). These data indicate that preservation of muscle mass and prevention of sarcopenia can help prevent the decrease in metabolic rate. While body weight increases with advancing age, an age-associated increase in relative body fat content has been demonstrated by a number of investigators. This increase in body fat results from a number of factors, but chief among these causes are a declining metabolic rate and activity level coupled with an energy intake that does not match this declining need for calories. Meredith et al. (32) demonstrated that endurance-trained men between 20 and 60 yr old consumed a diet very high in calories but that body fat levels were closely related to the total number of hours spent exercising per week. Age was not found to be a covariate in this study. More recently, Roberts and co-workers (37) examined the relationship between total energy use (using the doubly labeled water technique) and body composition in a group of sedentary young and old men and found that energy spent in daily activity accounted for 73% of the variability in body fat content.

In addition to its role in energy metabolism, skeletal muscle and its age-related decline may contribute to such age-associated changes as a reduction in bone density (6, 39, 40), insulin sensitivity (23), and aerobic capacity (13). For these reasons, strategies for preservation of muscle mass with advancing age and for increasing muscle mass and strength in the previously sedentary elderly may be an important way to increase functional independence and decrease the prevalence of many age-associated chronic diseases.

Protein Needs and Aging

Previous estimates of dietary protein needs of the elderly using nitrogen balance have ranged from 0.59 to 0.8 g · kg^{-1} · d^{-1} (18, 42, 45). However, the low value was reported by Zanni, Calloway, and Zezulka (45) who preceded their 10-d dietary protein feeding with a 17-d protein-free diet, which was likely to improve nitrogen retention during the 10-d balance period. Recently, we (9) reassessed the nitrogen balance studies previously mentioned using the currently accepted, 1985 WHO (43) nitrogen balance formula. These newly recalculated data were combined with nitrogen balance data collected on 12 healthy older men and women (age range 56-80 yr, 8 men and 4 women) consuming the current Recommended Dietary Allowance (RDA) for protein or double this amount (0.8 g · kg^{-1} · d^{-1} and 1.6 g · kg^{-1} · d^{-1}, respectively) in our laboratory. Our subjects consumed the diet for 11 consecutive days and nitrogen balance (mg N · kg^{-1} · d^{-1}) was measured during days 6 to 11. The estimated mean protein requirements from the three retrospectively assessed studies and the current study can be combined by weighted averaging to produce an overall protein requirement estimate of 0.91 ± 0.043 g · kg^{-1} · d^{-1}. The combined estimate, excluding the data from our 12 subjects, is 0.894 ± 0.048 g protein · kg^{-1} · d^{-1}. Figure 22.1 shows the mean values for achieving nitrogen equilibrium for the three retrospectively assessed studies as well as our most recent data.

The current RDA in the United States of 0.8 g · kg^{-1} · d^{-1} is based on data collected, for the most part, on young subjects. The RDA includes an upward adjustment based on the coefficient of variation (CV) of the average requirement established in these studies (0.6 g · kg^{-1} · d^{-1}). Based on the CV previously established for nitrogen balance studies, an adequate dietary protein level for 97.5% of the elderly population would be provided by an intake of 25% (twice the standard deviation [SD]) above the mean protein requirement. Our data suggest that the safe protein intake for elderly adults is 1.25 g · kg^{-1} · d^{-1}. On the basis of the current and recalculated short-term nitrogen balance results, a safe recommended protein intake for older men and women should be set at 1.0 to 1.25 g of high-quality protein · kg^{-1} · d^{-1}. Hartz (20) reported that approximately 50% of 946 healthy free-living men and women above the age of 60 living in the Boston, Massachusetts, area consume less than this amount of protein, and 25% of the elderly men and women in this survey consume less than 0.86 g and less than 0.81 g protein · kg^{-1} · d^{-1}, respectively. A large percentage of housebound elderly people consuming their habitual dietary protein intake (0.67 g mixed protein · kg^{-1} · d^{-1}) have been shown to be in negative nitrogen balance (8). Inadequate dietary protein intake may be an important cause of sarcopenia. The compensatory response to long-term decreased dietary protein intake is a loss in lean body mass.

Strength Training

Strength conditioning is generally defined as training in which the resistance against which a muscle generates force is progressively increased over time. Muscle strength has been shown to increase in response to training between 60% and 100%

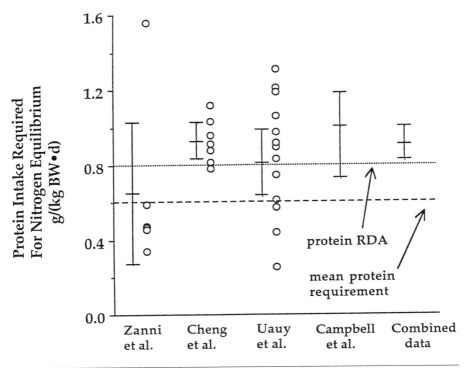

Figure 22.1   Dietary protein intakes required to achieve nitrogen equilibrium in elderly subjects. Individual subject (circles) and group mean protein intakes (±2 SEMs; solid bars) at nitrogen equilibrium were calculated from data by Zanni et al., Cheng et al., Uauy et al., and Campbell et al., based on the 1985 FAO/WHO/UNU nitrogen balance formula. The dashed line represents the current estimated mean protein requirement for all adults, and the dotted line represents the current suggested safe level of protein intake for elderly men and women.

of the one-repetition maximum (1-RM; 29). Strength conditioning results in an increase in muscle size, and this increase in size is largely the result of increased contractile proteins.

It is clear that when the intensity of the exercise is low, only modest increases in strength are achieved by elderly subjects (2, 26). A number of studies have demonstrated that, given an adequate training stimulus, older men and women show similar or greater strength gains compared with young individuals as a result of resistance training.

Frontera et al. (16, 17) showed that older men responded to a 12-wk progressive resistance training program (80% of the 1-RM, three sets of eight repetitions of the knee extensor and flexors, 3 d/wk) by more than doubling extensor strength and more than tripling flexor strength. The increases in strength averaged approximately 5% per training session, similar to strength gains observed by younger men. Total muscle area estimated by CT increased by 11.4%. Biopsies of the vastus lateralis muscle revealed similar increases in type I fiber area (33.5%) and type II fiber area (27.6%). Daily excretion of urinary 3-methyl-L-histidine increased with training ($p < .05$) by an average of 40.8%, indicating that increased muscle size and strength resulting from progressive resistance training is associated with an increased rate of myofibrillar protein turnover. Half of the men who participated in this study were given a daily protein-calorie supplement (S) providing an extra 560 ± 16 kcal $\cdot$ d^{-1} (16.6% as protein, 43.3% as carbohydrate, and 40.1% as fat) in addition to their normal ad lib diet. The rest of the subjects received no supplement (NS) and consumed an ad lib diet. By the 12th week of the study, dietary energy (2960 ± 230 kcal in S vs. 1620 ± 80 kcal in NS) and protein intake (118 ± 10 g $\cdot$ d^{-1} in S vs. 72 ± 11 g $\cdot$ d^{-1} in NS) were significantly different between the S and NS groups.

Composition of the midthigh was estimated by CT and showed that the S group had greater gains in muscle than did the NS men (31). In addition, urinary creatinine excretion at the end of the training was greater in the S group than in the NS group, indicating a greater muscle mass in the S group at the end of the 12 wk of training. The change in energy and protein intake (beginning vs. 12 wk) was correlated with the change in midthigh muscle area ($r = .69, p = .019$; $r = .63, p = .039$, respectively). There were no differences in the strength gains between the two groups. These data suggest that a change in total food intake, or perhaps in selected nutrients, in subjects beginning a strength training program can affect muscle hypertrophy. High-intensity resistance training appears to have profoundly anabolic effects in the elderly. Data from our laboratory demonstrate a 10% to 15% decrease in nitrogen excretion at the initiation of training that persists for 12 wk. That is, progressive resistance training improved nitrogen balance; thus, older subjects performing resistance training have a lower mean protein requirement than do sedentary subjects. These results are somewhat at variance to our previous research (32), demonstrating that regularly performed aerobic exercise causes an increase in the mean protein requirement of middle-aged and young endurance athletes. This difference is likely to result from increased oxidation of amino acids during aerobic exercise that may not be present during resistance training.

The very old and frail elderly experience skeletal muscle atrophy as a result of disuse, disease, undernutrition, and the effects of aging per se. Muscle weakness that accompanies advanced age has been positively related to the risk of falling and fracture in these older individuals (38). For this reason, we studied the effects of high-intensity, progressive resistance training on quadriceps muscle strength in a group of institutionalized elderly men and women (age range 87-96 yr). Initial strength levels were extremely low in these subjects, with a mean 1-RM of 8 kg for the quadriceps. The absolute amount of weight lifted by the subjects during the training increased from 8 to 21 kg. The average increase in strength after 8 wk of resistance training was $174 \pm 31\%$, and the mean increase in muscle cross-sectional area via CT was $10 \pm 8\%$. The substantial increases in muscle size and strength were accompanied by clinically significant improvements in tandem gait speed and in index of functional mobility. Repeat 1-RM testing in seven of the subjects after 4 wk of no training showed that quadriceps strength had declined 32%. This study demonstrates that frail elderly men and women, well into their 10th decade of life, retain the capacity to adapt to progressive resistance exercise training with significant and clinically relevant muscle hypertrophy and increases in muscle strength. Results from the resistance training studies performed in the young, middle-aged, elderly, and the oldest old indicate that it is the intensity of the stimulus, not the underlying fitness or frailty of the individual, that determines the magnitude of the gains in strength and muscle size. More recently, we (12) conducted a randomized, placebo-controlled trial comparing progressive resistance training, a protein-calorie supplement, both interventions, and neither in a similar group of 100 frail nursing home residents over a 10-wk period. The mean age of the 63 women and 37 men in the study was 87.1 ± 0.6 yr (range, 72 to 98). Muscle strength increased by $113 \pm 8\%$ in the exercising subjects compared with $3 \pm 9\%$ in the nonexercising subjects ($p < .001$). In the exercising subjects, there was a significant increase in gait velocity, stair-climbing power, and the level of spontaneous physical activity. However, unlike the effects seen in the younger group of men, the supplement had no effect on muscle strength or muscle size. Total energy intake was significantly increased only in the exercising subjects who also received nutritional supplementation. Those subjects who received the supplement and did not exercise decreased their habitual energy intake to compensate for the calories supplied in the supplement; thus there was no change in total energy intake in this group.

In conclusion, sarcopenia, defined as the age-related loss in skeletal muscle mass, results in decreased strength and aerobic capacity and thus in decreased functional capacity. Sarcopenia is also closely linked to age-related losses in bone mineral, decreases in basal metabolic rate, and increased body fat content. Through physical exercise and training, especially resistance training, it may be possible to prevent sarcopenia and the remarkable array of associated abnormalities, such as NIDDM, coronary artery disease, hypertension, osteoporosis, and obesity. Using an exercise program of sufficient frequency, intensity, and duration, it is quite possible to increase muscle strength and endurance at any age. Advancing age is associated with increased dietary protein requirements. This increased need for dietary protein by the elderly may be decreased with regularly performed resistance exercise. There is no pharmacological intervention that holds a greater promise of improving health and promoting independence in the elderly than does exercise.

References

1. Aniansson, A.; Grimby, G.; Hedberg, M.; Krotkiewski, M. Muscle morphology, enzyme activity and muscle strength in elderly men and women. Clin. Physiol. 1:73-86; 1981.
2. Aniansson, A.; Gustafsson, E. Physical training in elderly men with special reference to quadriceps muscle strength and morphology. Clin. Physiol. 1:87-98; 1981.
3. Bassey, E.J.; Bendall, M.J.; Pearson, M. Muscle strength in the triceps surae and objectively measured customary walking activity in men and women over 65 years of age. Clin. Sci. 74:85-89; 1988.
4. Bassey, E.J., Fiatarone, M.A.; O'Neill, E.F.; Kelly, M.; Evans, W.J.; Lipsitz, L.A. Leg extensor power and functional performance in very old men and women. Clin. Sci. 82:321-327; 1992.
5. Bassey, E.J.; Morgan, K.; Dallosso, H.M.; Ebrahim, S.B.J. Flexibility of the shoulder joint measured as a range of abduction in a large representative sample of men and women over 65 years of age. Eur. J. Appl. Physiol. 58:353-360; 1989.
6. Bevier, W.C.; Wiswell, R.A.; Pyka, G.; Kozak, K.C.; Newhall, K.M.; Marcus, R. Relationship of body composition, muscle strength, and aerobic capacity to

bone mineral density in older men and women. J. Bone Mineral Res. 4:421-432; 1989.

7. Bruce, S.A.; Newton, D.; Woledge, R.C. Effect of age on voluntary force and cross-sectional area of human adductor pollicis muscle. Q. J. Exp. Physiol. 74:359-362; 1989.

8. Bunker, V.W.; Lawson, M.S.; Stanfield, M.F.; Clayton, B.E. Nitrogen balance studies in apparently healthy elderly people and those who are housebound. Br. J. Nutr. 57:211-221; 1987.

9. Campbell, W.W.; Crim, M.C.; Dallal, G.E.; Young, V.R.; Evans, W.J. Increased protein requirements in the elderly: New data and retrospective reassessments. Am. J. Clin. Nutr. 60:S01-S09; 1994.

10. Cohn, S.H.; Vartsky, D.; Yasumura, S.; Savitsky, A.; Zanzi, I.; Vaswani, A.; Ellis, K.J. Compartmental body composition based on total-body, potassium, and calcium. Am. J. Physiol. 239:E524-E530; 1980.

11. Danneskoild-Samsoe, B.; Kofod, V.; Munter, J.; Grimby, G.; Schnohr, P. Muscle strength and functional capacity in 77-81 year old men and women. Eur. J. Appl. Physiol. 52:123-135; 1984.

12. Fiatarone, M.A.; O'Neill, E.F.; Ryan, N.D.; Clements, K.M.; Solares, G.R.; Nelson, M.E.; Roberts, S.B.; Kehayias, J.J.; Lipsitz, L.A.; Evans, W.J. Exercise training and nutritional supplementation for physical frailty in very elderly people. N. Engl. J. Med. 330:1769-1775; 1994.

13. Flegg, J.L.; Lakatta, E.G. Role of muscle loss in the age-associated reduction in VO_2max. J. Appl. Physiol. 65:1147-1151; 1988.

14. Flynn, M.A.; Nolph, G.B.; Baker, A.S.; Martin, W.M.; Krause, G. Total body potassium in aging humans: A longitudinal study. Am. J. Clin. Nutr. 50:713-717; 1989.

15. Frontera, W.R.; Hughes, V.A.; Evans, W.J. A cross-sectional study of upper and lower extremity muscle strength in 45-78 year old men and women. J. Appl. Physiol. 71:644-650; 1991.

16. Frontera, W.R.; Meredith, C.N.; O'Reilly, K.P.; Evans, W.J. Strength training and determinants of VO_2max in older men. J. Appl. Physiol. 68:329-333; 1990.

17. Frontera, W.R.; Meredith, C.N.; O'Reilly, K.P.; Knuttgen, H.C.; Evans, W.J. Strength conditioning in older men: Skeletal muscle hypertrophy and improved function. J. Appl. Physiol. 64:1038-1044; 1988.

18. Gersovitz, M.; Munro, H.; Scrimshaw, N.; Young, V. Human protein requirements: Assessment of the adequacy of the current recommended dietary allowance for dietary protein in elderly men and women. Am. J. Clin. Nutr. 35:6-14; 1982.

19. Harries, U.J.; Bassey, E.J. Torque-velocity relationships for the knee extensors in women in their 3rd and 7th decades. Eur. J. Appl. Physiol. 60:187-190; 1990.

20. Hartz, S.C. The NSS study population. In: Hartz, S.C.; Russell, R.M.; Rosenberg, I.H., editors. Nutrition in the elderly: The Boston Nutritional Status Survey. London: Smith-Gordon; 1992, p. 55-64.

21. Imamura, K.; Ashida, H.; Ishikawa, T.; Fujii, M. Human major psoas muscle and sacrospinalis muscle in relation to age: A study by computed tomography. J. Gerontol. 38:678-681; 1983.

22. Jette, A.M.; Branch, L.G. The Framingham disability study: 11. Physical disability among the aging. Am. J. Public Health 71:1211-1216; 1981.

23. Kolterman, O.G.; Insel, J.; Saekow, M.; Olefsky, J.M. Mechanisms of insulin resistance in human obesity. Evidence for receptor and postreceptor defects. J. Clin. Invest. 65:1272-1284; 1980.

24. Larsson, L. Histochemical characteristics of human skeletal muscle during aging. Acta Physiol. Scand. 117:469-471; 1983.

25. Larsson, L. Morphological and functional characteristics of the aging skeletal muscle in man. Acta Physiol. Scand. (suppl. 457):1-36; 1978.

26. Larsson, L. Physical training effects on muscle morphology in sedentary males at different ages. Med. Sci. Sports Exercise 14:203-206; 1982.

27. Larsson, L.G.; Grimby, G.; Karlsson, J. Muscle strength and speed of movement in relation to age and muscle morphology. J. Appl. Physiol. 46:451-456; 1979.

28. Lexell, J.; Henriksson-Larsen, K.; Wimblod, B.; Sjostrom, M. Distribution of different fiber types in human skeletal muscles: Effects of aging studied in whole muscle cross sections. Muscle Nerve 6:588-595; 1983.

29. MacDougall, J.D. Adaptability of muscle to strength training—A cellular approach. In: Saltin, B., ed. Biochemistry of exercise VI. Champaign, IL: Human Kinetics Publishers; 1986:501-513.

30. McGandy, R.B.; Barrows, C.H.; Spanias, A.; Meredith, A.; Stone, J.L.; Norris, A.H. Nutrient intake and energy expenditure in men of different ages. J. Gerontol. 21:581-587; 1966.

31. Meredith, C.N.; Frontera, W.R.; Evans, W.J. Body composition in elderly men: Effect of dietary modification during strength training. J. Am. Geriatr. Soc. 40:155-162; 1992.

32. Meredith, C.N.; Zackin, M.J.; Frontera, W.R.; Evans, W.J. Dietary protein requirements and body protein metabolism in endurance-trained men. J. Appl. Physiol. 66:2850-2856; 1989.

33. Murray, M.P.; Duthie, E.H.; Gambert, S.T.; Sepic, S.B.; Mollinger, L.A. Age-related differences in knee muscle strength in normal women. J. Gerontol. 40:275-280; 1985.

34. Novak, L.P. Aging, total body potassium, fat free-mass, and cell mass in males and females between ages 18 and 85 years. J. Gerontol. 27:438-443; 1972.

35. Ravussin, E.; Lillioja, S.; Anderson, T.E.; Cristin, L.; Bogardus, C. Determinants of 24-hour energy expenditure in man. J. Clin. Invest. 78:1568-1578; 1986.

36. Rice, C.L.; Cunningham, D.A.; Paterson, D.H.; Rechnitzer, P.A. Strength in an elderly population. Arch. Phys. Med. Rehabil. 70:391-397; 1989.

37. Roberts, S.B.; Young, V.R.; Fuss, P.; Heyman, M.B.; Fiatarone, M.A.; Dallal, G.E.; Cortiella, J.; Evans, W.J. What are the dietary energy needs of elderly adults? J. Obesity 16:969-976; 1992.

38. Scheibel, A. Falls, motor dysfunction, and correlative neurohistologic changes in the elderly. Clin. Geriatr. Med. 1:671-677; 1985.

39. Sinaki, M.; McPhee, M.C.; Hodgson, S.F. Relationship between bone mineral density of spine and strength of back extensors in healthy postmenopausal women. Mayo Clin. Proc. 61:116-122; 1986.

40. Snow-Harter, C.; Bouxsein, M.; Lewis, B.; Charette, S.; Weinstein, P.; Marcus, R. Muscle strength as a predictor of bone mineral density in young women. J. Bone Mineral Res. 5(6):589-595; 1990.

41. Tzankoff, S.P.; Norris, A.H. Longitudinal changes in basal metabolic rate in man. J. Appl. Physiol. 33:536-539; 1978.

42. Uauy, R.; Scrimshaw, N.; Young, V. Human protein requirements: Nitrogen balance response to graded levels of egg protein in elderly men and women. Am. J. Clin. Nutr. 31:779-785; 1978.
43. WHO/FAO/UNU. Energy and protein requirements. WHO Tech. Rep. Ser. 724; 1985.
44. Young, A.; Stokes, M.; Crowe, M. The size and strength of the quadriceps muscle of old and young women. Eur. J. Clin. Invest. 14:282-287; 1984.
45. Zanni, E.; Calloway, D.; Zezulka, A. Protein requirements of elderly men. J. Nutr. 109:513-524; 1979.

CHAPTER 23

Age-Related Fiber Type Changes in Human Skeletal Muscle

Eva Jansson

Huddinge University Hospital, Huddinge, Sweden

Muscle fiber type distribution, expressed as the proportion of type I (slow twitch) and type II (fast twitch) fibers in human skeletal muscle, varies a lot among individuals (32). This individual variation is explained to some extent by the endowment, level of physical activity, and sex of the individual (23, 24, 32, 54). Individuals with a high level of physical activity are known to have a high percentage of type I fibers (23), and women have also been shown to have a higher percentage of type I fibers than men (23, 54). In addition to these factors, some of the variation in fiber type distribution among individuals may be explained by the age of the individual. However, recent reviews of changes in skeletal muscle that occur with aging have pointed to large discrepancies found in the results of various studies describing age-related changes in muscle fiber type distribution (4, 51). For example, in a cross-sectional study by Larsson et al. (39) on sedentary men between the ages of 20 and 65, it was shown that the percentage of type I fibers in the vastus lateralis was higher in old age. Sato et al. (53), on the other hand, demonstrated that the percentage of type I fibers in the pectoralis minor muscle was similar in women between the ages of 26 and 80.

Many factors, however, have to be considered when comparing the results of different studies, including the biopsy technique, muscle group, physical activity, sex, and health. In this chapter, aimed at describing age-related changes in fiber type distribution in human skeletal muscle, an attempt was made to take all these factors into account.

Methods

Mean values and standard deviations (or standard errors) for the percentage of type I fibers (type I%) in m. quadriceps femoris vastus lateralis and for age were collected from 42 studies on 1,112 subjects without any known diseases. Studies on extremely well trained subjects or competitive athletes were not included. Most subjects had a low level of physical activity (no regular physical training) or a moderate level (1-4 h/wk in recreational sports). Biopsy specimens were taken by the Bergström needle technique in 33 studies, by an open surgical technique in 4 studies, and by a conchotome in 1 study. Autopsy specimens were taken in 4 studies.

To statistically evaluate the relationship between type I% and age, weighted means and pooled variances were calculated for different age groups. For younger subjects, sex and the level of physical activity were not always indicated in the selected studies. Therefore, weighted mean values were calculated for the age groups 0-0.8 mo and 1-4, 5-9, 10-14, and 15-19 yr without dividing the material into subgroups by sex and physical activity level. For the adult subjects, the following age groups were chosen for each sex and physical activity group (low or moderate): 20-29, 30-49, 50-69, and 70-89 yr. In addition, in a few studies sex and activity level were indicated for the ages of 10 and 16 yr, which made a separate calculation of means possible for each sex and activity group. The weighted means were compared using Student's t-test, and p values were corrected for multiple comparisons (29).

Results

Type I% in vastus lateralis as a function of age is presented in figures 23.1 and 23.2. There was a significant increase in type I% from the lowest age group of 0-0.8 mo to the age group 1-4 yr. Type I% in the age group 5-9 yr was of similar magnitude to that in the 1-4 yr group. Thereafter, type I% seemed to decrease and was significantly lower in the age groups 10-14 yr and 15-19 yr than in the age groups 1-4 and 5-9 yr. In the men with a low physical activity level, there was a significant decrease in type I% from the age of 16 to 20-29, with no further change from the age of 20-29 to 30-49. Thereafter, the type I% increased from the age of 50-69 to 70-89. A similar pattern was seen in the men with a moderate level of physical activity: Type I% decreased from the age of 16 to 20-29 and further to the age of 30-49. Thereafter, type I% at the ages of 50-69 and 70-89 was higher than the levels at the age of 20-29 and 30-49 yr.

No clear-cut relationship between the type I% and age could be demonstrated in the women, although there was a tendency for a pattern similar to that for the men. The women had a higher type I% than the men in the age group 20-29 yr. Both men and women with a moderate level of physical activity had a higher type I% than men and women with a low level of physical activity in the age groups 15-19 and 20-29 yr.

Discussion

Based on these results, it is suggested that the percentage of type I fibers in the vastus lateralis decreases in sedentary to moderately active men without any known diseases between the ages of 10 and 35 years and then increases. No clear age-related fiber type changes were observed in women. In most of the studies, the fiber type data were based on biopsy specimens obtained by a percutaneous needle biopsy

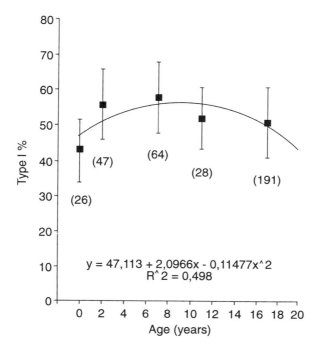

Figure 23.1 Fiber type distribution (type I%) in childhood and adolescence from 10 different studies (6, 18, 32, 35, 41-43, 49, 59, Dahlström et al., unpublished data) were pooled into five age groups (0-0.8 mo and 1-4, 5-9, 10-14, and 15-19 yr). Each point represents the weighted mean value in each age group and the standard deviation calculated from the pooled variances. The number of subjects in each age group is indicated in parentheses. Data were not grouped into males and females because information about the sex was not always available.

technique. In a few studies, open surgical biopsy specimens were taken or specimens were taken from autopsies: either small ones or whole vastus lateralis sections.

There are several theoretically possible explanations of the findings of altered fiber type distributions with age: (a) a systematic sampling error as a result of obtaining biopsy specimens from different depths by using different biopsy techniques, (b) fiber splitting or proliferation (new fibers from satellite cells), (c) motoneuron degeneration and death leading to denervation of muscle fibers followed by reinnervation by a neuron of another type or not followed by reinnervation due to loss of terminal sprouting, (d) transformation of one fiber type into another without motoneuron death (e.g, a fiber type transformation due to an altered impulse pattern in the neuron). In all probability, there are different explanations for different age ranges.

A number of studies have not been able to demonstrate any significant differences in fiber type distribution between biopsy specimens obtained from deep and from superficial portions of the vastus lateralis in humans (16, 17, 33, 44, 48). However, Lexell et al. (40), using whole vastus lateralis sections, showed

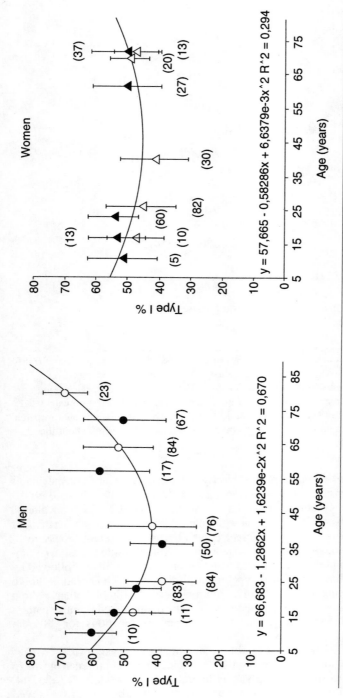

Figure 23.2 Fiber type distribution (type I%) in men and women from different studies (1-3, 8-14, 20-22, 24-27, 30, 34, 38, 39, 42, 45-47, 50, 52, 54-57, 60) were pooled into five age groups (15-19, 20-29, 30-49, 50-69, and 70-89 yr). Each point represents the weighted mean value in each age group and the standard deviation calculated from the pooled variances. The number of subjects in each age group is indicated in parentheses. Subjects with a low level of physical activity are indicated by open symbols and subjects with a moderate level of physical activity are indicated by filled symbols. For comparison, a few data from 10-year-old subjects were also included (Dahlström et al., unpublished data). Data from ref. 50 were recalculated from the relative type I fiber area to the relative number of type I fibers using a formula given in ref. 32.

a tendency to an increased percentage of type I fibers with increasing depth in the muscle. Thus, it cannot be completely ruled out that there may be a slight variation in fiber type distribution with the muscle depth. Thus, if there is a variation with the depth, biopsy specimens taken by the open surgical technique (samples are taken from the surface of the muscle) may give a lower percentage of type I fibers on average than needle biopsy specimens, which are usually taken from deeper portions of the muscle. Furthermore, theoretically, needle biopsy specimens obtained from a standardized depth in individuals with different muscle sizes may be sampled at different relative depths. First, however, on comparing data from two studies on children in which autopsy specimens were taken either from the surface of the muscle or from the center of the muscle belly, no differences could be seen in fiber type composition (49, 59). Second, considering only results from studies using the needle biopsy techniques, the same picture was obtained as shown in figure 23.2. Thus, the inclusion of some studies using biopsy techniques other than needle biopsy does not seem to have given rise to a systematic error. The precision of the depth from which the needle biopsy specimen is taken is very unlikely to be so high that any differences noted when comparing subjects with different muscle sizes could be due to a slight variation in fiber type distribution with depth, if any such variation exists at all.

The influence of such processes as fiber splitting and proliferation of satellite cells on the fiber type distribution is not known in any of the age groups studied. It could possibly occur to some extent in old age to counteract the reduced muscle mass. The increase in the percentage of type I fibers that was indicated in the very early age range (0-7 yr) could probably be explained by a transformation of fibers due to increased physical activity when learning to walk and run (49, 59).

In a second age range from approximately 10 to 35 yr, the percentage of type I fibers decreased in the men. Is this decrease in the percentage of type I fibers explained by a transformation of fibers due to a decreased level of physical activity? In a recent study by Glenmark (23), however, it was shown that a decrease in the percentage of type I fibers in the men between the ages of 16 and 27 occurred independently of the recorded change in the level of physical activity during leisure time. Therefore, some other possible explanations ought to be discussed. First, there is support from experiments both in the rat and in humans that testosterone may lower the percentage of type I fibers (36; Krotkiewski, personal communication). Second, the muscle mass in men seems to reach its highest value around the age of 30 yr (4, 41, 51), while the maximal oxygen uptake, a determining factor for walking and running intensity, reaches its maximum around the age of 20 yr (5). Therefore, in men there is a period in life between approximately 20 and 30 yr with decreasing maximal oxygen uptake and increasing muscle mass. This may result in a lower fraction of the muscle being activated at the age of 30 than at the age of 20 during running at the same relative intensity. Thus, the decrease in the percentage of type I fibers in men from childhood and adolescence to adulthood that seems to occur independently of the subject's level of physical activity may still be due to a reduced level of muscle fiber activation, as previously discussed.

The third age range that could be identified from the data covers the period between the ages of 40 and 80 yr. In that age range, the muscle mass starts to decline, and the maximal oxygen uptake continues to fall. The average reduction in muscle mass during this age range is approximately 40% (42). The relative fall in maximal oxygen uptake is of a magnitude similar to that of muscle mass (5). Therefore, during this third age range, there is probably no increased fractional activation of the leg muscles during walking and running due to changes in the relationship between muscle mass and maximal oxygen uptake. However, at the more advanced ages, the work load in relation to the maximal oxygen uptake may have to be increased to perform daily activities because of very low levels of maximal oxygen uptake (e.g., around 25 ml · kg^{-1} · min^{-1}). If this is the case, it will increase the relative activity of the muscle involved in physical activity, possibly leading to a transformation of type II into type I fibers. The importance of the relative load for fiber type changes was recently demonstrated by Esbjörnsson et al. (19) in a one-legged ischemic training model. In the age range between 40 and 80 yr, other mechanisms also probably help to explain the increased percentage of type I fibers. Endocrine hypofunction is known to develop during aging, and, in particular, the level of testosterone decreases (7, 58). A third possibility that may help to explain the increased percentage of type I fibers is the death of motoneurons, perhaps especially neurons that innervate type II fibers, and loss of terminal sprouting of the remaining neurons, leading to muscle fiber death of preferentially type II fibers (37, 42). However, nonselective neuron death might also result in an increased percentage of type I fibers, through a transformation of some of the remaining type II fibers into type I fibers.

The relative increase in type I fibers in old age, regardless of whether it is due to a selective muscle fiber death or some other mechanism, may be counteracted in a diseased state. This can be exemplified by comparing the muscle fiber composition data on healthy, sedentary to moderately active men with data from, for example, patients (50-81 yr old) with chronic obstructive lung disease who had on average only 29% type I fibers in the vastus lateralis (28). In fact, the patient with the most severe disease had only 10% type I fibers. This kind of patient is extremely sedentary, and that may partly explain the very low percentage of type I fibers. However, some other mechanisms are probably also operating, because a 10-d period with repeated hemodilutions increased the arterial oxygen pressure and also the percentage of type I fibers in these patients. This fiber type change probably was not related to an increased level of physical activity, as the patients were hospitalized during the observation period. Other diseases of old age such as hypertension and chronic heart failure seem also to be characterized by a decreased percentage of type I fibers (15, 31). All these diseases are systemic diseases accompanied by altered sympathoadrenergic activity, a factor that may also be involved in the determination of muscle fiber type composition (28).

Why the changes in fiber type distribution were more pronounced in men than in women is not known. It might be a methodological matter, because the number of women studied was smaller than that of men, especially in the age group 30-49 yr, for whom no results for women with a moderate level of physical activity were found in the literature. However, the lack of change in the percentage of type I fibers from adolescence to adulthood was supported by results from a longitudinal study between the ages of 16 and 27, referred to earlier in this paper (23, 24). This finding was significantly different from what was demonstrated for the men, in whom the percentage of type I fibers decreased from the age of 16 to 27. Even when the individual changes in leisure time physical activity levels were considered, there was still a significant sex-related difference in the response of the fiber types to increased age (23). Whether this sex-related difference is the result of divergent sex hormonal exposure, of differences in mechanical activation of the musculature, or of other factors is not clear. Speculation about muscle activation may be warranted, considering the fact that there is a sex difference in the time course for muscle growth during physical development: Men reach their peak muscle mass later (at about 30) than women (probably before 20). Thus, during the age range studied by Glenmark (23), the muscle mass may possibly be increasing in men while decreasing or remaining unchanged in women. Support for this view was evidenced by the sex difference in strength that increased markedly between the ages of 16 and 27 (23). Thus, if the sex difference in muscle mass is greater than the difference in maximal oxygen uptake at the age of 27, this may lead to a larger fraction of the muscle being activated in women than in men during running at the same relative intensity. This may result in a higher precentage of type I fibers in women than men through a transformation of type II into type I fibers.

The present comparisons among the results of different studies on subjects of different ages used a cross-sectional approach. The problem with a cross-sectional design is difficulty in selecting subjects who are similar in all respects except age. A special problem is that at the older ages, the "survivors" are studied, who are perhaps healthier and physically more active individuals than the average. Thus, it is not certain that the differences found among different age groups reflect individual changes. Only a few longitudinal studies on the present topic have been published. The longitudinal study mentioned earlier that followed subjects from the age of 16 to 27 showed that the percentage of type I fibers in the vastus lateralis decreased in the men but not in the women. Aniansson et al. (2) followed physicially active men from the age of 69 to 80 yr. No significant alteration in fiber type distribution was found. To the author's knowledge, there is no longitudinal study covering the age range between middle age and old age.

Conclusions

Assuming that the observed age group differences reflect individual changes over time, the following conclusions can be drawn. The increase in the percentage of type I fibers in vastus lateralis from the newborn state to childhood most likely represents an adaptation of the contractile characteristics to increased mechanical activity as the child learns to walk and run. The second phase that was identified, especially in the men, represents the period from childhood and adolescence to middle age, when a decrease in the percentage of type I fibers was found. This may also reflect, to some extent, an adaptation to an altered level of physical activity. However, as this change was more clear-cut in men than women, there might be a sex-related adaptation linked to sex hormone exposure and increased muscle mass in the men. The last phase that was identified from the data was the period from middle age to old age. It is known from other human studies (42) that a decrease in the number of muscle fibers occurs during this period, which may be an explanation of a change in fiber type distribution, on the assumping that a selective death of a certain fiber type occurs or else that the remaining fibers adapt to increased use because of a decreased muscle mass (both loss of fibers and decreased dimensions of the remaining fibers). Possibly, endocrine insufficiency in old age adds to a tranformation from type II to type I. The finding of a much lower percentage of type I fibers in some systemic diseases in old age such as cardiovascular or lung diseases indicates, however, that there is a potential for adaptive response of the muscle fibers to altered demands in old age also.

Acknowledgments

The author's research is supported by grants from the Swedish Medical Research Council (No. 4494) and the Swedish National Centre for Research in Sports. The author also wishes to thank Mrs. Elsie Rollvén for excellent secretarial support in preparing this manuscript.

References

1. Ama, P.F.; Simoneau, J.A.; Boulay, M.R.; Serresse, O.; Thériault, G.; Bouchard, C. Skeletal muscle characteristics in sedentary black and caucasian males. J. Appl. Physiol. 61(5):1758-1761; 1986.
2. Aniansson, A.; Grimby, G.; Hedberg, M. Compensatory muscle fiber hypertrophy in elderly men. J. Appl. Physiol. 73(3):812-816; 1992.
3. Aniansson, A.; Grimby, G.; Hedberg, M.; Krotkiewski, M. Muscle morphology, enzyme activity and muscle strength in elderly men and women. Clin. Physiol. 1:73-86; 1981.
4. Aoyagi, Y.; Shephard, R.J. Aging and muscle function. Sports Med. 14(6):376-396; 1992.
5. Åstrand, P.O.; Christensen, E.H. Aerobic work capacity. In: Dickens, F.; Neil, E.; Widdas, W.G., eds. Oxygen in the animal organism. New York: Pergamon Press; 1964; 295.
6. Bell, R.D.; MacDougall, J.D.; Billeter, R.; Howald, H. Muscle fiber types and morphometric analysis of skeletal muscle in six-year-old children. Med. Sci. Sports Exercise 12:28-31; 1980.
7. Björntorp, P. Endocrine insufficiency and nutrition in aging. Aging Clin. Exp. Res. 5 (suppl. 1):45-49; 1993.
8. Bouchard, C.; Simoneau, J.A.; Lortie, G.; Boulay, M.R.; Marcotte, M.; Thibault, M.C. Genetic effects in human skeletal muscle fiber type distribution and enzyme activities. Can. J. Physiol. Pharmacol. 64:1245-1251; 1986.
9. Bylund, A.-C.; Bjur, T.; Cederblad, G.; Holm, J.; Lundholm, K.; Sjöström, M.; Ängquist, K.A.; Scherstén, T. Physical training in man. Skeletal muscle metabolism in relation to muscle morphology and running ability. Eur. J. Appl. Physiol. 36:151-169; 1977.
10. Charette, S.L.; McEvoy, L.; Pyka, G.; Snow-Harter, C.; Guido, D.; Wiswell, R.A.; Marcus, R. Muscle hypertrophy response to resistance training in older women. J. Appl. Physiol. 70(5):1912-1916; 1991.
11. Cress, M.E.; Thomas, D.P.; Johnson, J.; Kasch, F.W.; Cassens, R.G.; Smith, E.L.; Agre, J.C. Effect of training on VO_2max, thigh strength, and muscle morphology in septuagenarian women. Med. Sci. Sports Exercise 23:752-758; 1991.
12. Danneskiold-Samsøe, B.; Grimby, G. The influence of prednisone on the muscle morphology and muscle enzymes in patients with rheumatoid arthritis. Clin. Sci. 71:693-701; 1986.
13. Denis, C.; Chatard, J.-C.; Dormois, D.; Linossier, M.-T.; Geyssant, A.; Lacour, J.-R. Effects of endurance training on capillary supply of human skeletal muscle on two age groups (20 and 60 years). J. Physiol. 81:379-383; 1986.

14. Doriguzzi, C.; Mongini, T.; Palmucci, L.; Gagnor, E.; Schiffer, D. Quantitative analysis of quadriceps muscle biopsy. Results in 30 healthy females. J. Neurol. Sci. 66:319-326; 1984.

15. Drexler, H.; Riede, U.; Münzel, T.; Knig, H.; Funke, E.; Just, H. Alterations of skeletal muscle in chronic heart failure. Circulation 85:1751-1759; 1992.

16. Edgerton, V.R.; Smith, J.I.; Simpson, D.R. Muscle fibre type populations of human leg muscles. Histochem. J. 7:259-266; 1975.

17. Elder, G.C.B.; Bradbury, K.; Roberts, R. Variability of fiber type distributions within human muscles. J. Appl. Physiol. 53:1473-1480; 1982.

18. Eriksson, B.O.; Friberg, L.-G.; Hanson, E.; Mellgren, G. Muscle substrate levels, muscle enzyme activities and muscle morphology in the vastus lateralis and deltoideus muscles in normal children and in children with coarctation of the aorta. Acta Paediatr. Scand. 72:843-847; 1983.

19. Esbjörnsson, M.; Jansson, E.; Sundberg, C.J.; Sylvén, C.; Eiken, O.; Nygren, A.; Kaijser, L. Muscle fibre types and enzyme activities after training with local leg ischaemia in man. Acta Physiol. Scand. 148:233-241; 1993.

20. Essén-Gustavsson, B.; Borges, O. Histochemical and metabolic characteristics of human skeletal muscle in relation to age. Acta Physiol. Scand. 126:107-114; 1986.

21. Froese, E.A.; Houston, M.E. Torque-velocity characteristics and muscle fiber type in human vastus lateralis. J. Appl. Physiol. 59(2):309-314; 1985.

22. Frontera, W.R.; Meredith, C.N.; O'Reilly, K.P.; Knuttgen, H.G.; Evans, W.J. Strength conditioning in older men: Skeletal muscle hypertrophy and improved function. J. Appl. Physiol. 64(3):1038-1044; 1988.

23. Glenmark, B. Skeletal muscle fiber types, physical performance, physical activity and attitude to physical activity in women and men. A follow-up from age 16 to 27. Acta Physiol. Scand. 151 (suppl. 623):1-47; 1994.

24. Glenmark, B.; Hedberg, G.; Jansson, E. Changes in muscle fibre type from adolescence to adulthood in women and men. Acta Physiol. Scand. 146:251-259; 1992.

25. Gollnick, P.D.; Armstrong, R.B.; Saubert, C.W.; Piehl, K.; Saltin, B. Enzyme activity and fiber composition in skeletal muscle of untrained and trained men. J. Appl. Physiol. 33:312-319; 1972.

26. Green, H.J.; Jones, S.; Ball-Burnett, M.E.; Smith, D.; Livesey, J.; Farrance, B.W. Early muscular and metabolic adaptations to prolonged exercise training in humans. J. Appl. Physiol. 70(5):2032-2038; 1991.

27. Hather, B.M.; Tesch, P.A.; Buchanan, P.; Dudley, G.A. Influence of eccentric actions on skeletal muscle adaptations to resistance training. Acta Physiol. Scand. 143:177-185; 1991.

28. Hildebrand, I.L.; Sylvén, C.; Esbjörnsson, M.; Hellström, K.; Jansson E. Does chronic hypoxaemia induce transformations of fiber types? Acta Physiol. Scand. 141:435-439; 1991.

29. Holm, S. A simple sequentially rejective multiple test procedure. Scand. J. Statist. 6:63-70; 1979.

30. Ingjer, F. Effects of endurance training on muscle fibre ATP-ase activity, capillary supply and mitochondrial content in man. J. Physiol. 294:419-432; 1979.

31. Isaksson, H.; Cederholm, T.; Jansson, E.; Nygren, A.; Östergren, J. Therapy-resistant hypertension associated with central obesity, insulin resistance, and large muscle fiber area. Blood Press. 2:46-52; 1993.

32. Jansson, E.; Hedberg, G. Skeletal muscle fiber types in teenagers: Relationship to physical performance and activity. Scand. J. Med. Sci. Sports 1:31-44; 1991.

33. Johnson, M.A.; Polgar, J.; Weightman, D.; Appleton, D. Data on the distribution of fibre types in thirty-six human muscles—An autopsy study. J. Neurol. Sci. 18:111-129; 1973.

34. Klausen, K.; Andersen, L.B.; Pelle, I. Adaptive changes in work capacity, skeletal muscle capillarization and enzyme levels during training and detraining. Acta Physiol. Scand. 113:9-16; 1981.

35. Komi, P.V.; Karlsson, J. Skeletal muscle fibre types, enzyme activities and physical performance in young males and females. Acta Physiol. Scand. 103:210-218; 1978.

36. Krotkiewski, M.; Kral, J.G.; Karlsson, J. Effects of castration and testosterone substitution on body composition and muscle metabolism in rats. Acta Physiol. Scand. 109:233-237; 1980.

37. Larsson, L. Aging in mammalian skeletal muscles. In: Mortimer, J.A.; Pirozzolo, F.J.; Maletta, G.J., eds. The aging motor system. New York: Praeger; 1982:60-97. (Adv. Neurogerontol.; vol 3).

38. Larsson, L.; Örlander, J. Skeletal muscle morphology, metabolism and function in smokers and non-smokers. A study on smoking-discordant monozygous twins. Acta Physiol. Scand. 120:343-352; 1984.

39. Larsson, L.; Sjödin, B.; Karlsson, J. Histochemical and biochemical changes in human skeletal muscle with age in sedentary males, age 22-65 years. Acta Physiol. Scand. 103:31-39; 1978.

40. Lexell, J.; Henriksson-Larsén, K.; Winblad, B.; Sjöström, M. Distribution of different fiber types in human skeletal muscles: Effects of aging studied in whole muscle cross-sections. Muscle Nerve 6:588-595; 1983.

41. Lexell, J.; Sjöström, M.; Nordlund, A.-S.; Taylor, C.C. Growth and development of human muscle: A quantitative morphological study of whole vastus lateralis from childhood to adult age. Muscle Nerve 15:404-409; 1992.

42. Lexell, J.; Taylor, C.C.; Sjöström, M. What is the cause of the ageing atrophy? Total number, size and proportion of different fiber types studied in whole vastus lateralis muscle from 15- to 83-year-old men. J. Neurol. Sci. 84:275-294; 1988.

43. Lundberg, A.; Eriksson, B.O.; Mellgren, G. Metabolic substrates, muscle fibre composition and fibre size in late walking and normal children. Eur. J. Pediatr. 130:79-92; 1979.

44. Mahon, M.; Toman, A.; Willan, P.L.; Bagnall, K.M. Variability of histochemical and morphometric data from needle biopsy specimens of human quadriceps femoris muscle. J. Neurol. Sci. 63:85-100; 1984.

45. Maughan, R.J.; Nimmo, M.A.; Harmon, M. The relationship between muscle myosin ATP-ase activity and isometric endurance in untrained male subjects. Eur. J. Appl. Physiol. 54:291-296; 1985.

46. Miller, A.E.; MacDougall, J.D.; Tarnopolsky, M.A.; Sale, D.G. Gender differences in strength and muscle fiber characteristics. Eur. J. Appl. Physiol. 66:254-262; 1993.

47. Nygaard, E. Skeletal muscle fiber characteristics in young women. Acta Physiol. Scand. 112:299-304; 1981.

48. Nygaard, E.; Sanchez, I. Intramuscular variation of fibre types in the brachial biceps and the lateral vastus muscles of elderly men. How representative is a small biopsy sample? Anat. Rec. 203:541-549; 1982.

49. Oertel, G. Morphometric analysis of normal skeletal muscles in infancy, childhood and adolescence. An autopsy study. J. Neurol. Sci. 88:303-313; 1988.

50. Poggi, P.; Marchetti, C.; Scelsi, R. Automatic morphometric analysis of skeletal muscle fibers in the aging man. Anat. Rec. 217:30-34; 1987.

51. Rogers, M.A.; Evans, W.J. Changes in skeletal muscle with aging: Effects of exercise training. Exercise Sports Sci. Rev. 21:65-102; 1993.

52. Saltin, B.; Nazar, K.; Costill, D.L.; Stein, E.; Jansson, E.; Essén, B.; Gollnick, P.D. The nature of the training response: Peripheral and central adaptations to one-legged exercise. Acta Physiol. Scand. 96:289-305; 1976.

53. Sato, T.; Akatsuka, H.; Kito, K.; Tokoro, Y.; Tauchi, H.; Kato, K. Age changes in size and number of muscle fibers in human minor pectoral muscle. Mech. Ageing Develop. 28:99-109; 1984.

54. Simoneau, J.A.; Lortie, G.; Boulay, M.R.; Thibault, M.-C.; Thériault, G.; Bouchard, C. Skeletal muscle histochemical and biochemical characteristics in sedentary male and female subjects. Can. J. Physiol. Pharmacol. 63:30-35; 1985.

55. Staron, R.S.; Hikida, R.S.; Hagerman, F.C.; Dudley, G.A.; Murray, T.F. Human skeletal muscle fiber type adaptability to various workloads. J. Histochem. Cytochem. 32:146-152; 1984.

56. Suominen, H.; Heikkinen, E.; Parkatti, T. Effect of eight weeks' physical training on muscle and connective tissue of the m. vastus lateralis in 69-year-old men and women. J. Gerontol. 32:33-37; 1977.

57. Svedenhag, J.; Henriksson, J.; Juhlin-Dannfelt, A. β-Adrenergic blockade and training in human subjects: Effects on muscle metabolic capacity. Am. J. Physiol. 247:E305-E311; 1984.

58. Swerdloff, R.; Wang, C. Androgenes and aging in men. Exp. Gerontol. 28:435-446; 1993.

59. Vogler, C.; Bove, K.E. Morphology of skeletal muscle in children. Arch. Pathol. Lab. Med. 109:238-242; 1985.

60. Wretling, M.L.; Gerdle, B.; Henriksson-Larsén, K. EMG: A non-invasive method for determination of fibre type proportion. Acta Physiol. Scand. 131:627-628; 1987.

CHAPTER 24

Programmed Cell Death and Aging: The Role of Mitochondria

Claudio Franceschi, Daniela Monti, Stefano Salvioli, Galina Kalachnikova, Daniela Barbieri, Paolo Salomoni, Emanuela Grassilli, Leonarda Troiano, Franco Tropea, Andrea Cossarizza
University of Modena School of Medicine, Modena, Italy

Aging and Longevity: A Unified Theory

Physiological aging is still a poorly understood phenomenon, and very little is known about environmental factors and genes that control aging. The problem is even more complicated if we consider longevity. Usually, hypotheses of aging do not account for longevity differences between species and between individuals within a species.

The theories proposed to explain the aging process may be schematically grouped in two main categories. The first suggests that aging is indirectly controlled by genes that have been selected for reproductive fitness before maturity. Such genes could exert pleiotropic undesirable effects later in life. Evidence favoring this hypothesis comes from studies in *Drosophila,* where selection for late fecundity increases life-span (25). The second type of theories proposes that aging is the consequence of a stochastic process of deterioration caused by the accumulation of unavoidable errors in the synthesis and processing of macromolecules, that is, DNA, RNA, and proteins. Probably the most elaborate theories of this kind are the somatic mutation theory of aging and the error hypothesis of aging (14, 25). At the DNA level, the aging process appears to be the result of a balance between mechanisms that tend to destabilize DNA information, and mechanisms that tend to maintain and preserve DNA integrity (11).

We recently proposed a unified hypothesis that will be summarized as follows. Cells continuously exposed to exogenous and endogenous stressors, such as heat, radiation, reducing sugars, and oxygen free radicals (OFRs), have developed a variety of defense and repair mechanisms, such as DNA repair mechanisms, antioxidant defense systems, and production of stress proteins. These mechanisms are interconnected and constitute a network of integrated cellular defense systems that must be considered all together, and not one by one (10).

In fact, when cells are exposed to a potential genotoxic agent such as OFRs, all the aforementioned defense mechanisms are triggered (10). The final result, that is, cell survival with or without heavy DNA damage or cell death, will depend on the coordinated capability of the network to cope with the attrition caused by the damaging agent.

Our hypothesis is that longevity determinant genes proposed by Cutler (9) are in fact the genes responsible for the aforementioned network of defense mechanisms and that the global level of efficiency of this network is genetically controlled. We assume that the efficiency of such genes has been evolutionarily set at different levels in different species, thus accounting for the different life-spans among them. We also assume that interindividual differences in life-span within a species depend on the different efficiencies of the network (13).

These considerations are particularly important for understanding the role of the immune and the neuroendocrine systems in maintaining the homeostasis and the integrity of the body. These systems, which are profoundly interconnected and probably share a common evolutionary origin, are composed of a variety of cells continuously exposed to damaging agents and could be severely impaired if a derangement occurs in their repair and defense mechanisms. Thus, we assume that the correct function of the network of defense mechanisms is essential for the performances of the immunoneuroendocrine system.

Age-related attrition of the network of defense mechanisms could alter the balance between DNA stability and instability, favoring the accumulation of mutations and rearrangements with time (11). Disastrous consequences can be predicted if different cells of the same organ or lineage accumulate different types of DNA lesions; cell heterogeneity is increased, and cell-cell interactions altered. These are particularly important in the immune and in the nervous systems.

We also assume that the network of cellular defense mechanisms that counteract the aging process and favor longevity is fundamentally the same as that which offsets the development of cancer, as its main purpose is to maintain the integrity of genetic information in somatic cells and eliminate damaged or mutated cells (20).

Mitochondria, Oxygen Free Radicals, and Aging

More than 30 years ago, D. Harman proposed the free radicals theory of aging. According to this theory, a major role has to be ascribed to reactive oxygen species in aging and senescence. Pros and cons of this theory have been reviewed (1). OFRs appear to play a crucial role, because they are continuously produced during normal metabolism. An inverse relationship between OFR-induced DNA damage and life-span has been observed in mammals. Moreover, antioxidant systems have been proposed as one of the most important longevity determinant mechanisms (8). It is usually taken for granted that oxidative stress increases with age and that the efficiency of antioxidant mechanisms declines with age. However, the data available are scant and contradictory, particularly as far as humans are concerned. The situation is probably much more complex. A balance between OFR production and processing is continuously taking place, and the age-related derangement may be the consequence of different factors. Moreover, we still do not know which is the most important type of damage(s) and the critical cellular target(s) of OFRs. A possible relevant target is mitochondrial DNA (mtDNA), and a mitochondrial theory of aging has been proposed (27). Mitochondria contain 2 to 10 copies of a small, double-stranded, circular DNA molecule of 16,659 base pairs (bp). The mitochondrial genome contributes about 1% of total cellular DNA and encodes 2 ribosomal RNAs, 22 transfer RNAs, and 13 of the 67 subunits of the mitochondrial respiratory chain and oxidative phosphorylation system. Thus, the mammalian mtDNA genome is very small and contains no introns, being one of the most tightly packed genomes in the biosphere. Mitochondria generate high levels of OFRs, and 2% of all oxygen used by mammalian cells does not form water but oxygen-activated species. In rats, a 15-fold increase of 8-hydroxy-2'-deoxy-guanosine (8-OH-dG), a hydroxyl-radical adduct of deoxyguanosine, in mtDNA compared with nuclear DNA has been demonstrated (24). In human heart mtDNA, the 8-OH-dG content increases exponentially with age up to 1.5% at age 97, with a clear correlation of the population of mtDNA with deletion (12). Damage to mitochondria and mtDNA during aging has been documented in several eukaryotes, including fungi, flies, mice, rats, and humans. The most studied damage has been the so-called common deletion, that is, a deletion of 4,977 bp found most frequently in Kearns-Sayre syndrome and in progressive external ophthalmoplegia. In muscle, this type of deletion accumulates by a factor of 10,000 over the course of the normal human life-span, reaching a level of approximately 0.1% to 1% of total muscle mtDNA in people over 80 yr of age (4, 22). Numerous other deletions and point mutations, as well as bases modified through oxidation, may accumulate with age in mtDNA, and thus the total number of deleted mtDNA may be significantly higher and may reach levels that could be important physiologically in contributing to a decline in mitochondrial function in normal human aging. All these observations only establish a correlation between mtDNA deletions and aging, and cannot be used to establish any kind of cause-and-effect relationship, which awaits further investigation (3). The central idea is that random mutations occurring throughout life in the population of mtDNA molecules in each cell are a major contributor to the gradual loss of cellular bioenergetic capacity within tissues and organs associated with senescence and diseases of aging. However, a direct correlation between mammalian mtDNA mutations and bioenergetic decline is yet to be definitely established (15).

Apoptosis and Aging

An integral part of our hypothesis is that an age-related derangement of the efficiency of the network may disturb the subtle and critical equilibrium between cell proliferation and cell death that appears to be present in most cells. In recent papers, we argued that an intriguing relationship exists among cellular senescence, tumor growth, and longevity and that all these phenomena are deeply related to programmed cell death, or apoptosis (20, 21). A possible scenario is the following: Cells may be equipped with genes that actively promote cellular senescence, thus controlling cell death in order to escape transformation. This situation is balanced by other genes responsible for survival and viability. Circumstantial evidence suggests that cellular senescence may be considered a peculiar type of cell differentiation whose biological function is to counteract uncontrolled cell proliferation. From this point of view, cellular senescence can be considered one of the most important mechanisms in avoiding the continuous onset of tumors. The most effective way for a cell to control neoplastic growth is to set up genes that promote apoptotic cell death. The data available in the literature point out that apoptosis is indeed a process devoted to the elimination (without inflammation) of damaged or virus-infected cells. Thus, a major role of this phenomenon can be envisaged in the aging process, when changes or alterations of cell proliferation and cell loss occur and when damaged cells can accumulate.

The energy-producing machinery of the cell is probably critical not only for cell proliferation, but also for cell death. Mitochondrial function and poly(ADP-ribose) polymerase are likely to play an important role in these phenomena (17-19, 21).

Apoptosis and Mitochondria

One of the major problems we are facing in research on mitochondrial function is that these organelles must be isolated from organs, tissues, or cell cultures. A relatively large amount of biological material is therefore necessary, and selection can occur during the procedure for the isolation and purification of the organelles. This has hampered the analysis of mitochondrial function in several biological conditions, including apoptosis. The biochemical and molecular mechanisms that mediate apoptosis are poorly understood. However, there is a general agreement that apoptosis is an active process requiring energy. Indeed, this assumption is mainly based on morphological evidence showing well-preserved mitochondria in cells undergoing apoptosis analyzed by electron microscopy. Further evidence has been hampered by the lack of reliable tests to measure mitochondrial function in single, intact cells. We recently described a new cytofluorometric method that allows the analysis of mitochondrial membrane potential in intact cells by using the lipophilic cation 5,5',6,6'-tetrachloro-1,1',3,3'-tetraethylbenzimidazol-carbocyanine iodide (JC-1) (5). This molecule, able to selectively enter into mitochondria (23), exists in a monomeric form emitting at 527 nm after excitation at 490 nm. However, depending on the membrane potential, JC-1 is able to form J-aggregates that are associated with a large shift in emission (590 nm). Thus, the color of the dye changes reversibly from green to greenish orange as the mitochondrial membrane becomes more polarized (26). Both colors can be detected using the filters commonly mounted in flow cytometers, so that the green emission can be analyzed in fluorescence channel 1 (FL1) and the greenish orange emission in channel 2 (FL2).

Using this method, we demonstrated that the incubation of human cells such as U937 cell line with valinomycin, a K^+ ionophore, decreases the mitochondrial membrane potential (MMP) in a dose-dependent manner (figure 24.1). A separate analysis of the fluorescence pattern in FL1 and FL2 is shown in figure 24.2. The method is sensitive enough to appreciate changes in MMP occurring after 1-h

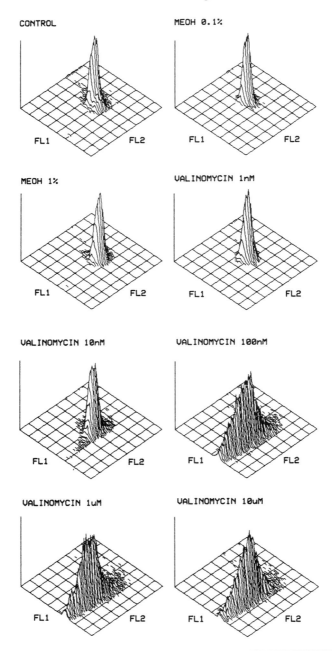

Figure 24.1   Cytofluorometric analysis of U937 cells stained with JC-1 and treated with different doses of valinomycin (1 nM to 10 µM), dissolved in methanol (MEOH 0.1% or 1%, vol/vol). FL1 indicates green fluorescence (log. scale), FL2 orange fluorescence (log. scale). The changes of the fluorescence emission (decrease in FL2 and increase in FL1) indicate the modifications of mitochondrial membrane potential.

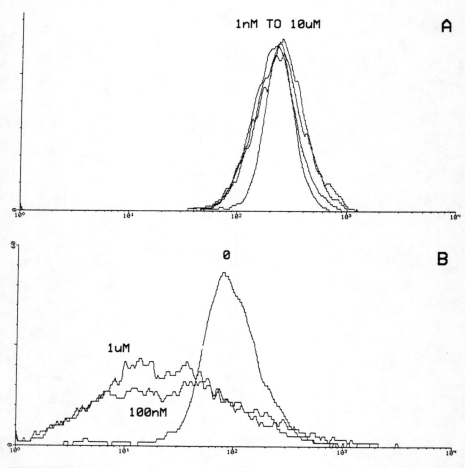

Figure 24.2 Separate analysis of JC-1 fluorescence emissions (A, FL1; B, FL2) in K562 cells treated with valinomycin (100 nM or 1 μM). Abscissa indicates fluorescence intensity, ordinate relative cell number.

exposure of human monocytes to an OFR-producing system formed by xanthine oxidase plus hypoxanthine (figure 24.3). A similar observation has been found with U937 cells exposed for 1 h to hydrogen peroxide (figure 24.4). The staining with JC-1 has also been performed in isolated mitochondria treated with a variety of depolarizing agents (valinomycin, FCCP, and ADP, among others) analyzed by flow cytometry. The data obtained show that a direct correlation exists between the variations of membrane potential detected biochemically or flow cytometrically (6).

Thus, the method is sensitive enough to show evidence of mitochondrial damage of different kinds. We asked whether mitochondrial alterations took place in apoptotic cells (7). First, we used a classical model of apoptosis, that is, rat thymocytes treated with glucocorticoids or heat shocked. The results showed that marked alterations of MMP are evident in apoptotic cells (figure 24.5, p. 317). Because one of

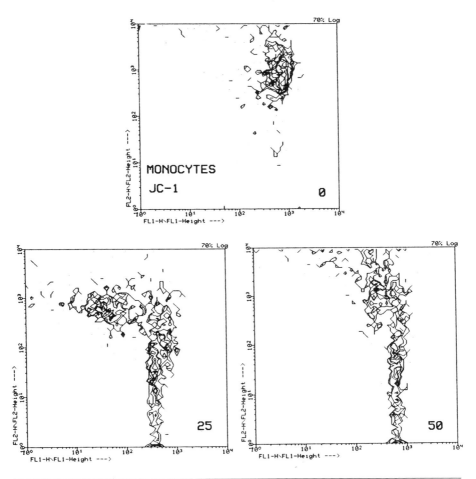

Figure 24.3   Modifications of mitochondrial membrane potential in human monocytes stained with JC-1 after a 1-h exposure at 37° C to an oxygen free radical–producing system constituted by xanthine oxidase (0.5 U/ml) plus hypoxanthine (0-50 μM).

the major hallmarks of apoptosis is DNA fragmentation, we tested whether MMP alteration preceded or followed DNA fragmentation. As shown in figures 24.6 through 24.9 (pp. 318, 319-321), DNA fragmentation, assessed by gel electrophoresis and evidenced by cytofluorometric analysis of propidium iodide–binding to DNA, preceded MMP alterations as well as alterations of mitochondrial mass, assessed by nonyl-acridine orange (16). The general interpretation of this is that the decreases of mitochondrial membrane potential and mass are not the first events that can be detected during thymocyte apoptosis. Consequently, apoptotic cells would require the functional integrity of this organelle to begin or continue the cell death program. MMP alterations would follow as an integral part of the apoptotic program.

Finally, we asked whether apoptosis is an age-dependent phenomenon and whether mitochondria play a role in it. First, we set up a method to induce

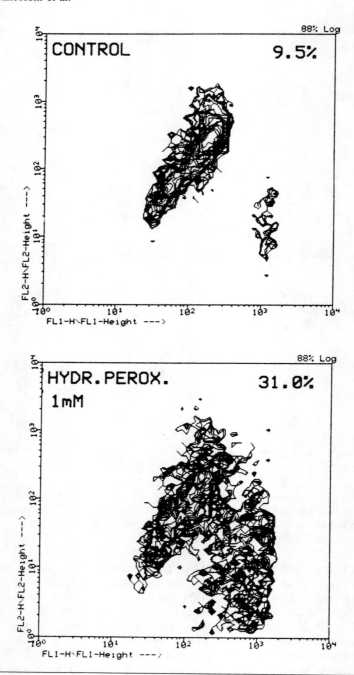

Figure 24.4 Modifications of mitochondrial membrane potential in U937 cell line after a 1-h exposure at 37° C to hydrogen peroxide (1 mM). Numbers indicate the percentage of cells with depolarized mitochondria.

RAT THYMOCYTES

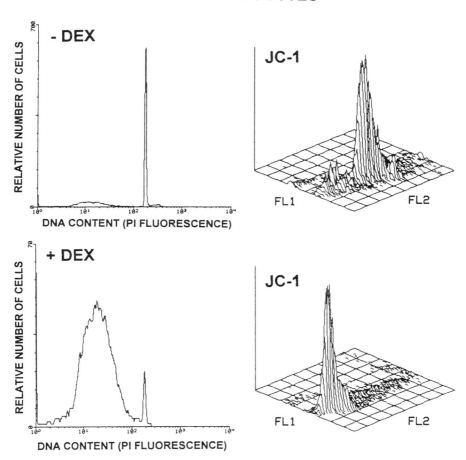

Figure 24.5 Cytofluorometric analysis of rat thymocytes after a 24-h incubation with dexamethasone (DEX, 10 μM). Graphs on left indicate the DNA content of apoptotic cells: Apoptosis is well evidenced by the presence of a marked hypodiploid peak (*lower left panel*). Graphs on right indicate the modifications of mitochondrial membrane potential analyzed by the probe JC-1. Data are from cells kept for 24 h without (*upper right panel*) or with DEX (*lower right panel*). Apoptotic cells show a clear alteration of mitochondrial membrane potential.

apoptosis in resting human peripheral blood mononuclear cells (HPBMC), which are relatively resistant to the induction of apoptosis. Figure 24.10 (p. 322) shows that two sugars, D-ribose and deoxy-D-ribose, are capable of inducing apoptosis in HPBMC (2). Moreover, we showed that this type of apoptosis is completely inhibited by *N*-acetyl-cysteine, suggesting that deoxy-D-ribose induces apoptosis by interfering with glutathione metabolism and perhaps by inducing an oxidative

TIME (hrs)

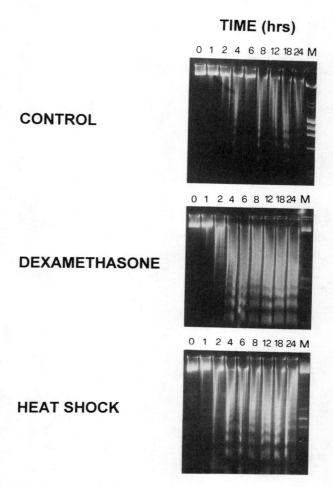

Figure 24.6   Agarose gel electrophoresis of DNA from rat thymocytes treated for 24 h with DEX (10 μM) or heat shocked (20 min at 43° C). Numbers over the lanes indicate the hours of culture. M = marker DNA (Lambda DNA-Hind III/fX-174 DNA-Hae III Digest, Pharmacia). DNA fragmentation is well evident at the fourth hour of culture.

stress (figure 24.11, p. 323). Using deoxy-D-ribose as the apoptotic agent and JC-1 to assess MMP, we tested the sensitivity of HPBMC from subjects of different ages. As shown in figure 24.12, p. 324, it is evident that an inverse correlation exists between donor age and sensitivity to deoxy-D-ribose–induced apoptosis. Moreover, mitochondria from elderly subjects, including centenarians (data not shown), appear to be more resistant than those from young subjects.

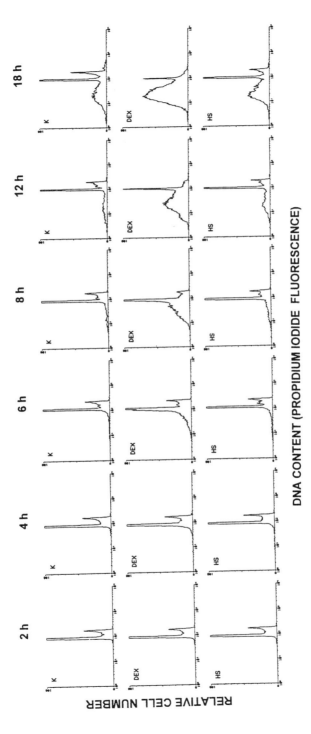

Figure 24.7 Cytofluorometric analysis of DNA content in rat thymocytes treated for 18 h with DEX (10 μM) or heat shocked (20 min at 43° C), as assessed by staining with propidium iodide. The presence of a hypodiploid population is evident starting from the sixth hour of culture. K = control; DEX = dexamethasone treated; HS = heat shocked.

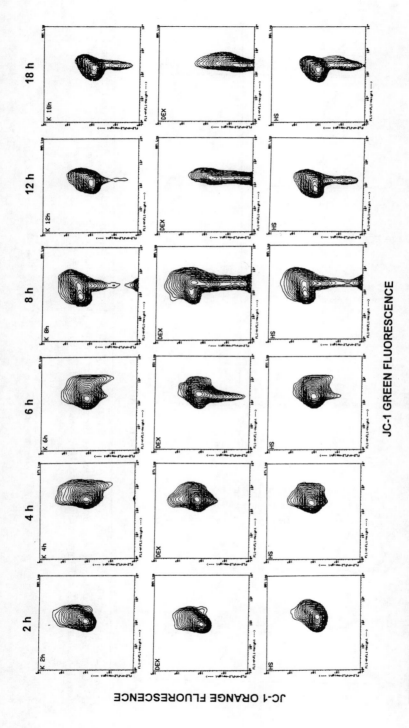

JC-1 GREEN FLUORESCENCE

Figure 24.8 Cytofluorometric analysis of mitochondrial membrane potential in rat thymocytes treated for 18 h with DEX (10 μM) or heat shocked (20 min at 43° C), as assessed by staining with JC-1. The first modifications of mitochondrial membrane potential are evident after 6 h of culture. K = control; DEX = dexamethasone treated; HS = heat shocked.

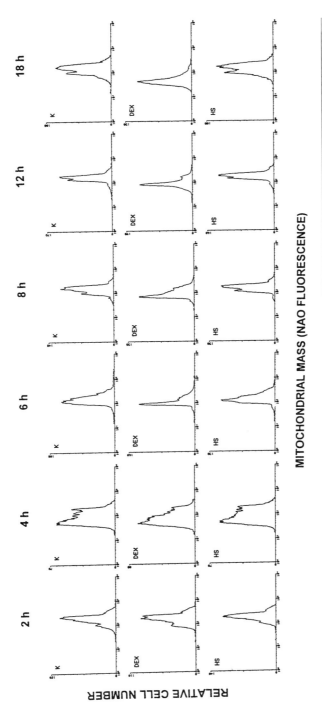

Figure 24.9 Cytofluorometric analysis of mitochondrial mass in rat thymocytes treated for 18 h with DEX or heat shocked (20 min at 43° C), as assessed by staining with nonyl-acridine orange (NAO). The first modifications of mitochondrial mass are evident after 8 h of culture. K = control; DEX = dexamethasone treated; HS = heat shocked.

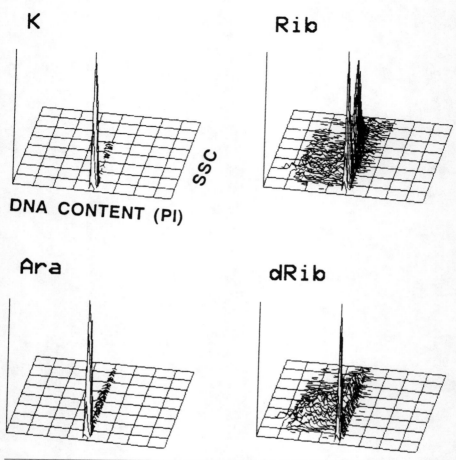

Figure 24.10 D-ribose (Rib) and deoxy-D-ribose (dRib), but not arabinose (Ara), are capable of inducing apoptosis in human peripheral blood mononuclear cells. Data represent the cytofluorometric analysis of DNA content and side scatter (SSC). The presence of nuclei with a hypodiploid DNA content is well evident in both of the right panels. K = control cells.

Conclusions

The data presented here suggest that:

1. MMP can be reliably assessed in intact HPBMC using flow cytometry and JC-1 as a probe;
2. apoptosis induces MMP alterations in cells undergoing apoptosis following treatment with a variety of apoptotic agents (glucocorticoids, heat shock);
3. deoxy-D-ribose is able to induce apoptosis in resting HPBMC and this phenomenon is inversely correlated to donor age; and

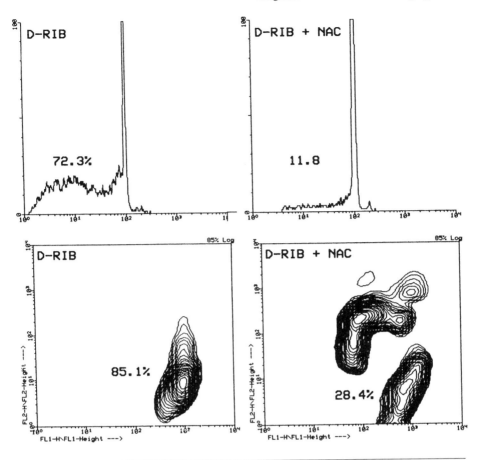

Figure 24.11 Upper panels show that *N*-acetyl-cysteine (NAC) completely inhibits apoptosis induced by deoxy-D-ribose (D-RIB), and lower panels indicate that NAC also preserves mitochondrial membrane potential. Numbers indicate the percentage of apoptotic cells (*upper panels*) or of cells with depolarized mitochondria (*lower panels*).

4. mitochondria from aged subjects, including centenarians, appear to be more resistant than organelles from young subjects during apoptosis induced by deoxy-D-ribose.

The relevance of these phenomena for the physiopathology of the aging process and of age-related diseases such as cancer, autoimmune diseases, and dementia of Alzheimer type deserves further investigation. In particular, the age-related increase in the resistance to the induction of apoptosis is an intriguing phenomenon. Indeed, it might favor the rescue of damaged cells, but it could also avoid cell loss in organs and tissues. This balance is probably the price humans have to pay for the maintenance of soma for more than 100 years.

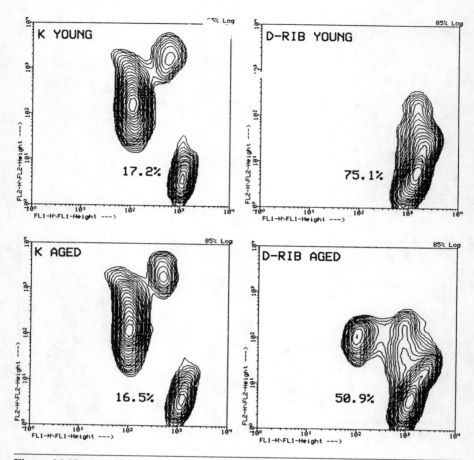

Figure 24.12 Peripheral blood mononuclear cells from subjects of different ages show a different sensitivity to deoxy-D-ribose (D-RIB). Data indicate the percentage of cells with depolarized mitochondria in control (K) or D-RIB-treated cells from a young (*upper panels*) or an aged donor (*lower panels*).

Acknowledgments

The authors gratefully acknowledge C.N.R. (PF ''Invecchiamento'') and AIRC (Associazione Italiana per la Ricerca sul Cancro), which supported the research whose results are reported in this review. Drs. Daniela Barbieri and Paolo Salomoni are recipients of an AIRC fellowship.

References

1. Balin, A.K. Testing the free radicals theory of aging. In: Adelman, R.C.; Roth, G.S., eds. Testing the theories of aging. Boca Raton, FL: CRC Press; 1982:137-182.

2. Barbieri, D.; Grassilli, E.; Monti, D.; Salvioli, S.; Franceschini, M.G.; Franchini, A.; Bellesia, E.; Salomoni, P.; Negro, P.; Capri, M.; Troiano, L.; Cossarizza, A.; Franceschi, C. D-ribose and deoxy-D-ribose induce apoptosis in human quiescent peripheral blood mononuclear cells. Biochem. Biophys. Res. Commun. 201:1109-1116; 1994.

3. Chen, X.; Simonetti, S.; Di Mauro, S.; Schon, E.A. Accumulation of mitochondrial DNA deletions in organisms with various lifespans. Bull. Mol. Biol. Med. 18:57-66; 1993.

4. Cortopassi, G.A.; Arnheim, N. Detection of a specific mitochondrial DNA deletion in tissues of older humans. Nucleic Acids Res. 18:6927-6933; 1990.

5. Cossarizza, A.; Baccarani Contri, M.; Kalashnikova, G.; Franceschi, C. A new method for the cytofluorimetric analysis of mitochondrial membrane potential using the J-aggregate forming lipophilic cation 5,5',6,6'-tetrachloro-1,1',3,3'-tetraethylbenzimidazolcarbocyanine iodide (JC-1). Biochem. Biophys. Res. Commun. 197:40-45; 1993.

6. Cossarizza, A.; Ceccarelli, D.; Masini, A. Functional heterogeneity of isolated mitochondrial population revealed by cytofluorimetric analysis at the single organelle level. Exp. Cell Res. 222:84-94; 1996.

7. Cossarizza, A.; Kalashnikova, G.; Grassilli, E.; Chiappelli, F.; Salvioli, S.; Capri, M.; Barbieri, D.; Troiano, L.; Monti, D.; Franceschi, C. Mitochondrial modifications during rat thymocyte apoptosis: A study at the single cell level. Exp. Cell Res. 214:323-330; 1994.

8. Cutler, R.G. Antioxidants and aging. Am. J. Clin. Nutr. 53:373S-379S; 1991.

9. Cutler, R.G. Longevity is determined by specific genes. In: Adelman, R.C.; Roth, G.S., eds. Testing the theories of aging. Boca Raton, FL: CRC Press; 1982:25-114.

10. Franceschi, C. Cell proliferation, cell death and aging. Aging Clin. Exp. Res. 1:1-13; 1989.

11. Franceschi, C. Genomic instability: A challenge for aging research. (Editorial). Aging Clin. Exp. Res. 2:101-104; 1990.

12. Hayakawa, M.; Hattori, K.; Sugiyama, S.; Ozawa, T. Age-associated oxygen damage and mutation in mitochondrial DNA in human hearts. Biochem. Biophys. Res. Commun. 189:979-985; 1992.

13. Kirkwood, T.B.L.; Franceschi, C. Is ageing as complex as it would appear? New perspectives in gerontological research. Ann. N.Y. Acad. Sci. 663:412-417; 1992.

14. Kirkwood, T.B.L.; Rose, M.R. Evolution of senescence: Late survival sacrificed for reproduction. Philosoph. Trans. Royal Soc. London, B., 332:15-24; 1991.

15. Linnane, A.W. Mitochondria and aging: The universality of bioenergetic disease. Aging Clin. Exp. Res. 4:267-271; 1992.

16. Maftah, A.; Petit, J.M.; Ratinaud, M.H.; Julien, R. 10-N nonyl-acridine orange: A fluorescent probe which stains mitochondria independently of their energetic state. Biochem. Biophys. Res. Commun. 164:185-190; 1989.

17. Malorni, W.; Rainaldi, G.; Straface, E.; Rivabene, R.; Cossarizza, A.; Salvioli, S.; Monti, D.; Franceschi, C. Cell death protection by 3-aminobenzamide: Impairment of cytoskeleton function in human NK cell-mediated killing. Biochem. Biophys. Res. Commun. 199:1250-1255; 1994.

18. Marini, M.; Zunica, G.; Tamba, M.; Cossarizza, A.; Monti, D.; Franceschi, C. Recovery of human lymphocytes damaged with gamma radiation or enzymatically-produced oxygen radicals: Different effects of poly(ADP-rybosil) transferase inhibitors. Int. J. Radiat. Biol. 58:279-291; 1990.

19. Monti, D.; Cossarizza, A.; Salvioli, S.; Franceschi, C.; Rainaldi, G.; Straface, E.; Rivabene, R.; Malorni, W. Cell death protection by 3-aminobenzamide and other poly(ADP-ribose)polymerase inhibitors: Different effects on human natural killer and lymphokine activated killer cell activities. Biochem. Biophys. Res. Commun. 199:525-530; 1994.

20. Monti, D.; Troiano, L.; Grassilli, E.; Agnesini, C.; Tropea, F.; Capri, M.; Ronchetti, I.; Bellomo, G.; Cossarizza, A.; Franceschi, C. Cell proliferation and cell death in immunosenescence. Ann. N.Y. Acad. Sci. 663:250-261; 1992.

21. Monti, D.; Troiano, L.; Tropea, F.; Grassilli, E.; Cossarizza, A.; Barozzi, D.; Pelloni, M.C.; Tamassia, M.G.; Franceschi, C. Apoptosis—Programmed cell death: A role in the aging process? Am. J. Clin. Nutr. 55:1208S-1214S; 1992.

22. Ozawa, T.; Tanaka, M.; Ikebe, S.; Ohno, K.; Kondo, T.; Mizuno, Y. Quantitative determination of deleted mitochondrial DNA relative to normal DNA in parkinsonian striatum by a kinetic PCR analysis. Biochem. Biophys. Res. Commun. 172:483-489; 1990.

23. Reers, M.; Smith, T.W.; Chen, L.B. J-aggregate formation of a carbocyanine as a quantitative fluorescent indicator of membrane potential. Biochemistry 30:4480-4486; 1991.

24. Richter, C.; Park, J.W.; Ames, B.N. Normal oxidative damage to mitochondrial and nuclear DNA is extensive. Proc. Natl. Acad. Sci. USA 85:6465-6467; 1988.

25. Rose, M.R. Evolutionary biology of aging. Oxford: Oxford University Press; 1991.

26. Smiley, S.T.; Reers, M.; Mottola-Hartshorn, C.; Lin, M.; Chen, A.; Smith, T.W.; Steele, G.D.; Chen, L.B. Intracellular heterogeneity in mitochondrial membrane potentials revealed by a J-aggregate-forming lipophilic cation JC-1. Proc. Natl. Acad. Sci. USA 88:3671-3675; 1991.

27. Viña, J.; Sastre, J.; Pallardò, F.V.; Plà, R.; Estrela, J.M.; Miquel, J. The mitochondrial theory of aging: Recent developments. Bull. Mol. Biol. Med. 18:81-87; 1993.

PART VII

Muscle Adaptation to Endurance Training

CHAPTER 25

Muscle Adaptation to Endurance Training: Impact on Fuel Selection During Exercise

Jan Henriksson
Department of Physiology and Pharmacology, The Karolinska Institute, Stockholm, Sweden

Skeletal muscle cells possess a quite remarkable capacity for adaptation to changes in metabolic demand, and it is well documented that endurance training induces marked adaptive changes in several structural components and metabolic variables in the engaged skeletal muscles. Among the observed changes with different training regimens are those involving the muscle's content of metabolic enzymes, the sensitivity to hormones, and the composition of the contracting filaments. Other adaptations affect membrane transport processes and the muscular capillary network. These adaptive changes have consequences for the fuel selection of the working muscle and hence for the whole-body metabolic homeostasis during exercise and probably also for a considerable time after an exercise bout.

Muscle Glucose Uptake

Oxidation of plasma-derived glucose may represent a significant portion of the fuel for muscular exercise. It may cover 10% to 30% of total substrate oxidation by the leg during light to moderate exercise, and during prolonged exercise it has been reported to cover up to 75% to 90% of the estimated carbohydrate oxidation by muscle (67). With endurance training, the importance of plasma glucose as an energy substrate decreases (8). This is not unexpected, since the reliance on fat metabolism is known to be increased in the trained state (discussed later). However, the recent reports (11, 14, 27, 29) that endurance training leads to an increased number of glucose transporters owing to an increased synthesis of transporter protein in skeletal muscle are difficult to reconcile with the evidence that the reliance on plasma glucose is decreased with training also when expressed as a percentage of total carbohydrate oxidation (8). Jansson and Kaijser (31) suggested that the decreased blood glucose extraction by the legs of trained subjects was secondary to the glycogen-sparing effect of training, resulting in higher muscle glycogen concentration during the later stages of the exercise session. However, a recent study showed that other adaptations also must be responsible for the decreased glucose utilization following training (44). As is evident from Dr. Ivy's chapter (see chapter 28), this is presently a very active research area, and the involvement of several previously unrecognized factors, such as insulinlike growth factor 1 and adenosine, have only recently started to be revealed.

Muscle Glycogen Utilization

Endogenous glycogen is the dominant fuel for the contracting muscle during the initial period of moderate to severe exercise. During sustained exercise at work rates around 60% to 80% of the maximal oxygen uptake, fatigue coincides with the depletion of muscle glycogen (3, 58). Glycogen depletion has been found to be reduced during prolonged exercise in trained compared with untrained individuals working at the same absolute rate (the same rate of oxygen consumption; 15), although the rate of glycogen depletion has been found to be both similar (22, 55) and reduced (31) if the subjects are exercising at the same relative intensity (same percentage of $\dot{V}O_2$max). Jansson and Kaijser (31), and also Green et al. (17), found that training exerts its greatest effect in reducing glycogen degradation early in exercise. Green et al. (17) were also able to show that this effect occurs in both fast- and slow-twitch fibers.

Training can result in reduced muscle glycogen utilization during exercise in several ways. It is conceivable that a major factor is the adaptive increase in muscle mitochondria. A hypothetical biochemical mechanism whereby a large concentration of mitochondrial oxidative enzymes (i.e., citric acid cycle enzymes, fat oxidation enzymes, and respiratory chain components) in trained muscle would lead to a greater reliance on fat metabolism, a lower rate of lactate formation, and sparing of muscle glycogen during exercise has been formulated by Holloszy and Booth (25). This is discussed in detail in this symposium by Dr. Green (see chapter 27).

Muscle Glycogen Storage

Apart from a lower rate of glycogenolysis during exercise, trained individuals also have an increased glycogen storage capacity in skeletal muscle and in all probability a capacity for faster replenishment of muscle glycogen stores following exercise bouts (33, 45). Particularly convincing evidence that local, and not only dietary, factors are responsible for this difference in storage capacity between trained and untrained muscle comes from studies of one-leg training (21, 56). This increased level of glycogen, however, is reduced to that of untrained muscle upon detraining or immobilization (19).

The increased storage capacity of muscle glycogen, which is found in trained skeletal muscle, is likely to be secondary to the improved insulin action (see next section). In addition, muscle glycogen synthase activity has been found to be higher in trained individuals than in untrained ones (14, 46, 53), and athletes have increased whole-body insulin-stimulated glucose metabolism associated with both pretranscriptional (mRNA) and posttranslational (enzyme activity) up-regulation of glycogen synthase (65). It is known that glycogen synthase is activated by insulin (4, 12).

Insulin Action

Insulin is the major hormone regulating carbohydrate and protein metabolism. Skeletal muscle is the principal site of insulin-mediated glucose disposal (10). This may be important, since impaired tissue sensitivity for insulin has been shown to be associated with several pathological conditions, such as obesity, type II diabetes, and cardiovascular disease. It has been shown that variations in the rate of insulin-mediated glycogen synthesis in muscle account for a large part of the observed interindividual variations in tissue insulin sensitivity or resistance with different normal or pathological conditions (40, 59).

Consistent with the reports showing increases in muscle GLUT4 protein with training (previously discussed), several studies have shown that endurance training results in increased insulin sensitivity and responsiveness in skeletal muscle, whereas insulin resistance accompanies inactivity (see references in 61). In healthy individuals, these changes in insulin action are not usually accompanied by similar changes in glucose tolerance (54), since the plasma insulin level during a glucose tolerance test changes in a reciprocal manner relative to the changes in insulin action. Most investigations performed to date have indicated that the enhanced glucose uptake at submaximal insulin concentrations (insulin sensitivity) noted in trained individuals is not a true training-induced adaptation but merely an effect of the last exercise bout, since it is lost within a few days following cessation of training (35, 46, 48, 54). Whether this also is true for the training-induced increase in insulin responsiveness is uncertain, because available data are conflicting (35, 36, 46). The question of whether or not the improved insulin action in skeletal muscle is to be regarded as a true adaptation to training may be purely academic, however, and the results demonstrate the importance of regularly performed exercise to protect against the development of insulin resistance (for example, with aging) or to improve insulin action in such pathological states as obesity and type II diabetes. It may also be noted that not all types of exercise are associated with increased insulin action, because one bout of eccentric exercise has been found to be associated with insulin resistance (13, 37).

Mechanisms for Enhanced Insulin Action With Endurance Training

Two important underlying factors are likely to be the training-induced increase in the number of glucose transporters and the higher muscle glycogen synthase activity in trained individuals than in untrained ones (previously discussed). This is discussed by Dr. Ivy in chapter 28. In this chapter, I will discuss some other mechanisms that may or may not be important in this respect, but that have not yet been subjected to closer examination.

Recent data in various patient groups suggest a novel mechanism for insulin resistance: a decreased effect of insulin to stimulate blood flow (39). We have recently presented some evidence that the opposite mechanism may enhance insulin sensitivity in aerobically trained individuals (14). In contrast, using the microdialysis ethanol technique (23) for blood flow determination in muscle, we failed to detect any blood flow increase during insulin stimulation with a euglycemic clamp (Hickner et al., unpublished results presented at the Ninth International Conference on the Biochemistry of Exercise). Clearly, more information is needed on this issue. Holmäng, Björntorp, and Rippe (26) found evidence for extensive binding of insulin to the vascular endothelium in muscle. This may indicate that the higher capillary content in trained muscle (2, 6) might improve insulin action in the trained state. It is well documented that trained individuals have a significantly higher fraction of slow-twitch fibers in their active muscles. Two studies suggest that this fiber type profile may be associated with significantly improved insulin action in skeletal muscle (51, 66).

Other newly proposed mechanisms that could be of importance for insulin action in skeletal muscle include changes in the fatty acid composition of muscle sarcolemma (5), in the hexosamine pathway as a glucose sensor, which may induce insulin resistance (41), and in glycogenin as a priming mechanism of muscle glycogen synthesis (62). Another novel factor is amylin (71), which is cosecreted with insulin and has potent actions on skeletal muscle glycogen metabolism opposing those of insulin. It remains to be shown whether any of these novel mechanisms are of significance for the insulin sensitivity of muscle subjected to acute exercise or training.

Utilization of Blood-Borne Nonesterified Fatty Acids

Nonesterified fatty acid (NEFA) is the dominant fuel in muscle at rest and has been estimated to correspond to 80% of the oxygen uptake in resting muscle (20). During exercise at low to moderate intensities, plasma NEFA may often cover more than half of the muscle's oxidative metabolism, especially during prolonged exercise (1), but its importance diminishes as the exercise intensity increases. The plasma levels of nonesterified fatty acids are often lower during exercise in endurance-trained than in control subjects (see 24), and it has been shown that the turnover of plasma NEFA during exercise is reduced in the trained state (43). In fact, Jansson and Kaijser (31) and Hurley et al. (30) concluded that the reduced reliance on carbohydrate metabolism in their trained, as compared to their untrained, subjects would have been covered by intramuscular triglycerides and not by an increased uptake by plasma NEFA.

In contrast, based on the results of a one-leg training study, Kiens et al. (34) concluded that the uptake of plasma NEFA during one-leg exercise was significantly higher in the trained than in the untrained leg. These authors present evidence for a carrier-mediated transport of free fatty acids across the sarcolemma and hypothesize that training might have induced a change in the structure or function of this membrane transport system. No information is presently available on this issue.

Utilization of Blood-Borne Triglycerides

Plasma triacylglycerol has been regarded to contribute very little to exercise metabolism (20, 32), but there is evidence in the literature that plasma triglycerides may not always be unimportant as a fuel for contracting skeletal muscle. Griffiths et al. (18) calculated that during an exercise bout 3 h following a meal, the uptake of plasma-derived triglycerides could, if completely oxidized, cover 40% of the energy demand. Studies of tissue lipoprotein lipase (LPL), which is located on the intraluminal surface of the capillaries and which catalyzes the hydrolysis of intravascular triglycerides (50), indicate that circulating triacylglycerol may be more important in the trained than in the untrained state. Simsolo, Ong, and Kern (60) found a marked reduction in muscle LPL activity with 2 wk of detraining, whereas that of adipose tissue increased. This is in accordance with several other studies showing increases in muscle LPL activity with training (49, 64), but not with all (63). This area needs more experimentation. Its importance is illustrated by the fact that exercise may lead to a decrease in plasma triglycerides, which persists for 1 to 5 d (50). A problem is that the small a-v differences for plasma triglycerides make it difficult to directly study the effect of training on the utilization of this fuel (34).

Utilization of Endogenous Triglycerides

Relatively little is known about endogenous triglycerides as a potential source of energy for the contracting muscle, but this fuel source seems likely to be important during exercise. Fröberg and Mossfeldt (16) calculated that the decrease in muscle triglycerides during the 7-h Swedish Wasa ski race corresponded to twice as much energy as the decrease in muscle glycogen. Hurley et al. (30) studied nine male subjects before and after a 12-wk program of endurance training. When exercising at the same absolute intensity after as compared with before training, muscle triglyceride utilization was found to be twice as great. From these data, they concluded, as did Jansson and Kaijser in an earlier study (31), that the greater utilization of fat in the trained state was completely fueled by increased lipolysis of intramuscular triglycerides.

Based on these findings, one might expect an increased resting level of intramuscular triglycerides in trained muscle. This has not been definitively demonstrated, however, in human muscle (28, 30, 47). Therefore, other changes must be responsible for the increased triglyceride utilization in the trained state. Such changes might include increases in the low-molecular-weight cytosolic fatty acid–binding proteins, which may play an important role in the intracellular transport and targeting of fatty acids (52), and a change in the activity of regulatory molecules, such as malonyl CoA (an inhibitor of carnitine acyltransferase I activity; 69). Whether malonyl CoA is reduced in trained skeletal muscle is not known at present. Because beta-receptor mechanisms regulate skeletal muscle triglyceride hydrolysis via hormone-sensitive lipase (50), it is possible that an increased beta-receptor density may at least partially oppose the lower sympathoadrenal activation during exercise in the trained state.

However, to date, increased density of beta-receptors has been found in response to training only in the rat (7, 68). Martin et al. (42) found no increase in beta-receptor density in human subjects following 12 wk of endurance training. Another potentially more important factor regulating intramuscular triglyceride utilization may be a training-induced increase in hormone-sensitive lipase. No information is currently available, however, on this issue.

Yki-Järvinen et al. (70) presented evidence of a feedback mechanism that could serve to maintain a certain rate of cellular fatty acid oxidation under conditions of changing inflow of plasma nonesterified fatty acids. This mechanism is supposed to involve stimulation of LPL at times of lowered intracellular fatty acid concentration, resulting from either insufficient hormone-sensitive lipase activity or lowered plasma NEFA concentrations (see also 50). Whether such mechanisms are important in explaining the increased fat reliance in endurance-trained muscle remains to be demonstrated.

Conclusion

The adaptive changes in muscle mitochondrial enzymes and capillaries are the best-described consequences of endurance training. They are accompanied by other changes, such as a possible increase in Na^+-K^+ pump activity, which would enhance reuptake of K^+ and thereby delay fatigue in the contraction process (38). After several years of endurance training, fiber type transformations from fast-twitch to slow-twitch (57), which would serve to increase the overall muscle oxidative capacity and possibly also reduce energy expenditure (9), would be expected to have a further positive influence on the endurance capacity of the muscle. Recombinant DNA techniques are now being used to explore the genetic mechanisms behind these different adaptive changes. Insight from this research area is given by Dr. Booth in chapter 26.

The increased insulin action in skeletal muscles of individuals regularly involved in endurance training demonstrates the importance of regular exercise to improve insulin action in pathological states such as obesity and type II diabetes and to protect against the development of insulin resistance with aging. Training-induced adaptations in other important metabolic systems in skeletal muscle await further exploration. These include the utilization of plasma-derived glucose with contractions or insulin, the utilization of plasma-derived NEFA, and the utilization of endogenous and plasma-derived triglycerides. The training-induced adaptations in skeletal muscle must be considered in the light of adaptations in all other organs of the body in order to obtain an accurate picture of how endurance training may influence the metabolic homeostasis of the organism as a whole.

References

1. Ahlborg, G.; Felig, P.; Hagenfeldt, L.; Hendler, R.; Wahren, J. Substrate turnover during prolonged exercise in man: Splanchnic and leg metabolism of glucose, free fatty acids and amino acids. J. Clin. Invest. 53:1080-1090; 1974.

2. Andersen, P.; Henriksson, J. Capillary supply of the quadriceps femoris muscle of man: Adaptive response to exercise. J. Physiol. 270:677-690; 1977.
3. Bergström, J.; Hermansen, L.; Hultman, E.; Saltin, B. Diet, muscle glycogen and physical performance. Acta Physiol. Scand. 71:140-150; 1967.
4. Bogardus, C.; Ravussin, E.; Robbins, D.C.; Wolfe, R.R.; Horton, E.S.; Sims, E.A.H. Effects of physical training and diet therapy on carbohydrate metabolism in patients with glucose intolerance and non-insulin-dependent diabetes mellitus. Diabetes 33:311-318; 1984.
5. Borkman, M.; Storlien, L.H.; Pan, D.A.; Jenkins, A.B.; Chisholm, D.J.; Campbell, L.V. The relation between insulin sensitivity and the fatty-acid composition of skeletal-muscle phospholipids. N. Engl. J. Med. 328(4):238-244; 1993.
6. Brodal, P.; Ingjer, F.; Hermansen, L. Capillary supply of skeletal muscle fibres in untrained and endurance-trained men. Am. J. Physiol. 232:H705-H712; 1977.
7. Buckenmeyer, P.J.; Goldfarb, A.H.; Partilla, J.S.; Pineyro, M.A.; Dax, E.M. Endurance training, not acute exercise, differentially alters β-receptors and cyclase in skeletal fiber types. Am. J. Physiol. 258:E71-E77; 1990.
8. Coggan, A.R.; Kohrt, W.M.; Spina, R.J.; Bier, D.M.; Holloszy, J.O. Endurance training decreases plasma glucose turnover and oxidation during moderate-intensity exercise in men. J. Appl. Physiol. 68(3):990-996; 1990.
9. Crow, M.; Kushmerick, M.J. Chemical energetics of slow- and fast-twitch muscles of the mouse. J. Gen. Physiol. 79:147-166; 1982.
10. DeFronzo, R.A.; Jacot, E.; Jequier, E.; Maeder, E.; Wahren, J.; Felber, J.P. The effect of insulin on the disposal of intravenous glucose: Results from indirect calorimetry and hepatic femoral venous catheterization. Diabetes 30:1000-1007; 1981.
11. Dela, F.; Handberg, A.; Mikines, K.J.; Vinten, J.; Galbo, H. GLUT 4 and insulin receptor binding and kinase activity in trained human muscle. J. Physiol. (London) 469:615-624; 1993.
12. Devlin, J.T.; Horton, E.S. Effects of prior high-intensity exercise on glucose metabolism in normal and insulin-resistant men. Diabetes 34:973-979; 1985.
13. Doyle, J.A.; Sherman, W.M.; Strauss, R.L. Effects of eccentric and concentric exercise on muscle glycogen replenishment. J. Appl. Physiol. 74(4):1848-1855; 1993.
14. Ebeling, P.; Bourey, R.; Koranyi, L.; Tuominen, J.A.; Groop, L.C.; Henriksson, J.; Mueckler, M.; Sovijärvi, A.; Koivisto, V.A. Mechanism of enhanced insulin sensitivity in athletes. Increased blood flow, muscle glucose transport protein (glut-4) concentration, and glycogen synthase activity. J. Clin. Inv. 92:1623-1631; 1993.
15. Fitts, R.H.; Booth, F.W.; Winder, W.W.; Holloszy, J.O. Skeletal muscle respiratory capacity, endurance, and glycogen utilization. Am. J. Physiol. 228(4):1029-1033; 1975.
16. Fröberg, S.O.; Mossfeldt, F. Effect of prolonged strenuous exercise on the concentration of triglycerides, phospholipids and glycogen in muscle of man. Acta Physiol. Scand. 82:167; 1971.
17. Green, H.J.; Smith, D.; Murphy, P.; Fraser, I. Training-induced alterations in muscle glycogen utilization in fibre-specific types during prolonged exercise. Can. J. Physiol. Pharmacol. 68:1372-1376; 1990.
18. Griffiths, A.J.; Humphreys, S.M.; Clark, M.L.; Frayn, K.N. Forearm substrate utilization during exercise after a meal containing both fat and carbohydrate. Clin. Sci. 86:169-175; 1994.

19. Häggmark, T. A study of morphologic and enzymatic properties of the skeletal muscles after injuries and immobilization in man. Stockholm: Karolinska Institutet; 1978. Thesis.

20. Havel, R.J.; Pernow, B.; Jones, N.L. Uptake and release of free fatty acids and other metabolites in the legs of exercising men. J. Appl. Physiol. 23:90-99; 1967.

21. Henriksson, J. Training induced adaptation of skeletal muscle and metabolism during submaximal exercise. J. Physiol. 270:661-675; 1977.

22. Hermansen, L.; Hultman, E.; Saltin, B. Muscle glycogen during prolonged severe exercise. Acta Physiol. Scand. 71:129-139; 1967.

23. Hickner, R.C.; Rosdahl, H.; Borg, I.; Ungerstedt, U.; Jorfeldt, L.; Henriksson, J. The ethanol technique of monitoring blood flow changes in rat skeletal muscle: Implications for microdialysis. Acta Physiol. Scand. 146(1):87-97; 1992.

24. Holloszy, J.O. Metabolic consequences of endurance exercise training. In: Horton, E.S., Terjung, R.L., eds. Exercise, nutrition and energy metabolism. New York: Macmillan; 1988:116-131.

25. Holloszy, J.O.; Booth, F.W. Biochemical adaptations to endurance exercise in muscle. Annu. Rev. Physiol. 38:273-291; 1976.

26. Holmäng, A.; Björntorp, P.; Rippe, B. Tissue uptake of insulin and inulin in red and white skeletal muscle in vivo. Am. J. Physiol. 263:H1-H7; 1992.

27. Houmard, J.A.; Egan, P.C.; Neufer, P.D.; Friedman, J.E.; Wheeler, W.S.; Israel, R.G.; Dohm, G.L. Elevated skeletal muscle glucose transporter levels in exercise-trained middle-aged men. Am. J. Physiol. 261(4, pt. 1):E437-E443; 1991.

28. Howald, H.; Hoppeler, H.; Claassen, H.; Mathieu, O.; Straub, R. Influences of endurance training on the ultrastructural composition of the different muscle fiber types in humans. Pflügers Arch. 403:369-376; 1985.

29. Hughes, V.A.; Fiatarone, M.A.; Fielding, R.A.; Kahn, B.B.; Ferrera, C.M.; Shepherd, P.; Fisher, E.C.; Wolfe, R.R.; Elahi, D.; Evans, W.J. Exercise increases muscle GLUT-4 levels and insulin action in subjects with impaired glucose tolerance. Am. J. Physiol. 264:E855-E862; 1993.

30. Hurley, B.F.; Nemeth, P.M.; Martin, W.H., III; Hagberg, J.M.; Dalsky, G.P.; Holloszy, J.O. Muscle triglyceride utilization during exercise: Effect of training. J. Appl. Physiol. 60(2):562-567; 1986.

31. Jansson, E.; Kaijser, L. Substrate utilization and enzymes in skeletal muscle of extremely endurance-trained men. J. Appl. Physiol. 62:999-1005; 1987.

32. Jones, N.L.; Heigenhauser, G.J.F.; Kuksis, A.; Matos, C.G.; Sutton, J.R.; Toews, C.J. Fat metabolism in heavy exercise. Clin. Sci. 59:469-478; 1980.

33. Kern, M.; Tapscott, E.B.; Downes, D.L.; Frisell, W.R.; Dohm, G.L. Insulin resistance induced by high-fat feeding is only partially reversed by exercise training. Pflügers Arch. 417:79-83; 1990.

34. Kiens, B.; Essén-Gustavsson, B.; Christensen, N.J.; Saltin, B. Skeletal muscle substrate utilization during submaximal exercise in man: Effect of endurance training. J. Physiol. (London) 469:459-478; 1993.

35. King, D.S.; Dalsky, G.P.; Clutter, W.E.; Young, D.A.; Staten, M.A.; Cryer, P.E.; Holloszy, J.O. Effects of exercise and lack of exercise on insulin sensitivity and responsiveness. J. Appl. Physiol. 64(5):1942-1946; 1988.

36. King, D.S.; Dalsky, G.P.; Staten, M.A.; Clutter, W.E.; Van Houten, D.R.; Holloszy, J.O. Insulin action and secretion in endurance-trained and untrained humans. J. Appl. Physiol. 63:2247-2252; 1987.

37. Kirwan, J.P.; Hickner, R.C.; Yarasheski, K.E.; Kohrt, W.M.; Wiethop, B.V.; Holloszy, J.O. Eccentric exercise induces transient insulin resistance in healthy individuals. J. Appl. Physiol. 72(6):2197-2202; 1992.

38. Kjeldsen, K.; Norgaard, A.; Hau, C. Exercise-induced hyperkalaemia can be reduced in human subjects by moderate training without change in skeletal muscle Na, K-ATPase concentration. Eur. J. Clin. Invest. 20:642-647; 1990.
39. Laakso, M.; Edelman, S.V.; Olefsky, J.M.; Brechtel, G.; Wallace, P.; Baron, A.D. Kinetics of in vivo muscle insulin-mediated glucose uptake in human obesity. Diabetes 39:965-974; 1990.
40. Lillioja, S.; Mott, D.M.; Zawadzki, J.K.; Young, A.A.; Abbott, W.G.; Bogardus, C. Glucose storage is a major determinant of in vivo "insulin resistance" in subjects with normal glucose tolerance. J. Clin. Endocrinol. Metab. 62:922-927; 1986.
41. Marshall, S.; Garvey, W.T.; Traxinger, R.R. New insights into the metabolic regulation of insulin action and insulin resistance: Role of glucose and amino acids. FASEB J. 5:3031-3036; 1991.
42. Martin, W.H., III; Coggan, A.R.; Spina, R.J.; Saffitz, J.E. Effects of fiber type and training on β-adrenoceptor density in human skeletal muscle. Am. J. Physiol. 257:E736-E742; 1989.
43. Martin, W.H., III; Dalsky, G.P.; Hurley, B.F.; Matthews, D.E.; Bier, D.M.; Hagberg, J.M.; Rogers, M.A.; King, D.S.; Holloszy, J.O. Effect of endurance training on plasma free fatty acid turnover and oxidation during exercise. Am. J. Physiol. 265:E708-E714; 1993.
44. Mendenhall, L.A.; Swanson, S.C.; Habash, D.L.; Coggan, A.R. Ten days of exercise training reduces glucose production and utilization during moderate-intensity exercise. Am. J. Physiol. 266:E136-E143; 1994.
45. Mikines, K.J.; Sonne, B.; Farrell, P.A.; Tronier, B.; Galbo, H. Effect of training on the dose-response relationship for insulin action in men. J. Appl. Physiol. 66(2):695-703; 1989.
46. Mikines, K.J.; Sonne, B.; Tronier, B.; Galbo, H. Effects of acute exercise and detraining on insulin action in trained men. J. Appl. Physiol. 66(2):704-711; 1989.
47. Morgan, T.E.; Short, F.A.; Cobb, L.A. Effect of long-term exercise on skeletal muscle lipid composition. Am. J. Physiol. 216(1):82-86; 1969.
48. Nagasawa, J.; Sato, Y.; Ishiko, T. Effect of training and detraining on in vivo insulin sensitivity. Int. J. Sports Med. 11:107-110; 1990.
49. Nikkilä, E.A.; Taskinen, M.-R.; Rehunen, S.; Härkönen, M. Lipoprotein lipase activity in adipose tissue and skeletal muscle of runners: Relation to serum lipoproteins. Metabolism 27(11):1661-1671; 1978.
50. Oscai, L.B.; Essig, D.A.; Palmer, W.K. Lipase regulation of muscle triglyceride hydrolysis. J. Appl. Physiol. 69(5):1571-1577; 1990.
51. Pagliassotti, M.J.; Shahrokhi, K.A.; Hill, J.O. Skeletal muscle glucose metabolism in obesity-prone and obesity-resistant rats. Am. J. Physiol. 264:R1224-R1228; 1993.
52. Paulussen, R.J.A.; Veerkamp, J.H. Intracellular fatty-acid-binding proteins. Characteristics and function. In: Hilderson, H.J., ed. Subcellular biochemistry. New York: Plenum Press; 1990:175-226.
53. Piehl, K.; Adolfsson, S.; Nazar, K. Glycogen storage and glycogen synthetase activity in trained and untrained muscle of man. Acta Physiol. Scand. 90:779-788; 1974.
54. Rogers, M.A.; King, D.S.; Hagberg, J.M.; Ehsani, A.A.; Holloszy, J.O. Effect of 10 days of physical inactivity on glucose tolerance in master athletes. J. Appl. Physiol. 68(5):1833-1837; 1990.

55. Saltin, B.; Karlsson, J. Muscle glycogen utilization during work of different intensities. In: Pernow, B.; Saltin, B., eds. Muscle metabolism during exercise. New York: Plenum Press; 1971:289-299.

56. Saltin, B.; Nazar, D.L.; Costill, D.L.; Stein, E.; Jansson, E.; Essén, B.; Gollnick, P. The nature of the training response: Peripheral and central adaptations to one-legged exercise. Acta Physiol. Scand. 96:289-305; 1976.

57. Schantz, P. Plasticity of human skeletal muscle. Acta Physiol. Scand. 128 (suppl. 558):1-62; 1986.

58. Sherman, W.M.; Costill, D.L. The marathon: Dietary manipulation to optimize performance. Am. J. Sports Med. 12(1):44-51; 1984.

59. Shulman, G.I.; Rothman, D.L.; Jue, T.; Stein, P.; DeFronzo, R.A.; Shulman, R.G. Quantitation of muscle glycogen synthesis in normal subjects and subjects with non-insulin-dependent diabetes by ^{13}C nuclear magnetic resonance spectroscopy. N. Engl. J. Med. 322:223-228; 1990.

60. Simsolo, R.B.; Ong, J.M.; Kern, P.A. The regulation of adipose tissue and muscle lipoprotein lipase in runners by detraining. J. Clin. Invest. 92:2124-2130; 1993.

61. Sinacore, D.R.; Gulve, E.A. The role of skeletal muscle in glucose transport, glucose homeostasis, and insulin resistance: Implications for physical therapy. Phys. Therapy 73:878-891; 1993.

62. Smythe, C.; Cohen, P. The discovery of glycogenin and the priming mechanism for glycogen biogenesis. Eur. J. Biochem. 200:625-631; 1991.

63. Stubbe, I.; Hansson, P.; Gustafson, A.; Nilsson-Ehle, P. Plasma lipoproteins and lipolytic enzymes activities during endurance training in sedentary men: Changes in high-density lipoprotein subfractions and composition. Metabolism 32(12):1120-1128; 1983.

64. Svedenhag, J.; Lithell, H.; Juhlin-Dannfelt, A.; Henriksson, J. Increased skeletal muscle lipoprotein lipase following endurance training in man. Atherosclerosis 49:203-207; 1983.

65. Vestergaard, H.; Andersen, P.H.; Lund, S.; Schmitz, O.; Junker, S.; Pedersen, O. Pre- and posttranslational upregulation of muscle-specific glycogen synthase in athletes. Am. J. Physiol. 266:E92-E101; 1994.

66. Wade, A.J.; Marbut, M.M.; Round, J.M. Muscle fibre type and aetiology of obesity. Lancet 335:805-808; 1990.

67. Wahren, J.; Felig, P.; Ahlborg, G.; Jorfeldt, L. Glucose metabolism during leg exercise in man. J. Clin. Invest. 50:2715-2725; 1971.

68. Williams, R.S.; Caron, M.G.; Daniel, K. Skeletal muscle β-adrenergic receptors: Variations due to fiber type and training. Am. J. Physiol. 246:E160-E167; 1984.

69. Winder, W.W.; Arogyasami, J.; Barton, R.J.; Elayan, I.M.; Vehrs, P.R. Muscle malonyl-CoA decreases during exercise. J. Appl. Physiol. 67(6):2230-2233; 1989.

70. Yki-Järvinen, H.; Puhakainen, I.; Saloranta, C.; Groop, L.; Taskinen, M.-R. Demonstration of a novel feedback mechanism between FFA oxidation from intracellular and intravascular sources. Am. J. Physiol. 260:E680-E689; 1991.

71. Young, A.A.; Carlo, P.; Smith, P.; Wolfe-Lopez, D.; Pittner, R.; Wang, M.W.; Rink, T. Evidence for release of free glucose from muscle during amylin-induced glycogenolysis in rats. FEBS Lett. 334(3):317-321; 1993.

CHAPTER 26

Molecular and Cellular Adaptations of Muscle in Response to Exercise

Frank W. Booth, James A. Carson, Zhen Yan
University of Texas-Houston Health Science Center, Houston, Texas, U.S.A.

Descriptive events concerning the plasticity of skeletal muscle to alterations in the inherent pattern of contractile activity have been documented in numerous reviews (3, 7, 12, 13). Recently, investigations have begun to outline the mechanisms for changes in gene expression when muscle adapts to a new level of contractile activity. Investigators are now applying molecular and cellular techniques as tools to delineate signaling pathways from the initial exercise signal (for example, from the sensing of load bearing or of the energy flux by the skeletal muscle) to the alteration in the quantity of a specific protein. To date, the most frequent measurement made in exercise studies using molecular biological techniques has been of the quantity of mRNAs in skeletal muscle in various exercise models. A recent review summarizes these responses (2). As a rule, if an mRNA changes in skeletal muscle because of a change in the inherent quantity of contractile activity, the direction of the change in the mRNA is similar to the direction of the change in its protein. However, changes in the quantities of mRNAs and their proteins do not always occur together. Numerous interpretations could explain this lack of synchrony; for example, sensitivities of assays for mRNAs and their proteins differ, or the timing of changes for mRNAs is truly different. Sufficient data now exist to support the hypothesis that changes in mRNAs and proteins do not occur on the same time scale. These observations permit the interpretation that adaptive changes in protein quantities of skeletal muscles during inherent alterations in contractile activity are due to changes at multiple sites of regulation (figure 26.1). Selected examples of changes in the regulation of these sites by alterations in the inherent level of contractile activity will be given in this review.

Transcriptional Regulation

Transcription rates of GLUT4 and citrate synthase, which were determined by nuclear run-on assays, were increased postexercise (11). GLUT4 transcription rate in rat fast red muscle was increased 3 h, but not 30 min or 24 h, after completing a 33-min bout of running either on the first or eighth day of training (11). The

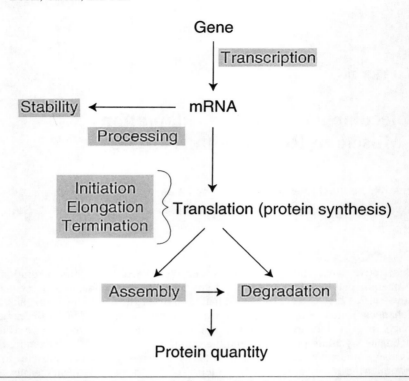

Figure 26.1   Regulatory sites of gene expression. Alterations in the inherent quantity of contractile activity can interact at multiple sites (shaded) in the determination of changes in protein quantity, which is the definition of changes in gene expression.

training protocol consisted of 3 × 33 min of treadmill running each day by rats. GLUT4 protein did not increase after 7 d of treadmill running. The transcription rate of citrate synthase increased after a single 33-min bout of running, but citrate synthase activity had not yet increased significantly after 7 d of training (11). These data imply that increases in transcription rate precede increases in protein and enzyme activity.

Increases in reporter gene activity driven by muscle-specific promoters indirectly imply an increased transcription rate from that promoter. Two models of exogenous gene expression have shown increased reporter gene activity in hypertrophic models. Carson et al. (5) noted increased luciferase activity driven from the −2090 promoter of the chicken skeletal α-actin gene in the anterior latissimus dorsi muscle on the sixth day of stretch-induced hypertrophy. Tsika and Gao (see chapter 17) observed a 10-fold increase in chloramphenicol acetyltransferase activities driven by the first 600 base pairs of the human β-myosin heavy chain promoter after 6 to 8 wk of overloading of the plantaris muscle of transgenic mice.

mRNA Stability

Connor and Hood (6) have determined that transcription can be blocked for only 6 h before the rat becomes too sick to allow differentiation of changes in transcription as due to the exercise model or due to an unhealthy rat. Therefore, this technique can only be used to estimate the decay of mRNAs with short half-lives. 5'-aminolevulinate synthase mRNA turnover was not significantly altered in tibialis anterior muscles that had undergone 10 d of chronic electrical stimulation (6).

mRNA Processing

We have found no studies employing exercise models in whole animals.

Translational Regulation

The initial decreases in synthesis rates of actin, cytochrome c, and myofibrillar proteins have been noted in atrophying skeletal muscles without decreases in their mRNAs at these early times. These data imply that translational regulation is decreased in muscle atrophy produced either by limb immobilization or by hindlimb unloading. During the first 5 to 6 h of hindlimb immobilization, the synthesis rates of actin and cytochrome c proteins in fast skeletal muscle decrease 50%, but their mRNA concentrations are unchanged at this time (10, 15). These findings are interpreted to mean that translation of cytochrome c and actin are decreased at the start of muscle atrophy in immobilized fast muscle of rats. Thomason, Biggs, and Booth (14) observed a decrease in myofibrillar protein synthesis rate during the first 5 h of unloading by the soleus muscle of rats, but no change in the concentration of β-myosin heavy chain mRNA for the first 7 d of unloading by the soleus muscle (14). These data imply that a decrease in protein translation is an early event producing adaptation of skeletal muscle to non–load bearing by a postural muscle.

Initiation of Translation

A decrease in the initiation of the synthesis of new proteins of mRNA has been noted in the heart of rats during unloading of the hindlimbs (see chapter 16).

Elongation of Translation

A prolongation of translation occurs in the unloaded soleus muscle. Polysomes isolated from 18-h unloaded soleus muscles are larger in size due to more ribosomes per mRNA (8). An increase in the amount of rRNA attached to polyribosomes occurs. In addition, α-actin mRNA shifts to the heavier polysomes without a change in the absolute amount of this message (8). Thus, a prolonged elongation of polypeptide synthesis on ribosomes explains, in part, the initial decrease in protein synthesis rate that occurs in the unloaded slow muscle.

Protein Assembly

During stretch-induced hypertrophy of skeletal muscle, the increase in the protein synthesis rate is greater than that required to produce new protein for hypertrophy. Since excess protein is synthesized, assembly of this new protein is the apparent rate-limiting factor for muscle growth. During stretch-induced growth of the anterior latissimus dorsi muscle of chickens, 72% of the increase in mixed protein synthesis rate over basal rate is estimated to be wasted (9). Millward (9) indicates that his estimation of protein wastage in hypertrophy is not novel, as others have shown that most newly synthesized collagen is degraded before it can become fully cross-linked. Booth found no increase in the synthesis rate of cytochrome c protein in skeletal muscles of rats that exhibit increases in cytochrome c protein concentration during daily bouts of treadmill running (1). One interpretation of these results is that cytochrome c protein is synthesized in excess of its assembly.

Protein Degradation

Protein degradation in skeletal muscles is decreased during short-duration aerobic exercise (4). However, longer durations of increased contractile activity have shown increases in the rate of protein degradation in skeletal muscles (4, 9). Booth has estimated that the turnover of cytochrome c protein in skeletal muscle increases during endurance training in rats (1).

Summary

Techniques adapted from molecular biology now permit the delineation of mechanisms by which alterations in the inherent level of contractile activity in skeletal muscle lead to changes in the quantities of muscle protein. These approaches will continue to provide insights into the cellular mechanisms causing the training adaptation. Nevertheless, the task of mapping the trail from the exercise signal to the sites of altered gene expression appears to be extremely complex. The map is likely to have multiple forks in the road as the exercise signal progresses from the exercise event to the multiple regulatory sites of gene expression, as shown in figure 26.1. These sites include transcription, mRNA stability, mRNA processing, polypeptide initiation, polypeptide elongation, polypeptide termination, protein assembly, and protein degradation. This review indicates that most, if not all, of these sites are regulated by inherent changes in contractile activity. The complexity of this regulation could also involve different types of exercise following completely different roads, since they exhibit differential gene expression. For example, endurance exercise increases mitochondrial density without enlarging contractile protein quantity. In contrast, resistance training increases contractile protein quantity while not enhancing mitochondrial density. Thus, different pathways must be followed by endurance and resistance exercises on the adaptation road map. The magnitude of the signaling pathways that cause alterations in protein expression leading to exercise adaptations is too large for any single laboratory and will require decades to complete.

Acknowledgment

This work was supported by U.S. Public Health Service Grant AR 19393.

References

1. Booth, F.W. Cytochrome c protein synthesis rate in rat skeletal muscle. J. Appl. Physiol. 71:1225-1230; 1991.
2. Booth, F.W.; Baldwin, K.M. Muscle plasticity: Energy demand/supply process. In: Rowell, L.B.; Shepherd, J.T., eds. Handbook of physiology, Section 12: Integration of motor, circulatory, respiratory, and metabolic control during exercise. Oxford: Oxford University Press; 1996:1075-1123.
3. Booth, F.W.; Thomason, D.B. Molecular and cellular adaptations in muscle in response to exercise: Perspectives of various models. Physiol. Rev. 71:541-585; 1991.
4. Booth, F.W.; Watson, P.A. Control of adaptations in protein levels in response to exercise. Fed. Proc. 44:2293-2300; 1985.
5. Carson, J.A.; Yan, Z.; Booth, F.W.; Coleman, M.E.; Schwartz, R.J.; Stump, C.S. Regulation of skeletal-actin promoter in young chickens during hypertrophy caused by stretch overload. Am. J. Physiol. 268:C918-C924, 1995.
6. Connor, M.K.; Hood, D.A. Tissue-specific regulation of mRNA stability. Med. Sci. Sports Exercise 26:S94; 1994.
7. Holloszy, J.O.; Booth, F.W. Biochemical adaptations to exercise in muscle. Annu. Rev. Physiol. 38:273-291; 1976.
8. Ku, Z.; Thomason, D.B. Soleus muscle nascent polypeptide chain elongation slows protein synthesis rate during non-weightbearing. Am. J. Physiol. 267:C115-C126, 1994.
9. Millward, D.J. Protein turnover in skeletal muscle and cardiac muscle during normal growth and hypertrophy. In: Wildenthal, K., ed. Degradative processes in heart and skeletal muscle. Amsterdam: Elsevier; 1980:188-189.
10. Morrison, P.R.; Montgomery, J.A.; Wong, T.S.; Booth, F.W. Cytochrome c protein-synthesis rates and mRNA contents during atrophy and recovery in skeletal muscle. Biochem. J. 241:257-263; 1987.
11. Neufer, P.D.; Dohm, G.L. Exercise induces a transient increase in transcription of the GLUT-4 gene in skeletal muscle. Am. J. Physiol. 265:C1597-C1603; 1993.
12. Pette, D., ed. The dynamic state of muscle fibers. Berlin: Walter de Gruyter; 1990.
13. Saltin, B.; Gollnick, P.D. Skeletal muscle adaptability: Significance for metabolism and performance. In: Peachey, L.D., ed. Handbook of physiology: Sect. 10. Skeletal muscle. Bethesda, MD: American Physiological Society; 1983:555-631.

14. Thomason, D.B.; Biggs, R.B.; Booth, F.W. Protein metabolism and β-myosin heavy-chain mRNA in unweighted soleus muscle. Am. J. Physiol. 257:R300-R305; 1989.
15. Watson, P.A.; Stein, J.P.; Booth, F.W. Changes in actin synthesis and α-actin-mRNA content in rat muscle during limb immobilization. Am. J. Physiol. 247:C39-C44; 1984.

CHAPTER 27

What Is the Physiological Significance of Training-Induced Adaptations in Muscle Mitochondrial Capacity?

Howard J. Green

University of Waterloo, Waterloo, Ontario, Canada

Whole-body exercise performed regularly induces extensive physiological adaptations in a variety of systems, tissues, and cells. These adaptations, which become most emphasized during the exercise state, include alterations in both energy metabolic behavior and substrate selection. During prolonged exercise following training at a given absolute oxygen consumption ($\dot{V}O_2$), individuals display a reduced carbohydrate dependency and an increased preference for fats. The reduction in carbohydrate dependency is readily illustrated by the glycogen reserves in the working muscle. At comparable periods of exercise, glycogen concentration is higher following training than before (35). Metabolic alterations are also evident in the working muscle. Exercise following training is accompanied by a smaller decrease in the phosphorylation potential as indicated by higher levels of high-energy phosphates (ATP and PCr) and by lower levels of free ADP (ADP$_f$) and inorganic phosphate (Pi; 17, 32). Training-induced reductions in muscle lactate also occur during exercise, strongly suggesting a decrease in glycolysis (17, 30, 32, 35). Collectively, these results indicate that following training a given level of oxidative phosphorylation, designed to satisfy the steady-state ATP requirements of the contracting cell, can be realized with less of an imbalance between ATP synthetic and ATP catalytic rates. The trained muscle exhibits a tighter metabolic control (31). The tighter metabolic control has been linked to a reduced glycolytic flux and a sparing of carbohydrate reserves (16, 32).

The metabolic and substrate alterations observed during moderate exercise following training raise several intriguing issues, not the least of which is the mechanism underlying the shift from loose to tight metabolic control. In addition, the apparent coupling of the reduction in glycogenolysis and glycolysis to the higher phosphorylation potential observed during exercise following training needs to be further explained, as does the relationship between phosphorylation potential and increased fat utilization. At least in long-term training, the observation that all of these behaviors occur concurrently suggests a common mechanism, dependent on some primary compositional adaptation in the muscle to the training.

A hypothesis that has long dominated our thinking is that the transition from loose to tight metabolic control that occurs with training is mechanistically linked to increases in mitochondrial potential (16, 32). According to this theory, changes in select metabolites of high-energy phosphate transfer reactions—such as ADP_f and Pi, both substrates for oxidative phosphorylation—are viewed as key regulators in the recruitment of mitochondrial respiration at a level necessary to increase ATP synthetic rates to meet ATP demands of the contractile activity. Since regular activity induces increases in both the size and number of mitochondria—and consequently the number of respiratory chains—at constant exercise VO_2, the flux in each respiratory chain would be decreased. Assuming recruitment of all mitochondria in the trained cell, the lower oxidative phosphorylation per respiratory chain could be accomplished with a lower level of the metabolites ADP_f and Pi.

The credibility of this hypothesis is supported by several lines of evidence. First, a role, however minor, has been established for ADP_f or the ratio of [ATP] to [ADP] and [Pi] in the control of mitochondrial respiratory rates (for review see 57). Second, cross-sectional studies comparing muscles differing in mitochondrial potential have established a close inverse correlation between the mitochondrial content and the change in phosphorylation potential over a broad range of work rates and ATP demands (31). These studies have also been extended to longitudinal studies where training (14) and hypothyroidism (14) have been used to manipulate the mitochondrial potential. All approaches have consistently and intimately linked the mitochondrial content of the cell to the sensitivity of respiratory control.

Skeletal muscle cells with tight metabolic control and consequently a high oxidative potential have also been used to explain the apparently lower glycolytic rate at a given level of oxidative phosphorylation. Changes in the high-energy phosphates (for example, ATP) and related by-products such as ADP_f and Pi have also been demonstrated to act as regulatory factors in the control of glycolysis, primarily at the level of phosphofructokinase (PFK), which is generally acknowledged as the rate-limiting step in glycolysis (52). Reductions in glycogenolysis with reductions in ADP and Pi have also been postulated to occur via regulation of the active and inactive forms of phosphorylase (7, 16). Collectively, a higher phosphorylation potential observed in working muscle following exercise is hypothesized to result in a coordinated down-regulation of both glycogenolysis and glycolysis and in less lactate production. Muscles with high mitochondrial content, whether compared cross-sectionally (31) or induced by some experimental manipulation such as training, have been repeatedly shown to result in less of an increase in lactate concentration when subjected to an increase in contractile activity either via voluntary exercise (35) or electrical stimulation (10, 15).

The mitochondrial content of the working muscle cell is also thought to act as a key regulatory mechanism in substrate selection. According to this theory, increases in the potential for β-oxidation and oxidative phosphorylation would allow, by virtue of Henri-Michaelis-Menton kinetics, a reduction in the K_m and consequently in the substrate level needed to attain a given flux rate (16). The preferential use of free fatty acids under such conditions has also been postulated to be encouraged by the depression in pyruvate availability that occurs consequent to a reduction in PFK activity. Reductions in PFK activity may also occur as a result of a higher cytosolic redox potential and higher citrate levels. Indeed, trained muscles have been shown to oxidize free fatty acids at a much higher level than untrained muscles (32). Moreover, whole-body activity performed after prolonged training has been repeatedly shown to increase fat utilization during exercise when evaluated by changes in both RER and specifically labeled isotopes (36).

It is of little wonder that the mitochondrial theory of metabolic control and substrate selection has received no serious challenge, given the apparent supporting evidence. However, a careful review of many of the earlier training papers reveals a major flaw in experimental design. Most of the earlier studies have examined the adaptive effects only after a prolonged period of training in which mitochondrial potential has been invariably increased. More recent studies using short-term training have suggested that most if not all of the adaptations may occur earlier, well before the expression in mitochondrial potential is observed.

Metabolism, Substrate Utilization, and Short-Term Training

Our studies during the last several years have focused on challenging the hypothesis that increases in mitochondrial potential are an essential prerequisite for the adaptations in metabolism and fuel utilization observed in the working muscle following training. To examine this hypothesis, we have employed a series of short-term training models, lasting for periods of 3 to 12 d, in an attempt to uncouple the metabolic adaptations from the adaptations in mitochondrial potential. The daily training stimulus has typically included 2 h of cycle exercise performed at moderate intensity. The vastus lateralis muscle was selected for examination, not only because of the ease with which repeated samples can be harvested by the biopsy technique, but because the vastus lateralis muscle is heavily recruited to perform the work of cycling (44). In all studies performed to date, only male university students, active but untrained, were used as participants.

Our results have repeatedly confirmed that short-term training results in a shift toward a tighter metabolic control. In one study, using 5 to 7 consecutive days of training, the decrease in phosphocreatine (PCr) was attenuated during moderate exercise, as was the increase in creatine (Cr), inorganic phosphate (Pi), and inosine monophosphate (IMP). These changes were also accompanied by reductions in the calculated concentrations of free ADP (ADP_f) and free AMP (AMP_f). No significant decreases were found in ATP concentration (21). Muscle mitochondrial capacity, as determined by measurements of both succinic dehydrogenase (SDH) and citrate synthase (CS), was unaltered. When the training period was extended for 10 to 12 d, essentially the same adaptations were observed in the high-energy phosphate transfer reactions (26). Again, no significant elevations in either SDH or CS were observed. In both of these studies, oxygen consumption ($\dot{V}O_2$) and consequently whole-body oxidative phosphorylation were unchanged during the prolonged exercise protocol following training (20, 21). Further, the inability to find elevations in aerobic power ($\dot{V}O_2max$) in the 5- to 7-d protocol indicates that the metabolic adaptations need not be accompanied by increases in the level of oxidative phosphorylation that can be realized during progressive exercise to fatigue. Using an exercise protocol consisting of three-step increases in power output, we have also been able to establish that the metabolic adaptations extend over a range of mitochondrial respiration rates (6). With this protocol, training-induced reductions in $\dot{V}O_2$ occur at the two intensities that extend beyond the lactate threshold.

Although the metabolic adaptations noted during exercise occur soon after the onset of training, there appears to be a threshold level of training necessary to induce the adaptation. Three days of training, for example, do not appear sufficient to promote a tighter metabolic control in the vastus lateralis muscle (22).

Other models have also been employed to demonstrate that the expression of tighter metabolic control over a range of submaximal work rates need not be accompanied by increases in oxidative potential. Both short-term (28) and long-term (37) acclimatization to altitude results in less of a reduction in phosphorylation potential during moderate exercise than exercise performed on acute exposure to altitude. These metabolic adaptations cannot be explained by increases in oxidative potential. During short-term acclimatization, maximal SDH activity remains unchanged when measured in homogenates of mixed fiber type and in specific fiber types (types I, IIa, IIb) using microphotometry (28). With more extended exposure to altitude, reductions in muscle oxidative potential appear to occur (33), possibly due to a loss of mitochondria from selective fiber types (48). High-altitude natives who display minimal disruption in phosphorylation potential with exercise (37) do not have elevated levels of mitochondrial enzyme activities. As with the short-term training model, increases in $\dot{V}O_2$ during submaximal exercise or in $\dot{V}O_2$max do not appear necessary for the acclimatization effect on energy metabolic behavior (28).

In the long-term training studies, the tighter metabolic control observed over a range of submaximal work rates has invariably been accompanied by a reduction in muscle lactate concentration (10, 15, 35). Such has also been the case with the short-term training studies. As an example, 3 d of training failed to alter either phosphorylation potential or lactate concentration in the working vastus lateralis (22). It was not until training was extended to 5 to 7 d that the coupling between these two parameters was observed (21). This coupling suggests a mechanistic basis, potentially occurring as a result of a depression in glycogenolysis and glycolysis induced by the more protected energy state. Alterations in substrate selection also appear to accompany short-term training. However, the time course for the expression in the adaptations in muscle metabolism and substrate selection do not appear to occur concurrently. With the 3-d training model, in which no change in metabolic behavior was observed (22), the respiratory exchange ratio (RER) also remained unchanged, suggesting no shift toward enhanced fat utilization during prolonged exercise (23). Of interest, muscle glycogen in the working muscle was not depleted as rapidly (22). When the work period was extended to 5 to 7 d, energy metabolic adaptations were conspicuous, but RER still remained undisturbed (21). It was not until the training period was extended for 10 to 12 d that indications of increased fat utilization, based on RER, were observed (20). The apparent increase in fat utilization did not appear to depend on increases in either the potential for oxidative phosphorylation or β-oxidation (26). In all short-term training studies, regardless of training duration, a pronounced sparing of muscle glycogen resulted. A summary of the proposed changes in substrate selection with short-term training is provided in figures 27.1 and 27.2.

Since the RER remained unchanged in the more abbreviated training models, it would appear that increases in fat utilization cannot account for the sparing of muscle glycogen that occurred with exercise. In the absence of reductions in carbohydrate utilization, a sparing of glycogen in the working muscle would have to be mediated by reductions in glycogenolysis and glycolytic flux rates or by an elevated utilization of glucose.

Reductions in lactate concentration consequent to reductions in glycogenolysis and glycolysis would mean that less carbohydrate in the form of lactate is removed from the muscle. Alternatively, extramuscular glucose might displace some of the

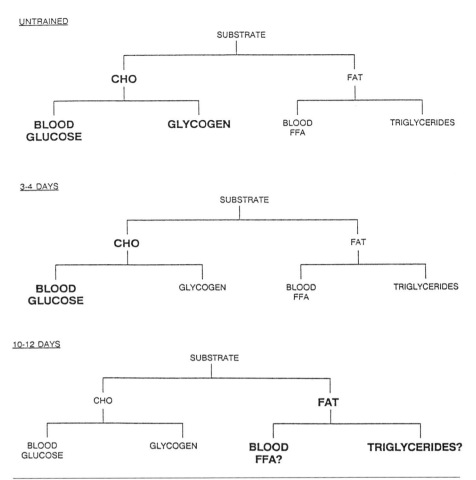

Figure 27.1   Prolonged exercise, substrate selection, and short-term training. The bold-face words indicate the postulated predominate substrates used during exercise of moderate intensity in the untrained and following 3 to 4 d and 10 to 12 d of training. Note that in the untrained, carbohydrate (CHO) in the form of blood glucose and muscle glycogen predominates as substrate. With 3 to 4 d of training, the CHO emphasis is maintained, but the dependency on muscle glycogen degradation is decreased, while the dependency on blood glucose is postulated to increase. By 10 to 12 d of training, fuel utilization is hypothesized to shift more toward fat oxidation, with the source of the substrate (blood FFA or muscle triglycerides) unknown.

glycogen as a substrate for pyruvate formation for subsequent use by the mitochondria (2) or for use directly in glycogenesis (1). If glycogenesis were elevated, the attenuation in glycogen loss could conceivably occur without an alteration in glycogenolytic flux rate.

Recently, we have initiated series of training studies of various durations using a number of stable isotopes to investigate alterations in substrate selection during

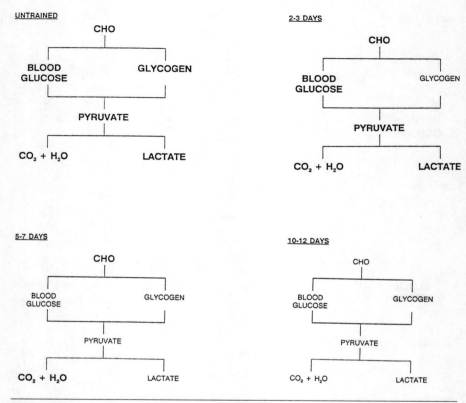

Figure 27.2 Prolonged exercise, muscle carbohydrate utilization, and short-term training. In the untrained, both blood glucose and muscle glycogen serve as important substrates for carbohydrate (CHO) utilization and pyruvate formation by muscle. In this schema, both oxidative phosphorylation and lactate formation are important fates of pyruvate. With 2 to 3 d of training, pyruvate formation is postulated to remain constant, but the source of substrate tends more toward blood glucose. Lactate formation and pyruvate utilization by mitochondria are unchanged. By 5 to 7 d of training, pyruvate utilization by mitochondria remains unaltered; however, lactate production is decreased or clearance is increased. This period of training is accompanied by a reduction in CHO utilization as a consequence of depression in glucose utilization. By 10 to 12 d of training, total CHO utilization is reduced, resulting in lower rates of blood glucose and muscle glycogen utilization. The reduction in CHO utilization corresponds to a decrease in pyruvate utilization by mitochondria as a result of increased fat utilization.

prolonged exercise. Using a 10-d training model and a primed continuous infusion of $[6,6-^2H_2]$glucose, we have found that training decreased plasma glucose turnover and presumably the oxidation of glucose (45). As has been noted earlier, using 10 consecutive days of training (20), we found depressions in RER, suggestive of an increase in fat oxidation, and no change in the level of $\dot{V}O_2$. This finding has also been confirmed in a recent paper by Mendenhall et al. (41) using essentially the same training program. Although these authors continue to speculate that increases in muscle respiratory capacity are necessary for the training-induced reduction in glucose utilization during the prolonged exercise, we have reconfirmed, based on the measurement of the maximal activity of citrate synthase, that mitochondrial potential remains unchanged (45). It would appear, at least after 10 consecutive days of training, that increases in fat utilization result in a sparing of carbohydrate utilization and specifically of blood-borne glucose. In addition, the reduced depletion of muscle glycogen utilization would occur not because of enhanced glycogenesis, but, at least in part, because of a reduction in glycogenolysis and glycolysis. It is not clear, however, if training periods shorter than 10 d result in a reduction in glucose utilization, since RER appears to be unchanged even though a tighter metabolic control is induced (21). Under these conditions, an increase in glucose utilization might be expected to underlie the slower glycogen depletion rate observed during exercise. This scenario would not be without precedent. Short-term acclimatization to altitude results in an enhanced utilization of glucose during submaximal exercise (4). As with the short-term training model, a tighter metabolic control is indicated in the absence of change in mitochondrial potential (28).

A tighter metabolic control noted previously with both short-term (21, 26) and long-term training studies (10, 15) has been invariably accompanied by reductions in muscle lactate concentration. The reductions in muscle lactate concentration could occur consequent to an increased removal of lactate or a decreased glycolysis. We have recently examined these possibilities using a primed, continuous infusion of the isotope [3-^{13}C]lactate and found that with 10 d of training, lactate clearance was enhanced in the absence of changes in lactate production (46). These results support the findings of Donovan and Brooks (13) using rats subjected to a much longer duration of training. Although increased lactate clearance rates appear to be an important mechanism for the depression in muscle lactate noted during prolonged exercise following training, we feel that a reduction in glycolytic flux is also implicated. Since the depression in muscle lactate concentration occurs early in the exercise (19), a depressed flux is indicated, which would be difficult to detect with the tracer protocol used. Previous studies have also noted decreased lactate early in stimulation following long-term training and have attributed the decrease to lower lactate production (10, 15). With acclimatization, lactate production is also decreased during moderate exercise (3). However, in contrast to the long-term training studies, the reduction occurs in the absence of an increase in muscle respiratory capacity (28).

Assuming a reduction in glycolytic flux, the most likely mechanism would be inhibition of the nonequilibrium reaction between fructose-6-phosphate (F6P) and fructose-1,6-phosphate (F-1,6-P) mediated by phosphofructokinase (PFK). The reduction in PFK activity could occur as a result of a depression of several of the metabolic effectors of the enzyme, such as ADP, AMP, and Pi, which accompanies the tighter metabolic control noted with training (6, 21, 26). Our short-term training studies have not provided a clear indication of PFK control as indicated by the ratio of F6P to F-1,6-P. We attribute this to the window that we have selected for sampling the tissue for measurement of glycolytic intermediates during exercise. Since the major burst of glycolysis occurs during the transition phase to steady-state exercise, PFK control should be more emphasized during this time period. Sampling later in exercise, for example at 15 min, would mean that removal processes would be much more important. Since many of the modulators of PFK also modulate phosphorylase activity (7), it is possible that both enzymes coordinate to reduce both glycogenolysis and glycolysis.

At least in the voluntarily exercising human, the results seem clear, namely, that an increase in muscle respiratory capacity is not required to induce significant adaptations in muscle energy metabolism and substrate preference over a range of submaximal work rates. What then are the underlying mechanisms? Several possibilities exist. These possibilities address the locus of control as being either within the working muscle itself (peripheral) or external to the muscle (central).

Central Versus Peripheral Regulation of Metabolism

One appealing hypothesis is that the adaptations, at least at the level of the high-energy phosphate transfer reactions, occur because of adjustments in events during the non-steady-state phase of submaximal exercise. To examine this possibility, we have sampled the working vastus lateralis muscle at the transition point between non-steady-state and steady-state exercise and at 15 and 98 min of exercise, prior to and following 4 d of training (19). These results indicate that the tighter metabolic control induced by training was expressed by 3 min of exercise and persisted for the remainder of the exercise period. In addition, lower muscle lactate concentrations were also observed at the transition to steady-state exercise. These findings support previous studies that phosphorylation potential, at least over a spectrum of power outputs below the lactate threshold, is established very early in the exercise and persists during an extended period during the steady-state phase (43, 49). It would appear that short-term training alters one or more events within the window, resulting in less of an imbalance between ATP utilization and ATP synthesis.

Increases in ATP availability could be mediated by altered flux rates in one or more of the ATP-regenerating pathways. Since glycolysis appears to be depressed during the non-steady-state phase following short-term training and therefore would not contribute to elevations in ATP availability, increases in oxidative phosphorylation remain a likely alternative. To examine this possibility, we have measured $\dot{V}O_2$ using an open circuit system with gas collections performed over 30-s intervals during the non-steady-state phase of the exercise. With this measurement system we were not able to detect any alterations in $\dot{V}O_2$ kinetics (19). In subsequent work (unpublished) using a much more sensitive breath-by-breath measurement system, we have been able to detect decreases in the mean response time during moderate intensity cycle exercise following short-term training. Alterations in $\dot{V}O_2$ kinetics have previously been shown to occur in the absence of change in steady-state $\dot{V}O_2$ with β-blockers (34).

Increases in $\dot{V}O_2$ kinetics during the non-steady-state phase of moderate exercise could be mediated either by increases in blood flow to the working muscles or by increases in oxygen extraction. To date, we have examined only the possibility that blood flow has been altered and only in one-leg dynamic exercise (unpublished). Using the noninvasive Doppler procedure to measure blood velocity, we have found decreases in mean response time, indicating a more rapid adjustment in blood flow to steady state. These findings provide further collaborative evidence that adjustments in blood flow may promote an enhancement in oxidative phosphorylation, creating less of a disturbance in energy homeostasis during the non-steady-state phase of moderate exercise. At present, we have no evidence to explain the early adaptation in blood flow; however, additional observations may seem pertinent. The short-term training model is invariably accompanied by alterations in cardiodynamics (20, 23). Heart rate is also depressed concomitantly with the altered metabolic response during the early phase of exercise following training. The reductions in blood norepinephrine levels would suggest a reduction in sympathetic drive and possibly a relief of some of the α-mediated vasoconstriction in skeletal muscle that opposes the dilatory stimulation (42). Another interesting possibility is that the endothelial-derived relaxing factors, in particular nitric oxide, have been increased. Nitric oxide (NO), which has been demonstrated to be a powerful vasodilator in a number of vascular beds, including skeletal muscle, has been shown to be readily adaptable during short-term training in dogs (53).

Changes in the recruitment pattern to the muscles involved in cycling also remain as a distinct possibility to explain the early metabolic adaptations observed following exercise. Cycling involves the recruitment of at least seven different limb muscles, including the anterior group (rectus femoris, vastus medialis, and vastus lateralis) and posterior group (gluteus maximus, biceps femoris, semimembranosus) of the upper leg (44). Since tissue is only harvested from the vastus lateralis muscle, it is possible that the tighter metabolic control following short-term training could have occurred as a result of shifting some of the mechanical load to other synergistic muscles (trade-off and coactivation; 44). Recently, using EMG techniques, we have monitored the activation profiles of the muscles used in cycling at selected times during moderate cycle exercise before and after 6 d of training (50). Activation levels obtained with full-wave-rectified EMG techniques, normalized to the first minute of exercise, were unchanged with training. At 1 min of exercise, no difference existed between the absolute level of activation. In addition, phasic patterns of recruitment evaluated by cross-correlation techniques were unchanged. These results provide convincing evidence that, at least at the level of the whole muscle, the adaptations cannot be explained by alterations in neuromuscular recruitment. It remains possible, however, that compensatory changes could have occurred in recruitment of the different motor units with training, since the vastus lateralis muscle contains a mixture of the different fiber types. At present, we have no direct evidence of this possibility. However, glycogen depletion profiles obtained during exercise indicate higher glycogen levels posttraining in the type I and type IIa fibers, which represent the majority of muscle fiber types within the vastus lateralis (27).

Adaptations external to the muscle that could also mediate the training-induced reduction in glucose preference during prolonged exercise in the absence of changes in oxidative potential remain unclear. With the 10-d training model, pronounced reductions are observed in the concentrations of plasma norepinephrine and epinephrine (25, 41) that could alter both substrate availability to the muscle and utilization of substrate by the working muscle (5, 11). As an example, the reduction in sympathoadrenal drive might be expected to blunt liver glucose production, reducing glucose availability (11). Alternatively, reductions in the catecholamines might blunt muscle glycogenolysis and glycolysis (7). Given the lower lactate and the lower pyruvate utilization by the mitochondria as a consequence of increased free fatty acid utilization during exercise after training, control could conceivably occur at some nonequilibrium step, such as phosphofructokinase (PFK). Increased inhibition to glucose transport does not appear feasible, since we have observed (47), as have others (8, 12), increases in hexokinase and in the glucose transporter GLUT4 with more extended training periods. Since glucose-6-phosphate is unchanged during exercise following training (26), cellular transport would be expected to be facilitated. At least with the 10-d training model, changes in plasma insulin and glucagon concentrations do not appear to be implicated, since no differences were found during exercise prior to and following training (25). This conclusion is also supported by others (41).

The mechanism controlling the increased utilization of fat noted during exercise following short-term training also remains poorly defined. Recent work using stable isotopes (36) has shown that muscle triglycerides not only account for the increase in fat utilization but also partially replace the use of adipose tissue–derived plasma fatty acids during exercise following extended training. Although it is unclear what lipid source—extramuscular versus intramuscular—becomes more emphasized during exercise with short-term training, intramuscular selection appears more probable. As noted with longer duration training models, increases in vascular transport of free fatty acids to the contracting muscle do not seem to occur, since both blood glycerol and serum free fatty acids are unchanged during prolonged exercise following training (25). As has been hypothesized for glucose, the reductions in the catecholamines observed following training could depress adipose tissue lipolysis (5). Since the catecholamines also appear to have some regulatory influence in intramuscular lipolysis, other mechanisms of control would apparently have to occur (18).

One obstacle to assigning a mechanistic role for the catecholamines in mediating a shift toward increased fat utilization following short-term training is the disparate time courses noted between the changes in RER and the change in the catecholamines during exercise. Decreases in catecholamine concentration are observed in the first 3 to 4 d of training in the absence of changes in RER (22), whereas increases in fat utilization occur later, but within 10 d of training (26, 41). It is unknown whether continued training beyond 3 to 4 d further exaggerates the depression in sympathoadrenal drive or whether tissue sensitivity to the catecholamines is altered.

Training-induced decreases in plasma catecholamines conceivably also could account for the lower muscle lactate noted during exercise. Based on the observation that the catecholamines, and in particular plasma epinephrine, have been shown to correlate with blood lactate changes (39), reductions in epinephrine could depress glycogenolysis and glycolysis (7), resulting in less lactate production. However, recent work using altitude acclimatization, in which depressions in muscle lactate (28) also are observed during exercise in the absence of altered muscle respiratory capacity, suggests that other mechanisms are involved (38). In this study, β-blockade was unable to prevent the lactate increase during exercise after acclimatization.

Another central factor of potential importance in altering peripheral metabolic events is the increase in plasma volume noted with short-term training. Plasma volume has been observed to increase by as much as 20% (23). This elevation in plasma volume in theory could account for the reductions in blood catecholamines noted with exercise or could alter peripheral resistance and blood flow (42). Excessive increases in plasma volume, however, could obviate any potential advantage due to the dilution effect and reductions in arterial oxygen content.

The possibility remains that adaptations in metabolic behavior in short-term-trained muscles could have an intramuscular locus even in the absence of changes in respiratory capacity. The tighter metabolic control that is expressed during the non-steady-state adjustment to moderate exercise would appear to represent an increased mitochondrial sensitivity to the effectors of mitochondrial respiration such as ADP_f or Pi, since mitochondrial flux rates were either unchanged or increased as indicated by $\dot{V}O_2$ kinetics (19). An increase in mitochondrial sensitivity could have occurred as a consequence of increased availability of O_2 or of an increase in mitochondrial redox potential (57). As previously noted, increases in O_2 availability to the mitochondria might have occurred because of increased blood flow (unpublished). Mitochondrial respiratory rate also appears to be very sensitive to the intramitochondrial $[NAD^+]/[NADH]$ ratio (57).

Increases in the mitochondrial sensitivity could occur because of increases in glycolytically generated H^+ and transport into the mitochondria (9) or because of increases in intramitochondrial free calcium (40). During increased contractile activity, the increase in cytosolic free Ca^{2+} (Ca^{2+}_f) needed to activate the myofibrillar apparatus is believed to be transmitted to the mitochondria by specific uptake and release pathways, resulting in activation of three separate mitochondrial dehydrogenase reactions and increases in H^+ production and redox potential (29, 40). In the absence of changes in mitochondrial H^+ transport processes, increases in cytosolic H^+ production do not appear to be a viable hypothesis, because glycolysis appears to be depressed early in exercise with short-term training (19). It is also unclear how increased mitochondrial Ca^{2+} levels would occur with moderate exercise following short-term training. Direct measurements of cytosolic Ca^{2+}_f levels during moderate exercise support a decrease, at least in fast-twitch fibers (55). Although force levels are depressed at low frequencies of stimulation following repetitive stimulation, no force decrements apparently occur in moderate-intensity exercise, due to the presence of myosin light chain phosphorylation (54). Conceivably, myosin light chain phosphorylation might represent a mechanism for maintaining the integrity of force levels at lower levels of Ca^{2+} activation. Maximal force levels are not compromised because of supersaturating levels of Ca^{2+}_f. A dampening of the cytosolic Ca^{2+}_f levels during acute exercise could conceivably attenuate glycogenolysis and glycolysis, since Ca^{2+}_f has been implicated in the control of phosphorylase and PFK (51). Whether the Ca^{2+} sensitivity of the actomyosin complex is altered with training, permitting similar force levels and lower Ca^{2+}_f, is unknown (56).

To examine whether the metabolic adaptations noted in the vastus lateralis muscle with voluntary cycle activity result from changes within the muscle, we have used electrical stimulation to elevate the activity level. Previous studies (10, 14, 15) have demonstrated a tighter metabolic control and a reduced muscle lactate concentration in stimulated muscles of rats subjected to long-term training using treadmill exercise. Our results with the vastus lateralis of humans indicate no effect of the training on phosphorylation potential but an increase in lactate concentration (unpublished). We attribute the increase in lactate concentration to mass action effects mediated by the elevated resting glycogen levels that occur with the training. These results suggest that, at least in the stimulated muscle, increases in mitochondrial potential are indeed necessary for the metabolic adaptations to be realized. It is possible that increases in $\dot{V}O_2$ kinetics and blood flow kinetics, as examples, are potential adaptations to the short-term training and can only be realized with voluntary, dynamic activity.

Significance of Mitochondrial Potential in Metabolic Regulation

If the classic adaptations in metabolism and fuel utilization can be imposed with short-term training in the absence of changes in mitochondrial potential, the question is presented of the role of increases in mitochondrial potential. Two hypotheses appear possible. On the one hand, increases in mitochondrial potential that occur later in training may act to further exaggerate the adaptations realized early in training. Conversely, the increases in respiratory capacity may represent another mechanistic strategy serving to replace the mechanism that occurred early in training. To investigate these hypotheses, we have performed an 8-wk training study with measurements performed prior to training and at 4 and 8 wk of training. All adaptations were fully realized by 4 wk. When these results were compared to a 5- to 7-d training program, we found that no further adaptation in phosphorylation potential, lactate concentration, or RER had occurred (24). Recently, however, Mendenhall et al. (41), using the same subject pool tested after both 10 d and 12 wk of endurance training, found further decreases in RER and glucose utilization. It is not clear why the two studies produced different results. However, the training progression may be significant. Training was much more progressive in the Mendenhall et al. study (41) than in our study (25).

Summary

The results of the short-term training experiments completed to date strongly suggest that, at least in the voluntarily exercising human, increases in mitochondrial potential are not required to elicit at least qualitative adaptations in metabolism and substrate selection. This would suggest that other adaptive strategies may prevail soon after the initiation of training. What these strategies are remains to be elucidated.

Acknowledgment

This work was supported by the Natural Sciences and Engineering Research Council of Canada (NSERC).

References

1. Bonen, A.; McDermott, J.C.; Hutber, C.A. Carbohydrate metabolism in skeletal muscle: An update of current concepts. Int. J. Sports Med. 10:385-401; 1989.
2. Brooks, G.A. Current concepts in lactate exchange. Med. Sci. Sports Exercise 23:895-906; 1991.
3. Brooks, G.A.; Butterfield, G.E.; Wolfe, R.R.; Groves, B.M.; Mazzeo, R.S.; Sutton, J.R.; Wolfel, E.E.; Reeves, J.T. Decreased reliance on lactate during exercise after acclimatization to 4,300 m exercise. J. Appl. Physiol. 71:333-341; 1991.
4. Brooks, G.A.; Butterfield, G.E.; Wolfe, R.R.; Groves, B.M.; Mazzeo, R.S.; Sutton, J.R.; Wolfel, E.E.; Reeves, J.T. Increased dependence on blood glucose after acclimatization to 4,300 m. J. Appl. Physiol. 70:919-927; 1991.
5. Brooks, G.A.; Mercer, J. Balance of carbohydrate and lipid utilization during exercise: The "crossover concept." J. Appl. Physiol. 76:2253-2261; 1994.
6. Cadefau, J.; Green, H.J.; Cussó, R.; Ball-Burnett, M.; Jamieson, G. Coupling of muscle phosphorylation potential to glycolysis during submaximal exercise

of varying intensity following short term training. J. Appl. Physiol. 76:2586-2593; 1994.

7. Chasiotis, D.; Sahlin, K.; Hultman, E. Regulation of glycogenolysis in human skeletal muscle at rest and during exercise. J. Appl. Physiol. 53:708-715; 1982.

8. Coggan, A.R.; Spina, R.J.; Kohrt, W.M.; Bier, D.M.; Holloszy, J.O. Effect of prolonged exercise on muscle citrate concentration before and after endurance training in men. Am. J. Physiol. 264:E215-E220; 1993.

9. Connett, R.J.; Honig, C.R.; Gayeski, T.E.J.; Brooks, G.A. Defining hypoxia: A systems view of VO_2, glycolysis, energetics and intracellular PO_2. J. Appl. Physiol. 68:833-842; 1990.

10. Constable, S.H.; Favier, R.J.; McLane, J.A.; Fell, R.D.; Chen, M.; Holloszy, J.O. Energy metabolism in contracting rat skeletal muscle: Adaptation to exercise training. Am. J. Physiol. 253:C316-C322; 1987.

11. Cryer, P.E. Glucose counterregulation: Prevention and correction for hypoglycemia in humans. Am. J. Physiol. 264:E149-E155; 1993.

12. Dela, F.; Handberg, A.; Mikines, K.J.; Vinten, J.; Galbo, H. Glut4 and insulin receptor binding and kinase activity in trained human muscle. J. Physiol. (London) 469:610-615; 1993.

13. Donovan, C.M.; Brooks, G.A. Endurance training affects lactate clearance not lactate production. Am. J. Physiol. 244:E83-E92; 1983.

14. Dudley, G.A.; Tullson, P.C.; Terjung, R.L. Influence of mitochondrial content on the sensitivity of respiratory control. J. Biol. Chem. 262:9109-9114; 1987.

15. Favier, R.J.; Constable, S.H.; Chen, M.; Holloszy, J.O. Endurance training reduces lactate production. J. Appl. Physiol. 61:885-889; 1986.

16. Gollnick, P.D. Metabolic regulation in skeletal muscle. Influence of endurance training as exerted by mitochondrial protein concentration. Acta Physiol. Scand. 128:53-66; 1986.

17. Gollnick, P.D.; Saltin, B. Significance of skeletal muscle oxidative enzyme enhancement with endurance training. Clin. Physiol. 2:1-12; 1982.

18. Gorski, J. Muscle triglyceride metabolism during exercise. Can. J. Physiol. Pharmacol. 70:123-131; 1992.

19. Green, H.J.; Cadefau, J.; Cussó, R.; Ball-Burnett, M.; Jamieson, G. Metabolic adaptations to short term training are expressed early in exercise. Can. J. Physiol. Pharmacol. 73:474-482; 1995.

20. Green, H.J.; Coates, G.; Sutton, J.R.; Jones, S. Early adaptations in gas exchange, cardiac function and hematology to prolonged exercise training in man. Eur. J. Appl. Physiol. 63:17-23; 1991.

21. Green, H.; Helyar, R.; Ball-Burnett, M.; Kowalchuk, N.; Symon, S.; Farrance, B. Metabolic adaptations to training precede changes in muscle mitochondrial capacity. J. Appl. Physiol. 72:484-491; 1992.

22. Green, H.J.; Jones, L.L.; Houston, M.E.; Ball-Burnett, M.E.; Farrance, B.W. Muscle energetics during prolonged cycling after exercise hypervolemia. J. Appl. Physiol. 66(2):622-631; 1989.

23. Green, H.J.; Jones, L.L.; Hughson, R.L.; Painter, D.C.; Farrance, B.W. Training-induced hypervolemia: Lack of an effect on oxygen utilization during exercise. Med. Sci. Sports Exercise 19(3):202-206; 1987.

24. Green, H.J.; Jones, S.; Ball-Burnett, M.; Farrance, B.; Ranney, D. Adaptations in muscle metabolism to prolonged exercise and training. J. Appl. Physiol. 78:138-145; 1995.

25. Green, H.J.; Jones, S.; Ball-Burnett, M.; Fraser, I. Early adaptations in blood substrates, metabolites, and hormones to prolonged exercise training in man. Can. J. Physiol. Pharmacol. 69:1222-1229; 1991.

26. Green, H.J.; Jones, S.; Ball-Burnett, M.E.; Smith, D.; Livesey, J.; Farrance, B.W. Early muscular and metabolic adaptations to prolonged exercise training in man. J. Appl. Physiol. 70:2032-2038; 1991.

27. Green, H.J.; Smith, D.; Murphy, P.; Fraser, I. Training-induced alterations in muscle glycogen utilization in fibre-specific types during prolonged exercise. Can. J. Physiol. Pharmacol. 68:1372-1376; 1990.

28. Green, H.J.; Sutton, J.R.; Wolfel, E.E.; Reeves, J.T.; Butterfield, G.E.; Brooks, G.A. Altitude acclimatization and energy metabolic adaptations in skeletal muscle during submaximal exercise. J. Appl. Physiol. 73:2701-2708; 1992.

29. Hansford, R.G. Role of calcium in respiratory control. Med. Sci. Sports Exercise 26:44-51; 1994.

30. Henriksson, J. Training induced adaptation of skeletal muscle and metabolism during submaximal exercise. J. Appl. Physiol. (London) 270:661-675; 1977.

31. Hochachka, P.W. The lactate paradox. Analysis of underlying mechanisms. Ann. Sports Med. 4:184-188; 1988.

32. Holloszy, J.O.; Coyle, E.F. Adaptations of skeletal muscle to endurance exercise and their metabolic consequences. J. Appl. Physiol. 56:831-838; 1984.

33. Howald, H.; Pette, D.; Simoneau, J.A.; Uber, A.; Hoppeler, H.; Ceretelli, P., III. Effect of chronic hypoxia on muscle enzyme activities. Int. J. Sports Med. 11 (suppl. 1):510-514; 1990.

34. Hughson, R.L. Alterations in the oxygen deficit–oxygen debt relationships with β-adrenergic receptor blockade in man. J. Physiol. 349:375-387; 1984.

35. Karlsson, J.; Nordesjo, L.-O.; Jorfeldt, L.; Saltin, B. Muscle lactate, ATP and CP levels during exercise after physical training in man. J. Appl. Physiol. 33:199-203; 1972.

36. Martin, W.H., III; Dalsky, G.P.; Hurley, B.F.; Mathews, D.E.; Bier, D.M.; Hagberg, J.M.; Rogers, M.A.; King, D.S.; Holloszy, J.O. Effect of endurance training on free fatty acid turnover and oxidation during exercise. Am. J. Physiol. 265:E708-E714; 1994.

37. Matheson, G.O.; Allen, P.S.; Ellinger, D.C.; Hanstock, C.C.; Gheorghiu, D.; McKenzie, D.C.; Stanley, C.; Parkhouse, W.S.; Hochachka, P.W. Skeletal muscle metabolism and work capacity—A ^{31}P-NMR study of Andean natives and lowlanders. J. Appl. Physiol. 70:1963-1976; 1991.

38. Mazzeo, R.S.; Brooks, G.A.; Butterfield, G.E.; Cymerman, A.; Roberts, A.C.; Selland, M.; Wolfel, E.E.; Reeves, J.T. β-Adrenergic blockade does not prevent the lactate response to exercise after acclimatization to high altitude. J. Appl. Physiol. 76:610-615; 1994.

39. Mazzeo, R.S.; Marshall, P. Influence of plasma catecholamines on the lactate threshold during graded exercise. J. Appl. Physiol. 67:1319-1322; 1989.

40. McCormack, J.G.; Denton, R.M. Signal transduction by intramitochondrial Ca^{2+} in mammalian energy metabolism. Trends Physiol. Sci. 9:71-76; 1994.

41. Mendenhall, L.A.; Swanson, S.C.; Hobosh, D.L.; Coggan, A.R. Ten days of exercise training reduces glucose production and utilization during moderate-intensity exercise. Am. J. Physiol. 266:E136-E143; 1994.

42. Mitchell, J.H.; Raven, P.B. Cardiovascular adaptation to physical activity. In: Bouchard, C.; Shephard, R.J.; Stephens, T., eds. Physical activity, fitness and health. Champaign, IL: Human Kinetics Publishers; 1994:286-301.

43. Norman, B.; Solleui, A.; Kaijser, L.; Jansson, E. ATP breakdown products in human skeletal muscle during prolonged exercise to exhaustion. Clin. Physiol. 7:503-509; 1987.
44. Patla, A.E. Some neuromuscular strategies characterizing adaptation process during prolonged activity in humans. Can. J. Sport Sci. 12(3):33S-44S; 1982.
45. Phillips, S.M.; Green, H.J.; Tarnopolsky, M.A.; Grant, S.M. Decreased glucose turnover following short term training. Amer. J. Physiol. 269:E222-E230; 1995.
46. Phillips, S.M.; Green, H.J.; Tarnopolsky, M.A.; Grant, S.M. Increased lactate clearance following endurance training in humans. J. Appl. Physiol. 79:1862-1869; 1995.
47. Phillips, S.M.; Green, H.J.; Tarnopolsky, M.A.; Grant, S.M.; Han, X.; Bonen, A. Short term training: Effects on muscle and whole-body substrate turnover. Can. J. Appl. Physiol. 19(Supplement):37; 1994.
48. Rosser, B.W.C.; Hochachka, P.W. Metabolic capacity of muscle fibers from high-altitude natives. Eur. J. Appl. Physiol. 67:513-517; 1993.
49. Sahlin, K.; Katz, A.; Broberg, S. Tricarboxylic acid cycle intermediates in human skeletal muscle during prolonged exercise. Am. J. Physiol. 259:C834-C841; 1990.
50. Simpson, M.; Green, H.; Patla, A.; Tate, C.; Grant, S. Adaptations in the neuromuscular system to prolonged exercise following short term training. Can. J. Appl. Physiol. 19(Supplement):44; 1994
51. Spriet, L.L. Anaerobic metabolism in human skeletal muscle during short-term intensity activity. Can. J. Physiol. Pharmacol. 70:157-165; 1992.
52. Spriet, L.L. Phosphofructokinase activity and acidosis during short-term tetanic contractions. Can. J. Physiol. Pharmacol. 69:298-304; 1991.
53. Sun, D.; Huang, A.; Koller, A.; Kaley, G. Short-term daily exercise activity enhances endothelial NO synthesis in skeletal muscle arterioles in rats. J. Appl. Physiol. 76:2241-2247; 1994.
54. Sweeney, H.L.; Bowman, B.F.; Stull, J.T. Myosin light chain phosphorylation in vertebrate striated muscle: Regulation and function. Am. J. Physiol. 264:C1085-C1095; 1993.
55. Westerblad, H.; Duty, S.; Allen, D.G. Intracellular calcium concentration during low-frequency fatigue in isolated single fibers of mouse skeletal muscle. J. Appl. Physiol. 75:382-388; 1993.
56. Westerblad, H.; Lee, J.A.; Lännergren, J.; Allen, D.G. Cellular mechanisms of fatigue in skeletal muscle. Am. J. Physiol. 261:C195-C209; 1991.
57. Wilson, D.F. Factors affecting the rate and energetics of mitochondrial oxidative phosphorylation. Med. Sci. Sports Exercise 26:37-43; 1994.

CHAPTER 28

The Effect of Exercise Training on Insulin-Stimulated Glucose Uptake in Rat Skeletal Muscle

John L. Ivy
University of Texas, Austin, Texas, U.S.A.

Blood glucose is maintained within narrow limits by opposing forces: those adding glucose to and those removing glucose from the circulation. In the postabsorptive state, glucose release from the liver is balanced with glucose clearance by the nervous system and peripheral tissues. However, postprandial glucose entry via the digestive system disrupts this balance, resulting in a rise in blood glucose. The blood glucose concentration is returned to within the normal range through the actions of the pancreatic hormone insulin. Sensing the elevation in circulating glucose, the pancreas increases insulin secretion, resulting in reduced glucose output from the liver and enhanced glucose uptake of insulin-sensitive peripheral tissues. Although the reduction in glucose output by the liver is beneficial in lowering blood glucose, the increase in glucose clearance is quantitatively more important. The tissue most responsible for the clearance of blood glucose following a glucose challenge is skeletal muscle, which accounts for 65% to 90% of the clearance of an oral or intravenous glucose load (10, 28).

Exercise training is associated with a lowering of the postabsorptive plasma insulin concentration and an attenuation of the insulin response to an oral or intravenous glucose load (4, 5, 32). Despite the lower insulin concentration, glucose tolerance is unchanged or improved in the trained state. As a result of the predominant role of skeletal muscle in the decrease of a postprandial glucose load, it has been assumed that the improvements in insulin action and glucose tolerance following exercise training result from changes in skeletal muscle. In this chapter the evidence for an exercise training effect on insulin-stimulated glucose uptake in non-insulin-resistant and insulin-resistant skeletal muscle of the rat will be reviewed.

Non-Insulin-Resistant Muscle

Using the perfused hindlimb technique, Berger et al. (4) and Mondon, Dolkas, and Rearen (33) found that hindlimb glucose uptake at the same insulin concentration was greater in exercise-trained than in sedentary rats. These findings were interpreted as evidence that exercise training induces adaptations resulting in enhanced skeletal muscle insulin sensitivity and that this adaptation is primarily responsible for improvements in total body glucose tolerance. In support of these findings, James, Kraegen, and Chisholm (25) observed that glucose clearance in exercise-trained rats was significantly greater than that in sedentary rats during a euglycemic clamp. Furthermore, using tritiated 2-deoxyglucose as a tracer, it was also demonstrated that the increased glucose clearance in the trained rats was associated with a greater rate of skeletal muscle glucose uptake.

In an attempt to better characterize the effects of prolonged training on insulin-stimulated muscle glucose uptake, however, we were unable to confirm the findings of Berger et al. (4), Mondon, Dolkas, and Rearen (33), and James, Kraegen, and Chisholm (25). We trained rats on a motor-driven treadmill up a 15% grade 5 d/ wk. The speed and duration of the training were progressively increased until after 12 wk the rats were running continuously at 32 m/min for 2 h/d. This is an intense training program that induces large changes in endurance, mitochondrial content of muscle, body composition, and metabolic response to exercise. When subjected to hindlimb perfusion following this training regimen, insulin-stimulated glucose uptake was approximately 50% higher in trained rats than in untrained rats on the day after their last training session (24). However, by the second day after the last training session, there were no significant differences in hindlimb glucose uptake rates between the trained and the sedentary rats either in the absence of insulin, at a physiological insulin concentration, or at a maximally effective insulin concentration. Of interest, a single bout of exercise, consisting of swimming to fatigue on the day before perfusion, resulted in a similar increase in insulin-stimulated hindlimb glucose uptake for trained and untrained rats (24).

Subsequent studies by Idström et al. (21) and Goodyear et al. (16), also using the perfused hindlimb procedure, confirmed our findings. In addition, Idström et al. (21) found that varying perfusate glucose concentrations from 2 to 25 mM increased insulin-stimulated glucose uptake; however, there were still no differences between trained and untrained rats. From these studies, it was concluded that the increased rate of muscle glucose uptake at the same insulin concentration in trained as compared with sedentary rats is primarily due to persistent effects of the last bout of exercise rather than to a long-term effect of training.

Recent advances in our understanding of how insulin controls muscle glucose uptake, however, renewed the interest in the effects of exercise training on this process. Evidence suggests that maximal insulin-stimulated glucose transport capacity is directly related to the concentration of glucose transporters (specifically the GLUT4 isoform) in a given muscle (2, 18, 29, 35). When the ability of insulin to stimulate glucose uptake is reduced in muscle, as after streptozotocin treatment (26, 38), denervation (19, 37), or physical inactivity (15), the GLUT4 protein concentration has also been found to be reduced. Conversely, Ploug et al. (34) and Rodnick et al. (35) found significant increases in total GLUT4 protein of selected muscles from exercise-trained rats examined within 24 h of the last exercise session. These results immediately led to speculation that a training response, and not just the acute effect of the last exercise bout, is responsible for the increase in insulin-stimulated glucose uptake observed within 24 h of the cessation of training. It must be emphasized, however, that these effects were examined within 7 to 24 h of the last exercise session, and thus the persistence of exercise-induced increases in skeletal muscle GLUT4 protein remained to be determined.

As a result of these findings, we found it necessary to repeat our initial study in order to resolve the question of whether exercise training has an effect independent of the last exercise bout on insulin-stimulated glucose uptake. In our previous study (24), it was possible that subtle alterations in individual muscles were overlooked, since we examined glucose uptake across the active hindlimb. Therefore, in addition to determining hindlimb glucose uptake, we used the nonmetabolizable glucose analog 3-O-methyl-D-glucose (3-MG) to examine rates of glucose uptake in individual muscles (12). We also determined the GLUT4 protein concentration in the individual muscles of the hindlimb.

Maximal insulin-stimulated hindlimb glucose uptake was approximately 30% above sedentary levels in trained rats examined within 24 h of their last exercise session. However, in confirmation of our previous study (24), when rats were examined 48 h after their last exercise session, hindlimb glucose uptake was not different from sedentary levels. The examination of individual muscles revealed that maximal 3-MG uptake was enhanced above sedentary levels in red (fast-twitch, oxidative) and white (fast-twitch, glycolytic) gastrocnemius and plantaris (mixed) muscles, but not soleus (slow-twitch, oxidative) muscles of rats perfused 24 h after exercise. In addition, GLUT4 protein concentration was significantly elevated in those muscles that exhibited enhanced 3-MG uptake. Taken alone, these results may be interpreted to suggest that exercise training enhances muscle GLUT4 protein, resulting in increased insulin-stimulated glucose uptake. However, we also observed that GLUT4 protein was significantly elevated 48 h after the last exercise session, yet despite this increase in glucose transporters, 3-MG uptake was not different from sedentary controls (12). Therefore, we thought it possible that the increased GLUT4 protein may not be contributing as much as previously hypothesized to the enhanced insulin-stimulated glucose uptake observed 24 h after the cessation of training, especially when it was considered that acute exercise has a protracted effect on insulin-stimulated glucose uptake under certain conditions.

Cartee et al. (8) demonstrated that maximal insulin-stimulated 3-MG uptake remains elevated for up to 18 h following an acute exercise bout only when rats are fasted or deprived of carbohydrate following the exercise session. Therefore, since our rats perfused 24 h after exercise were fasted from the time of their last exercise session until perfusion, it was possible that the results we observed for these rats were due to the acute effects of exercise followed by fasting. To test this hypothesis, we performed a separate experiment on another group of trained rats (12). These rats were subjected to the same protocol as the rats perfused 24 h after exercise, except they were provided access to food and water for 3 h immediately after their last exercise session. If the enhanced insulin responsiveness we observed in our fasted rats perfused 24 h after exercise was an acute, exercise-induced effect as demonstrated by Cartee et al. (8), it would be expected that glucose uptake and transport in muscles of our fed rats would be no different from that of our sedentary rats. However, the results of this experiment were no different from our previous findings. The fed rats perfused 24 h after exercise had glucose uptake rates similar to that of fasted rats perfused 24 h after exercise. As a result of these findings, our initial hypothesis was modified. We now believe that exercise training enhances maximal insulin-stimulated glucose uptake independently of the effects of the last exercise session, because the training response is not influenced by fasting or feeding. Like acute exercise, this effect is short lived, lasting less than 48 h.

The role of the increased GLUT4 protein concentration with regard to the enhanced insulin-stimulated glucose uptake is not immediately clear. Figure 28.1 depicts the

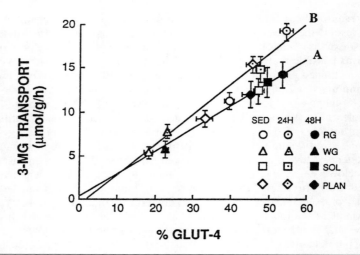

Figure 28.1   Relationship between percentage GLUT4 protein and 3-MG uptake in red (RG) and white (WG) gastrocnemius, soleus (SOL), and plantaris (PLAN) for sedentary control (SED) and trained rats perfused either 24 h (24H) or 48 h (48H) after last exercise session. (A), regression line for SED and 48H rats. (B), regression line for 24H rats. Based on results from Etgen et al. 1993 (12).

relationship we observed between GLUT4 protein concentration and 3-MG uptake. As illustrated by line A of figure 28.1, which represents the regression line of sedentary values, it is apparent that maximal insulin-stimulated 3-MG uptake is positively related with GLUT4 protein concentration. However, if the difference in 3-MG uptake that we observed between sedentary muscle and muscle from rats perfused 24 h after exercise were due solely to enhanced GLUT4 protein concentration, then values for the exercised rats would be located approximately on line A. This, however, is not what we observed. For a given increase in GLUT4 protein concentration in muscle of rats perfused 24 h after exercise, the magnitude of the corresponding increase in 3-MG uptake was greater than could be explained solely by the increase in GLUT4 protein, resulting in a significant increase in the slope of the regression line, as illustrated by line B. This shift in the slope of the regression line indicates that some factor(s) other than increased GLUT4 protein contributed to the enhanced rate of 3-MG uptake observed. This conclusion is further supported by the finding that the 3-MG uptake rates of sedentary rats and rats perfused 48 h after exercise were similar despite differences in muscle GLUT4 protein concentration.

The GLUT4 transporter is sequestered in a unique intracellular vesicular compartment under basal conditions (11, 20, 27). In response to insulin, these GLUT4-containing vesicles are translocated to and fuse with the plasma membrane, which results in an increased ability to transport glucose (11, 20, 27; figure 28.2). Therefore, other possible mechanisms through which exercise training may alter glucose transport include redistribution of GLUT4 protein between intracellular storage compartments and the plasma membrane, increased GLUT4 protein functional activity, and alterations in the insulin signal transduction process or glucose transporter translocation process.

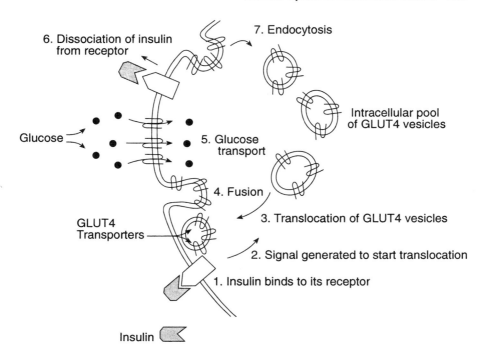

Figure 28.2   A hypothetical model of the stimulatory action of insulin on glucose transport. Insulin binds to its receptor on the plasma membrane and generates an intracellular signal that results in the exocytotic movement of membrane vesicles containing GLUT4 from an intracellular pool to the plasma membrane. The vesicles then fuse with the plasma membrane, exposing GLUT4 transporters to the extracellular medium and increasing the glucose transport process. Once insulin dissociates from its receptor the process is reversed. Modified from the model by Karnieli et al. 1981 (27).

Recently, Goodyear et al. (17) reported that exercise training increased the plasma membrane GLUT4 protein concentration of rat skeletal muscle and that this increase persisted for several days. Training, however, had no effect on the functional activity of the transporter as assessed by vesicle transport or insulin-stimulated translocation of the transporter from its intracellular pool to the plasma membrane. It was concluded that increased rates of glucose uptake in the endurance-trained skeletal muscle results primarily from an increase in the number of plasma membrane glucose transporters and not from an increase in their functional activity. The findings of Goodyear et al. (17), however, do not explain the reversal of this training response that we observed 48 h after the last exercise bout, nor do their results explain the increase in glucose transport that was not associated with an increased number of glucose transporters.

In general, it can be concluded that exercise training of normal rats results in an elevated muscle insulin responsiveness. These results are not dependent on feeding status and thus can be attributed to exercise training rather than to acute exercise effects. Associated with the enhanced insulin-stimulated glucose uptake is an increase in GLUT4 protein concentration. However, within 48 h of the cessation of exercise training, glucose uptake reverts back to a level not different from that of sedentary rats despite an elevated GLUT4 protein concentration. These results suggest that exercise training induces a short-lived increase in maximal insulin-stimulated glucose uptake in normal rats and that this increase is only partially explained by an increase in total muscle GLUT4 protein concentration.

Insulin-Resistant Muscle

The effects of exercise training on muscle insulin resistance has been evaluated in many different rodent models, including streptozotocin-treated rats, immobilized limb models, and muscle denervation models, to name a few. However, the most extensively studied model is the obese Zucker rat. The obese Zucker rat appeared as the result of a spontaneous mutation in a cross between Merck stock M and Sherman rats (1). The condition is thought to be due to a single recessive gene. The obesity can be partially explained by hyperphagia and decreased activity levels, but obese rats pair-fed with lean rats still become obese. Besides its obesity, this rat is glucose intolerant and highly insulin resistant (1, 9). The muscle of the obese Zucker rat displays both decreased insulin sensitivity and responsiveness (22, 36). By comparing the rates of insulin-stimulated glucose uptake in the hindlimb muscles of obese and lean Zucker rats, we demonstrated that the locus of their muscle insulin resistance is associated with a defect in the glucose transport process and that this defect is common to the three basic skeletal muscle fiber types: fast-twitch, red oxidative; fast-twitch, white glycolytic; and slow-twitch, red oxidative.

Becker-Zimmermann et al. (3) were the first to show that exercise training could improve insulin-stimulated hindlimb glucose uptake in obese Zucker rats. We confirmed the results of Becker-Zimmermann et al. (3) when we demonstrated that exercise training of obese Zucker rats resulted in a 46% increase in insulin-stimulated hindlimb glucose uptake 48 h after their last exercise session (23). We also investigated glucose uptake in various fiber types of trained and untrained obese Zucker rats over a range of insulin concentrations (0, 0.15, 1.5, and 15.0 mU/ml; 22). Training resulted in an increase in basal and insulin-stimulated glucose uptake in the red gastrocnemius. No improvement in insulin-stimulated glucose uptake was seen in the extensor digitorum longus (EDL, mixed fiber type composition), soleus, or white gastrocnemius. Furthermore, the increase in glucose uptake in the red gastrocnemius was due to an increase in responsiveness and not an increase in sensitivity (22). This suggested that the improvement was due to a post-insulin-receptor adaptation related directly to the transport process (movement of glucose across the plasma membrane).

Because no improvement in insulin-stimulated glucose uptake was noted in the white gastrocnemius or EDL and because these muscles demonstrated little if any increase in oxidative capacity with training, it was suggested that muscle recruitment is required for improvement in insulin-stimulated glucose uptake. Furthermore, the soleus, which was recruited during exercise as evidenced by an increase in oxidative capacity, did not demonstrate an improvement in insulin responsiveness. Therefore, the results also suggested that the training-induced increase in insulin-stimulated glucose uptake is fiber type specific and that slow-twitch, oxidative fibers do not increase insulin-stimulated glucose uptake in response to exercise training.

Because it was observed that the improvements in insulin-stimulated glucose uptake were restricted to those muscles that were active during exercise, we examined whether increasing the amount of muscle that was active during exercise training would further increase insulin-stimulated glucose uptake. This was accomplished by exercising rats either at a low intensity, which required an oxygen consumption of 65% to 70% of $\dot{V}O_2$max, or at a high intensity, which required an oxygen consumption of 80% to 85% $\dot{V}O_2$max. The total amount of work and caloric expenditure were held constant for the exercise-trained rats (9, 39).

We observed that the increases in hindlimb glucose uptake in the presence of a submaximal and maximal insulin concentration were further enhanced with increasing intensity of training (9, 39). As previously observed, low-intensity exercise training only resulted in an increase in insulin-stimulated glucose uptake in the red gastrocnemius (9). High-intensity exercise training, however, resulted in an increase in insulin-stimulated glucose uptake in the red gastrocnemius, plantaris, and white gastrocnemius (9). The increases in insulin-stimulated glucose uptake in the different muscle types closely paralleled increases in citrate synthase activity, except in the soleus. Although the soleus demonstrated a significant increase in citrate synthase activity following the low- and high-intensity training protocols, exercise training had no effect on the insulin-stimulated glucose uptake in this muscle.

These findings confirmed our hypothesis that the improvement in insulin-stimulated glucose uptake in the muscle of the obese rat is exercise-intensity specific and only occurs in muscles substantially recruited during training. It also suggested that training-induced improvements in insulin-stimulated glucose uptake are fiber type specific. That is, only fast-twitch fibers demonstrate an improved insulin action after an exercise training program. This phenomenon does not appear to be unique to the obese Zucker rat. Studies by Ploug et al. (34) and Rodnick et al. (35) as well as from our laboratory (12) have failed to demonstrate an increase in insulin-stimulated glucose uptake in the soleus of non-insulin-resistant rats.

Initial studies using various models of insulin resistance had suggested that muscle insulin resistance was due to a reduced GLUT4 protein concentration (19, 38). On the other hand, Kahn et al. (26) found that streptozotocin-treated rats displayed in vivo insulin resistance before a decline in skeletal muscle GLUT4 protein concentration. In addition, Friedman et al. (14) found that the GLUT4 protein concentrations of gastrocnemius muscles from obese and lean Zucker rats were similar. In fact, muscle insulin resistance without a deficient concentration of GLUT4 protein is not unique to the Zucker rat. The muscle of the db/db mouse, another model of obesity and insulin resistance, also expresses normal GLUT4 protein concentrations (31), and recently it was observed that the insulin resistance of NIDDM patients cannot be attributed to a reduced muscle GLUT4 protein concentration (13). These findings are in agreement with more recent observations from our laboratory that the GLUT4 protein concentration in the red gastrocnemius and soleus muscle of the obese rat is similar to that of its lean littermate (2, 6, 7). Only the white gastrocnemius of the obese rat was found to have a lower GLUT4 protein concentration than that of its lean littermate, but the difference was small and could not account for the insulin-resistant state of this muscle.

Since the muscle insulin resistance of the obese Zucker rat could not be explained by a deficient GLUT4 protein concentration, it was hypothesized that this condition may stem from an inability to recruit glucose transporters to the plasma membrane or from a defect in the activity of the transporter. King et al. (30) investigated these possibilities by comparing the effects of an intraperitoneal insulin injection on muscle GLUT4 protein distribution and intrinsic activity in lean and obese Zucker rats. They found that the insulin treatment increased the plasma membrane GLUT4 protein concentration 1.4-fold in lean rats but had no significant effect on obese Zucker rats. It was also found, by measuring glucose uptake in membrane vesicles under equilibrium exchange conditions, that insulin resulted in a doubling of the average carrier turnover number (intrinsic activity) in lean rats. A similar carrier turnover number was found in obese rats. It was concluded that the insulin resistance of the obese Zucker rat is due to an inability to translocate glucose transporters, while average carrier turnover number is normal. With the use of this in vivo model, however, it is not possible to compare the direct effects of insulin on GLUT4 protein translocation or transporter intrinsic activity between lean and obese Zucker rats because responses of counterregulatory hormones to the insulin injection may differ between these phenotypes. We therefore used the hindlimb perfusion technique to investigate the effects of insulin on GLUT4 protein distribution in muscle of lean and obese Zucker rats.

In agreement with King et al. (30), we found that GLUT4 protein translocation was significantly less in obese than in lean Zucker rats (6). However, examination of the functional activity of GLUT4 protein in the plasma membrane, as assessed by the ratio of glucose uptake to plasma membrane GLUT4 protein concentration, indicated that there was also a defect in the ability of insulin to activate or increase the functional activity of the GLUT4 protein in the obese rats (6). The differences in the results could be related to the fact that the glucose uptake measurements in the study by King et al. (30) were made in isolated membrane vesicles in vitro, whereas in our study glucose uptake was measured in situ during hindlimb perfusion. This would suggest that factors that modulate the functional activity of GLUT4 protein may be removed during the membrane isolation procedure. Nevertheless, the results from each of these studies provide good evidence that insulin-stimulated GLUT4 protein translocation is defective in the muscle of the obese rat and that glucose uptake is a multistep process involving both GLUT4 protein translocation and activation.

From our previous work, we knew that exercise training improved the muscle insulin resistance of the obese Zucker rat. Now it was apparent that the insulin resistance stemmed not from a reduced transporter number, but rather from a defective GLUT4 protein translocation process. Thus, it was reasonable to hypothesize that exercise training somehow modified that glucose transporter translocation process or the functional activity of the transporter. We therefore exercise trained obese Zucker rats and investigated the effects of insulin on GLUT4 protein distribution and functional activity following hindlimb perfusion (7). Rat hindlimbs were perfused in the absence and presence of a maximally effective insulin concentration. Under basal conditions, plasma membranes from the trained rats had a 2.5-fold greater GLUT4 protein concentration than plasma membranes from untrained rats (figure 28.3a). Insulin stimulation significantly increased plasma membrane GLUT4 protein concentration only in the untrained rats. However, GLUT4 protein concentration in insulin-stimulated plasma membranes from trained rats remained 53% greater than that from untrained rats. Basal glucose uptake was not different between untrained and trained obese rats, but the insulin-stimulated glucose uptakes of trained rats were about 90% greater than those of untrained rats (figure 28.3b). GLUT4 transporter functional activity was the same for untrained and trained rats under basal and insulin-stimulation conditions; however, insulin increased GLUT4 activity approximately

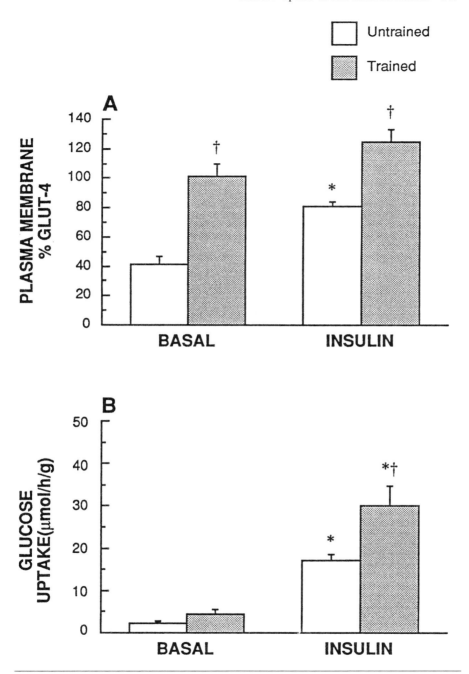

Figure 28.3   (A) Plasma membrane GLUT4 protein concentration and (B) hindlimb glucose uptake of trained and untrained obese Zucker rats. GLUT4 is expressed as a percentage of a heart standard. Values are means ± *SE*. * Significantly different from basal.
† Significantly different from untrained ($p < .05$). Based on results from Brozinick et al. 1993 (7).

fivefold above basal. These results suggest that the training-induced increase in insulin-stimulated glucose uptake is not the result of an adaptation in the GLUT4 protein translocation process or the functional activity of the GLUT4 transporter. Rather, the results indicate that defects in GLUT4 protein translocation and activation are compensated for by an increased expression of GLUT4 protein, which inherently becomes associated with the plasma membrane.

Summary

Exercise training improves the insulin-stimulated skeletal muscle glucose uptake of non-insulin-resistant and insulin-resistant muscle. The improvements with exercise training are both exercise-intensity and fiber type specific and appear to occur only in muscles or muscle fibers that are substantially recruited during exercise. In non-insulin-resistant muscle, the improvement in insulin-stimulated glucose uptake is related to the increased expression of GLUT4 protein concentration, although other factors may be involved. The improvement in insulin-stimulated glucose uptake is very short lived, lasting between 24 and 48 h after the last exercise session. In insulin-resistant muscle, the effects of exercise training are present at least 48 h after the last exercise session. Exercise training does not appear to affect the GLUT4 transporter translocation process or functional activity of the GLUT4 transporter in insulin-resistant muscle. Defects in GLUT4 transporter translocation and activation are simply compensated for by an increased expression of GLUT4 protein in the plasma membrane.

Acknowledgments

Grateful appreciation is extended to Gary Etgen and Ben Yaspelkis for their thoughtful comments and review of this manuscript.

References

1. Argiles, J. The obese Zucker rat: A choice for fat metabolism. 1969-1988: Twenty years of research on the insights of the Zucker mutation. Prog. Lipid Res. 28:53-66; 1989.
2. Banks, E.A.; Brozinick, J.T., Jr.; Yaspelkis, B.B., III; Kang, H.Y.; Ivy, J.L. Muscle glucose transport, GLUT-4 content, and degree of exercise training in obese Zucker rats. Am. J. Physiol. 263 (Endocrinol. Metab. Physiol. 26):E1015-E1020; 1992.
3. Becker-Zimmermann, K.; Berger, M.; Berchtold, P.; Gries, F.A.; Herberg, L.; Schwenen, M. Treadmill training improves intravenous glucose tolerance and insulin sensitivity in fatty Zucker rats. Diabetologia 22:468-474; 1982.
4. Berger, M.; Kemmer, F.W.; Becker, K.; Herberg, L.; Schwenen, M.; Gjinavci, A.; Berchtold, P. Effect of physical training on glucose tolerance and on glucose metabolism of skeletal muscle in anesthetized normal rats. Diabetologia 16:179-184; 1979.

5. Björntorp, P.; Fahlen, M.; Grimby, G.; Gustafson, A.; Holm, J.; Renstrom, P.; Schersten, T. Carbohydrate and lipid metabolism in middle-aged physically well trained men. Metabolism 21:1037-1044; 1972.

6. Brozinick, J.T., Jr.; Etgen, G.J., Jr.; Yaspelkis, B.B., III; Ivy, J.L. Glucose uptake and GLUT-4 protein distribution in skeletal muscle of the obese Zucker rat. Am. J. Physiol. 267 (Regulat. Integrat. Comp. Physiol. 36):R236-R243; 1994.

7. Brozinick, J.T., Jr.; Etgen, G.J., Jr.; Yaspelkis, B.B., III; Kang, H.Y.; Ivy, J.L. Effects of exercise training on muscle GLUT-4 protein content and translocation in obese Zucker rats. Am. J. Physiol. 265 (Endocrinol. Metab. Physiol. 28):E419-E427; 1993.

8. Cartee, G.D.; Young, D.A.; Sleeper, M.D.; Zierath, J.; Walberg-Henriksson, H.; Holloszy, J.O. Prolonged increase in insulin-stimulated glucose transport in muscle after exercise. Am. J. Physiol. 256 (Endocrinol. Metab. Physiol. 19):E494-E499; 1989.

9. Cortez, M.Y.; Torgan, C.E.; Brozinick, J.T., Jr.; Ivy, J.L. Insulin resistance of obese Zucker rats exercise trained at two different intensities. Am. J. Physiol. 261 (Endocrinol. Metab. Physiol. 24):E613-E619; 1991.

10. DeFronzo, R.A.; Jacot, E.; Jequier, E.; Macder, E.; Wahren, J.; Felber, J.P. The effect of insulin on the disposal of intravenous glucose: Results from indirect calorimetry and hepatic and femoral venous catheterization. Diabetes 30:1000-1007; 1981.

11. Douen, A.G.; Ramal, T.; Cartee, G.D.; Klip, A. Exercise modulates the insulin-induced translocation of glucose transporters in rat skeletal muscle. FEBS Lett. 261:256-260; 1990.

12. Etgen, G.J., Jr.; Brozinick, J.T., Jr.; Kang, H.Y.; Ivy, J.L. Effects of exercise training on skeletal muscle glucose uptake and transport. Am J. Physiol. 264 (Cell Physiol. 33):C727-C733; 1993.

13. Friedman, J.E.; Dohm, G.L.; Leggett-Frazier, N.; Elton, C.W.; Tapscott, E.B.; Pories, W.P.; Caro, J.F. Restoration of insulin responsiveness in skeletal muscle of morbidly obese patients after weight loss. J. Clin. Invest. 89:701-705; 1992.

14. Friedman, J.E.; Sherman, W.M.; Reed, M.J.; Elton, C.W.; Dohm, G.L. Exercise training increases glucose transporter protein GLUT-4 in skeletal muscle of obese Zucker (fa/fa) rats. FEBS Lett. 268:13-16; 1990.

15. Fushiki, T.; Kano, T.; Inoue, K.; Sugimoto, E. Decrease in muscle glucose transporter number in chronic physical inactivity in rats. Am. J. Physiol. 260 (Endocrinol. Metab. Physiol. 23):E403-E410; 1991.

16. Goodyear, L.J.; Hirshman, M.F.; Knutson, S.M.; Horton, E.D.; Horton, E.S. Effect of exercise training on glucose homeostasis in normal and insulin-deficient diabetic rats. J. Appl. Physiol. 65:844-851; 1988.

17. Goodyear, L.J.; Hirshman, M.F.; Valyou, P.M.; Horton, E.S. Glucose transporter number, function, and subcellular distribution in rat skeletal muscle after exercise training. Diabetes 41:1091-1099; 1992.

18. Henriksen, E.J.; Bourey, R.E.; Rodnick, K.J.; Koranyi, L.; Permutt, M.A.; Holloszy, J.O. Glucose transporter protein content and glucose transport capacity in rat skeletal muscles. Am. J. Physiol. 259 (Endocrinol. Metab. Physiol. 22):E593-E598; 1990.

19. Henriksen, E.J.; Rodnick, K.J.; Mondon, C.E.; James, D.E.; Holloszy, J.O. Effect of denervation or unweighting on GLUT-4 protein in rat soleus muscle. J. Appl. Physiol. 70:2322-2327; 1991.

20. Hirshman, M.F.; Goodyear, L.J.; Wardzala, L.J.; Horton, E.D.; Horton, E.S. Identification of an intracellular pool of glucose transporters from basal and insulin-stimulated rat skeletal muscle. J. Biol. Chem. 265:987-991; 1990.

21. Idström, J.P.; Rennie, M.J.; Schersten, T.; Bylund-Fellenius, A.C. Membrane transport in relation to net glucose uptake in the perfused rat hindlimb. Biochem. J. 233:131-137; 1986.

22. Ivy, J.L.; Brozinick, J.T., Jr.; Torgan, C.E.; Kastello, G.M. Skeletal muscle glucose transport in obese Zucker rats after exercise training. J. Appl. Physiol. 66:2635-2641; 1989.

23. Ivy, J.L.; Sherman, W.M.; Cutler, C.L.; Katz, A.L. Exercise and diet reduce muscle insulin resistance in obese Zucker rat. Am. J. Physiol. 251 (Endocrinol. Metab. Physiol. 14):E299-E305; 1986.

24. Ivy, J.L.; Young, J.C.; McLane, J.A.; Fell, R.D.; Holloszy, J.O. Exercise training and glucose uptake by skeletal muscle in rats. J. Appl. Physiol. 55:1393-1396; 1983.

25. James, D.E.; Kraegen, E.W.; Chisholm, D.J. Effects of exercise training on in vivo insulin action in individual tissues of the rat. J. Clin. Invest. 76:657-666; 1985.

26. Kahn, B.B.; Rossetti, L.; Lodish, H.F.; Charron, M.J. Decreased in vivo glucose uptake but normal expression of GLUT 1 and GLUT 4 in skeletal muscle of diabetic rats. J. Clin. Invest. 87:2197-2206; 1991.

27. Karnieli, E.; Zarnowski, M.J.; Hissin, P.J.; Simpson, I.A.; Salans, L.B.; Cushman, S.W. Insulin-stimulated translocation of glucose transport systems in the isolated rat adipose cell: Time course, reversal, insulin concentration-dependency and relationship to glucose transport activity. J. Biol. Chem. 256:4772-4777; 1981.

28. Katz, L.D.; Glickman, M.G.; Rapoport, S.; Ferrannini, E.; DeFronzo, R.A. Splanchnic and peripheral disposal of oral glucose in man. Diabetes 32:675-679; 1983.

29. Kern, M.; Wells, J.A.; Stephens, J.M.; Elton, C.W.; Friedman, J.E.; Tapscott, E.G.; Pekala, P.H.; Dohm, G.L. Insulin responsiveness in skeletal muscle is determined by glucose transporter (GLUT-4) protein level. Biochem. J. 270:397-400; 1990.

30. King, P.A.; Horton, E.D.; Hirshman, M.F.; Horton, E.S. Insulin resistance in obese Zucker rat (fa/fa) skeletal muscle is associated with a failure of glucose transporter translocation. J. Clin. Invest. 90:1568-1575; 1992.

31. Koranyi, L.; James, D.; Mueckler, M.; Permutt, M.A. Glucose transporter levels in spontaneously obese (db/db) insulin-resistant mice. J. Clin. Invest. 85:962-967; 1990.

32. LeBlanc, J.; Nadeau, A.; Richard, D.; Tremblay, A. Studies on the sparing effect of exercise on insulin requirements in human subjects. Metabolism 30:1119-1124; 1981.

33. Mondon, C.E.; Dolkas, C.B.; Reaven, G.M. Site of enhanced insulin sensitivity in exercise-trained rats at rest. Am. J. Physiol. 239 (Endocrinol. Metab. Physiol. 2):E169-E177; 1980.

34. Ploug, T.; Stallkhecht, B.M.; Pedersen, O.; Kahn, B.B.; Ohkuwa, T.; Vinten, J.; Galbo, H. Effects of endurance training on glucose transport capacity and glucose transporter expression in rat skeletal muscle. Am. J. Physiol. 259 (Endocrinol. Metab. Physiol. 22):E778-E786; 1990.

35. Rodnick, K.J.; Henriksen, E.J.; James, D.E.; Holloszy, J.O. Exercise training, glucose transporters, and glucose transport in rat skeletal muscle. Am. J. Physiol. 262 (Cell Physiol. 31):C9-C14; 1992.
36. Sherman, W.M.; Katz, A.L.; Cutler, C.L.; Withers, R.T.; Ivy, J.L. Glucose transport: Locus of muscle insulin resistance in obese Zucker rats. Am. J. Physiol. 255 (Endocrinol. Metab. Physiol. 18):E374-E382; 1988.
37. Sowell, M.O.; Dutton, S.L.; Buse, M.G. Selective in vitro reversal of the insulin resistance of glucose transport in denervated rat skeletal muscle. Am. J. Physiol. 257 (Endocrinol. Metab. Physiol. 20):E418-E425; 1989.
38. Strout, H.V.; Vicario, P.P.; Biswas, C.; Saperstein, R.; Brady, E.J.; Pilch, P.F.; Burger, J. Vanadate treatment of streptozotocin diabetic rats restores expression of the insulin-responsive glucose transporter in skeletal muscle. Endocrinology 126:2728-2732; 1990.
39. Willems, M.E.T.; Brozinick, J.T., Jr.; Torgan, C.E.; Cortez, M.Y.; Ivy, J.L. Muscle glucose uptake of obese Zucker rats trained at two different intensities. J. Appl. Physiol. 70:36-42; 1991.

PART VIII

Exercise and the Immune System

CHAPTER 29

Acute, Time-Limited Exercise Stress and the Immune System: Role of Stress Hormones

Bente Klarlund Pedersen

Copenhagen Muscle Research Centre, Copenhagen, Denmark

The human body is permanently influenced by an environment that contains several infectious microbial agents: viruses, bacteria, fungi, and parasites. These microorganisms have the potential to cause pathological damage, to multiply unchecked and eventually kill their host. However, most infections are of limited duration and leave very little permanent damage. This is due to the individual's immune system, which combats infectious agents. However, if the delicate balance between the invasiveness of microorganisms and the immune system is disturbed, infections may occur. This balance can be disturbed by the presence of large amounts of infectious agents (inoculum) or by suppression of the function of the immune system. It is currently under debate as to whether disturbances in the function of the immune system may also influence the ability of malignant cells to establish as metastases.

In the past few years, numerous studies have focused on the role of physical stress as an immunomodulatory stimulus. A large body of evidence suggests that the immunological effects of physical exercise are a subset of physical stress reactions, which include thermal and traumatic injury, surgery, acute myocardial infarction, and hemorrhagic shock (3, 9).

This part will focus on infections, cancer, and the acute phase response in relation to exercise. My task is to summarize how acute, time-limited exercise stress influences various components of the immune system and to present some hypotheses regarding underlying mechanisms of action.

Acute, Time-Limited Exercise Stress

Leukocyte Subpopulations

The "violent leukocytosis" first reported in an English language publication was experienced by a group of runners immediately following the 1902 Boston Marathon

(9). Neutrophil concentration increases during exercise and continues to increase following exercise. During exercise, natural killer (NK) cells, but also B and T cells, are recruited to the blood, and the total lymphocyte count thus increases. Simultaneously, the composition of T cells is altered with a decrease in the CD4/CD8 ratio. Following severe exercise, the lymphocyte concentration decreases below its initial value. The duration of this suppression depends on the intensity and duration of the exercise (2, 10).

Natural Killer and Lymphokine-Activated Killer Cells

During physical exercise, the absolute concentrations and the relative fraction of blood mononuclear cells (BMNC) expressing characteristic NK cell markers as CD16 and CD56 are increased. Simultaneously, the NK cell activity increases. The exercise-induced enhancement of NK cell activity is mainly due to a redistribution into the blood of recirculating NK cells. Following intense, acute, time-limited exercise stress, the NK cell activity is suppressed. When BMNC were incubated with interleukin-2 (IL-2) for 3 d, the lymphokine-activated killer (LAK) cell activity of cells from blood sampled at the end of the exercise period was very significantly increased. These data indicate that during exercise NK cells with a high IL-2 response capacity are recruited to the blood (11).

In relation to acute, time-limited bicycle exercise (1 h at 25%, 50%, and 75% of $\dot{V}O_2max$), the NK and LAK cell activities were enhanced at all intensities, but suppressed following the severe exercise only. Furthermore, only this intense exercise produced a postexercise monocytosis (15).

Proliferative Responses

The ability of lymphocytes to proliferate in vitro decreases following stimulation with T-dependent mitogens, whereas the proliferative response increases after stimulation with IL-2, lipopolysaccharide (LPS), and concanavalin A (ConA). Decreased phytohemagglutinin (PHA) response during bicycle exercise was not due to a changed proliferative response per $CD4^+$ cell, but to a decreased fraction of the $CD4^+$ subgroup (3).

B Cell Function

Exercise causes suppression of immunoglobulin production (13). To study the mechanism behind the suppression of immunoglobulins, a plaque-forming cell assay was used (14), allowing identification of individual immunoglobulin-secreting cells. Stimulation of cells with pokeweed mitogen (PWM), IL-2, and Epstein-Barr virus (EBV) resulted in significant decreases in the fraction of IgG-, IgA-, and IgM-secreting blood cells during, as well as 2 h after, bicycle exercise, with reversal to preexercise levels 24 h later. Since the percentage of $CD19^+$ B cells did not change in relation to exercise, the suppression of immunoglobulin-secreting cells was not likely to be due to concurrent changes in numbers of B cells. Purified B cells produce plaques only after stimulation with EBV, and in these cultures no exercise-induced suppression was found. Addition of indomethacin to IL-2-stimulated cultures of BMNC partly reversed the postexercise suppressed B cell function, suggestive of a role for monocytes in the B cell suppression (14).

Mechanisms of Action

Stress Hormones

In response to exercise, the concentrations in the blood of a number of stress hormones, including adrenaline, noradrenaline, growth hormone (GH), β-endorphin, and cortisol, are increased. Furthermore, bicycle exercise induces a rise in body temperature. The immunomodulatory role of individual stress factors such as stress hormones can be investigated by controlled infusion of any of the hormones to obtain concentrations in the blood identical with those obtained by exercise or by pharmacological or anesthesiological blocking of the hormones or their receptors.

When volunteers were given intravenous infusion of adrenaline to obtain plasma concentrations sevenfold greater than control levels (identical to those observed during bicycle exercise at 75% of $\dot{V}O_2$max for 1 h), the exercise-induced changes in BMNC subsets, NK activity, LAK activity, and proliferative responses were closely mimicked (7). However, adrenaline caused a significantly smaller increase in the concentration of neutrophils. Noradrenaline infusion to obtain noradrenaline levels 15 times above resting levels (mimicking that obtained during 75% of $\dot{V}O_2$max, 1 h) enhanced the NK cell activity but did not cause post-noradrenaline suppression (Kappel et al., unpublished data). Infusion of GH into human subjects at physiological concentrations characteristic of exercise had no effect on BMNC subsets, NK activity, cytokine production, or lymphocyte function but induced a significant increase in neutrophil concentration (5).

Administration of naloxone (an opioid antagonist) to young women who underwent a maximal bicycle ergometer test blocked the rise in NK cell activity, although the number of cells expressing the CD16 marker (NK cells) was not different from the group receiving placebo (1). Employing a different model, the exercise-induced rise in β-endorphin and ACTH was blocked by an epidural analgesia that blocked the afferent impulses. The exercise-induced increases in NK cell function, percentage of NK cells, and NK cell concentration were significantly increased (8).

During acute, time-limited exercise stress, only a minor increase in cortisol concentration is found, and it is still debatable whether this minor increase in cortisol concentration can account for the exercise-induced immunomodulation (see chapter 30). Infusion of insulin, while maintaining a stable plasma glucose level such that plasma insulin levels were increased 150 times above normal values, had only a minor influence on the immune system. However, a significant correlation existed between the NK cell activity and the insulin level (Kappel, unpublished observation).

Intense or prolonged exercise induces a rise in body temperature, a condition known as hyperthermia, which has numerous effects on the immune system. The in vivo effects of hyperthermia have been studied by immersing healthy volunteers in a hot water bath, whereby their rectal temperature increased to 39.5° C. On another day they served as their own control and were immersed into thermoneutral water. Hyperthermia induced immune alterations that resembled the changes observed in relation to exercise. However, unlike with acute exercise, only minor increases in plasma adrenaline and noradrenaline concentrations were observed (6). Recent data from our laboratory show that infusion of adrenaline to double the control values enhances the NK cell activity, whereas infusion of small doses of noradrenaline does not have this effect.

The mechanisms behind exercise-induced changes in immunity are not fully understood, but it was shown that adrenaline could account for the effect of physical exercise on NK activity, LAK activity, BMNC subsets, and proliferative responses, while adrenaline together with growth hormone may be responsible for the increase in neutrophil concentration following exercise. Whether stress hormones are responsible for changes in plasma cytokines or whether exercise-induced increases in plasma cytokines cause modulation of the immune system remain to be elucidated. Furthermore, it is unclear whether the increase in body temperature during exercise can explain part of the immunomodulation in relation to exercise.

Energy Supply of Lymphocytes

In vitro studies show that the proliferation of lymphocytes and the production of some cytokines are highly dependent on the presence of glutamine (6, 12). It has been proposed that the glutamine pathway in lymphocytes may be under external regulation and that this may be related to the supply of glutamine itself (12). The major tissue involved in glutamine production is skeletal muscle. In theory, therefore, the activity of the skeletal muscle may directly influence the immune system. The glutamine theory says that factors that influence glutamine synthesis or release may influence the function of lymphocytes and monocytes. It has been hypothesized that under intense physical exercise, the demands on muscle and other organs for glutamine are such that the lymphoid system may be forced into a glutamine debt that temporarily affects its function. The weak point in this hypothesis is that if the lowest concentrations of glutamine obtained in plasma after exercise are added to the lymphocytes in vitro, these will proliferate as well as they do at glutamine concentrations obtained before exercise. However, we do not have information about local concentrations of glutamine in relation to exercise.

Chronic Exercise Stress

The influence of training or fitness level on the immune system is dealt with by Nieman in the next chapter. In general, however, cross-sectional comparisons of athletes' and nonathletes' immune system resting levels have shown no effect of fitness level on leukocyte, lymphocyte, and neutrophil concentrations; proliferative responses; or antibody production. However, a rather constant finding has been an increased NK cell function in trained compared with untrained subjects.

During moderate as well as severe acute exercise, the immune system is enhanced, but only severe exercise is followed by immunodepression. Elite athletes have increased NK cell activity at rest. However, due to frequent, severe, acute exercise, the NK cell function is often temporarily severely suppressed. During the time of immunodepression, referred to as the "open window," microbacterial agents, especially viruses, may invade the host, and infections can be established. However, in those who perform regular, moderate exercise, the immune system will often be enhanced, and this will protect these individuals from infectious and maybe also malignant diseases. To further support this hypothesis, epidemiological and experimental studies are required.

Future Prospectives

Systematic research into exercise and immunology has been performed only during the last decade. This research has revealed that exercise alters the distribution and trafficking of mononuclear cells and induces an acute phase response. Future research should look for immune changes not only in the blood, but also in the muscle cells, since myoblasts have interesting biological and immunological cellular properties. Furthermore, muscle cells provide the microenvironment for many clinically important immune reactions (4). Future research should also elucidate the clinical role of exercise in preventing infectious and malignant diseases. The following chapters will deal with exercise and infections, exercise and cancer, and the acute phase response and cytokines in blood and in muscles.

Acknowledgment

This work was supported by the Danish National Research Foundation #504-14.

References

1. Fiatarone, M.A.; Morley, J.E.; Bloom, E.T.; Donna, M.; Makinodan, T.; Solomon, G.F. Endogenous opioids and the exercise-induced augmentation of natural killer cell activity. J. Lab. Clin. Med. 112:544-552; 1988.
2. Fitzgerald, L. Exercise and the immune system. Immunol. Today 9:337-339; 1988.
3. Hoffman-Goetz, L.; Pedersen, B.K. Exercise and the immune system: A model of the stress response? Immunol. Today 15:345-392; 1994.
4. Hohlfeld, R.; Engel, A.G. The immunobiology of muscle. Immunol. Today 15:269-274; 1994.
5. Kappel, M.; Hansen, M.B.; Diamant, M.; Jørgensen, J.O.; Gyhrs, A.; Pedersen, B.K. Effects of an acute bolus growth hormone infusion on the human immune system. Horm. Metab. Res. 11:593-602; 1993.
6. Kappel, M.; Stadeager, C.; Tvede, N.; Galbo, H.; Pedersen, B.K. Effect of in vivo hyperthermia on natural killer cell activity, in vitro proliferative responses and blood mononuclear cell subpopulations. Clin. Exp. Immunol. 84:175-180; 1991.

7. Kappel, M.; Tvede, N.; Galbo, H.; Haahr, P.M.; Kjær, M.; Linstouw, M.; Klarlund, K.; Pedersen, B.K. Epinephrine can account for the effect of physical exercise on natural killer cell activity. J. Appl. Physiol. 70(6):2530-2534; 1991.

8. Klokker, M.; Kjær, M.; Secher, N.H.; Hanel, B.; Worm, L.; Kappel, M.; Pedersen, B.K. Natural killer cell response to exercise in humans: Effect of hypoxia and epidural anesthesia. J. Appl. Physiol. 78:709-716; 1995.

9. Larrabee, R.C. Leukocytosis after violent exercise. J. Med. Res. 7:76-82; 1902.

10. Pedersen, B.K.; Kappel, M.; Klokker, M. The immune system during exposure to extreme physiologic conditions. Int. J. Sports Med. 15:S116-S121 (Supplement 3); 1994.

11. Pedersen, B.K.; Ullum, H. NK cell response to physical activity: Possible mechanisms of action. Med. Sci. Sports Exercise 26:140-146; 1994.

12. Rohde, T.; Newsholme, E.; Ullum, H.; Palmø, J.; Halkjær Kristensen, J.; Pedersen, B.K. Effects of glutamine concentrations on the cellular immune system at rest and at muscular exercise in HIV positive and negative subjects. J. Appl. Physiol. 79:146-150; 1995.

13. Tomasi, F.; Trudeau, D.; Czerqinski, D.; Erredge, S. Immune parameters in athletes before and after strenuous exercise. J. Clin. Immunol. 2:173-178; 1982.

14. Tvede, N.; Heilmann, C.; Halkjær-Kristensen, J.; Pedersen, B.K. Mechanisms of B lymphocyte suppression induced by acute physical exercise. J. Clin. Lab. Immunol. 30:169-173; 1989.

15. Tvede, N.; Kappel, M.; Halkjær-Kristensen, J.; Galbo, H.; Pedersen, B.K. The effect of light, moderate and severe exercise on lymphocyte subsets, natural and lymphokine activated killer cells, lymphocyte proliferative response and interleukin 2 production. Int. J. Sports Med. 14:275-282; 1993.

CHAPTER 30

Effect of Long-Term Training on the Immune System and on Resistance to Infectious Diseases

David C. Nieman

Appalachian State University, Boone, North Carolina, U.S.A.

Among elite athletes and their coaches, a common perception is that heavy exertion lowers resistance and is a predisposing factor to upper respiratory tract infections (2, 13). For example, Liz McColgan blamed overtraining, "which led to a cold and two subsequent illnesses," as the major reason for her poor performance in the 1992 World Cross-Country Championships (63). Uta Pippig, winner of the 1994 Boston Marathon, caught a cold the week before the race after training 140 mi (225 km) per week for 10 wk at high altitude. Pippig claimed, "when you are on such a high level you can so quickly fall off" (64). During the Winter and Summer Olympic Games, it has been regularly reported by clinicians that "upper respiratory infections abound" (21) and that "the most irksome troubles with the athletes were infections" (26).

On the other hand, there is also a common belief among many individuals that regular exercise confers resistance against infection. For example, a 1989 *Runner's World* subscriber survey revealed that 61% of 700 runners reported fewer colds since beginning to run, while only 4% felt they had experienced more (82). In a survey of 170 non-elite marathon runners (average personal best time of 3 h 25 min) who had been training for and participating in marathons for an average of 12 yr, 90% reported that they definitely or mostly agreed with the statement that they "rarely get sick" (unpublished observations).

The U.S. Centers for Disease Control and Prevention have estimated that over 425 million upper respiratory tract infections (URTI) occur annually in the United States, resulting in $2.5 billion in lost school and work days and in medical costs (57). The National Center for Health Statistics reports that acute respiratory conditions (primarily the common cold and influenza) have an annual incidence rate of 90 per 100 persons (1). Understanding the relationship between exercise and infection has potential implications for public health, and for the athlete it may mean the difference between being able to compete or performing at a subpar level or missing the event altogether because of illness (41, 53).

In this chapter, emphasis will be placed on the relationship between exercise and URTI in humans and on potential changes in the immune system that might explain the altered risk of infection. Research on the potential for skin infections and other infections in athletes (e.g., from hepatitis B and human immunodeficiency viruses) has been reviewed elsewhere (41, 53).

Exercise and Upper Respiratory Tract Infection in Humans

It has been proposed that the relationship between exercise and URTI may be modeled in the form of a J curve (41; figure 30.1). This model suggests that although the risk of URTI may decrease below that of a sedentary individual when one engages in moderate exercise training, risk may rise above average during periods of excessive high-intensity exercise.

At present, there is more evidence, primarily epidemiological in nature, exploring the relationship between heavy exertion and infection, and these data will be reviewed first, followed by a brief section on moderate exercise training and infection. Much more research using larger subject pools and improved research designs is necessary before this model can be wholly accepted or rejected.

Heavy Exertion and URTI: Epidemiological Evidence

Several epidemiological reports suggest that athletes engaging in marathon-type events or very heavy training are at increased risk of URTI (48, 71-73). Nieman et

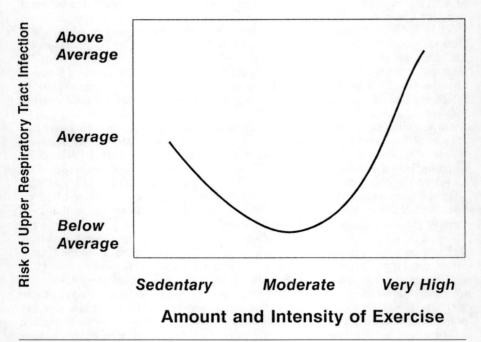

Figure 30.1   J-shaped model of relationship between varying amounts of exercise and risk of URTI. This model suggests that moderate exercise may lower risk of respiratory infection, while excessive amounts may increase the risk.

al. (48) researched the incidence of URTI in a group of 2,311 marathon runners who varied widely in running ability and training habits. Runners retrospectively self-reported demographic, training, and URTI episode and symptom data for the 2-mo period (January and February) prior to and for the 1-wk period immediately following the 1987 Los Angeles Marathon race. During the week following the race, 12.9% of the marathoners reported a URTI, compared with only 2.2% of control runners who did not participate (odds ratio = 5.9; figure 30.2). Forty percent of the runners reported at least one URTI episode during the 2-mo winter period prior to the marathon race. Controlling for various confounders, it was determined that runners training more than 96 km/wk doubled their odds for sickness compared with those training less than 32 km/wk (figure 30.3).

Other epidemiological data support these findings. Linde (32) studied URTI in a group of 44 elite orienteers and 44 nonathletes of the same age, sex, and occupational distribution during a 1-yr period. The orienteers experienced significantly more URTI episodes during the year than the control group (2.5 vs. 1.7 episodes, respectively).

Peters and Bateman (72) studied the incidence of URTI in 150 randomly selected runners who took part in a 56-km Cape Town race in comparison with matched controls who did not run. Symptoms of URTI occurred in 33.3% of runners compared with 15.3% of controls during the 2-wk period following the race and were most common in those who achieved faster race times. Two subsequent studies from this group of researchers have confirmed this finding (71, 73). During the 2-wk period

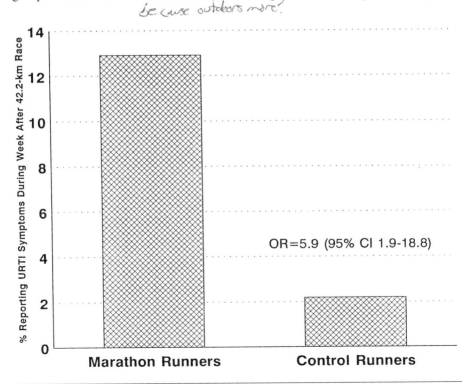

Figure 30.2   Self-reported URTI in 2,311 Los Angeles Marathon runners during the week following the 1987 Los Angeles Marathon. Data from Nieman et al. 1990 (48).

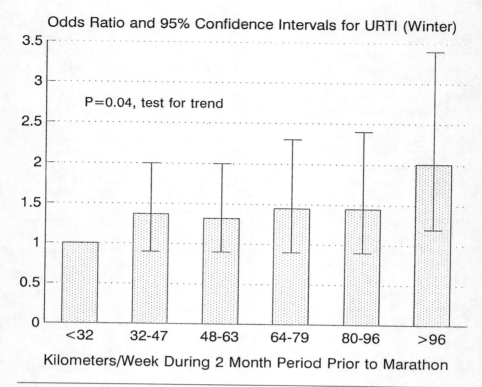

Figure 30.3   Self-reported URTI in 2,311 Los Angeles Marathon runners during the 2-mo period prior to the 1987 Los Angeles Marathon according to average weekly training distances. Data from Nieman et al. 1990 (48).

following the 56-km Milo Korkie Ultramarathon in Pretoria, South Africa, 28.7% of the 108 subjects who completed the race reported non-allergy-derived URTI symptoms as compared with 12.9% of controls (71). In the most recent report from Peters et al. (73), 68% of runners reported the development of symptoms of URTI within 2 wk after the 90-km Comrades Ultramarathon. Using a double-blind placebo research design, it was determined that only 33% of runners taking a 600-mg vitamin C supplement daily for 3 wk prior to the race developed URTI symptoms. The authors suggested that because heavy exertion enhances the production of free oxygen radicals, vitamin C, which has antioxidant properties, may be required in increased quantities.

URTI risk following a race event may depend on the distance, with an increased incidence conspicuous only following marathon or ultramarathon events. For example, Nieman, Johanssen, and Lee (47) were unable to establish any increase in prevalence of URTI in 273 runners during the week following 5-km, 10-km, and 21.1-km events as compared with the week before. URTI incidence was also measured during the 2-mo winter period prior to the three races, and in this group of recreational runners, 25% of those running 25 km/wk or more (average of 42 km/wk) reported at least one URTI episode, as opposed to 34% who trained less than 25 km/wk (average of 12 km/wk; $p = .09$). These findings suggest that in recreational running an average weekly distance of 42 versus 12 km is associated with either no change in or even a slight reduction of URTI incidence. Further, they suggest that racing 5 to 21.1 km is not related to an increased risk of sickness during the ensuing week.

Together, these epidemiological studies imply that heavy acute or chronic exercise is associated with an increased risk of URTI (24). The risk appears to be especially high during the 1- or 2-wk period following marathon-type race events. Among runners varying widely in training habits, the risk for URTI is slightly elevated for the highest distance runners, but only when several confounding factors are controlled.

Moderate Exertion and URTI

What about the common belief that moderate physical activity is beneficial in decreasing URTI risk? Very few studies have been carried out in this area, and more research is certainly warranted to investigate this interesting question.

At present, there are no published epidemiological reports that have retrospectively or prospectively compared incidence of URTI in large groups of moderately active and sedentary individuals. Two randomized experimental trials using small numbers of subjects have provided important preliminary data in support of the viewpoint that moderate physical activity may reduce URTI symptomatology. In one randomized, controlled study of 36 women (mean age 35 yr), exercising subjects walked briskly for 45 min, 5 d/wk, and experienced one-half the number of days with URTI symptoms during the 15-wk period compared with the sedentary control group (5.1 ± 1.2 vs. 10.8 ± 2.3 d; $p = .039$; figure 30.4; 55). The number of separate URTI episodes did not vary between groups, but the number of symptom days per URTI episode was significantly lower in the exercise group ($p = .049$).

In a study of elderly women, the incidence of the common cold during a 12-wk period in fall was measured to be lowest in highly conditioned, lean subjects who exercised moderately each day for about 1.5 h (8%). Elderly subjects who walked 40 min, 5 times/wk, had an incidence of 21%, as compared with 50% for the sedentary control group ($\chi^2 = 6.36$, $p = .042$; figure 30.5; 45). These data suggest that elderly women not engaging in cardiorespiratory exercise are more likely than those who do exercise regularly to experience a URTI during the fall season.

Acute and Chronic Effects of Exercise on the Immune System

It naturally follows that if heavy and fatiguing exertion leads to an increased risk of URTI, various measures of immune function should be negatively affected. And conversely, if moderate exercise decreases URTI risk, there should be some aspect of immune function that is chronically or at least transiently improved. Despite intense investigation during the last 10 years on this issue, however, there is no clear consensus. The wide variety of research designs, exercise protocols, subject characteristics, and methodologies combined with the innate complexity of the immune system have made interpretation of published findings extremely formidable and equivocal.

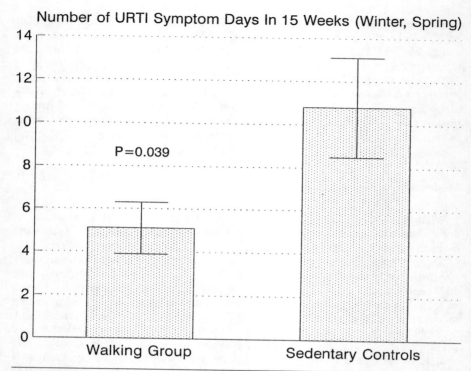

Figure 30.4   Number of URTI symptom days in 18 walkers versus 18 sedentary controls during a 15-wk randomized, controlled study. Data from Nieman et al. 1990 (55).

The Acute Immune Response to Exercise

A growing number of published reports on exercise immunology provide evidence that the immune system is profoundly affected by acute exercise. The clinical significance of these large but transient alterations is disputed, however.

High-intensity endurance exercise is associated with a unique biphasic perturbation of the circulating leukocyte count (12, 16, 17, 22, 33, 49). Immediately post-exercise, total leukocytes increase by 50% to 100%, represented equally by lymphocytes and neutrophils with a small contribution from monocytes. Following prolonged endurance exercise such as marathon race events, the leukocytosis is even larger (200-300%) but is represented more by neutrophils than lymphocytes (23, 42, 52, 75). All of the lymphoid tissues appear to contribute cells, with the spleen considered to be of primary importance (69, 83).

Within 30 min of recovery from exercise, however, the lymphocyte count dips 30% to 50% below preexercise levels, remaining low for 3 to 6 h, during which there is a sustained neutrophilia. There is no clear consensus regarding the tissue site to which the blood lymphocytes are transferred; some investigators provide evidence that peripheral lymphoid tissues (e.g., the thymus and spleen) are also depleted (11). Moderate-intensity exercise has been demonstrated to induce much smaller leukocytosis, lymphocytosis, neutrophilia, and lymphocytopenia (27, 40,

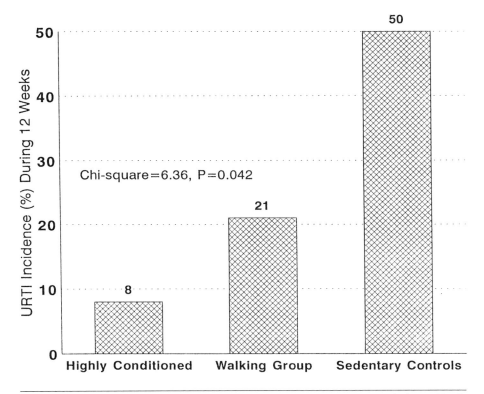

Figure 30.5   Incidence of URTI (expressed as a percentage of the group) during a 12-wk study period in highly conditioned, walking, and sedentary control groups of elderly women. Data from Nieman et al. 1993 (45).

49, 54). The extent and duration of the alterations in leukocyte subset counts are very much dependent on the exercise-induced changes in epinephrine and cortisol, which begin to increase strongly when the exercise intensity rises above 60% $\dot{V}O_2$max (8, 14, 36, 49). Figure 30.6 summarizes the cortisol and neutrophil data from several studies using different exercise modalities and work loads. Notice the close parallel between the overall cortisol response and recovery neutrophilia.

Of the three major lymphocyte subpopulations (T, B, and natural killer cells), natural killer (NK) cells are by far most responsive to exercise (16, 50). It is typical for NK cells to increase 150% to 300% within minutes of initiating high-intensity exercise, contributing substantially to the overall lymphocytosis (4, 5, 16, 27, 50, 67, 68). Circulating numbers of T cytotoxic-suppressor cells also increase markedly (50-100%) after high-intensity exercise, while T helper-inducer and B cells are relatively unaffected (16, 17, 49). However, the effect is transient, and within 30 min lymphocytes from each of the subpopulation groups exit the circulation in large numbers under the influence of cortisol (8).

A common finding immediately following high- but not moderate-intensity exercise is that mitogen-stimulated proliferation of separated mononuclear cells is decreased by 35% to 50%, returning to preexercise levels within 2 h (12, 14, 15, 18,

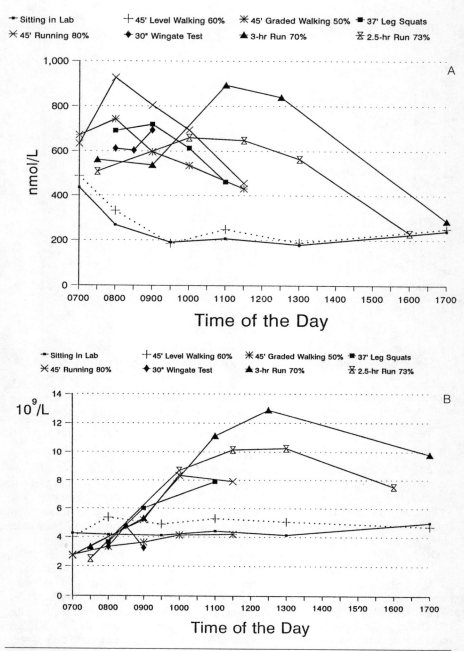

Figure 30.6 (A) Change in serum cortisol concentration in response to different exercise modalities and work loads. (B) Change in concentrations of circulating neutrophils in response to different exercise modalities and work loads. Notice the parallel between the exercise-induced changes in cortisol and neutrophils. Data from unpublished observations, Nieman et al. 1989 (42), Nieman et al. (49), Nieman et al. 1993 (50), and Nieman et al. 1991 (54).

49, 76). Several researchers have provided evidence that elevation of both plasma cortisol and epinephrine following intensive exercise inhibits mitogen-induced lymphocyte proliferation (8, 36, 49, 65, 83). However, others reason that the decrease in mitogen response is most likely due to the large, exercise-induced increase in NK cells that occurs immediately following sessions of vigorous exercise. Since a constant number of peripheral blood mononuclear cells are utilized in the pre- and postexercise in vitro assays, the large increase in NK cells relative to T cells means that a smaller percentage of cells that respond to mitogens are available (NK cells do not divide in response to mitogens; 49, 76). Thus the drop in T cell function after exercise has been challenged as not being clinically important (14, 15, 76). However, even though the function of each T cell may be unaltered by intense exercise, the blood and peripheral lymphoid compartments may have fewer T cells than normal for several hours of recovery from exercise, which may have the same impact on host protection as having fewer soldiers on the front lines of a battlefield. Research to settle these issues is certainly warranted and may improve our understanding of the acute immune response and its link with epidemiological findings.

Investigators have also consistently reported that immediately following high-intensity exercise, NK cell cytotoxic activity (NKCA) is increased by 40% to 100% before falling 25% to 35% below preexercise levels by 1 h and 2 h of recovery (4, 5, 50, 67, 68, 76). Although most researchers agree that the immediate postexercise increase in NKCA is due to the recruitment of NK cells into the circulation (50), they tend to disagree on the reasons for the transient NKCA decrease during recovery. Although some researchers reason that the drop in NKCA can be ascribed to numerical shifts in NK cells (34, 76), others report that prostaglandins from activated monocytes and neutrophils (65, 67, 68) or elevated stress hormone levels (5) suppress the ability of NK cells to function appropriately. This issue has not yet been resolved and will require further investigation. Nonetheless, most researchers would agree that the NKCA of the blood compartment is significantly reduced for several hours after heavy exertion primarily because of the transfer of NK cells to other tissues (50). Whether this is a reflection of NKCA in other lymphoid compartments remains to be determined, but there are some animal data to support this supposition (35, 77).

Neutrophils, among the body's best phagocytes, are considered to be a part of the innate functional division of the immune system (as are NK cells), acting as a first line of defense against infectious agents. There is growing evidence that both moderate and intense endurance exercise are associated with a prolonged improvement in the killing capacity of blood neutrophils and peritoneal macrophages (9, 20, 28, 59, 60, 74, 78). In contrast, immediately following a 20-km race, neutrophils in a nasal lavage taken from 12 male runners were less able to ingest bacteria, an effect that lasted for 3 d (37). Prolonged impairment of lung neutrophil antimicrobial function has also been reported in race horses following a single strenuous event (85). Although blood neutrophils are easier to study, data from these two studies suggest that neutrophils from the respiratory area may respond differently to intense exercise than do those from the blood compartment.

In general, there are no convincing data at this time that exercise-induced changes in the lymphocyte proliferative response to mitogens in vitro, in natural killer cell cytotoxic activity, or in neutrophil-macrophage function explain the increased risk of URTI suggested by epidemiological data. Researchers disagree on the mechanistic interpretation of their findings, and none have provided follow-up data of large numbers of subjects to determine whether various changes in immunity translate to altered host protection. Further research is needed to settle these issues and to determine if the large but transient perturbations in leukocyte cell concentrations in both blood and peripheral lymphoid tissue (which often underlie reported in vitro functional alterations) are important from a clinical viewpoint.

Immune Response to Chronic Exercise

Numerous studies have made cross-sectional comparisons of the immune systems of athletes and nonathletes (5, 7, 19, 29, 30, 36, 43, 46, 56, 62, 66, 81) or have followed sedentary individuals as they initiate exercise programs, comparing pre- and postexercise training immunity measurements with those of control groups (3, 39, 44, 45, 55, 79, 84). Most of these studies have failed to demonstrate any important effects of regular exercise training on concentrations of circulating total leukocytes, lymphocyte subsets, or immunoglobulins (51, 52).

Several studies on animals and humans, however, have shown significant improvements in natural killer cell cytotoxic activity (NKCA) with exercise training (7, 29, 35, 45, 55, 66, 77, 81). In cross-sectional studies, NKCA has been reported to be significantly higher in physically active versus inactive Japanese men (29), in highly conditioned versus sedentary elderly women (7, 45), and in elite cyclists versus untrained subjects (66, 81). Researchers disagree, however, whether the higher NKCA is due to a greater concentration of circulating NK cells or to an enhanced cytotoxic capacity of these cells (45, 66, 81). Additionally, the positive association between NKCA and exercise training has not been consistently demonstrated, especially in randomized, controlled studies with special population groups such as the elderly or subjects with rheumatoid arthritis or breast cancer (3, 5, 38, 44-46). Thus, the positive effect of chronic exercise training on resting NKCA remains an inconsistent finding, despite the growing consensus that acute exercise has a strong but transient influence on concentrations of circulating NK cells.

In cross-sectional and prospective studies of animals and humans, exercise training has been reported to have a positive (38, 45, 70, 80, 84), negative (10, 31, 38, 61, 62), or neutral (6, 19, 25, 36, 45, 81) relationship to mitogen-stimulated lymphocyte proliferation (T cell function). Studies differ widely on the type of subject, volume of exercise training, and methodology employed, with several of these studies not providing information on T cell enumeration. Nonetheless, if there is an exercise training effect on T cell function, it is likely to be small and probably not clinically significant except for elderly subjects (45).

The literature is equally divergent on the effect of exercise training on neutrophil killing capacity, with investigators reporting lower (78), higher (58), or similar (20, 30) function when comparing elite athletes and untrained controls.

Conclusions

Although further research is needed, present epidemiological findings suggest that heavy exertion is associated with an increased URTI risk, while moderate activity lowers this risk. Other than the potential effect of chronic training on NKCA, there is little agreement in the literature as to consistent changes in immune function.

Although the immune system is affected profoundly by acute exercise bouts, interpretation of the findings is heavily based on the intensity and duration of the exercise bout and on the type of immunity measurements and assays used. Most investigators have demonstrated that exercise stimulates phagocytic function of blood neutrophils and peripheral macrophages, but it is uncertain whether this is related more to an involvement of the immune system in the acute phase response or to enhanced host protection from pathogens. Lymphocyte function is often reported to be transiently decreased following high-intensity exercise, but researchers disagree on whether the changes reflect alterations in circulating numbers of lymphocytes or real immune suppression. Further research is warranted to establish the clinical importance of exercise-induced changes in immune function and whether a physiological rationale can be provided in support of preliminary epidemiological findings.

References

1. Adams, P.F.; Benson, V. Current estimates from the National Health Interview Survey. National Center for Health Statistics. Vital Health Stat. 10(181); 1991.
2. Baetjer, A.M. The effect of muscular fatigue upon resistance. Physiol. Rev. 12:453-468; 1932.
3. Baslund, B.; Lyngberg, K.; Andersen, V.; Dristensen, J.H.; Hansen, M.; Klokker, N.; Pedersen, B.K. Effect of 8 wk of bicycle training on the immune system of patients with rheumatoid arthritis. J. Appl. Physiol. 75:1691-1695; 1993.
4. Berk, L.S.; Nieman, D.C.; Youngberg, W.S.; Arabatzis, K.; Simpson-Westerberg, M.; Lee, J.W.; Tan, S.A.; Eby, W.C. The effect of long endurance running on natural killer cells in marathoners. Med. Sci. Sports Exercise 22:207-212; 1990.
5. Brahmi, Z.; Thomas, J.E.; Park, M.; Park, M.; Dowdeswell, I.A.G. The effect of acute exercise on natural killer-cell activity of trained and sedentary human subjects. J. Clin. Immunol. 5:321-328; 1985.
6. Campbell, S.A.; Hughes, H.C.; Griffin, H.E.; Landi, M.S.; Mallon, F.M. Some effects of limited exercise on purpose-bred beagles. Am. J. Vet. Res. 49:1298-1301; 1988.
7. Crist, D.M.; Mackinnon, L.T.; Thompson, R.F.; Atterbom, H.A.; Egan, P.A. Physical exercise increases natural cellular-mediated tumor cytotoxicity in elderly women. Gerontology 35:66-71; 1989.
8. Cupps, T.R.; Fauci, A.S. Corticosteroid-mediated immunoregulation in man. Immunol. Rev. 65:133-155; 1982.
9. Fehr, H.G.; Lötzerich, H.; Michna, H. Human macrophage function and physical exercise: Phagocytic and histochemical studies. Eur. J. Appl. Physiol. 58:613-617; 1989.
10. Ferry, A.; Rieu, P.; Laziri, F.; Guezennec, C.Y.; Elhabazi, A.; Le Page, C.; Rieu, M. Immunomodulations of thymocytes and splenocytes in trained rats. J. Appl. Physiol. 71:815-820; 1991.
11. Ferry, A.; Rieu, P.; Le Page, C.; Elhabazi, A.; Laziri, F.; Rieu, M. Effect of physical exhaustion and glucocorticoids (dexamethasone) on T-cells of trained rats. Eur. J. Appl. Physiol. 66:455-460; 1993.

12. Field, C.J.; Gougeon, R.; Marliss, E.B. Circulating mononuclear cell numbers and function during intense exercise and recovery. J. Appl. Physiol. 71:1089-1097; 1991.
13. Fitzgerald, L. Overtraining increases the susceptibility to infection. Int. J. Sports Med. 12 (suppl. 1):S5-S8; 1991.
14. Fry, R.W.; Morton, A.R.; Crawford, G.P.M.; Keast, D. Cell numbers and in vitro responses of leucocytes and lymphocyte subpopulations following maximal exercise and interval training sessions of different intensities. Eur. J. Appl. Physiol. 64:218-227; 1992.
15. Fry, R.W.; Morton, A.R.; Keast, D. Acute intensive interval training and T-lymphocyte function. Med. Sci. Sports Exercise 24:339-345; 1992.
16. Gabriel, H.; Schwarz, L.; Born, P.; Kindermann, W. Differential mobilization of leucocyte and lymphocyte subpopulations into the circulation during endurance exercise. Eur. J. Appl. Physiol. 65:529-534; 1992.
17. Gabriel, H.; Urhausen, A.; Kindermann, W. Circulating leukocyte and lymphocyte subpopulations before and after intensive endurance exercise to exhaustion. Eur. J. Appl. Physiol. 63:449-457; 1991.
18. Gmünder, F.K.; Lorenzi, G.; Bechler, B.; Joller, P.; Müller, J.; Ziegler, W.H.; Cogoli, A. Effect of long-term physical exercise on lymphocyte reactivity: Similarity to spaceflight reactions. Aviat. Space Environ. Med. 59:146-151; 1988.
19. Green, R.L.; Kaplan, S.S.; Rabin, B.S.; Stanitski, C.L.; Zdziarski, U. Immune function in marathon runners. Ann. Allergy 47:73-75; 1981.
20. Hack, V.; Strobel, G.; Rau, J.-P.; Weicker, H. The effect of maximal exercise on the activity of neutrophil granulocytes in highly trained athletes in a moderate training period. Eur. J. Appl. Physiol. 65:520-524; 1992.
21. Hanley, D.F. Medical care of the US Olympic team. JAMA 12:147-148; 1976.
22. Hansen, J.B.; Wilsgård, L.; Osterud, B. Biphasic changes in leukocytes induced by strenuous exercise. Eur. J. Appl. Physiol. 62:157-161; 1991.
23. Haq, A.; Al-Hussein, K.; Lee, J.; Al-Sedairy, S. Changes in peripheral blood lymphocyte subsets associated with marathon running. Med. Sci. Sports Exercise 25:186-190; 1993.
24. Heath, G.W.; Macera, C.A.; Nieman, D.C. Exercise and upper respiratory tract infection: Is there a relationship? Sports Med. 14:353-365; 1992.
25. Jensen, M. The influence of regular physical activity on the cell-mediated immunity in pigs. Acta Vet. Scand. 30:19-26; 1989.
26. Jokl, E. The immunological status of athletes. J. Sports Med. 14:165-167; 1974.
27. Kendall, A.; Hoffman-Goetz, L.; Houston, M.; MacNeil, B.; Arumugam, Y. Exercise and blood lymphocyte subset responses: Intensity, duration, and subject fitness effects. J. Appl. Physiol. 69:251-260; 1990.
28. Kokot, K.; Schaefer, R.M.; Teschner, M.; Gilge, U.; Plass, R.; Heidland, A. Activation of leukocytes during prolonged physical exercise. Adv. Exp. Med. Biol. 240:57-63; 1988.
29. Kusaka, Y.; Kondou, H.; Morimoto, K. Healthy lifestyles are associated with higher natural killer cell activity. Prevent. Med. 21:602-615; 1992.
30. Lewicki, R.; Tchórzewski, H.; Denys, A.; Kowalska, M.; Golinska, A. Effect of physical exercise on some parameters of immunity in conditioned sportsmen. Int. J. Sports Med. 8:309-314; 1987.
31. Lin, Y.S.; Jan, M.S.; Chen, H.I. The effect of chronic and acute exercise on immunity in rats. Int. J. Sports Med. 14:86-92; 1993.

32. Linde, F. Running and upper respiratory tract infections. Scand. J. Sports Sci. 9:21-23; 1987.
33. Linden, A.; Art, T.; Amory, H.; Massart, A.M.; Burvenich, C.; Lekeux, P. Quantitative buffy coat analysis related to adrenocortical function in horses during a three-day event competition. Zentralblatt Veterinärmed. 38:376-382; 1991.
34. Mackinnon, L.T.; Chick, T.W.; Van As, A.; Tomasi, T.B. Effects of prolonged intense exercise on natural killer cell number and function. Exercise Physiol. Curr. Select. Res. 3:77-89; 1988.
35. MacNeil, B.; Hoffman-Goetz, L. Chronic exercise enhances in vivo and in vitro cytotoxic mechanisms of natural immunity in mice. J. Appl. Physiol. 74:388-395; 1993.
36. MacNeil, B.; Hoffman-Goetz, L.; Kendall, A.; Houston, A.M.; Arumugam, Y. Lymphocyte proliferation responses after exercise in men: Fitness, intensity, and duration effects. J. Appl. Physiol. 70:179-185; 1991.
37. Muns, G. Effect of long-distance running on polymorphonuclear neutrophil phagocytic function of the upper airways. Int. J. Sports Med. 15:96-99; 1993.
38. Nasrullah, I.; Mazzeo, R.S. Age-related immunosenescence in Fischer 344 rats: Influence of exercise training. J. Appl. Physiol. 73:1932-1938; 1992.
39. Nehlsen-Cannarella, S.L.; Nieman, D.C.; Balk-Lamberton, A.J.; Markoff, P.A.; Chritton, D.B.W.; Gusewitch, G.; Lee, J.W. The effects of moderate exercise training on immune response. Med. Sci. Sports Exercise 23:64-70; 1991.
40. Nehlsen-Cannarella, S.L.; Nieman, D.C.; Jessen, J.; Chang, L.; Gusewitch, G.; Blix, G.G.; Ashley, E. The effects of acute moderate exercise on lymphocyte function and serum immunoglobulin levels. Int. J. Sports Med. 12:391-398; 1991.
41. Nieman, D.C. Physical activity, fitness and infection. In: Bouchard, C.; Shephard, R.J.; Stephens, T., eds. Physical activity, fitness, and health: International proceedings and consensus statement. Champaign, IL: Human Kinetics Books; 1994:796-813.
42. Nieman, D.C.; Berk, L.S.; Simpson-Westerberg, M.; Arabatzis, K.; Youngberg, W.; Tan, S.A.; Eby, W.C. Effects of long endurance running on immune system parameters and lymphocyte function in experienced marathoners. Int. J. Sports Med. 10:317-323; 1989.
43. Nieman, D.C.; Brendle, D.; Henson, D.A.; Suttles, J.; Cook, V.D.; Warren, B.J.; Butterworth, D.E.; Fagoaga, O.R.; Nehlsen-Cannarella, S.L. Immune function in athletes versus nonathletes. Int. J. Sports Med. 16:329-333; 1995.
44. Nieman, D.C.; Cook, V.D.; Henson, D.A.; Suttles, J.; Rejeski, W.J.; Ribisl, P.M.; Fagoaga, O.R.; Nehlsen-Cannarella, S.L. Moderate exercise training and natural killer cell cytotoxic activity in breast cancer patients. Int. J. Sports Med. 16:334-337; 1995.
45. Nieman, D.C.; Henson, D.A.; Gusewitch, G.; Warren, B.J.; Dotson, R.C.; Butterworth, D.E.; Nehlsen-Cannarella, S.L. Physical activity and immune function in elderly women. Med. Sci. Sports Exercise 25:823-831; 1993.
46. Nieman, D.C.; Henson, D.A.; Sampson, C.; Herring, J.L.; Suttles, J.; Conley, M.; Stone, M.H. Natural killer cell cytotoxic activity in weight lifters and sedentary controls. J. Strength Cond. Res. 8:251-254; 1994.
47. Nieman, D.C.; Johanssen, L.M.; Lee, J.W. Infectious episodes in runners before and after a roadrace. J. Sports Med. Phys. Fitness 29:289-296; 1989.

48. Nieman, D.C.; Johanssen, L.M.; Lee, J.W.; Arabatzis, K. Infectious episodes in runners before and after the Los Angeles Marathon. J. Sports Med. Phys. Fitness 30:316-328; 1990.
49. Nieman, D.C.; Miller, A.R.; Henson, D.A.; Warren, B.J.; Gusewitch, G.; Johnson, R.L.; Davis, J.M.; Butterworth, D.E.; Herring, J.L.; Nehlsen-Cannarella, S.L. Effects of high- versus moderate-intensity exercise on circulating lymphocyte subpopulations and proliferative response. Int. J. Sports Med. 15:199-206; 1994.
50. Nieman, D.C.; Miller, A.R.; Henson, D.A.; Warren, B.J.; Gusewitch, G.; Johnson, R.L.; Davis, J.M.; Butterworth, D.E.; Nehlsen-Cannarella, S.L. The effects of high- versus moderate-intensity exercise on natural killer cell cytotoxic activity. Med. Sci. Sports Exercise 25:1126-1134; 1993.
51. Nieman, D.C.; Nehlsen-Cannarella, S.L. The effects of acute and chronic exercise on immunoglobulins. Sports Med. 11:183-201; 1991.
52. Nieman, D.C.; Nehlsen-Cannarella, S.L. Effects of endurance exercise on immune response. In: Shephard, R.J.; Astrand, P.O., eds. Endurance in sport. Oxford, England: Blackwell Scientific Publications Ltd.; 1992.
53. Nieman, D.C.; Nehlsen-Cannarella, S.L. Exercise and infection. In: Eisinger, M.; Watson, R.W., eds. Exercise and disease. Boca Raton, FL: CRC Press, Inc.; 1992.
54. Nieman, D.C.; Nehlsen-Cannarella, S.L.; Donohue, K.M.; Chritton, D.B.W.; Haddock, B.L.; Stout, R.W.; Lee, J.W. The effects of acute moderate exercise on leukocyte and lymphocyte subpopulations. Med. Sci. Sports Exercise 23:578-585; 1991.
55. Nieman, D.C.; Nehlsen-Cannarella, S.L.; Markoff, P.A.; Balk-Lamberton, A.J.; Yang, H.; Chritton, D.B.W.; Lee, J.W.; Arabatzis, K. The effects of moderate exercise training on natural killer cells and acute upper respiratory tract infections. Int. J. Sports Med. 11:467-473; 1990.
56. Nieman, D.C.; Tan, S.A.; Lee, J.W.; Berk, L.S. Complement and immunoglobulin levels in athletes and sedentary controls. Int. J. Sports Med. 10:124-128; 1989.
57. Office of Disease Prevention and Health Promotion, U.S. Public Health Service, U.S. Department of Health and Human Services. Disease prevention/health promotion: The facts. Palo Alto, CA: Bull Publishing Co.; 1988.
58. Ortega, E.; Barriga, C.; De la Fuente, M. Study of the phagocytic process in neutrophils from elite sportswomen. Eur. J. Appl. Physiol. 66:37-42; 1993.
59. Ortega, E.; Collazos, M.E.; Barriga, C.; De la Fuente, M. Stimulation of the phagocytic function in guinea pig peritoneal macrophages by physical activity stress. Eur. J. Appl. Physiol. 64:323-327; 1992.
60. Ortega, E.; Collazos, M.E.; Maynar, M.; Barriga, C.; De la Fuente, M. Stimulation of the phagocytic function of neutrophils in sedentary men after acute moderate exercise. Eur. J. Appl. Physiol. 66:60-64; 1993.
61. Pahlavani, M.A.; Cheung, T.H.; Chesky, J.A.; Richardson, A. Influence of exercise on the immune function of rats of various ages. J. Appl. Physiol. 64:1997-2001; 1988.
62. Papa, S.; Vitale, M.; Mazzotti, G.; Neri, L.M.; Monti, G.; Manzoli, F.A. Impaired lymphocyte stimulation induced by long-term training. Immunol. Lett. 22:29-33; 1989.
63. Patrick, D. McColgan sets world best in Nike. USA Today. 1992 May 11.
64. Patrick, D. Pippig eyes world record. USA Today. 1994 April 19.
65. Pedersen, B.K. Influence of physical activity on the cellular immune system: Mechanisms of action. Int. J. Sports Med. 12 (suppl. 1):S23-S29; 1991.

66. Pedersen, B.K.; Tvede, N.; Christensen, L.D.; Klarlund, K.; Kragbak, S.; Halkjær-Kristensen, J. Natural killer cell activity in peripheral blood of highly trained and untrained persons. Int. J. Sports Med. 10:129-131; 1989.

67. Pedersen, B.K.; Tvede, N.; Hansen, F.R.; Anderson, V.; Bendix, T.; Bendixen, G.; Bendtzen, K.; Galbo, H.; Haahr, P.M.; Klarlund, K.; Sylvest, J.; Thomsen, B.; Halkjær-Kristensen, J. Modulation of natural killer cell activity in peripheral blood by physical exercise. Scand. J. Immunol. 27:673-678; 1988.

68. Pedersen, B.K.; Tvede, N.; Klarlund, K.; Christensen, L.D.; Hansen, F.R.; Galbo, H.; Kharazmi, A.; Halkjær-Kristensen, J. Indomethacin in vitro and in vivo abolishes post-exercise suppression of natural killer cell activity in peripheral blood. Int. J. Sports Med. 11:127-131; 1990.

69. Peters, A.M.; Allsop, P.; Stuttle, A.W.J.; Arnot, R.N.; Gwilliam, M.; Hall, G.M. Granulocyte margination in the human lung and its response to strenuous exercise. Clin. Sci. 82:237-244; 1992.

70. Peters, B.A.; Sothmann, M.; Wehrenberg, W.B. Blood leukocyte and spleen lymphocyte immune responses in chronically physically active and sedentary hamsters. Life Sci. 45:2239-2245; 1989.

71. Peters, E.M. Altitude fails to increase susceptibility of ultramarathon runners to post-race upper respiratory tract infections. S. Afr. J. Sports Med. 5:4-8; 1990.

72. Peters, E.M.; Bateman, E.D. Respiratory tract infections: An epidemiological survey. S. Afr. Med. J. 64:582-584; 1983.

73. Peters, E.M.; Goetzsche, J.M.; Grobbelaar, B.; Noakes, T.D. Vitamin C supplementation reduces the incidence of postrace symptoms of upper-respiratory-tract infection in ultramarathon runners. Am. J. Clin. Nutr. 57:170-174; 1993.

74. Rodriguez, A.B.; Barriga, C.; De la Fuente, M. Phagocytic function of blood neutrophils in sedentary young people after physical exercise. Int. J. Sports Med. 12:276-280; 1991.

75. Shinkai, S.; Kurokawa, Y.; Hino, S.; Hirose, M.; Torii, J.; Watanabe, S.; Watanabe, S.; Shiraishi, S.; Oka, K.; Watanabe, T. Triathlon competition induced a transient immunosuppressive change in the peripheral blood of athletes. J. Sports Med. Phys. Fitness 33:70-78; 1993.

76. Shinkai, S.; Shore, S.; Shek, P.N.; Shephard, R.J. Acute exercise and immune function: Relationship between lymphocyte activity and changes in subset counts. Int. J. Sports Med. 13:452-461; 1992.

77. Simpson, J.R.; Hoffman-Goetz, L. Exercise stress and murine natural killer cell function. Proc. Soc. Exp. Biol. Med. 195:129-135; 1990.

78. Smith, J.A.; Telford, R.D.; Mason, I.B.; Weidemann, M.J. Exercise, training and neutrophil microbicidal activity. Int. J. Sports Med. 11:179-187; 1990.

79. Soppi, E.; Varjo, P.; Eskola, J.; Laitinen, L.A. Effect of strenuous physical stress on circulating lymphocyte number and function before and after training. J. Clin. Lab. Immunol. 8:43-46; 1982.

80. Tharp, G.D.; Preuss, T.L. Mitogenic response of T-lymphocytes to exercise training and stress. J. Appl. Physiol. 70:2535-2538; 1991.

81. Tvede, N.; Steensberg, J.; Baslund, B.; Halkjær-Kristensen, J.; Pedersen, B.K. Cellular immunity in highly-trained elite racing cyclists and controls during periods of training with high and low intensity. Scand. J. Sports Med. 1:163-166; 1991.

82. Up with people. Runner's World, (April):77; 1990.

83. Van Tits, L.J.; Michel, M.C.; Grosse-Wilde, H.; Happel, M. Catecholamines increase lymphocyte beta 2-adrenergic receptors via a beta 2-adrenergic, spleen-dependent process. Am. J. Physiol. 258:E191-202; 1990.

84. Watson, R.R.; Moriguchi, S.; Jackson, J.C.; Werner, L.; Wilmore, J.H.; Freund, B.J. Modification of cellular immune functions in humans by endurance exercise training during β-adrenergic blockade with atenolol or propranolol. Med. Sci. Sports Exercise 18:95-100; 1986.

85. Wong, C.W.; Smith, S.D.; Thong, Y.H.; Opdebeeck, J.P.; Thornton, J.R. Effects of exercise stress on various immune functions in horses. Am. J. Vet. Res. 53:1414-1417; 1992.

CHAPTER 31

Exercise, Natural Immunology, and Cancer

Laurie Hoffman-Goetz
University of Waterloo, Waterloo, Ontario, Canada

There is a common perception among the general public that, unlike other prevalent chronic diseases such as heart disease or diabetes mellitus, cancer is not influenced by behavioral or lifestyle risk factors. For example, despite an enormous body of scientific evidence linking cigarette smoking (a very common, addictive behavior) with lung cancer, smoking onset rates continue to increase among North American female adolescents. Cancer has a strange place in our cultural perspective. Although cancer is a relatively prevalent disease, there is a widespread impression that it is both random and outside of individual control. Heart disease, which is the number one killer in terms of chronic diseases, does not seem to carry with it the gloomy overtones of a diagnosis of cancer. There is also a tendency to look for miracle cures and wonder drugs that will alleviate or even reverse cancer; in contrast, for other chronic conditions a preventive approach may be stressed through changes in diet or exercise patterns.

It is incontrovertible that the primary prevention of chronic disease is a more effective and less expensive approach than treatment. This is especially true of cancer given the morbidity, emotional anguish, and financial burden associated with active disease.

This chapter will focus on exercise as a preventive approach in the cancer equation. The relationship between exercise and immunological defenses against cancer, the role exercise might play in immunoprophylaxis, and possible biological mechanisms for an exercise-immune cancer will be discussed.

Cancer Prevention Research: Where Are We?

Are we making progress in either the battle or the war against cancer? However this is defined, a substantial reduction in total cancer mortality is essential. While it may be too optimistic to expect a rapid breakthrough against all cancers simultaneously (since cancer comprises more than 100 different diseases ranging from acute lymphoblastic leukemia to Wilms' tumor), it is not unrealistic to expect that the higher mortality for some cancers is balanced by reduced mortality for others.

The age-adjusted cancer mortality trends for North America indicate that the rates have steadily increased since 1950. When lung cancer is excluded from the picture, there is a small decline in the mortality rates. Most of this decrease in cancer mortality occurred before 1975. For example, from 1975 to 1989, the age-adjusted cancer death rate in Canada declined from 134 to 133.8 per 100,000—an extremely small reduction. Despite intensive research efforts, cancer epidemiologists and health promotion experts argue that the cancer mortality patterns are largely unchanged over the last two decades.

The conclusions reached are that the strong emphasis on progress in treatment of cancer may not have been as successful as one would have hoped. The failure to significantly reduce cancer incidence is all the more striking once national recommendations for cancer control are considered. In Canada the (Ontario) Premier's Council on Health Strategy lists as a target objective "a reduction in mortality from cancer by 10% in people under 65 years by the year 2000" (34). Similar policy documents with various targets for reduction in cancer mortality are found in many countries.

Against this backdrop of why cancer prevention has become so important as we enter the 21st century, there is increasing evidence for exercise as a prevention strategy in the war against cancer. A potential mechanism for the anticancer role of exercise may be through exercise-induced changes in natural immune function. The remainder of this paper reviews evidence for an inverse relationship between exercise and cancer development and how exercise-induced changes in immune function influence one aspect of the cancer process, namely that of metastasis.

Exercise and the Prevention of Cancer

In order to evaluate the relationship between exercise and cancer, it is helpful to consider some differences between physical activity, exercise, and physical fitness, since each of these terms has been used in the exercise-cancer literature. Caspersen (4) defined *physical activity* as any activity that results from muscular contraction and is best thought of as the total energy expenditure throughout a day, including sleep, occupational activity, and leisure activity. Most of the epidemiological studies on exercise and cancer examine physical activity to varying degrees. *Exercise* differs from the broader category of physical activity in that it involves the intention of those engaging in the activity to improve or maintain some aspect of physical fitness. The vast majority of studies on immune function examine responses to exercise only and not to the broader category of physical activity. Finally, *physical fitness* is a set of characteristics including cardiovascular and muscular endurance, strength, flexibility, and body composition. Physical fitness is determined in part by a genetic or inherited element. Some of the confusion in this area may be due to the different uses of the terms exercise, physical activity, and fitness. Better methods of determining physical activity and its subsets in human population studies would help in interpreting results and arriving at a true measure of the strength of the association.

Similarly, in considering the link between exercise and cancer, it is important to appreciate that cancer is not a unitary process. Neoplasia has been described as an evolving process: initiation, promotion, progression, and metastasis. Initiation, which occurs first in the natural history of neoplasia, is characterized by a permanent and irreversible change in the initiated cell; this change encompasses mutational alterations in the cellular genome (28). The second stage of cancer development is referred to as promotion. Promotion is characterized by operational reversibility (1); promoting agents typically alter gene expression in target cells and can selectively stimulate mitosis or inhibit apoptosis (programmed cell death) in initiated cells. Neoplastic progression involves the continuing destabilization and chromosomal deviation of initiated and promoted cells (29). For example, the increasing karyotypic deviation relates to patterns of increased growth and invasiveness of the neoplastic cell. The final stage, that of metastasis, involves the spread of malignant cells to distant sites with establishment of multiple tumor foci (19).

Similarly, the process of metastasis can be divided into a number of steps (6, 21). These steps include the detachment of specific tumor subpopulations from the primary mass with invasion of surrounding host tissue; the escape of tumor emboli into the vascular or lymphatic circulation (intravasation); the arrest of tumor cells or emboli in capillary beds of distant organs; the movement of tumor cells from the vasculature or lymphatics through the extracellular matrix; and the invasion of tissue or organ parenchyma and establishment of secondary growths or metastases. The process of metastasis involves the capacity of tumor cells to invade the extra-cellular matrix by secreting a variety of serine, aspartyl and cysteinyl proteases, metalloproteinases, and heparinases (3, 31). The expression of adhesion molecules by tumor cells is also essential for attachment and detachment of the tumor cells (39, 42). The expression of some adhesion molecules by tumor cells may not change; it may be that the distribution on cell membranes is more diffuse rather than localized to sites of focal adhesion (33). Moreover, there is increasing evidence to show that various cytokines and growth regulatory factors influence the expression of intercellular adhesion molecules on the membrane of immune and inflammatory cells (8). Many other factors—including mechanical stress caused by blood turbulence, by the capacity to resist or evade recognition by host immune defenses, by the presence of host hormones and growth factors, or by angiogenic capability of a given tissue—have important roles in the survival of tumor cells in the circulation and lymphatics. Indeed, most neoplastic cells that metastasize never form secondary foci. For example, even in the highly metastatic B16-BL6 mouse melanoma tumor, only 0.1% of injected cells ever produce final metastases (30).

Trying to isolate the impact of exercise on the cancer process is difficult, given the multifactorial process of carcinogenesis and the difficulty in measurement of physical activity in human populations. Nevertheless, there are some data from experimental models suggestive of a protective effect of exercise or training at various stages of cancer development. The majority of the evidence comes from postinitiation manipulations (i.e., promotional, progressional, or metastatic considerations). For example, Roebuck, McCaffrey, and Baumgartner (32) demonstrated in rats that voluntary wheel running, after initiation of pancreatic neoplastic foci with azaserine, was associated with a smaller size and reduced growth rate of the foci at 4 mo postinitiation. The antipromotional effects of exercise on hepatocarcino-genesis (38) and mammary adenocarcinogenesis (5) have also been described.

There are only a limited number of epidemiological studies that have investi-gated the relationship between exercise and cancer development. These studies have been recently reviewed (14, 37). For the most part, the data speak of a protective effect of physical activity or exercise for colon cancer. With the notable exception of colon cancer and exercise, there are simply an insufficient number of human studies on the relationship between exercise and other site-specific cancers to permit generalization.

Exercise and Natural Immunity

The immune system consists of a network of lymphoid organs, tissues, cells, and the secreted products of these cells. Most broadly, the immune system can be envisioned as being divided into three main components: the specific immune component; the innate, nonspecific, natural immune component; and the physical barriers of the body.

Nonspecific, innate, or natural immunity includes those cells and cell products of the immune system that do not stimulate immunological memory, are inducible, show self-nonself discrimination, and play an important role in inflammation and disease resistance (23). Three of the best-studied components of natural immunity are the natural killer (NK) cell, the lymphokine-activated killer (LAK) cell, and the macrophage, along with their cytokine products. Other chapters in this volume deal with macrophage and cytokine products of the innate immune system. The focus here will be on NK and LAK cells.

NK cells are a subpopulation of lymphocytes that exhibit spontaneous cytotoxicity against tumor targets without prior sensitization and in a manner that is independent of the major histocompatibility complex (11). Cell killing occurs by one of two mechanisms: necrosis and apoptosis. NK cellular cytotoxicity utilizes an apoptotic mechanism with the delivery of lethal damage to target cells by a regulated secretory pathway in NK cells (20). The granule exocytosis model of cell killing is a two-step process involving a group of closely related serine proteases (granzymes) and the lytic protein perforin (cytolysin). Perforin exocytosis results in target cell transmembrane pores, leading to osmotic instability and lysis (40); granzymes act synergistically with perforin to produce DNA fragmentation and apoptotic cell death (36, 37).

In vitro culture of NK cells with interleukin-2 (IL-2), IL-2 and tumor necrosis factor-α (TNF-α), or interferons (IFNs) induces differentiation into enhanced killer cells, known as LAK cells (2); LAK cells are able to kill a variety of tumor targets that are normally resistant to NK-mediated cytolysis. LAK cells may represent a functionally, rather than morphologically, discrete population of activated killers.

Evidence that NK (and LAK) cells have a major role in the control of tumor metastasis comes from studies on beige (T and B lymphocytes intact but NK cell deficient) and wild-type C57BL mice (9); animals were compared for experimental lung metastases as a function of basal NK activity. In the beige strain, tumor growth was significantly higher than in the wild-type strain. Mice injected with polyinosinic:polycytidylic acid (poly I:C), an IFN inducer that stimulates LAK cell generation, showed fewer tumor metastases if the injection occurred 24 h before tumor exposure than mice injected with vehicle control (10). Provocative work by Levy and colleagues (22) demonstrated that NK activity was significantly associated with axillary nodal status in 75 women with primary breast disease: lower NK cytolytic activity at the time of primary treatment was correlated with greater numbers of axillary lymph nodes positive for neoplastic cells. These studies point to a potentially important role for NK and LAK cells in the control of tumor distribution.

The effect of exercise on NK function is well documented in humans and has been reviewed by Hoffman-Goetz and Pedersen (18). After an acute bout of exercise, NK cytolytic activity increases markedly, drops abruptly, and then returns to levels observed before exercise. The biological basis for the pronounced, but transient, changes in NK cytolytic activity have been attributed to epinephrine and prostaglandin E; rapid demargination of NK cells from tissue reservoirs and entry into the circulation likely contribute to the initial increase in NK cytolytic activity. There are far fewer studies on training and NK cell functions. Although most tend to show an enhancement of NK cell cytolytic activity at rest in trained individuals, there are contradictory findings as well. Moreover, the mechanisms for the observed increase have not been characterized. The discrepancies are likely to be due to variations in the length of the training history, fitness levels of the subjects, time of sampling, and uncertainty about the degree of normal variation in NK cellular responses in the population. LAK activity has been shown to increase in response to acute exercise (13).

Exercise, Natural Immunity, and Metastasis

The complexity of the relationships among exercise, the natural immune system, and tumor metastasis is best illustrated by two tumor models that show differing resistance to cytolysis by natural immune effector cells. In a recent study of voluntary wheel running activity and forced treadmill exercise (15 m/min, 0% grade, 30 min/d, 5 times/wk for 9 wk), trained male C3H/He mice had higher in vitro splenic natural killer cell activity and in vivo clearance from the pulmonary vasculature of ^{51}Cr-labeled CIRAS tumor cells than did sedentary mice (24). An elevated natural killer cell activity was maintained in tumor-bearing mice who experienced detraining over 3 wk (25). Pretreatment of the animals with anti–asialo GM$_1$ antibody (anti-ASGM$_1$) eliminated the in vitro elevation in NK activity observed in the trained animals and partially blocked the clearance of radiolabeled tumor cells. Of clinical relevance was the observation that wheel-trained mice had fewer CIRAS tumors in the lungs than did the sedentary mice (trial 1: sedentary = 35 ± 5 vs. wheel runners = 25 ± 5; trial 2: sedentary = 117 ± 22 vs. wheel runners = 65 ± 18). The reduced tumor counts in the wheel-exercised mice were not due to a concomitant increase, at rest, in plasma tumor necrosis α concentrations in these mice (26).

In contrast to the preceding findings on the metastasis of the CIRAS 3 fibrosarcoma and exercise training are studies using an NK-resistant adenocarcinoma cell line (17). The MMT line 66 tumor is a cloned subpopulation originally derived from a single, spontaneously arising mammary tumor of a BALB/cfC3H mouse (7, 27). Similar to CIRAS 3, intravenous injection of MMT 66 produces pulmonary metastases within 3 wk. Female BALB/c mice that were sedentary (S), that were trained to run on a treadmill (T; 18 m/min, 0% grade, 30 min/d, 5 times/wk for 8 wk), or that had free access to in-cage running wheels (W) were injected with 5×10^4 tumor cells; the mice were then randomized into continuation of exercise (TT, WW), sedentary continuation (SS), cessation of exercise (TS, WS), or initiation of exercise (ST, SW) for a further 3 wk. Splenic LAK activity (a measure of primed or immunoenhanced NK cells) was significantly higher in the WS (44 ± 3%) and TS (49 ± 3%) mice compared with the sedentary (SS; 30 ± 3%) mice ($p < .05$ and .003, respectively). Despite higher LAK activities in the WS and TS mice, there was no difference in tumor burden among the groups. However, those mice that had the lowest LAK activity (TT mice: 18 ± 3%) also had the highest tumor yields (162 ± 22). These data suggest that the impact of exercise-induced changes in natural cytotoxic mechanisms on experimental tumor metastasis is determined (at least in part) by the sensitivity of the tumor to lysis by cells of the natural immune system (macrophages, natural killer cells, lymphokine activated killers, neutrophils). In other words, although exercise may modulate immune functions, the clinical relevance of the modulation is dependent on the specific sensitivity of tumor metastases to control by the immune system.

The timing of exercise in relation to tumor exposure appears to be critical in modulating the natural immune responses. In the C3H/He mice, exercise before CIRAS tumor exposure was associated with higher NK activity and in the BALB/c mice before MMT 66 tumor exposure with higher LAK activity relative to the other groups. Exercise begun after tumor exposure was associated with both lower natural immune activity and higher density of tumor foci than exercise before tumor exposure. Thus, the timing of exercise onset influences the extent of experimental tumor metastases.

Biological Mechanisms

By what mechanisms could exercise or training enhance NK cell activity against tumor targets and lead to reduced metastasis? Recent work from my laboratory points to several potential mechanisms, including differential expression of intracellular adhesion molecules (ICAMs) and activity of serine proteases.

The evidence for ICAMs is both direct and indirect. In one study (16), C3H/He and (C3H/He × BALB/c)F$_1$ mice were given free access to running wheels for 9 wk or were sedentary, after which time they were injected with radiolabeled CIRAS tumor cells. Lungs and other organs were collected at various time intervals after injection for remaining radioactivity. The data showed that trained mice had a lower retention of labeled tumor cells even at 5 min (59 ± 4%) after intravenous injection than sedentary mice (75 ± 3%). At 30 min (32 ± 3%), but not at 24 h (9 ± 1%), the trained mice still differed from sedentary animals (69 ± 3% at 30 min, 9 ± 1% at 24 h). Since exercise is known to elevate soluble serum ICAM (41), it was suggested that if training resulted in a greater expression of ICAMs by NK cells, this would lead to more efficient or rapid effector:tumor conjugates. Alternatively, if the expression of adhesion molecules expressed on vascular endothelium is altered in trained animals, this could lead to changes in the "traction" of the tumor cells, and hence extravasation. Studies are currently under way to find out whether NK cells from exercised and trained mice show greater ICAM-1 (i.e., LFA-1) and CD2 expression on NK cells or differences in target cell killing following adhesion blockade than those of sedentary controls and point to ICAM differences due to exercise (13).

A second approach used to determine mechanisms for enhanced NK cell cytotoxicity in trained animals and implications for tumor metastasis has been to evaluate granule exocytosis of serine esterases by NK cells. Preliminary work from my lab found that phorbol myristate acetate (PMA) and calcium ionophore–induced exocytosis of maximal BLT-esterase from splenic nonadherent cells did not differ in healthy mice trained to run on a treadmill versus sedentary controls (14). Splenic NK cytotoxicity measured at rest was significantly higher in the trained subjects. Surprisingly, this lack of effect for serine esterase activity was also characteristic of trained animals with tumors present. Thus, despite a small increase in NK cytolytic activity in vitro, serine esterase activity was not significantly affected by activity condition in mice bearing CIRAS tumors (figure 31.1). These data suggest that the

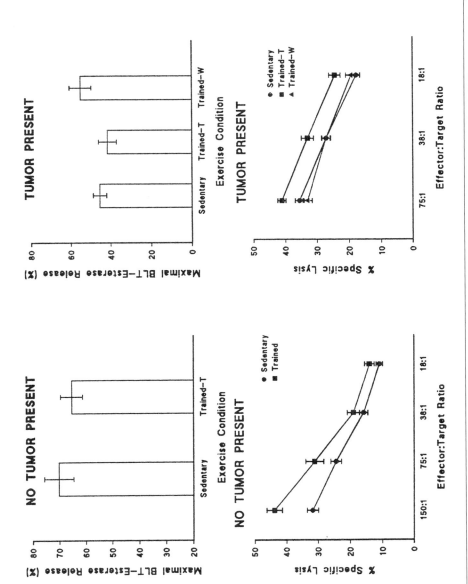

Figure 31.1   Effect of exercise on C3H/He mice without and with tumor present on splenic nonadherent maximal BLT-esterase release and on percentage specific lysis of ^{51}Cr-labeled YAC-1 target cells.

increase in NK cytolysis in trained individuals (with and without CIRAS tumors) is not due to a concomitant increase in the activity of BLT-esterase in NK cells. However, since the cells were maximally stimulated, a submaximal stimulus may yield different results; alternatively, other granzymes (non-BLT-esterases) or perforin may be influenced by training.

Future Directions

The mechanisms by which physiological changes induced by exercise or long-term adaptations with training alter cancer risk have not been well studied. Although descriptive studies of exercise and cancer are important for establishing epidemiological associations, parallel work is needed to isolate biologically credible mechanisms within a framework of theories of carcinogenesis. Each step in the multistep model of carcinogenesis represents distinct processes involved ultimately in the formation of a malignant tumor mass; depending on when exercise is administered in the cycle, acceleration or slowing of the tumorigenic process may occur. A partial list of factors in the design of studies on exercise, natural immunity, and carcinogenesis is shown in figure 31.2. This list covers aspects of the host biology rather than the tumor biology (i.e., immunogenicity, metastatic potential, route of metastasis).

Given that cancer is a constellation of diseases having complex interactive origins involving genetic, epigenetic, and environmental factors, a single unifying role for exercise or exercise immunology in the etiology of cancer is doubtful. And, although it is unlikely that changes in natural immune parameters associated with exercise or arising from training constitute a major factor in cancer development, even a small change in the population attributable risk would result in substantial economic and public health benefits.

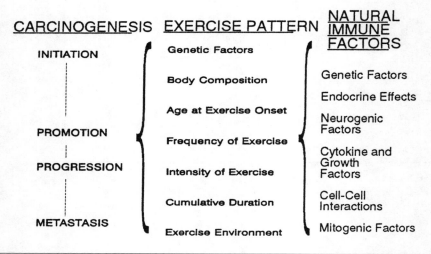

Figure 31.2   Factors to consider in design of exercise, natural immunity, and carcinogenesis studies.

Acknowledgment

The author acknowledges the research support from NSERC of Canada.

References

1. Berenblum, I. The cocarcinogenic action of croton resin. Cancer Res. 1:44-50; 1941.
2. Bonavida, B.; Lebow, L.T.; Jewett, A. Natural killer cell subsets: Maturation, differentiation and regulation. Natural Immun. 12:194-208; 1993.
3. Boyer, M.J.; Tannock, I.F. Lysosomes, lysosomal enzymes and cancer. Adv. Cancer Res. 60:269-291; 1993.
4. Caspersen, C.J.; Powell, K.E.; Christenson, G.M. Physical activity, exercise, and physical fitness: Definitions and distinctions for health related research. Public Health Rep. 100:126-131; 1985.
5. Cohen, L.A.; Choi, K.; Wang, C.-X. Influence of dietary fat, caloric restriction, and voluntary exercise on N-nitrosomethylurea-induced mammary tumorigenesis in rats. Cancer Res. 48:4276-4283; 1988.
6. Fidler, I.J. Cancer metastasis. Br. Med. Bull. 47:157-177; 1991.
7. Fulton, A.M.; Heppner, G.H. Relationships of prostaglandin E and natural killer sensitivity to metastatic potential in murine mammary adenocarcinomas. Cancer Res. 45:4779-4784; 1985.
8. Goebeler, M.; Roth; J.; Kunz, M.; Sorg, C. Expression of intercellular adhesion molecule-1 by murine macrophages is up-regulated during differentiation and inflammatory activation. Immunobiology 188:159-171; 1993.
9. Gorelik, E.; Wiltrout; R.H.; Okumura, K.; Habu, S.; Herberman, R.B. Role of NK cells in the control of metastatic spread and growth of tumor cells in mice. Int. J. Cancer 30:107-112; 1982.
10. Hanna, N. Expression of metastatic potential of tumor cells in young nude mice is correlated with low levels of natural killer cell–mediated cytotoxicity. Int. J. Cancer 26:675-680; 1980.
11. Herberman, R.B.; Ortaldo, J.R. Natural killer cells: Their role in defense against disease. Science 214:24-30; 1981.
12. Hoffman-Goetz, L. Effect of acute treadmill exercise on LFA-1 antigen expression in murine splenocytes. Anticancer Res. 15:1981-1984; 1995.
13. Hoffman-Goetz, L.; Arumugam, Y.; Sweeney, L. Lymphokine activated killer cell activity following voluntary physical activity in mice. J. Sports Med. Phys. Fitness 34:83-90; 1994.
14. Hoffman-Goetz, L.; Arumugam, Y.; Woolcott, C. Training alters serine esterase activity of mouse splenic nonadherent cells. Med. Sci. Sports Exercise 26: S182; 1994.
15. Hoffman-Goetz, L.; Husted, J.A. Exercise and breast cancer: Review and critical analysis of the literature. Can. J. Appl. Physiol. 19:237-252; 1994.
16. Hoffman-Goetz, L.; MacNeil, B.; Arumugam, Y. Tissue distribution of radio-labelled tumor cells in wheel exercised and sedentary mice. Int. J. Sports Med. 15:249-253; 1994.

17. Hoffman-Goetz, L.; May, K.M.; Arumugam, Y. Exercise training and mouse mammary tumour metastasis. Anticancer Res. 14:2627-2632; 1994.
18. Hoffman-Goetz, L.; Pedersen, B.K. Exercise and the immune system: A model of the stress response? Immunol. Today 15:382-387; 1994.
19. Ioachim, H.L. Immunobiology of metastases. Cancer Detect. Prevent. 15:127-131; 1991.
20. Joag, S.; Zychlinsky, A.; Young, J.D. Mechanisms of lymphocyte-mediated lysis. J. Cell. Biochem. 39:239-252; 1989.
21. Kerbel, R.S. Growth dominance of the metastatic cancer cell: Cellular and molecular aspects. Adv. Cancer Res. 55:87-132; 1990.
22. Levy, S.; Herberman, R.; Lippman, M.; d'Angelo, T. Correlation of stress factors with sustained depression of natural killer cell activity and predicted prognosis in patients with breast cancer. J. Clin. Oncol. 5:348-353; 1987.
23. Lotzová, E. Effector immune mechanisms in cancer. Natural Immun. Cell Growth Regul. 4:293-304; 1985.
24. MacNeil, B.; Hoffman-Goetz, L. Chronic exercise enhances in vivo and in vitro cytotoxic mechanisms of natural immunity in mice. J. Appl. Physiol. 74:388-395; 1993.
25. MacNeil, B.; Hoffman-Goetz, L. Effect of exercise on natural cytotoxicity and pulmonary tumor metastases in mice. Med. Sci. Sports Exercise 26:157-163; 1993.
26. MacNeil, B.; Hoffman-Goetz, L. Exercise training and tumour metastasis in mice: Influence of time of exercise onset. Anticancer Res. 13:2085-2088; 1993.
27. Miller, F.R.; Miller, B.E.; Heppner, G.H. Characterization of metastatic heterogeneity among subpopulations of a single mouse mammary tumor: Heterogeneity in phenotypic stability. Invasion Metast. 3:22-31; 1983.
28. Pitot, H.C. Multistage carcinogenesis—Genetic and epigenetic mechanisms in relation to cancer prevention. Cancer Detect. Prevent. 17:570-573; 1993.
29. Pitot, H.C. Progression: The terminal stage in carcinogenesis. Japan. J. Cancer Res. 808:599-607; 1989.
30. Price, J.E.; Aukerman, S.L.; Fidler, I.J. Evidence that the process of murine melanoma metastasis is sequential and selective and contains stochastic elements. Cancer Res. 46:5172-5178; 1986.
31. Reich, R.; Thompson, E.W.; Iwamoto, Y.; Martin, G.R.; Deason, J.R.; Fuller, G.C. Effects of inhibitors of plasminogen activator, serine proteinases, and collagenase IV on the invasion of basement membranes by metastatic cells. Cancer Res. 48:3307-3312; 1988.
32. Roebuck, B.D.; McCaffrey, J.; Baumgartner, K.J. Protective effects of voluntary exercise during the postinitiation phase of pancreatic carcinogenesis in the rat. Cancer Res. 50:6811-6816; 1990.
33. Roman, J.; LaChance, R.M.; Brockelmann, T.J.; Kennedy, C.J.R.; Wayner, E.A.; Carter, W.G. The fibronectin receptor is organized by extracellular matrix fibronectin: Implications for oncogenic transformation and for recognition of fibronectin matrices. J. Cell Biol. 108:2529-2543; 1989.
34. Shamley, M.; Dirks, J.; Marshall, V.; Carswell, A.O.; Pipe, A.; Rossi, M.; Scott, E.W. Towards health outcomes: Goals 2 and 4: Objectives and targets. Premier's Council on Health Strategy. Toronto: Government of Ontario; 1991:2-33.
35. Shi, L.; Kam, C.-M.; Powers, J.C.; Aebersold, R.; Greenberg, A.H. Purification of three cytotoxic lymphocyte granule serine proteases that induce apoptosis through distinct substrate and target cell interactions. J. Exp. Med. 176:1521-1529; 1992.

36. Shi, L.; Kraut, R.P.; Aebersold, R.; Greenberg, A.H. A natural killer cell granule protein that induces DNA fragmentation and apoptosis. J. Exp. Med. 175:553-566; 1992.

37. Sternfeld, B. Cancer and the protective effect of physical activity: The epidemiological evidence. Med. Sci. Sports Exercise 24:1195-1209; 1992.

38. Sugie, S.; Reddy, B.S.; Lowenfels, A.; Tanaka, T.; Mori, H. Effect of voluntary exercise on azoxymethane-induced hepatocarcinogenesis in male F344 rats. Cancer Lett. 63:67-72; 1992.

39. Takeichi, M. Cadherins: A molecular family important in selective cell-cell adhesion. Annu. Rev. Biochem. 59:237-252; 1990.

40. Thia, K.Y.T.; Smyth, M.J.; Trapani, J.A. Expression of human perforin in a mouse cytotoxic T lymphocyte cell line: Evidence for perturbation of granule-mediated cytotoxicity. J. Leuk. Biol. 54:528-533; 1993.

41. Tilz, G.P.; Domej, W.; Diez-Ruiz, A.; Weiss, G.; Breszinschek, R.; Breszinschek, H.; Huttel, E.; Pristautz, H.; Wachter, H.; Fuchs, D. Increased immune activation during and after physical exercise. Immunobiology 188:194-202; 1993.

42. Yamada, K.M. Adhesive recognition structures. J. Biol. Chem. 226:1209-1212; 1991.

CHAPTER 32

Age, Gender, and Nutritional Influences on Stress-Induced Cytokine Production

Joseph G. Cannon, Maria A. Fiatarone, William J. Evans
Pennsylvania State University, University Park, Pennsylvania, U.S.A.;
Tufts University, Boston, Massachusetts, U.S.A.; Pennsylvania State University,
University Park, Pennsylvania, U.S.A.

The Role of Cytokines in Metabolism and Host Defense

Cytokines such as interleukin-1 (IL-1), tumor necrosis factor (TNF), and IL-6 are now recognized as fundamental mediators of host responses to infection and trauma (27). In addition to augmenting immune responses and promoting other nonspecific antimicrobial mechanisms, these proteins have widespread influences on metabolic processes, including those highlighted in table 32.1.

Cytokine-mediated cytotoxic and inflammatory responses are beneficial to the host when effectively directed against invading microorganisms (26). However, in extreme circumstances such as septic shock, overexpression of these cytokines may damage host tissues and organs and actually contribute to morbidity and mortality (28). In addition, inflammatory diseases such as rheumatoid arthritis appear to be caused in part by cytokine dysregulation.

Survival rates in sepsis and in severe trauma and incidence rates for rheumatoid arthritis are age related. Therefore, there is current interest in determining if age-associated changes in cytokine production or action may underlie these clinical relationships.

Furthermore, there is considerable evidence that women are more resistant to infection than men (2, 12). However, a consequence of this superior immune responsiveness is that women are also more susceptible to autoimmune diseases (1). Lynch et al.

Table 32.1 Metabolic Processes Influenced by Interleukin-1

Thermoregulation	Anorexia	Glucose metabolism
Muscle proteolysis	Sleep	Lipid metabolism
Vascular resistance	HPA-axis alterations	Hepatic protein synthesis

have shown that IL-1 secretion is higher in women than men (24). Since IL-1 augments immune responsiveness, it may contribute to the gender differences in resistance to infection. Moreover, dysregulated IL-1-induced cytotoxicity and antibody production may be involved in the etiology of certain autoimmune diseases.

A better understanding of how cytokine production is affected by age and gender and of the extent to which cytokine production can be manipulated by diet may lead to more effective therapies for patients suffering from acute sepsis as well as chronic inflammatory or autoimmune diseases. Safe, controlled experimental models for inflammation or trauma in humans are needed to gain this understanding.

Eccentric Muscle Stress as an Experimental Model for Trauma

An eccentric action occurs when a muscle is forced to lengthen as it develops tension. For example, the quadriceps muscles perform eccentric actions when one walks down a flight of stairs. Because this type of action is less common, muscles are usually not well trained for such activity. As a result, an experimental protocol involving eccentric actions of high intensity or extended duration causes overload of muscle sarcomeres with limited, well-tolerated muscle damage and soreness. This sets into motion a sequence of responses qualitatively similar to a phenomenon observed during infection called the *acute phase response.*

The response is consistent with a scenario in which muscle damage liberates cellular fragments that in turn activate the complement system. This system comprises 20 plasma proteins that circulate in latent forms. Upon activation, a cascade of proteolytic cleavage reactions culminates in the formation of a variety of active complement components that have antibacterial and inflammatory properties. Following eccentric exercise, increases in activated complement components preceded and were proportional to increases in circulating neutrophils. These in turn preceded and were proportional to increases in muscle membrane permeability, as manifested by increased plasma creatine kinase levels (5). Both neutrophils and monocytes become activated, as evidenced by increases in plasma elastase and IL-1β, respectively (6). Table 32.2 shows the magnitude of the responses of young subjects to

Table 32.2   Comparison of Responses to Two Inflammatory Stresses

	Endotoxin infusion (%)		Eccentric stress (%)	
Complement activation	65	(32)	21	(5)
Plasma elastase	215	(25)	86	(6)
Neutrophilia	175	(36)	80	(9)
Plasma IL-1β	100	(10)	100	(8)
Plasma TNF	1,000	(10)	< 10	(8)

Values represent percentage increase. References in parentheses.

a classical inflammatory stress (endotoxin infusion) compared with eccentric stress. Although endotoxin infusion has been an important in vivo model for studying inflammatory/host defense mechanisms in young subjects, the potential cardio-vascular stresses of the procedure have restrained its use with older subjects.

Effects of Age and Nutrition on Cytokines and Inflammation

As mentioned, the age of a patient is a strong predictor of survival in critical care. Research regarding the influence of age on cytokine production and action has been conflicting (summarized in table 32.3). Considering the diversity of in vitro and in vivo approaches, stimuli, species differences, and measurement methods, these conflicting results are not surprising.

The eccentric stress model allows us to make measurements before and after an endogenous, in vivo inflammatory stress in humans. The benign nature of the stress (running downhill for 45 min at 75% of maximal heart rate) allows studies to be carried out in older human subjects. Thus, we are able to compare responses in older versus younger subjects as well as to compare the influence of dietary factors.

Complement

Eccentric stress-induced complement activation was similar in magnitude in groups of subjects younger than 33 yr as well as older than 60 yr (5). These results are in line with other studies showing that concentrations of circulating complement precursors do not decline with age.

Table 32.3   The Influence of Age on Cytokine Production and Action

Cytokine	Influence of aging	System	Species	Assay	Reference
IL-1	↔LPS-induced synthesis	In vitro	Human	Bioassay	(29)
	↓LPS-induced synthesis	In vitro	Mouse	Bioassay	(4)
	↓Sensitivity to IL-1	In vitro	Mouse	—	(4)
	↓LPS-induced synthesis	In vitro	Mouse	Bioassay	(19)
	↓Sensitivity to IL-1	In vitro	Human	—	(21)
	↑Urinary levels	In vivo	Human	Immunoassay	(22)
	ConA-induced synthesis	In vitro	Rat	Bioassay	(29)
TNF	↑Circulatory concentration after LPS infusion	In vivo	Rat	Bioassay	(16)
IL-6	↑Circulatory concentration, spontaneous synthesis	Both	Human	Immunoassay	(13)

LPS = lipopolysaccharide; ConA = concanavalin A.

Circulating Neutrophils

The increase in circulating neutrophils in older subjects following eccentric stress was approximately half that observed in younger subjects (5, 9). Dietary supplementation of older subjects with the antioxidant vitamin E brought the neutrophil response of the older subjects up to the level observed in the younger group (9). Vitamin E supplementation had no effect on the neutrophil responses of the younger subjects. It has been postulated that an age-related decline in endogenous antioxidant defenses may cause loss of leukocyte function. The restoration of response with vitamin E in our experiments supports this contention.

Elastase

Elastase, a proteolytic enzyme, is stored in cytosolic granules within neutrophils. Upon neutrophil activation by microbial products, activated complement, or other inflammatory mediators, elastase is released into the plasma. Thus, plasma elastase concentrations provide a marker for neutrophil activation in vivo. Increases in plasma elastase following eccentric stress were significantly smaller in older subjects than in younger subjects (6). However, when the diets of older subjects were supplemented with fish oil, the post–eccentric exercise elastase response was indistinguishable from that of the younger subjects. Fish oil provides an increased intake of eicosapentaenoic acid (EPA) and tends to cause a reduction of plasma and tissue levels of arachidonic acid (AA). The in vivo EPA/AA ratio affects leukotriene synthesis, which in turn regulates neutrophil degranulation.

Cytokine Production

Exercise (both concentric and eccentric) causes increases in circulating cytokines (7, 34), cytokine production (8, 17), and urinary cytokine (31) levels. However, the magnitude and temporal development of these increases have been extremely variable. Recently, we found that eccentric exercise–induced increases in IL-1β and TNF-α production in both young and old subjects taking dietary supplements of vitamin E were significantly less than in those taking a soybean oil "placebo" (8). In further studies involving dietary supplementation with fish oil or no dietary oil supplement whatsoever, a large degree of interindividual variability was observed (6). Upon closer examination, it was determined that the variability in cytokine production could be explained in large part by an individual's AA and lipid peroxide levels. AA is the precursor for prostaglandin E_2 (PGE$_2$), which inhibits cytokine production in vitro. Other in vitro studies have shown that reactive oxygen species and lipid peroxides augment cytokine production. Thus, the eccentric stress model has provided in vivo data in support of these previous in vitro findings. Subsequent to our studies employing soybean oil as a placebo, it has been shown that diets supplemented with soybean oil actually promote the formation of lipid peroxides (18). Therefore the pronounced postexercise increases in cytokine production observed in our soybean oil–supplemented groups did not represent a placebo-controlled basal condition, but rather diet-induced augmentation of cytokine production.

Dietary Modulation of Inflammatory Processes

The foregoing sections (summarized in figure 32.1) indicate that certain aspects of neutrophil function that diminish with age are apparently restored through dietary modifications. Cytokine production can be modulated through diet as well. Such dietary control may have important clinical ramifications for counteracting excessive cytokine production during sepsis or rheumatoid arthritis.

As consideration is given to modulating cytokine production and action through dietary (or other) means, it is important to understand that patients may benefit from correction of cytokine levels, but not from total blockade of cytokine production. Kampschmidt and Pulliam (20) first demonstrated in 1975 that products of activated leukocytes enhance resistance to infection. Subsequently, van der Meer et al. (33) identified IL-1 as one of the leukocyte products able to reduce mortality from potentially lethal infection. Others have gone on to demonstrate similar results for other cytokines. On the other hand, administration of antibodies and antagonists to IL-1 and TNF have been shown to reduce mortality in several models of severe sepsis (3, 35). To add to the complexity, total circulating IL-1β and the capacity

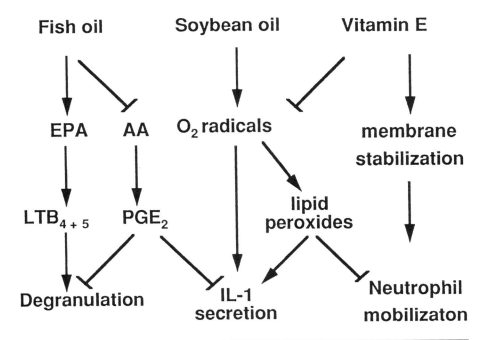

Figure 32.1   Schematic representation of the influence of diet on the intermediate factors that regulate the inflammatory responses. Arrowheads signify augmentation; crossbars signify inhibition. LTB = Leukotriene B.

for monocytes to make IL-1 correlated positively with survival in septic patients (10, 23). However, using an immunoassay that only detected unbound IL-1β, an inverse relationship was observed (11). Thus, not only do we need to develop the means to modulate cytokine levels in vivo, but we need to learn what constitutes an optimal cytokine level and how to best measure it (14).

Gender-Related Differences in Cytokine Responses

There is growing evidence that the production and disposition of IL-1 and other cytokines are markedly different between women and men. The eccentric stress model allows us to compare cytokine responses between genders and to relate these to other physiological responses that result from eccentric stress. For example, we have found that women, regardless of age, have a higher rate of IL-1 receptor antagonist (IL-1Ra) excretion than men before eccentric stress, which significantly increases in the 24-h period after the stress (15). IL-1Ra is an endogenous inhibitor of IL-1 that competes for the same binding sites on target cells but does not induce a biological response.

During infection, IL-1 contributes (possibly indirectly) to increased muscle protein breakdown. In a previous study of only male subjects, we found that cellular production of IL-1 significantly correlated with eccentric exercise-induced increases in urinary 3-methylhistidine (8). In more recent studies, women exhibited no significant increase in 3-methylhistidine following eccentric exercise (15). A possible explanation for these results is that higher levels of IL-1Ra in women inhibited the proteolytic activity of IL-1. Clearly, further studies are needed to fully quantify IL-1 agonist and antagonist responses in men and women following eccentric stress. Furthermore, other hormones that influence the proteolytic response need to be carefully considered.

The eccentric stress model has potential utility not only for examining gender-related differences in healthy subjects, but also to determine if inappropriate inflammatory responses are the basis for certain disease states. For example, studies are underway to determine if patients with chronic fatigue syndrome exhibit exaggerated cytokine responses following eccentric stress. Overproduction of cytokines such as IL-1 could account for the low-grade fevers and myalgias experienced by these patients.

Acknowledgments

This work was supported by NIH grants AR39595 and AI33414.

References

1. Ahmed, S.A.; Penhale, W.J.; Talal, N. Sex hormones, immune responses, and autoimmune diseases. Am. J. Pathol. 121:531-551; 1985.

2. Allen, E.V. The relationship of sex to disease. Ann. Intern. Med. 7:1000-1012; 1934.

3. Beutler, B.; Milsark, I.W.; Cerami, A.C. Passive immunization against cachectin/tumor necrosis factor protects mice from the lethal effect of endotoxin. Science 229:869-871; 1985.

4. Bruley-Rosset, M.; Vergnon, I. Interleukin-1 synthesis and activity in aged mice. Mech. Ageing Develop. 24:247-264; 1984.

5. Cannon, J.G.; Fiatarone, M.A.; Fielding, R.A.; Evans, W.J. Aging and stress-induced changes in complement activation and neutrophil mobilization. J. Appl. Physiol. 76:2616-2620; 1994.

6. Cannon, J.G.; Fiatarone, M.A.; Meydani, M.; Scott, L.; Blumberg, J.B.; Evans, W.J. Aging and dietary modulation of elastase and interleukin-1β secretion. Am. J. Physiol. 268:R208-R213; 1995.

7. Cannon, J.G.; Kluger, M.J. Endogenous pyrogen activity in human plasma after exercise. Science 220:617-619; 1983.

8. Cannon, J.G.; Meydani, S.N.; Fielding, R.A.; Fiatarone, M.A.; Meydani, M.; Farhangmehr, M.; Orencole, S.F.; Blumberg, J.B.; Evans, W.J. Acute phase response in exercise. II. Associations between vitamin E, cytokines and muscle proteolysis. Am. J. Physiol. 260:R1235-R1240; 1991.

9. Cannon, J.G.; Orencole, S.F.; Fielding, R.A.; Meydani, M.; Meydani, S.N.; Fiatarone, M.A.; Blumberg, J.B.; Evans, W.J. Acute phase response in exercise: Interaction of age and vitamin E on neutrophils and muscle enzyme release. Am. J. Physiol. 259:R1214-R1219; 1990.

10. Cannon, J.G.; Tompkins, R.G.; Gelfand, J.A.; Michie, H.R.; Stanford, G.G.; van der Meer, J.W.M.; Endres, S.; Lonnemann, G.; Corsetti, J.; Chernow, B.; Wilmore, D.W.; Wolff, S.M.; Burke, J.F.; Dinarello, C.A. Circulating interleukin-1 and tumor necrosis factor in septic shock and experimental endotoxin fever. J. Infect. Dis. 161:79-84; 1990.

11. Casey, L.C.; Balk, R.A.; Bone, R.C. Plasma cytokine and endotoxin levels correlate with survival in patients with the sepsis syndrome. Ann. Intern. Med. 119:771-778; 1993.

12. Centers for Disease Control. Mortality patterns—United States, 1989. Morbid. Mortal. Weekly Rep. 41:121-124; 1992.

13. Daynes, R.A.; Araneo, B.A.; Ershler, W.B.; Maloney, C.; Li, G.-Z.; Ryu, S.-Y. Altered regulation of IL-6 production with normal aging. J. Immunol. 150:5219-5230; 1993.

14. Dinarello, C.A.; Cannon, J.G. Cytokine measurements in septic shock. Ann. Intern. Med. 119:853-854; 1993.

15. Fielding, R.A.; Manfredi, T.J.; Parzick, A.D.; Fiatarone, M.A.; Evans, W.J.; Cannon, J.G. Eccentric exercise-induced muscle injury in humans: Effects on muscle cytokines, ultrastructure, and size. (Submitted for publication.)

16. Foster, K.D.; Conn, C.A.; Kluger, M.J. Fever, tumor necrosis factor, and interleukin-6 in young, mature and aged Fischer 344 rats. Am. J. Physiol. 262:R211-R215; 1992.

17. Haahr, P.M.; Pedersen, B.K.; Fomsgaard, A.; Tvede, N.; Diamant, M.; Klarlund, K.; Halkjær-Kristensen, J.; Bendtzen, K. Effect of physical exercise on in vitro production of interleukin-1, interleukin-6, tumor necrosis factor, interleukin-2 and interferon-γ. Int. J. Sports Med. 12:223-227; 1991.

18. Huang, C.-J.; Fwu, M.-L. Protein insufficiency aggravates the enhanced lipid peroxidation and reduced activities of antioxidant enzymes in rats fed diets high in polyunsaturated fat. J. Nutr. 122:1182-1189; 1992.

19. Inamizu, T.; Chang, M.P.; Makinodan, T. Influence of age on the production and regulation of interleukin-1 in mice. Immunology 55:447-455; 1985.
20. Kampschmidt, R.F.; Pulliam, L.A. Stimulation of antimicrobial activity in the rat with leukocyte endogenous mediator. J. Reticuloendothelial Soc. 17:162-168; 1975.
21. Lee, M.A.; Segal, G.M.; Bagby, G.C. The hematopoietic microenvironment in the elderly: Defects in IL-1-induced CSF expression in vitro. Exp. Hematol. 17:952-956; 1989.
22. Liao, Z.; Tu, J.H.; Small, C.B.; Schnipper, S.M.; Rosenstreich, D.L. Increased urine interleukin-1 levels in aging. Gerontology 39:19-27; 1993.
23. Luger, A.; Graf, H.; Schwartz, H.P.; Stummvoll, H.K.; Luger, T.A. Decreased serum interleukin-1 activity and monocyte interleukin-1 production in patients with fatal sepsis. Crit. Care Med. 14:458-461; 1986.
24. Lynch, E.A.; Dinarello, C.A.; Cannon, J.G. Gender differences in IL-1α, IL-1β and IL-1 receptor antagonist secretion from mononuclear cells and urinary excretion. J. Immunol. 153:300-306; 1994.
25. Meyer, J.; Yurt, R.W.; Duhaney, R.; Hesse, D.G.; Tracey, K.J.; Fong, Y.; Richardson, D.; Calvano, S.; Dineen, P.; Shires, G.T.; Lowry, S.F.; Davis, J.M. Differential neutrophil activation before and after endotoxin infusion in enterally versus parenterally fed volunteers. Surg. Gyn. Obst. 167:501-509; 1988.
26. Neta, R.; Oppenheim, J.J. Why should internists be interested in interleukin-1? Ann. Intern. Med. 109:1-3; 1988.
27. Oppenheim, J.J.; Rossio, J.L.; Gearing, A.J.H., eds. Clinical applications of cytokines: Role in pathogenesis, diagnosis and therapy. New York: Oxford University Press; 1993:379.
28. Parrillo, J.E.; Parker, M.M.; Natanson, C.; Suffredini, A.F.; Danner, R.L.; Cunnion, R.E.; Ognibene, F.P. Septic shock in humans. Ann. Intern. Med. 113:227-242; 1990.
29. Rosenberg, J.S.; Gilman, S.C.; Feldman, J.D. Effects of aging on cell cooperation and lymphocyte responsiveness to cytokines. J. Immunol. 130:1754-1758; 1983.
30. Rudd, A.G.; Banerjee, D.K. Interleukin-1 production by human monocytes in ageing and disease. Age Ageing 18:43-46; 1989.
31. Sprenger, H.; Jacobs, C.; Nain, M.; Gressner, A.M.; Prinz, H.; Wesemann, W.; Gemsa, D. Enhanced release of cytokines, interleukin-2 receptors, and neopterin after long-distance running. Clin. Immunol. Immunopathol. 63:188-195; 1992.
32. Suffredini, A.F.; Harpel, P.C.; Parrillo, J.E. Promotion and subsequent inhibition of plasminogen activation after administration of intravenous endotoxin to normal subjects. N. Engl. J. Med. 320:1165-1172; 1989.
33. van der Meer, J.W.M.; Barza, M.; Wolff, S.M.; Dinarello, C.A. A low dose of recombinant interleukin 1 protects granulocytopenic mice from lethal Gram-negative infection. Proc. Natl. Acad. Sci. USA 85:1620-1623; 1988.
34. Viti, A.; Muscettola, M.; Paulesa, L.; Bocci, V.; Almi, A. Effect of exercise on plasma interferon levels. J. Appl. Physiol. 59:426-428; 1985.
35. Wakabayashi, G.; Gelfand, J.A.; Burke, J.F.; Thompson, R.C.; Dinarello, C.A. A specific receptor antagonist for interleukin-1 prevents E. coli-induced shock in rabbits. FASEB J. 5:338-343; 1991.
36. Wolff, S.M.; Rubenstein, M.; Mulholland, J.H.; Alling, D.W. Comparison of hematologic and febrile response to endotoxin in man. Blood 26:190-201; 1965.

PART IX

Nutritional Influences on Fatigue

CHAPTER 33

Metabolic Responses to Carbohydrate and Lipid Supplementation During Exercise

Mark Hargreaves
The University of Melbourne, Parkville, Australia

Since the early part of this century, the importance of carbohydrates and lipids for exercise metabolism has been recognized (7, 8, 34). In the intervening years, many studies have examined the metabolic effects and potential ergogenic benefits of carbohydrate supplementation before, during, and after exercise. Although most attention has focused on carbohydrate metabolism and exercise performance, there has also been interest in the potential performance-enhancing effects of lipid supplementation. This paper will briefly review the metabolic effects of carbohydrate and lipid supplementation during exercise.

Carbohydrate Supplementation

Carbohydrate ingestion during prolonged, strenuous exercise is associated with enhanced performance, as measured either by an ability to maintain or increase work output during exercise (31, 40, 42, 54) or by an increased exercise time to fatigue (9, 13, 14, 17, 52). The increase in exercise performance is thought to be due in large part to maintenance of blood glucose levels and a high rate of carbohydrate oxidation late in exercise when muscle glycogen levels are reduced (9, 10, 13). Carbohydrate depletion results in reduced availability of pyruvate (48), a substrate for both acetyl CoA formation and anaplerotic reactions responsible for production of various tricarboxylic acid cycle intermediates (TCAI). Indeed, glycogen depletion is associated with reduced TCAI levels, a slight (approximately 10%) reduction in intramuscular [ATP] and increases in [IMP], suggesting an imbalance between rates of ATP utilization and resynthesis (48). The changes in [TCAI] and [IMP] are attenuated by ingestion of carbohydrate (52). In contrast, we have recently observed that muscle [ATP] and [IMP] following, and estimated carbohydrate oxidation during, exercise to fatigue were similar with and without carbohydrate ingestion, despite a 33% increase in endurance performance when carbohydrate was ingested (Hargreaves, Snow, McConell, and Proietto, unpublished data). This suggests that factors other than, or in addition to, carbohydrate supply to contracting skeletal muscle may have contributed to the enhanced exercise tolerance. For example, it is possible that the maintenance of blood glucose levels prevents, or at least attenuates, the negative effects of hypoglycemia on central nervous system function (6, 17). The potential role of central fatigue during prolonged exercise and the effect of carbohydrate ingestion have been discussed by others (see chapter 35). Since carbohydrate ingestion delays fatigue rather than preventing it, there are likely to be many factors involved in the etiology of fatigue during prolonged exercise (22).

A number of studies have failed to observe any effect of increased blood glucose availability on net muscle glycogen utilization during prolonged cycling exercise at 70% to 75% $\dot{V}O_2$max (4, 13, 15, 24, 40). In contrast, during variable-intensity, intermittent exercise, carbohydrate ingestion results in a reduction in net muscle glycogen utilization (25, 61). The periods of relatively low intensity exercise may allow for increased blood glucose and insulin levels (61), which facilitate muscle glucose uptake and utilization and perhaps even promote glycogen synthesis (35). During prolonged treadmill exercise at 70% $\dot{V}O_2$max, carbohydrate supplementation has been shown to reduce net glycogen utilization in vastus lateralis (56). In a subsequent study from the same group, this reduction in muscle glycogen use was observed to be restricted to type I muscle fibers and could account for the 27% improvement in endurance capacity during treadmill running to exhaustion (55). The reasons for a differential effect of carbohydrate ingestion on muscle glycogen utilization during prolonged cycling and running are not readily apparent. One possibility is that vastus lateralis is not recruited as much as other leg muscles during treadmill running, and increased glucose availability may result in enhanced glucose uptake by, and reduced glycogen degradation in, this muscle. However, the vastus lateralis glycogen levels at fatigue were quite low (55), suggesting extensive recruitment of this muscle.

Studies using ^{13}C-labeled glucose have demonstrated that glucose ingestion during exercise results in a decrease in the oxidation of endogenous carbohydrate stores (37, 43, 45, 60). As previously discussed, glucose ingestion has little effect on muscle glycogen utilization, at least during prolonged, strenuous cycling exercise. Thus, it is likely that mobilization of the liver glycogen reserves is inhibited by carbohydrate ingestion. We have recently completed a study examining this question (39). Six trained men exercised for 2 h at approximately 70% $\dot{V}O_2$max with and without glucose ingestion. Glucose turnover was measured using a primed, continuous infusion of 6,6-^{2}H-glucose, and hepatic glucose production was determined from the rate of appearance of glucose, corrected for gut-derived glucose obtained from the appearance of [^{3}H]glucose added to the 10% glucose drink. Over the 2 h of exercise, there was a 51% reduction in total hepatic glucose production when glucose was ingested (figure 33.1). This value is almost identical to that observed in another recent report (4). Although our tracer method cannot distinguish between liver glycogenolysis and gluconeogenesis as sources of hepatic glucose production, it is likely that both processes were inhibited by glucose ingestion. The increases in plasma glucose and insulin during exercise with glucose ingestion are the likely causes of the reduced hepatic glucose production. In addition, it is possible that the lower plasma glucagon and adrenaline levels observed in the latter stages of the exercise bout may have played a role.

Despite the reduction in hepatic glucose production, plasma glucose levels were higher throughout exercise when glucose was ingested, and this resulted in an increased tracer-determined glucose uptake (glucose R_d). Over the 2 h of exercise,

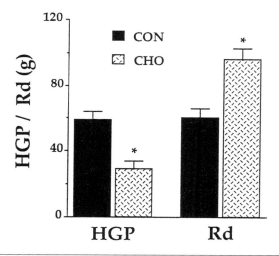

Figure 33.1   Total hepatic glucose production (HGP) and glucose uptake (R_d) during 2 h of cycling exercise at 70% $\dot{V}O_2$max with (CHO) and without (CON) glucose inges-tion. Values are means $\pm$ *SE* ($n = 6$). * denotes different from CON, $p < .05$. Data from McConell et al. 1994 (39).

there was a 60% increase in glucose R_d (figure 33.1). This increase in glucose R_d is consistent with previous observations of increased leg glucose uptake during low-intensity exercise with glucose ingestion (2) and of elevated rates of glucose disposal and oxidation during prolonged, strenuous exercise when blood glucose availability is increased (4, 10, 15, 28). As mentioned, the increase in blood glucose is a major factor contributing to the increase in muscle glucose uptake and oxidation; however, since metabolic clearance rate (glucose R_d/[glucose]) was also elevated during exer-cise with glucose ingestion (39), the increase in plasma insulin is also important. In addition, in the second hour of exercise, plasma FFA levels were lower when glucose was ingested, and this may have contributed in part to increased muscle glucose uptake (26). The highest glucose R_d during the latter stages of exercise was 1.18 ± 0.12 g $\cdot$ min^{-1}, and this agrees with peak values for glucose uptake or oxidation during prolonged, strenuous exercise obtained from a-v glucose differences (5), intravenous glucose infusion rates (9), or tracer methods (10, 29, 60). Thus, the maximal rate of oxidation of ingested carbohydrate appears to be in the range of 1 to 1.2 g $\cdot$ min^{-1} and is similar regardless of which type of carbohydrate is ingested (23, 29, 30, 36, 37, 41, 49, 60), although fructose is oxidized to a lesser extent than other carbohydrates (23, 36, 37).

Soluble corn starch is oxidized to a greater extent than insoluble starch during exercise (49). This is most likely due to the higher amylopectin/amylose ratio in the soluble starch, since the rate of digestion of amylopectin is more rapid than that of amylose (49). Increasing the concentration of ingested carbohydrate above about 8% has little effect on exogenous carbohydrate oxidation (figure 33.2; 41, 60). The potential factors limiting exogenous carbohydrate oxidation are glucose delivery (gastric emptying and intestinal absorption) and the ability of contracting muscle to take up and oxidize glucose. It has been suggested that the limit lies within the muscle (45); however, prior glycogen depletion, which might be expected to increase

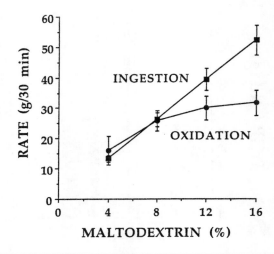

Figure 33.2   Rates of exogenous carbohydrate ingestion and oxidation during 90 to 120 min of cycling exercise at 65% Wmax with increasing beverage carbohydrate concentration. Values are means ± *SE* (*n* = 6). Data from Wagenmakers et al. 1993 (60).

muscle glucose uptake (27), was not associated with a greater exogenous [¹³C]glucose oxidation during exercise (44). Furthermore, in our own study (39), total glucose R_d was higher than the total amount of gut-derived glucose (34% of total glucose ingested), indicating that the contracting muscle took up all of the exogenous glucose that was presented to it. While some of the ingested glucose is absorbed and removed by the liver on first pass, it is likely that some remains within the gastrointestinal tract. Since gastric emptying does not appear to be a limiting factor (29, 41), the rate-limiting step may be intestinal absorption. Of interest, co-ingestion of glucose and fructose, which are absorbed by different mechanisms, results in greater exogenous carbohydrate oxidation than the ingestion of either glucose or fructose alone (1). Increasing blood glucose levels by intravenous infusion, above those obtained by carbohydrate ingestion, also results in higher rates of exogenous glucose oxidation (28). Nevertheless, even under these circumstances, a large proportion of the exogenous carbohydrate load cannot be accounted for by oxidation within contracting muscle (15). The metabolic fate of the "extra" carbohydrate (glycogen/lipid synthesis?) and the factors limiting oxidation of ingested carbohydrate warrant further investigation.

In addition to the aforementioned effects of carbohydrate supplementation on glycogen and glucose metabolism, there are also alterations in lipid and protein metabolism. Carbohydrate ingestion results in lower plasma FFA levels during prolonged, strenuous exercise (13, 14, 17), and this may account in part for lower rates of lipid oxidation. In addition, increased glucose availability results in higher muscle malonyl CoA (19), an inhibitor of FFA oxidation in contracting muscle. The effect of carbohydrate ingestion on intramuscular triglyceride utilization during exercise has not been examined. Increased blood glucose availability has also been observed to inhibit leucine oxidation (16), an effect that is likely to be due to an attenuation of the exercise-induced activation of the branched-chain oxoacid dehydrogenase by increased carbohydrate availability (59). In keeping with an inhibitory effect on amino acid catabolism, we have recently observed an attenuation of muscle and plasma ammonia accumulation during prolonged, nonfatiguing exercise when carbohydrate is ingested (Snow, Febbraio, Stathis, Carey, and Hargreaves, unpublished data).

Lipid Supplementation

As discussed, carbohydrate supplementation enhances endurance exercise performance, in part by maintaining carbohydrate availability and oxidation. Another approach has been to increase plasma FFA availability with the intention of enhancing fat oxidation and reducing carbohydrate utilization in contracting skeletal muscle, thereby delaying the onset of carbohydrate depletion. This is based largely upon the so-called glucose–fatty acid cycle (see chapter 12) and the view that muscle FFA oxidation during strenuous exercise is limited by FFA availability (46). Indeed, increased plasma FFA availability during strenuous exercise, as a consequence of intravenous Intralipid and heparin infusion, results in increased FFA oxidation (47). However, FFA oxidation was not fully restored to levels seen during less intense exercise (46), suggesting that the ability of muscle to take up and oxidize FFA at higher exercise intensities may also be a limiting factor. Nevertheless, total carbohydrate oxidation was lower when plasma FFA levels were elevated, without any effect of glucose R_d, suggesting a reduction in muscle glycogen utilization (47). This is in keeping with earlier observations that increased plasma FFA availability as a result of fat feeding or Intralipid infusion in combination with heparin administration resulted in a reduction in net muscle glycogen utilization during exercise at 70% to 85% $\dot{V}O_2$max (11, 18, 58). In contrast, increased plasma FFA availability had no effect on muscle glycogen utilization during dynamic knee extension exercise at 80% maximal power output (Wmax), but did result in a 30% to 40% reduction in muscle glucose uptake (26). The discrepancy between experimental results is difficult to explain but may be related in part to differences in the exercise mode and the methodology used to examine carbohydrate metabolism.

While Intralipid and heparin infusion has proved useful in studying the underlying mechanisms of lipid-carbohydrate interactions during exercise, it is not a practical way of elevating plasma FFA levels and oxidation during exercise. Carnitine is involved in the transport of fatty acids across the mitochondrial membrane and may represent a limiting step in FFA oxidation; however, carnitine supplementation has no effect on lipid metabolism during exercise (51). Caffeine ingestion has been shown to increase plasma FFA levels (12), intramuscular triglyceride utilization (20), and lipid oxidation (12, 20) during exercise and to enhance endurance performance (12, 21). Muscle glycogen utilization during exercise is reduced by prior caffeine ingestion (20, 53), although this may be more a consequence of a direct effect on phosphorylase activity (53) than of increased plasma FFA and lipid oxidation. Lipid ingestion during exercise has generally not been considered a useful means of reducing the reliance on endogenous carbohydrate, due to the relatively slow absorption of ingested fat and the potential inhibitory effects on gastric emptying. However, medium-chain triglyceride ingestion has attracted some interest, since medium-chain fatty acids are water soluble and more rapidly absorbed from the intestine, do not inhibit gastric emptying (3), and can enter the mitochondria independently of carnitine. Furthermore, since carbohydrate ingestion suppresses the mobilization of fatty acids, it has been suggested that co-ingestion of carbohydrate and medium-chain triglycerides may result in higher plasma FFA levels, thereby providing an optimal supply of substrate to contracting muscle (3). Medium-chain free fatty acids are oxidized to a greater extent than ingested long-chain fatty acids (50), but less (50) or only slightly less (38) than ingested glucose. Whether medium-chain triglyceride ingestion significantly alters carbohydrate metabolism or improves exercise performance remains unclear (32, 33, 38, 57) but no doubt will be the subject of further investigation.

Acknowledgments

The author's work has been supported by the National Health and Medical Research Council of Australia, the Australian Research Council, and Ross Australia.

References

1. Adopo, E.; Peronnet, F.; Massicotte, D.; Brisson, G.R.; Hillaire-Marcel, C. Respective oxidation of exogenous glucose and fructose given in the same drink during exercise. J. Appl. Physiol. 76:1014-1019; 1994.
2. Ahlborg, G.; Felig, P. Influence of glucose ingestion on fuel-hormone responses during prolonged exercise. J. Appl. Physiol. 41:683-688; 1976.
3. Beckers, E.J.; Jeukendrup, A.E.; Brouns, F.; Wagenmakers, A.J.M.; Saris, W.H.M. Gastric emptying of carbohydrate–medium chain triglyceride suspensions at rest. Int. J. Sports Med. 13:581-584; 1992.
4. Bosch, A.N.; Dennis, S.C.; Noakes, T.D. Influence of carbohydrate ingestion on fuel substrate turnover and oxidation during prolonged exercise. J. Appl. Physiol. 76:2364-2372; 1994.
5. Broberg, S.; Sahlin, K. Adenine nucleotide degradation in human skeletal muscle during prolonged exercise. J. Appl. Physiol. 67:116-122; 1989.
6. Burgess, M.L.; Robertson, R.J.; Davis, J.M.; Norris, J.M. RPE, blood glucose, and carbohydrate oxidation during exercise: Effects of glucose feedings. Med. Sci. Sports Exercise 23:353-359; 1991.
7. Christensen, E.H.; Hansen, O. III. Arbeitsfahigkeit und Ernahrung. Skand. Arch. Physiol. 81:161-171; 1939a.
8. Christensen, E.H.; Hansen, O. IV. Hypoglykamie, Arbeitsfahigkeit und Ermudung. Skand. Arch. Physiol. 81:172-179; 1939b.
9. Coggan, A.R.; Coyle, E.F. Reversal of fatigue during prolonged exercise by carbohydrate infusion and ingestion. J. Appl. Physiol. 63:2388-2395; 1987.
10. Coggan, A.R.; Spina, R.J.; Kohrt, W.M.; Bier, D.M.; Holloszy, J.O. Plasma glucose kinetics in a well-trained cyclist fed glucose throughout exercise. Int. J. Sports Nutr. 1:279-288; 1991.
11. Costill, D.L.; Coyle, E.; Dalsky, G.; Evans, W.; Fink, W.; Hoopes, D. Effects of elevated plasma FFA and insulin on muscle glycogen usage during exercise. J. Appl. Physiol. 43:695-699; 1977.

12. Costill, D.L.; Dalsky, G.P.; Fink, W.J. Effects of caffeine ingestion on metabolism and exercise performance. Med. Sci. Sports 10:155-158; 1978.
13. Coyle, E.F.; Coggan, A.R.; Hemmert, M.K.; Ivy, J.L. Muscle glycogen utilization during prolonged strenuous exercise when fed carbohydrate. J. Appl. Physiol. 61:165-172; 1986.
14. Coyle, E.F.; Hagberg, J.M.; Hurley, B.F.; Martin, W.H.; Ehsani, A.A.; Holloszy, J.O. Carbohydrate feeding during prolonged strenuous exercise can delay fatigue. J. Appl. Physiol. 55:230-235; 1983.
15. Coyle, E.F.; Hamilton, M.T.; Gonzalez-Alonso, J.; Montain, S.J.; Ivy, J.L. Carbohydrate metabolism during intense exercise when hyperglycemic. J. Appl. Physiol. 70:834-840; 1991.
16. Davies, C.T.M.; Halliday, D.; Millward, D.J.; Rennie, M.J.; Sutton, J.R. Glucose inhibits CO_2 production from leucine during whole-body exercise in man. J. Physiol. 332:40P-41P; 1982.
17. Davis, J.M.; Bailey, S.P.; Woods, J.A.; Galiano, F.J.; Hamilton, M.T.; Bartoli, W.P. Effects of carbohydrate feedings on plasma free tryptophan and branched-chain amino acids during prolonged cycling. Eur. J. Appl. Physiol. 65:513-519; 1992.
18. Dyck, D.J.; Putman, C.T.; Heigenhauser, G.J.F.; Hultman, E.; Spriet, L.L. Regulation of fat-carbohydrate interaction in skeletal muscle during intense aerobic cycling. Am. J. Physiol. 265:E852-E859; 1993.
19. Elayan, I.M.; Winder, W.W. Effect of glucose infusion on muscle malonyl-CoA during exercise. J. Appl. Physiol. 70:1495-1499; 1991.
20. Essig, D.; Costill, D.L.; Van Handel, P.J. Effects of caffeine ingestion on utilization of muscle glycogen and lipid during leg ergometer cycling. Int. J. Sports Med. 1:86-90; 1980.
21. Graham, T.E.; Spriet, L.L. Performance and metabolic responses to a high caffeine dose during prolonged exercise. J. Appl. Physiol. 71:2292-2298; 1991.
22. Green, H.J. How important is endogenous muscle glycogen to fatigue in prolonged exercise? Can. J. Physiol. Pharmacol. 69:290-297; 1991.
23. Guezennec, C.Y.; Satabin, P.; Duforez, F.; Merino, D.; Peronnet, F.; Koziet, J. Oxidation of corn starch, glucose, and fructose ingested before exercise. Med. Sci. Sports Exercise 21:45-50; 1989.
24. Hargreaves, M.; Briggs, C.A. Effect of carbohydrate ingestion on exercise metabolism. J. Appl. Physiol. 65:1553-1555; 1988.
25. Hargreaves, M.; Costill, D.L.; Coggan, A.; Fink, W.J.; Nishibata, I. Effect of carbohydrate feedings on muscle glycogen utilization and exercise performance. Med. Sci. Sports Exercise 16:219-222; 1984.
26. Hargreaves, M.; Kiens, B.; Richter, E.A. Effect of increased plasma free fatty acid concentrations on muscle metabolism in exercising men. J. Appl. Physiol. 70:194-201; 1991.
27. Hargreaves, M.; Meredith, I.; Jennings, G.L.. Muscle glycogen and glucose uptake during exercise in humans. Exp. Physiol. 77:641-644; 1992.
28. Hawley, J.A.; Bosch, A.N.; Weltan, S.M.; Dennis, S.C.; Noakes, T.D. Glucose kinetics during prolonged exercise in euglycemic and hyperglycemic subjects. Eur. J. Appl. Physiol. 426:378-386; 1994.
29. Hawley, J.A.; Dennis, S.C.; Noakes, T.D. Oxidation of carbohydrate ingested during prolonged endurance exercise. Sports Med. 14:27-42; 1992.
30. Hawley, J.A.; Dennis, S.C.; Nowitz, A.; Brouns, F.; Noakes, T.D. Exogenous carbohydrate oxidation from maltose and glucose ingested during prolonged exercise. Eur. J. Appl. Physiol. 64:523-527; 1992.

31. Ivy, J.L.; Costill, D.L.; Fink, W.J.; Lower, R.W. Influence of caffeine and carbohydrate feedings on endurance performance. Med. Sci. Sports 11:6-11; 1979.
32. Ivy, J.L.; Costill, D.L.; Fink, W.J.; Maglischo, E. Contribution of medium and long chain triglyceride intake to energy metabolism during prolonged exercise. Int. J. Sports Med. 1:15-20; 1980.
33. Jeukendrup, A.E.; Saris, W.M.H.; Schrauwen, P.; Brouns, F.; Wagenmakers, A.J.M. Metabolic availability of medium-chain triglycerides coingested with carbohydrates during prolonged exercise. J. Appl. Physiol. 79:756-762; 1995.
34. Krogh, A.; Lindhard, J. The relative value of fat and carbohydrate as sources of muscular energy. Biochem. J. 14:290-298; 1920.
35. Kuipers, H.; Keizer, H.A.; Brouns, F.; Saris, W.H.M. Carbohydrate feeding and glycogen synthesis in exercise in man. Pflügers Arch. 410:652-656; 1987.
36. Massicotte, D.; Peronnet, F.; Allah, C.; Hillaire-Marcel, C.; Ledoux, M.; Brisson, G. Metabolic response to [^{13}C]glucose and [^{13}C]fructose ingestion during exercise. J. Appl. Physiol. 61:1180-1184; 1986.
37. Massicotte, D.; Peronnet, F.; Brisson, G.; Bakkouch, K.; Hillaire-Marcel, C. Oxidation of a glucose polymer during exercise: Comparison with glucose and fructose. J. Appl. Physiol. 66:179-183; 1989.
38. Massicotte, D.; Peronnet, F.; Brisson, G.; Hillaire-Marcel, C. Oxidation of exogenous medium-chain free fatty acids during prolonged exercise: Comparison with glucose. J. Appl. Physiol. 73:1334-1339; 1992.
39. McConell, G.; Fabris, S.; Proietto, J.; Hargreaves, M. Effect of carbohydrate ingestion on glucose kinetics during exercise. J. Appl. Physiol. 77:1537-1541; 1994.
40. Mitchell, J.B.; Costill, D.L.; Houmard, J.A.; Fink, W.J.; Pascoe, D.D.; Pearson, D.R. Influence of carbohydrate dosage on exercise performance and glycogen metabolism. J. Appl. Physiol. 67:1843-1849; 1989.
41. Moodley, D.; Noakes, T.D.; Bosch, A.N.; Hawley, J.A.; Schall, R.; Dennis, S.C. Oxidation of exogenous carbohydrate during prolonged exercise: The effects of the carbohydrate type and its concentration. Eur. J. Appl. Physiol. 64:328-334; 1992.
42. Neufer, P.D.; Costill, D.L.; Flynn, M.G.; Kirwan, J.P.; Mitchell, J.B.; Houmard, J. Improvements in exercise performance: Effects of carbohydrate feedings and diet. J. Appl. Physiol. 62:983-988; 1987.
43. Pirnay, F.; Lacroix, M.; Mosora, F.; Luyckx, A.; LeFebvre, P. Effect of glucose ingestion on energy substrate utilization during prolonged muscular exercise. Eur. J. Appl. Physiol. 36:247-254; 1977.
44. Ravussin, E.; Pahud, P.; Dorner, A.; Arnaud, M.J.; Jequier, E. Substrate utilization during prolonged exercise preceded by ingestion of ^{13}C-glucose in glycogen depleted and control subjects. Pflügers Arch. 382:197-202; 1979.
45. Rehrer, N.J.; Wagenmakers, A.J.M.; Beckers, E.J.; Halliday, D.; Leiper, J.B.; Brouns, F.; Maughan, R.J.; Westerterp, K.; Saris, W.H.M. Gastric emptying, absorption, and carbohydrate oxidation during prolonged exercise. J. Appl. Physiol. 72:468-475; 1992.
46. Romijn, J.A.; Coyle, E.F.; Sidossis, L.S.; Gastaldelli, A.; Horowitz, J.F.; Endert, E.; Wolfe, R.R. Regulation of endogenous fat and carbohydrate metabolism in relation to exercise intensity and duration. Am. J. Physiol. 265:E380-E391; 1993.
47. Romijn, J.A.; Coyle, E.F.; Sidossis, L.S.; Zhang, X.-J.; Wolfe, R.R. Relationship between fatty acid delivery and fatty acid oxidation during strenuous exercise. J. Appl. Physiol. 79:1939-1945; 1995.

48. Sahlin, K.; Katz, A.; Broberg, S. Tricarboxylic acid cycle intermediates in human muscle during prolonged exercise. Am. J. Physiol. 259:C834-C841; 1990.

49. Saris, W.H.M.; Goodpaster, B.H.; Jeukendrup, A.E.; Brouns, F.; Halliday, D.; Wagenmakers, A.J.M. Exogenous carbohydrate oxidation from different carbohydrate sources during exercise. J. Appl. Physiol. 75:2168-2172; 1993.

50. Satabin, P.; Portero, P.; Defer, G.; Bricout, J.; Guezennec, C.Y. Metabolic and hormonal responses to lipid and carbohydrate diets during exercise in man. Med. Sci. Sports Exercise 19:218-223; 1987.

51. Soop, M.; Björkman, O.; Cederblad, G.; Hagenfeldt, L.; Wahren, J. Influence of carnitine supplementation on muscle substrate and carnitine metabolism during exercise. J. Appl. Physiol. 64:2394-2399; 1988.

52. Spencer, M.K.; Yan, Z.; Katz, A. Carbohydrate supplementation attenuates IMP accumulation in human muscle during prolonged exercise. Am. J. Physiol. 261:C71-C76; 1991.

53. Spriet, L.L.; MacLean, D.A.; Dyck, D.J.; Hultman, E.; Cederblad, G.; Graham, T.E. Caffeine ingestion and muscle metabolism during prolonged exercise in humans. Am. J. Physiol. 262:E891-E898; 1992.

54. Tsintzas, O.K.; Liu, R.; Williams, C.; Campbell, I.; Gaitanos, G. The effect of carbohydrate ingestion on performance during a 30-km race. Int. J. Sports Nutr. 3:127-139; 1993.

55. Tsintzas, O.K.; Williams, C.; Boobis, L. Muscle glycogen in different fibre types during running with and without carbohydrate ingestion. (Abstract). Proceedings of the Ninth International Conference on the Biochemistry of Exercise; 1994 July 21-26; Aberdeen, Scotland. 1994:28.

56. Tsintzas, O.K.; Williams, C.; Boobis, L.; Greenhaff, P. Carbohydrate ingestion and glycogen utilization in different muscle fiber types in man. J. Physiol. 489:243-250; 1995.

57. Van Zyl, C.G.; Lambert, E.V.; Hawley, J.A.; Noakes, T.D.; Dennis, S.C. Effects of medium-chain triglyceride on fuel metabolism and cycling performance. J. Appl. Physiol. (In press.)

58. Vukovich, M.D.; Costill, D.L.; Hickey, M.S.; Trappe, S.W.; Cole, K.J.; Fink, W.J. Effect of fat emulsion infusion and fat feeding on muscle glycogen utilization during cycle exercise. J. Appl. Physiol. 75:1513-1518; 1993.

59. Wagenmakers, A.J.M.; Beckers, E.J.; Brouns, F.; Kuipers, H.; Soeters, P.B.; Van Der Vusse, G.J.; Saris, W.H.M. Carbohydrate supplementation, glycogen depletion, and amino acid metabolism during exercise. Am. J. Physiol. 260: E883-E890; 1991.

60. Wagenmakers, A.J.M.; Brouns, F.; Saris, W.H.M.; Halliday, D. Oxidation rates of orally ingested carbohydrates during prolonged exercise in men. J. Appl. Physiol. 75:2774-2780; 1993.

61. Yaspelkis, B.B.; Patterson, J.G.; Anderla, P.A.; Ding, Z.; Ivy, J.L. Carbohydrate supplementation spares muscle glycogen during variable-intensity exercise. J. Appl. Physiol. 75:1477-1485; 1993.

CHAPTER 34

Branched-Chain Amino Acids: Nutrition and Metabolism in Exercise

Anton J.M. Wagenmakers, Gerrit van Hall
University of Limburg, Maastricht, The Netherlands

The branched-chain amino acids (BCAA)—leucine, valine, and isoleucine—are three of the nine essential amino acids in mammals. Together they make up 40% of the daily requirement for essential amino acids in humans. Most of the essential amino acids are degraded by the liver. However, after ingestion of a protein-containing meal the BCAA escape from hepatic uptake and are largely handled by the peripheral skeletal muscles. In the late 1970s, it was suggested that the BCAA were the third fuel for skeletal muscle beside fatty acids and carbohydrates and contributed substantial amounts of energy (up to 15% of total energy expenditure in incubated muscles; 11, 30). It furthermore was shown that addition of BCAA to the incubation medium or perfusion medium stimulated protein synthesis and inhibited protein degradation in muscle in vitro (18). These early scientific observations have awakened the interest of athletes and the sport nutrition market, and today BCAA-containing supplements are used by athletes and others to reduce net protein breakdown during exercise, to accelerate recovery following exercise, and to improve physical and mental performance. A critical review of the rationale behind the use of BCAA is given here based on the current knowledge of BCAA metabolism.

The Oxidative Pathways of BCAA and Tissue Distribution of Enzymes

Knowledge of the activities and tissue distribution of the various enzymes involved in the catabolism of BCAA is important for understanding the interactions with other pathways and for understanding the inter-organ relationships in the handling of BCAA and their products. The oxidative pathways were first elucidated in studies on rat liver preparations and are generally well established. For a recent detailed review and references we refer to Davis (6).

The first step in the degradation of BCAA is a reversible aminotransferase (transamination) reaction in which the BCAA are converted to their respective branched-chain 2-oxoacids (BCOA) and the amino group acceptor 2-oxoglutarate is converted to glutamate. High activities of the BCAA aminotransferase among others are present in pancreas and stomach; intermediate activities in heart, skeletal muscle, brain, and lung; and low activities in gut and liver.

The second step in the degradation of BCAA is an irreversible oxidative decarboxylation reaction. This is the rate-limiting reaction in many tissues, which decides whether the carbon skeleton of the BCAA remains available for protein synthesis or is broken down in the oxidative pathway. The BCOA formed in the BCAA aminotransferase reaction are decarboxylated by the branched-chain 2-oxoacid dehydrogenase complex (BC complex). The BC complex is a multienzyme complex, in structure very similar to pyruvate dehydrogenase, located on the inner surface of the inner mitochondrial membrane. A single enzyme exists that oxidatively decarboxylates all three BCOA. In the early 1980s, the activity of the BC complex was shown to be regulated by a phosphorylation-dephosphorylation cycle, with phosphorylation causing inactivation. Several laboratories (30) had measured the activity of this enzyme before it was realized that the enzyme was present in active and inactive forms; they came to the conclusion that, due to an intermediate activity and large mass (40-50% of whole-body mass), the combined skeletal muscle compartment contained by far the largest whole-tissue activity of this enzyme in rats. However, when taking the phosphorylation state into consideration (table 34.1), it is clear that liver and kidney contain a higher whole-tissue activity than the skeletal muscle compartment. Liver and kidney have a high total activity and high activity state, whereas skeletal muscle has an intermediate activity and low activity state.

The third step in the oxidative pathway of BCAA is dehydrogenation of the saturated acyl CoA esters by two specific branched-chain acyl CoA dehydrogenases.

Table 34.1   Activities of the Branched-Chain 2-Oxoacid Dehydrogenase Complex (BC Complex) in Tissues of Rat and Humans

	Activity of BC complex (nmol/g tissue per min)		Percentage active enzyme
	Actual	Total	
Rat			
Liver	200-1,000	200-1,000	93-100
Kidney	100-250	200-350	47-77
Skeletal muscle	0.6-2.2	29-63	1.5-6.0
Heart	20-30	220-570	7-12
Human			
Skeletal muscle	0.4-1.6	5-30	4.0-11

These data were obtained in fed and postabsorptive rats and human subjects by various authors using different methods. As substrate, the 2-oxoacid of leucine or valine was used in concentrations of ≤0.2 mM. Higher activities are observed at higher substrate concentrations.

The highest activities of these enzymes are present in the mitochondria of rat liver and heart, followed by kidney. Lower activities are present in skeletal muscle and brain.

After this step, the metabolic pathways for the individual BCAA diverge. The oxidation of leucine leads to formation of acetyl CoA and acetoacetate. Valine produces the TCA cycle intermediate succinyl CoA, and isoleucine produces both acetyl CoA and succinyl CoA. Little is known about the activity of the enzymes involved in these steps and their tissue distribution. It is believed that the degradation route in muscle and most other tissues is similar to that in liver, although the evidence is not yet complete. It is also believed that degradation routes and the tissue distribution of the enzymes in rats and humans are similar, but again the evidence is not yet complete.

Inter-Organ Relationships in the Handling of BCAA After Consumption of Protein- and BCAA-Containing Meals

Following consumption and digestion of a protein-containing meal, most of the resulting amino acids are absorbed by the gut and appear in the portal vein. A large proportion of these amino acids are extracted and metabolized by the liver (9). The remainder will enter the main circulation for subsequent use for protein synthesis in all tissues of the body. However, the BCAA largely escape hepatic uptake, due to the fact that liver has a low BCAA aminotransferase activity, and measurements of arteriovenous differences of amino acids have shown that they are mainly extracted by the peripheral tissues (1, 8, 9, 18). Two tissues appear to be important candidates for the handling of BCAA in the periphery: skeletal muscle and maybe adipose tissue, as suggested by Goodman and Frick (12).

Skeletal muscle, as indicated, has a high BCAA aminotransferase activity and an intermediate total activity of the BC complex, but a low activity state (table 34.1). However, the activity state of the BC complex in rats increased from 2% in the postabsorptive state to 8% 3 h after consumption of a meal containing 25% casein and even to 17% 3 h after consumption of a meal containing 50% casein (2). Oral ingestion of BCAA also activates the BC complex in human muscle. A doubling of the percentage of active BC complex was observed (from 10.5 ± 1.8% to 22.1 ± 3.1%) 30 min after ingestion of 20 g of BCAA by postabsorptive human subjects (45).

The Metabolic Fate of BCAA in Muscle

Rat and human muscles have a high BCAA aminotransferase activity, exceeding by far the activity of the BC complex. Skeletal muscle may not be able to oxidize all the BCOA produced by transamination, as evidenced by a release of BCOA from in vivo muscle in rats (19) and humans (8). In vitro skeletal muscle not only releases substantial amounts of BCOA, but even larger quantities of the branched-chain fatty acids and hydroxylated branched-chain fatty acids derived from the respective BCAA (17, 42). It is not known whether (hydroxylated) branched-chain fatty acids are also released from skeletal muscle in vivo. If they are, then they most likely will be further oxidized in liver and kidney, since both of these tissues contain higher activities of the branched-chain acyl CoA dehydrogenases than skeletal muscle. This may imply that the first steps of BCAA metabolism occur in muscle, with further metabolism in liver and kidney, and that an active shunt of the carbon skeletons exists between these tissues. *interesting*

Ruderman and Lund (26) were the first to observe that addition of BCAA to the perfusion medium of rat hindquarters increases the release of alanine and glutamine. The relationship between BCAA metabolism and alanine and glutamine has since been the subject of many studies (for reviews see 11 and 32). Most of this relationship has now been firmly established (figure 34.1). In the BCAA aminotransferase reaction, the amino group is donated to 2-oxoglutarate to form glutamate and the BCOA. In the reaction catalyzed by glutamine synthase, glutamate reacts subsequently with ammonia to give glutamine. Alternatively, glutamate may donate the amino group to pyruvate to form alanine and regenerate 2-oxoglutarate. These reactions provide a tool to eliminate amino groups from muscle in the form of nontoxic nitrogen carriers (alanine and glutamine). It is assumed that the BCAA also contribute carbon skeletons for the synthesis of glutamine (17, 42, 47). Carbon from the BCAA enters the TCA cycle as acetyl CoA (leucine and isoleucine) and as succinyl CoA (isoleucine and valine) and is then converted to glutamate and glutamine via 2-oxoglutarate.

BCAA as a Fuel During Exercise

Exercise leads to activation of the BC complex in skeletal muscle by an increase of the percentage of active muscle enzyme. This was shown first in studies with rats (13, 14, 43) and more recently also in humans (38, 39). Increased oxidation of BCAA during exercise also was observed in studies with L-[1-^{13}C]leucine (15, 25, 46), and this was used as a rationale to support claims that athletes needed BCAA as an additional energy source (beside carbohydrates and fatty acids). However, methodological problems with the oxidation of [^{13}C]leucine during exercise (changes in background $^{13}CO_2$ enrichment when going from rest to exercise) have led to an overestimation of leucine oxidation (for a more detailed discussion see 39 and 41). It furthermore has become clear that the nutritional state and the muscle glycogen content influence activation of the BC complex during exercise. Carbohydrate loading and carbohydrate ingestion, such as athletes practice during competition, prevented activation (1.3-fold, not significant) of the BC complex in trained human subjects studied during 2 h of cycle exercise at 70% to 75% of the maximal workload, whereas a 3.6-fold activation was observed when the same subjects were studied with low resting muscle glycogen concentrations and without carbohydrate ingestion at a lower exercise intensity (38). This implies that the oxidation of BCAA is not significantly increased in competitive endurance events of about 2 h at $\leq 75\%$ $\dot{V}O_2$max compared with the resting situation and that the contribution of amino acid oxidation to total energy expenditure will remain small, since the metabolic rate of the exercising muscle is accelerated much more (up to 20-fold) than BCAA oxidation. The contribution of BCAA oxidation to total energy expenditure in fact seems to be lower during exercise than at rest and can be estimated to be $\leq 1\%$ of total

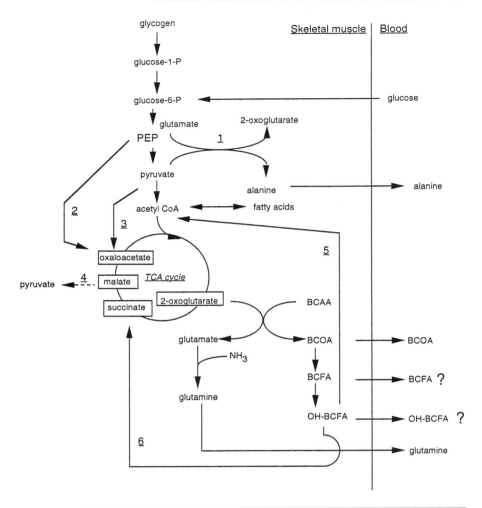

Figure 34.1   Central role of BCAA metabolism in the regulation of the ambient level of tricarboxylic acid (TCA) cycle intermediates in skeletal muscle (37). BCAA metabolism is accelerated during exercise. The BCAA aminotransferase reaction is draining the carbon flux in the TCA cycle by using 2-oxoglutarate as an amino group acceptor. The draining effect of the BCAA aminotransferase reaction is normally counteracted by the anaplerotic conversion of glycogen and glucose to TCA cycle intermediates and glutamine. Muscle glycogen, therefore, acts as a precursor for the synthesis of TCA cycle intermediates and glutamine. In exercise leading to glycogen depletion, this mechanism will lead to a fall in the concentration of TCA cycle intermediates and fatigue (27). 1, alanine aminotransferase; 2, reversal of the phosphoenolpyruvate carboxykinase; 3, pyruvate kinase; 4, NADP-dependent malic enzyme (flux assumed to be insignificant); 5, acetyl CoA is formed from the carbon skeletons of leucine and isoleucine; 6, succinyl CoA is formed from the carbon skeletons of valine and isoleucine. ? indicates that it is not known whether the branched-chain fatty acids (BCFA) and hydroxylated branched-chain fatty acids (OH-BCFA) are released by skeletal muscle in vivo as they are in vitro.

energy expenditure in subjects exercising for 2 h at 70% to 80% of $\dot{V}O_2$max while ingesting carbohydrate drinks. The BCAA, in other words, do not seem to play a role as alternative fuel during exercise of light, moderate, and high intensity, and from this point of view there is no reason for supplementation of BCAA prior to, during, or following exercise.

BCAA Supplementation, Ammonia Production, and the Maximal Aerobic Capacity in Muscle

Previously we have suggested (37, 38, 40) that oral ingestion of BCAA may interfere with fatigue mechanisms in skeletal muscle. This hypothesis is primarily based on observations made in patients with McArdle's disease (myophosphorylase deficiency). Due to the glycogen breakdown defect in muscle, these patients have a limited exercise capacity; during incremental exercise, the maximal power output is between 40 and 100 W. An excessive activation of the BC complex was observed in the muscle of these patients during exercise and also an excessive muscle production of ammonia (plasma ammonia may rise up to 500 μM in the patients and to 150 μM in healthy individuals). When 20 g of BCAA were given to two of these patients 30 min before an incremental exercise test, plasma ammonia increased even further, and exercise performance deteriorated (40). Both time to exhaustion and the maximal power output reached during incremental exercise were reduced by administration of the BCAA.

On the basis of these observations it has been hypothesized (37, 38, 40) that acceleration of BCAA metabolism in muscle during exercise may put a carbon drain on the TCA cycle and may limit maximal oxidative capacity of the muscle, especially in conditions of limited glycogen availability. The degradation routes of the BCAA clearly imply that the metabolism of the BCAA may have an impact on the ambient level of TCA cycle intermediates in skeletal muscle. The BCAA aminotransferase reaction uses 2-oxoglutarate as an amino group acceptor and therefore removes carbon from the TCA cycle (figure 34.1). The following mechanisms may replete TCA cycle intermediates: (a) Valine and isoleucine are metabolized to succinyl CoA, so that the level of intermediates would be maintained if complete degradation of these amino acids takes place in muscle itself; on the other hand, if BCOA, branched-chain fatty acids, and hydroxylated branched-chain fatty acids are released by muscle for further metabolism in liver and kidney (17, 42), then the BCAA aminotransferase reaction would put a net drain on the TCA cycle pool (figure 34.1). Leucine metabolism always is coupled to net removal of TCA cycle intermediates, since its degradation does not lead to synthesis of TCA cycle intermediates. (b) If the formation of glutamate in the BCAA aminotransferase reaction is coupled to alanine formation (glutamate + pyruvate → 2-oxoglutarate + alanine) then no drain exists on the TCA cycle pool; however, glutamine and not alanine appears to be the main product of BCAA metabolism in humans (8). (c) If the purine nucleotide cycle is functioning, then fumarate and ammonia can be formed from aspartate, but its activity is assumed to be low in muscle, both at rest and during exercise. (d) If glutamate dehydrogenase is active, then glutamate can be deaminated under formation of 2-oxoglutarate, but again its activity is assumed to be low. (e) Direct synthesis of oxaloacetate from pyruvate via carboxylation of pyruvate (7) or from reversal of the phosphoenolpyruvate carboxykinase reaction (16) therefore seem to be required for net repletion of TCA cycle intermediates (figure 34.1).

In healthy individuals with full glycogen stores, these mechanisms apparently allow for an acceleration of BCAA degradation during exercise, without net loss of TCA cycle intermediates and with maintenance of oxidative capacity. However, in patients with McArdle's disease, no pyruvate will be available due to the glycogen breakdown defect, and compensation of the draining effect of the BCAA aminotransferase reaction by mechanisms b and e will be reduced or absent. Deamination of aspartate (mechanism c) and glutamate (mechanism d) may then be required to prevent a substantial loss of TCA cycle intermediates but will lead to ammonia production (40). A net reduction of the anaplerotic carbon flow into the TCA cycle also will limit the availability of 2-oxoglutarate and glutamate for subsequent glutamine synthesis and, by this mechanism, will also lead to accumulation of ammonia. These mechanisms seem to explain the large ammonia production of patients with McArdle's disease and the negative effect of BCAA supplements on performance (40).

The same mechanism may come into operation in healthy individuals during endurance exercise leading to glycogen depletion (38). Glycogen depletion, among other effects, leads to greater activation of the BC complex, to higher plasma ammonia concentrations (38), and to a decrease of the level of TCA cycle intermediates in muscle (27). When this mechanism occurs in healthy individuals, oral ingestion of BCAA could have a negative effect on performance. The oral administration of 20 g BCAA prior to exercise has been reported to increase the activity of the BC complex in muscle both at rest and during exercise (45), and ingestion of BCAA also increases plasma ammonia concentrations in healthy individuals during exercise both before and after glycogen depletion (21, 33, 44). However, administration of sucrose drinks containing 6 g and 18 g BCAA per liter did not have an effect on time to exhaustion at 70% to 75% maximal power output (Wmax; 33) in comparison with the sucrose drink alone, most probably due to the fact that the draining effect of the BCAA aminotransferase reaction could be compensated by anaplerotic mechanisms b and e.

In conclusion, oral ingestion of BCAA prior to and during exercise enhances the increase in plasma ammonia concentration that is usually seen during exercise in both healthy individuals and patients with McArdle's disease. Oral ingestion of BCAA leads to a deterioration of performance in patients with McArdle's disease, most likely via a draining action of the BCAA aminotransferase reaction on the TCA cycle under conditions of zero glycogen availability. Ingestion of mixed carbohydrate-BCAA solutions has no effect (negative or positive) on time to exhaustion in endurance exercise of healthy individuals.

Effect of Infusion or Ingestion of BCAA on Rates of Protein Synthesis and Degradation in Vivo

The idea that BCAA may have an anticatabolic effect is based not only on the observed in vitro effects on protein synthesis and degradation (18). Early therapeutic trials in small groups of traumatized and septic patients also claimed that BCAA prevented protein catabolism in vivo (5). However, more recent controlled clinical trials in large groups of patients did not show improvements of nitrogen balance or clinical outcome (35). Many in vivo studies have also been done on healthy individuals, in whom rates of protein synthesis and degradation have been measured with stable isotope techniques in the presence and absence of an intravenous BCAA infusion (1-2 g/h). In none of these studies (10, 20, 22) could stimulation of protein synthesis rates by BCAA be demonstrated either at the whole-body level or in skeletal muscle. However, protein degradation rates could be reduced both at whole-body level and in skeletal muscle when the studies were performed in the post-absorptive state in the presence of leucine. Net anabolism only could be reached by infusion of insulin and an "appropriate" dose of all physiological amino acids (10). Data on a potential effect of BCAA on protein synthesis and degradation in humans in the fed state—when by definition there is an appropriate supply of amino acids and insulin—to the best of our knowledge are not available. It also has not been investigated with stable isotope methodology whether intravenous or oral administration of BCAA may have a positive effect on the balance between protein synthesis and degradation during exercise. However, claims have been made that oral supplementation of BCAA may prevent muscle wasting (loss of lean body mass) as usually observed during trekking at high altitude (28), but the design of this study and the methods used have been questioned (36). Blomstrand and Newsholme (4) have suggested that oral supplementation of BCAA may reduce net protein degradation in endurance exercise (marathon and cross country). Their suggestion was based on the observation that the postexercise concentration of aromatic amino acids (phenylalanine and tyrosine, amino acids that are not metabolized in muscle by processes other than protein synthesis and degradation) was reduced in plasma and muscle by BCAA supplementation. However, changes in the concentration of these amino acids can be caused by other metabolic events (e.g., increased uptake in other tissues, fluid shifts during exercise) and therefore do not provide qualitative or quantitative information on rates of protein synthesis and degradation in muscle. Also, collection of the postexercise samples 90 min after the end of exercise (4) was not ideal. In conclusion, there is no valid scientific evidence to support claims that intravenous or oral BCAA administration has an anticatabolic effect in patients, healthy individuals, or athletes.

BCAA, Tryptophan, and Central Fatigue

In 1987, Newsholme, Blomstrand, and colleagues (3, 23, 24) proposed the central fatigue hypothesis (for more details see chapters 15 and 35). One of the implications of the central fatigue hypothesis is that BCAA supplementation would reduce the increase in the plasma concentration ratio of free tryptophan to BCAA during prolonged exercise and, via this mechanism, could reduce increases in brain uptake of tryptophan and subsequent increases in brain concentrations of 5-hydroxytryptamine and central fatigue. Physical performance has been studied by Blomstrand and colleagues (3), and improvements have been claimed in subjects receiving oral BCAA supplements. However, the design of this study and interpretation of the data are questionable. Blomstrand et al. (3) studied male subjects running a marathon race (193 subjects). Subjects were randomly divided into two groups. One group, the experimental group, was given 16 g of BCAA in plain water (divided in four aliquots) during the race, the placebo group received flavored water. The subjects were allowed any other drink provided (including carbohydrate drinks). No difference was observed in the marathon time of the group receiving BCAA and of those receiving placebo. However, when subjects were divided into fast (≤ 3 h 5 min) and slower runners, then a small but significant reduction in performance time was observed in the slower runners only. Three main criticisms can be raised against this design and interpretation: First, in a performance test investigating a potential ergogenic effect, subjects in the treatment and placebo groups should have been matched for performance. Second, carbohydrate intake and nutritional status before and during the marathon should have been controlled and should have been the same in the treatment and placebo groups. Third, division of subjects in a group into fast and slower runners, taking an arbitrary marathon time as selection criterion, is not in accordance with accepted statistical methods. In the same study, no effect of BCAA supplementation (in combination with carbohydrate) was found on physical performance in subjects participating in a 30-km cross-country race.

A recent controlled performance study in the laboratory in Maastricht (33) failed to show an effect of BCAA supplementation on time to fatigue during cycle exercise at 70% to 75% Wmax. Subjects ($n = 10$) ingested one of four drinks, which were given in double-blind fashion and random order (4 ml per kg body weight during warm-up and then 2 ml per kg body weight every 15 min during exercise). Drinks were control (6% sucrose), low-dose BCAA (6% sucrose + 6 g per liter BCAA), high-dose BCAA (6% sucrose + 18 g per liter BCAA), and tryptophan (6% sucrose + 3 g per liter tryptophan). No difference was observed among these four drinks in time to exhaustion (mean time to exhaustion was about 2 h) or on any of the measured variables (heart rate and perceived exertion) during exercise and at exhaustion. In rats running on a motor-driven treadmill at 5% gradient and a speed of 16 m/min, intragastric BCAA supplementation also failed to improve time to exhaustion in comparison with the water control (34).

If the central fatigue mechanisms suggested by Newsholme and colleagues have a physiological impact on physical performance, then another implication would be that supplements of tryptophan would have a negative effect. No such effect has been observed in three human studies. Segura and Ventura (29) reported that 1.2 g of L-tryptophan supplementation taken in 300-mg doses over a 24-h period before exercise increased total exercise time by 49% in 12 subjects who were running at 80% of maximal oxygen uptake. The results of this study were questioned by Stensrud et al. (31). They studied 49 well-trained males in a randomized, double-blind, placebo-controlled experiment. Subjects in the tryptophan group ($n = 24$) and placebo group ($n = 25$) were matched for performance (maximal oxygen uptake, anaerobic threshold, and speed during an all-out run). Tryptophan ingestion (again 1.2 g over a 24-h period prior to the run) had no effect on running performance, when subjects ran until exhaustion at a speed corresponding to 100% of their $\dot{V}O_2$max. Van Hall et al. (33) did not see an effect of L-tryptophan ingestion on time to exhaustion during cycle exercise at 70% to 75% Wmax (for details of supplementation see the preceding paragraph; total tryptophan intake was 3-5 g during exercise).

In conclusion, performance studies from various laboratories so far have failed to show that manipulation of the plasma concentration ratio of free tryptophan to BCAA by means of supplementation of BCAA or tryptophan influences performance. This may imply that the central fatigue mechanisms suggested by Newsholme and colleagues cannot be manipulated by oral ingestion of the involved amino acids.

Alternatively, it may be that the suggested central fatigue mechanism is of little importance for physical performance (time to exhaustion) in endurance exercise.

Conclusions

A review of the performance research fails to show either a positive or negative effect of BCAA supplementation on time to exhaustion in healthy individuals. However, BCAA supplementation increases plasma ammonia during exercise in healthy individuals and has a negative effect on performance in patients with a glycogen breakdown defect in muscle. BCAA most likely have no effect on protein synthesis and protein degradation at the whole-body level or in muscle of healthy individuals in the fed state and do not improve nitrogen retention in catabolic patients. No evidence is available that BCAA have a positive effect on the balance between protein synthesis and degradation during exercise. A critical evaluation of the physiology of the BCAA does not provide a sound rationale for the use of these compounds as a nutritional supplement before, during, or following exercise.

References

1. Aoki, T.T.; Brennan, M.F.; Fitzpatrick, G.F.; Knight, D.C. Leucine meal increases glutamine and total nitrogen release from forearm muscle. J. Clin. Invest. 68:1522-1528; 1981.
2. Block, K.P.; Aftring, R.P.; Mehard, W.B.; Buse, M.G. Modulation of rat skeletal muscle branched-chain α-keto acid dehydrogenase in vivo. Effects of dietary protein and meal consumption. J. Clin. Invest. 79:1349-1358; 1987.
3. Blomstrand, E.; Hassmén, P.; Ekblom, B.; Newsholme, E.A. Administration of branched-chain amino acids during sustained exercise—Effects on performance and on plasma concentration of some amino acids. Eur. J. Appl. Physiol. 63:83-88; 1991.
4. Blomstrand, E.; Newsholme, E.A. Effect of branched-chain amino acid supplementation on the exercise-induced change in aromatic amino acid concentration in human muscle. Acta Physiol. Scand. 146:293-298; 1992.
5. Cerra, F.B.; Mazuski, J.E.; Chute, E.; Nuwer, N.; Teasley, K.; Lysne, J.; Shronts, E.P.; Konstantinides, F.N. Branched chain metabolic support. A prospective, randomized, double blind trial in surgical stress. Ann. Surg. 199:286-291; 1984.
6. Davis, E.J. Pathways of branched-chain amino acid metabolism in mammals. In: Odessey, R., ed. Problems and potential of branched-chain amino acids in physiology and medicine. Amsterdam: Elsevier Science Publishers; 1986:3-29.
7. Davis, E.J.; Spydevold, Ø.; Bremer, J. Pyruvate carboxylase and propionylCoA carboxylase as anaplerotic enzymes in skeletal muscle mitochondria. Eur. J. Biochem. 110:255-262; 1980.
8. Elia, M.; Livesey, G. Effects of ingested steak and infused leucine on forelimb metabolism in man and the fate of the carbon skeletons and amino groups of branched-chain amino acids. Clin. Sci. 64:517-526; 1983.

9. Felig, P. Inter-organ amino acid exchange. In: Waterlow, J.C.; Stephen, J.M.L, eds. Nitrogen metabolism in man. London: Applied Science Publishers; 1981: 45-61.

10. Frexes-Steed, M.; Brooks Lacy, D.; Collins, J.; Abumrad, N.N. Role of leucine and other amino acids in regulating protein metabolism in vivo. Am. J. Physiol. 262:E925-E935; 1992.

11. Goldberg, A.L.; Chang, T.W. Regulation and significance of amino acid metabolism in skeletal muscle. Fed. Proc. 37:2301-2307; 1978.

12. Goodman, H.M.; Frick, G.P. The metabolism of branched-chain amino acids in adipose tissue. In: Odessey, R., ed. Problems and potential of branched-chain amino acids in physiology and medicine. Amsterdam: Elsevier Science Publishers; 1986:173-198.

13. Kasperek, G.J.; Dohm, G.L.; Snider, R.D. Activation of branched-chain keto acid dehydrogenase by exercise. Am. J. Physiol. 248:R166-R171; 1985.

14. Kasperek, G.J.; Snider, R.D. Effect of exercise intensity and starvation on activation of branched-chain keto acid dehydrogenase by exercise. Am. J. Physiol. 252:E33-E37; 1987.

15. Knapik, J.; Meredith, C.; Jones, B.; Fielding, R.; Young, V.; Evans, W. Leucine metabolism during fasting and exercise. J. Appl. Physiol. 70:43-47; 1991.

16. Krebs, H.A. The role of chemical equilibrium in organ function. Adv. Enzyme Regul. 15:449-472; 1975.

17. Lee, S.-H.C.; Davis, E.J. Amino acid catabolism by perfused rat hindquarter. The metabolic fates of valine. Biochem. J. 233:621-630; 1986.

18. Li, J.B.; Odessey, R. Regulation of protein turnover in heart and skeletal muscle by branched-chain amino acids and the keto acids. In: Odessey, R., ed. Problems and potential of branched-chain amino acids in physiology and medicine. Amsterdam: Elsevier Science Publishers; 1986:83-106.

19. Livesey, G.; Lund, P. Enzymatic determination of branched-chain amino acids and 2-oxoacids in rat tissues. Transfer of 2-oxoacids from skeletal muscle to liver in vivo. Biochem. J. 188:705-713; 1980.

20. Louard, R.J.; Barrett, E.J.; Gelfand, R.A. Effect of infused branched-chain amino acids on muscle and whole-body amino acid metabolism in man. Clin. Sci. 79:457-466; 1990.

21. MacLean, D.A.; Graham, T.E. Branched-chain amino acid supplementation augments plasma ammonia responses during exercise in humans. J. Appl. Physiol. 74:2711-2717; 1993.

22. Nair, K.S.; Schwartz, R.G.; Welle, S. Leucine as a regulator of whole body and skeletal muscle protein metabolism in humans. Am. J. Physiol. 263:E928-E934; 1992.

23. Newsholme, E.A.; Acworth, I.N.; Blomstrand, E. Amino acids, brain neurotransmitters and a functional link between muscle and brain that is important in sustained exercise. In: Benzi, G., ed. Advances in myochemistry. London: John Libby Eurotext; 1987:127-138.

24. Newsholme, E.A.; Blomstrand, E.; Ekblom, B. Physical and mental fatigue: Metabolic mechanisms and importance of plasma amino acids. Br. Med. Bull. 48:477-495; 1992.

25. Rennie, M.J.; Edwards, R.H.T.; Krywawych, S.; Davies, C.T.M.; Halliday, D.; Waterlow, J.C.; Millward, D.J. Effect of exercise on protein turnover in man. Clin. Sci. 61:627-639; 1981.

26. Ruderman, N.B.; Lund, P. Amino acid metabolism in skeletal muscle. Regulation of glutamine and alanine release in the perfused rat hindquarter. Israel J. Med. Sci. 8:295-302; 1972.

27. Sahlin, K.; Katz, A.; Broberg, S. Tricarboxylic acid cycle intermediates in human muscle during prolonged exercise. Am. J. Physiol. 259:C834-C841; 1990.

28. Schena, F.; Guerrini, F.; Tregnaghi, P.; Kayser, B. Branched-chain amino acid supplementation during trekking at high altitude. The effects on loss of body mass, body composition and muscle power. Eur. J. Appl. Physiol. 65:394-398; 1992.

29. Segura, R.; Ventura, J.L. Effect of L-tryptophan supplementation on exercise performance. Int. J. Sports Med. 9:301-305; 1988.

30. Shinnick, F.L.; Harper, A.E. Branched-chain amino acid oxidation by isolated rat tissue preparations. Biochim. Biophys. Acta 437:477-486; 1976.

31. Stensrud, T.; Ingjer, F.; Holm, H.; Strømme, S.B. L-Tryptophan supplementation does not improve running performance. Int. J. Sports Med. 13:481-485; 1992.

32. Tischler, M.E. Relationship of branched-chain amino acids to the synthesis of alanine and glutamine. In: Odessey, R., ed. Problems and potential of branched-chain amino acids in physiology and medicine. Amsterdam: Elsevier Science Publishers; 1986:107-134.

33. Van Hall, G.; Raaymakers, J.S.H.; Saris, W.H.M.; Wagenmakers, A.J.M. Effect of branched-chain amino acid supplementation on performance during prolonged exercise. J. Physiol. 486:789-794; 1995.

34. Verger, P.; Aymard, P.; Cynobert, L.; Anton, G.; Luigi, R. Effect of administration of branched-chain amino acids versus glucose during acute exercise in the rat. Physiol. Behav. 55:523-526; 1994.

35. Von Meyenfeldt, M.F.; Soeters, P.B.; Vente, J.P.; Van Berlo, C.L.H.; Rouflart, M.M.J.; De Jong, K.P.; Van der Linden, C.J.; Gouma, D.J. Effect of branched chain amino acid enrichment of total parenteral nutrition on nitrogen sparing and clinical outcome of sepsis and trauma: A prospective randomized double blind trial. Br. J. Surg. 77:924-929; 1990.

36. Wagenmakers, A.J.M. Branched-chain amino acid supplementation during trekking at high altitude. Eur. J. Appl. Physiol. 67:92-93; 1993.

37. Wagenmakers, A.J.M. Role of amino acids and ammonia in mechanisms of fatigue. In: Marconnet, P.; Komi, P.V.; Saltin, B.; Sejersted, O.M., eds. Muscle fatigue mechanisms in exercise and training. Basel: Karger; 1992:69-86. (Med. Sport Sci.; vol. 34).

38. Wagenmakers, A.J.M.; Beckers, E.J.; Brouns, F.; Kuipers, H.; Soeters, P.B.; van der Vusse, G.J.; Saris, W.H.M. Carbohydrate supplementation, glycogen depletion, and amino acid metabolism during exercise. Am. J. Physiol. 260: E883-E890; 1991.

39. Wagenmakers, A.J.M.; Brookes, J.H.; Coakley, J.H.; Reilly, T.; Edwards, R.H.T. Exercise-induced activation of the branched-chain 2-oxo acid dehydrogenase in human muscle. Eur. J. Appl. Physiol. 59:159-167; 1989.

40. Wagenmakers, A.J.M.; Coakley, J.H.; Edwards, R.H.T. Metabolism of branched-chain amino acids and ammonia during exercise: Clues from McArdle's disease. Int. J. Sports Med. 11:S101-S113; 1990.

41. Wagenmakers, A.J.M.; Rehrer, N.J.; Brouns, F.; Saris, W.H.M.; Halliday, D. Breath $^{13}CO_2$ background enrichment at rest and during exercise: Diet-related differences between Europe and America. J. Appl. Physiol. 74:2353-2357; 1993.

42. Wagenmakers, A.J.M.; Salden, H.J.M.; Veerkamp, J.H. The metabolic fate of branched-chain amino acids and 2-oxo acids in rat muscle homogenates and diaphragms. Int. J. Biochem. 17:957-965; 1985.

43. Wagenmakers, A.J.M.; Schepens, J.T.G.; Veerkamp, J.H. Effect of starvation and exercise on actual and total activity of the branched-chain 2-oxo acid dehydrogenase complex in rat tissues. Biochem. J. 223:815-821; 1984.

44. Wagenmakers, A.J.M.; Smets, K.; VandeWalle, L.; Brouns, F.; Saris, W.H.M. Deamination of branched-chain amino acids: A potential source of ammonia production during exercise. Med. Sci. Sports Exercise 23:S116; 1991.

45. Wagenmakers, A.J.M.; Van Hall, G.; MacLean, D.A.; Graham, T.E.; Saltin, B. Effect of ingestion of branched-chain amino acids and exercise on activation of the branched-chain α-keto acid dehydrogenase in human muscle. J. Physiol. 479:15P; 1994.

46. Wolfe, R.R.; Goodenough, R.D.; Wolfe, M.H.; Royle, G.T.; Nadel, E.R. Isotopic analysis of leucine and urea metabolism in exercising humans. J. Appl. Physiol. 52:458-466; 1982.

47. Yoshida, S.; Lanza-Jacoby, S.; Stein, T.P. Leucine and glutamine metabolism in septic rats. Biochem. J. 276:405-409; 1991.

CHAPTER 35

Nutritional Influences on Central Mechanisms of Fatigue Involving Serotonin

J. Mark Davis

University of South Carolina, Columbia, South Carolina, U.S.A.

The decrease in muscle performance that occurs with various forms of exercise, termed *muscle fatigue,* has been defined as a failure to maintain the required or expected force or power output (23). Investigators have traditionally concentrated on mechanisms within the muscle fiber that result in dysfunction of the contraction process. However, voluntary muscular contractions require a series of steps from the brain to the contractile machinery.

Mechanisms of fatigue that occur within the muscle fiber include specific impairments of neuromuscular transmission and impulse propagation (36, 39), dysfunction within the sarcoplasmic reticulum involving calcium release and uptake (26), various metabolic factors that disrupt contraction (30), and substrate depletion (20). Muscle fatigue during short-duration, high-intensity exercise is thought to be due to perturbations in electrochemical coupling and calcium regulation that are at least partly mediated by excess protons (H) and inorganic phosphate (Pi; 26, 39), whereas fatigue during prolonged endurance exercise is most commonly related to depletion of body carbohydrate stores reflected in a depletion of muscle glycogen and decreased blood glucose (20).

Much less effort has been focused on the potential role of the central nervous system (CNS) in muscular fatigue, though it has been well documented for over a century that "psychological factors" can affect exercise performance (4). Recent studies also support an important role of the CNS in exercise fatigue (10, 35), but most investigations are limited, since they generally fail to provide plausible biological mechanisms. Recently, however, interesting new theories have been proposed that implicate the neurotransmitters serotonin (5-hydroxytryptamine [5-HT]) and dopamine (DA) as potential mediators of central fatigue during prolonged exercise. This paper will focus primarily on the evidence regarding a possible role of brain 5-HT in central fatigue during prolonged exercise and on the possibility that nutrition may play an important role in delaying central fatigue. Central fatigue is defined in this chapter as a subset of fatigue (failure to maintain the required or expected force or power output) associated with specific alterations in CNS function that cannot reasonably be explained by dysfunction within the muscle itself.

Brain 5-HT and Central Fatigue

Recent research involving brain 5-HT and fatigue has generated the most interest. This neurotransmitter was first proposed as a potential mediator of central fatigue by Newsholme, Acworth, and Blomstrand in 1987 (34). There is a large body of literature linking brain 5-HT and various psychological responses—including arousal, lethargy, sleepiness, and mood—that could be linked to alterations in perceived exertion and muscular fatigue (43). This, along with the understanding that the mechanisms controlling 5-HT metabolism are likely to be affected by exercise, makes it a particularly attractive candidate as a mediator of fatigue during prolonged exercise (figure 35.1).

The rate of 5-HT synthesis in the brain is explained by the availability of its precursor, tryptophan (Trp), since none of the enzymes involved in 5-HT synthesis are saturated under physiological conditions (34). The amino acid Trp exists in the blood bound and unbound to albumin, and it is the unbound or free Trp (f-Trp) that is transported across the blood-brain barrier. This transport occurs via a specific mechanism that Trp shares with other large neutral amino acids, predominately the branched-chain amino acids (BCAA; valine, leucine, isoleucine). Consequently, the entry of Trp into the brain is largely regulated by the f-Trp/BCAA ratio (18, 19, 34). Newsholme (34) proposed that this ratio would increase during prolonged exercise due to an increased uptake of branched-chain amino acids into working muscle (decreased plasma BCAA) and increased mobilization of free fatty acids that can displace Trp from albumin (increased f-Trp). Investigators have begun to test the validity of this hypothesis in experiments involving the effects of exercise on brain 5-HT metabolism, the effects of various 5-HT agonist and antagonist drugs on exercise fatigue, and the influence of various nutritional strategies that may affect the transport of Trp into the brain and alter central fatigue during exercise.

Effect of Exercise on Brain 5-HT Synthesis and Turnover in Rats

The most extensive series of investigations into the effects of acute treadmill exercise on brain serotonin have been performed by Chaouloff and associates (16-19). They have shown that 1 to 2 h of treadmill running at 20 m/min caused marked increases in plasma free (but not total) Trp, roughly proportional rises in brain Trp concentration, and a small but significant increase in 5-hydroxyindoleacetic acid (5-HIAA, primary metabolite of 5-HT; 16, 18). They later showed that similar increases in Trp and 5-HIAA occur in cerebrospinal fluid (CSF) during exercise and return to basal levels by about 1 h thereafter (18). These data, along with their subsequent data showing increases in both 5-HT and 5-HIAA in various brain regions following 90 min of treadmill running (17), suggest quite strongly that prolonged, moderate-intensity exercise in rats increases 5-HT synthesis and turnover in various brain regions and that this increase is likely to be due to increases in plasma f-Trp.

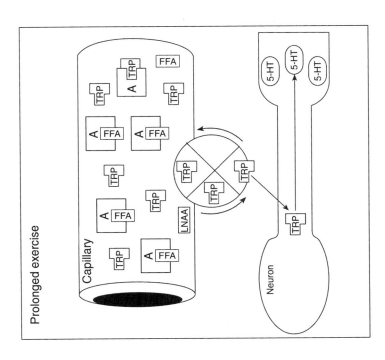

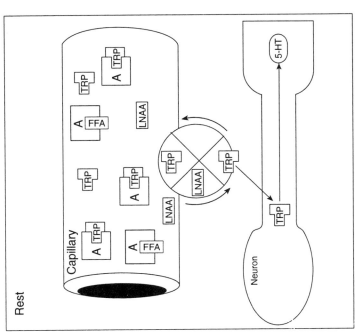

Figure 35.1 Illustration of the changes from rest to prolonged exercise in plasma concentrations of tryptophan (TRP) and free fatty acids (FFA) bound and unbound to albumin (A), in transport of TRP and large neutral amino acids (LNAA) into the brain, and in synthesis of serotonin (5-HT) in serotonergic neurons in the brain.
Adapted from Fernstrom 1994.

Effects of Fatigue on Brain 5-HT Metabolism

Blomstrand et al. (14) have also studied the effects of running to exhaustion on brain 5-HT metabolism. They found increases in plasma free (but not total) Trp and regional brain Trp and in 5-HT and 5-HIAA concentrations immediately after a treadmill run to exhaustion in both trained ($\approx$ 180 min) and untrained ($\approx$ 72 min) rats.

We have extended these observations to include a study of the effects of both moderate and fatiguing exercise on neurotransmitters in various regions of the rat brain (7). Measurements of 5-HT, 5-HIAA, DA, and DOPAC (major metabolite of dopamine) were made in the midbrain, striatum, hypothalamus, and hippocampus of rats sacrificed at rest, after 1 h of exercise, and after exhaustive exercise (20 m $\cdot$ min^{-1}, 5% grade). After 1 h of exercise, the concentrations of 5-HT and 5-HIAA were higher in all brain regions studied except the hippocampus, where only 5-HIAA was elevated. At exhaustion 5-HT leveled off, but 5-HIAA increased even further in the midbrain and striatum. DA and DOPAC also increased in the midbrain, striatum, and hypothalamus after 1 h but then decreased back to baseline levels in rats run to exhaustion. The results indicated that 5-HT synthesis and turnover increased at 1 h and was even higher at fatigue, especially in the midbrain and striatum. Alternatively, DA metabolism was higher at 1 h but then dropped at fatigue.

Drug-Induced Alterations of Brain 5-HT and Fatigue

The experimental results just described suggest that a good relationship exists between prolonged exercise to fatigue and elevated brain 5-HT synthesis and turn-over. However, they do not directly address the question of whether alterations in brain 5-HT activity cause decrements in endurance performance via central fatigue. In order to approach this problem more directly, we completed a series of experiments investigating the effects of pharmacological manipulation of 5-HT activity on endurance performance (run time to exhaustion at 20 m $\cdot$ min^{-1}, 5% grade, in rats). In a preliminary experiment, the administration of a specific 5-HT$_{1c}$ receptor agonist (*m*-chlorophenyl piperazine) reduced endurance performance in a dose-response manner (5). This was followed by an experiment in which a more general 5-HT agonist (quipazine dimaleate, QD) and a 5-HT antagonist (LY-53,857; a 5-HT$_{1c}$ and 5-HT$_2$ receptor antagonist) were used at various doses to determine their effects on performance (6). In this experiment, run time to exhaustion was reduced in a dose-dependent manner by increasing dosages of the 5-HT agonist, whereas run time was extended by the highest dose of the antagonist. The likelihood that the agonist drug was working within the central nervous system is supported by the observation that prior administration of a peripherally restricted 5-HT antagonist (xylamidine tosylate) did not attenuate this effect.

These results using a pharmacological approach in a rat model have recently been supported by two investigations in which 5-HT activity was pharmacologically increased in humans (21, 42). When brain 5-HT activity was increased by prior oral administration of a 5-HT reuptake blocker (20 mg paroxetine or 70 mg fluoxetine), exercise time to fatigue occurred earlier (42), and perceived exertion was higher (21) during prolonged cycling at 70% $\dot{V}O_2$max. It is important to note that the subjects did not report any strange side effects when they were on the drug, and there were no treatment differences in various markers of cardiovascular, thermo-regulatory, and metabolic function. Therefore, these studies would suggest that increased brain 5-HT activity can impair endurance performance perhaps through an effect on central fatigue.

Potential Mechanisms of Fatigue
Associated With Increased Brain 5-HT Activity

The studies previously described in both rats and humans appear to provide good evidence that brain 5-HT increases during prolonged exercise and that changes in brain 5-HT activity can affect fatigue. However, the strength of these findings will continue to be questioned until more direct methods are available to directly measure central fatigue during dynamic exercise and until the potential biological mechanisms of such an effect are determined.

Investigators have begun to explore possible biological mechanisms whereby increased brain 5-HT might be involved in fatigue. The serotonergic system is associated with numerous brain functions that could positively or negatively affect endurance performance. Increased serotonergic activity may induce fatigue through inhibition of the dopaminergic system (7, 19), by reducing arousal and motivation to perform (32, 43), or both. Furthermore, serotonergic activity can affect the hypothalamic-pituitary-adrenal axis, thermoregulation, pain, and mood, which may positively or negatively influence endurance performance, depending on the specific situation and the species studied (2, 3, 24, 43).

5-HT/Dopamine Interactions

We have observed that fatigue during prolonged exercise in the rat appears to be associated with an increase in brain 5-HT metabolism and an attenuation in brain dopamine metabolism (5, 7). This relationship was found in both control animals and those that were administered a 5-HT agonist in our study. It also appears that fatigue hastened by administration of a 5-HT agonist could not be reasonably explained by altered hypothalamic-pituitary-adrenal axis activity, sympatho-adrenal-medullary activity, or metabolic dysfunction involving substrate mobilization and utilization (7). Altered thermoregulatory function is also not a likely limiting factor in this experimental paradigm (unpublished data). Therefore it would appear that, at least in the rat model, alterations in dopamine metabolism might explain some of the effects of altered 5-HT activity on fatigue.

Dopamine (DA) was the first neurotransmitter to be investigated for its potential role in exercise performance. This is probably due to the previously established role of DA in controlling movements in general (27) and to the reported use of amphetamine-like drugs by athletes to improve performance (15).

Others have also shown that DA metabolism is increased during exercise in the midbrain, hippocampus, striatum, and hypothalamus (7, 18, 19, 31) but is apparently reduced as fatigue develops, at least in the midbrain and brain stem (7). In addition, it is known that endurance performance is impaired following partial destruction of dopaminergic neurons by 6-hydroxydopamine (6-OHDA; 31) and that endurance performance can be improved following increased dopaminergic activation by amphetamine (9, 29). An explanation for a possible interaction between brain 5-HT and DA in central fatigue remains to be determined. However, it is possible that a low 5-HT/DA ratio in various brain areas favors increased arousal, motivation, and neuromuscular coordination, whereas a high 5-HT/DA ratio favors lethargy, fatigue, and loss of coordination (central fatigue).

Nutritional Effects on 5-HT and Central Fatigue

For obvious ethical reasons, investigators have used the rat model to study the effects of fatigue on regional brain concentrations of 5-HT and its metabolites. Investigations in human subjects have focused primarily on factors that affect Trp availability to the brain (i.e., proposed markers of central fatigue).

Blomstrand, Celsing, and Newsholme (11) were the first to approach the problem in humans. They studied 22 subjects before and after a marathon race. After the race, plasma f-Trp was 2.4 times higher, and branched-chain amino acids (BCAA) were slightly lower ($\approx$ 19%). This drop in the f-Trp/BCAA ratio was consistent with their hypothesis that Trp availability to the brain is increased by prolonged exercise and that increased brain 5-HT activity and central fatigue may occur under these conditions. They also reported similar responses following a soccer match (45% increase in f-Trp, 29% decrease in BCAA) and prolonged cross-country skiing (f-Trp not reported, 28% decrease in BCAA; 12, 13). These data are in general agreement with the rat data and support the basic tenets of the central fatigue hypothesis.

The theoretical possibility that central fatigue could be delayed by nutritional strategies that alter the f-Trp/BCAA ratio is intriguing. Investigations have centered primarily around two strategies involving supplementation of BCAA, carbohydrates, or both during exercise. Both of these strategies would theoretically decrease the f-Trp/BCAA ratio and thereby decrease the availability of f-Trp to the brain and delay central fatigue.

Blomstrand, Newsholme, and colleagues have focused on the administration of BCAA as a way to delay central fatigue. They reported that the administration of 7.5 to 21 g of BCAA prior to and during a marathon, a cross-country ski race, or a soccer match was associated in some subjects with small improvements in both physical (marathon running and cross-country skiing) and mental performance (12, 13). However, it should be noted that while field studies such as these are designed to mimic the real world situation in which athletes find themselves, they are often limited in scientific value. For example, subjects are often not matched or randomly divided into control and treatment groups; the treatments are usually not administered in a blind experimental design to the subjects; very few, if any, blood samples are collected; and perhaps more important, exercise intensity and nutrition are usually not well controlled. These limitations increase the likelihood that the observed benefits of a particular supplement may not have been due to the supplement but to one or more of the uncontrolled variables (false positive). Indeed, no benefits of BCAA supplementation have been found in recent well-controlled laboratory experiments. Varnier et al. (37) infused approximately 20 g BCAA or saline throughout a 70-min period prior to exercise using a double-blind, crossover design and found no differences in performance of a graded incremental exercise test to fatigue. We also performed a double-blind, crossover study in the laboratory to determine the effects of a smaller, more palatable supplement of BCAA (approximately 0.5 g · h⁻¹ added to a carbohydrate-electrolyte drink) during cycling exercise at 70% $\dot{V}O_2$max to fatigue (28). This amount of BCAA was designed to replace the calculated maximal amount of BCAA catabolism that might occur during this type of exercise. The results showed that the supplement prevented the slight drop in plasma BCAA concentration during exercise, but there was no effect on ride time to fatigue, perceived exertion, or various measures of cardiovascular and metabolic function. Finally, Verger et al. (38) recently reported that ingestion of BCAA by rats caused a reduction in run time to exhaustion as compared with rats fed either water or glucose.

One must also not overlook the possible negative side effects of giving a large amount of BCAA during exercise, including the accumulation of ammonia, which can be toxic to the brain and may also negatively affect muscle metabolism (8, 40, 41). Acute ammonia toxicity, although transient and reversible, may be severe enough in critical regions of the central nervous system to impair performance (coordination, motor control) or produce severe symptoms of fatigue (8). The buffering of ammonia could also cause fatigue in the muscle by depleting glycolytically derived carbon skeletons (pyruvate) and by draining intermediates of the tricarboxylic acid cycle, which are coupled to glutamine production by transamination reactions (40, 41). This could conceivably impair oxidative metabolism in the muscle and lead to early fatigue. When we administered ammonium acetate (which does not affect acid-base balance) to rats prior to treadmill exercise in doses calculated to elicit physiologically relevant levels of blood ammonia, it caused a dose-related reduction in time to fatigue. Furthermore, the effect was partially blocked by co-administration of aspartate, which is known to buffer increases in ammonia. Aspartate is thought to work by increasing the removal of ammonia via stimulation of the urea cycle (1).

Finally, it could be argued that the magnitude of changes in f-Trp/BCAA reported in these studies are much too small to be physiologically relevant. Indeed, it has been shown that 8- to 16-fold increases in the Trp/BCAA ratio are required to effect a change in 5-HT and 5-HIAA in the brains of monkeys (33).

We reasoned, therefore, that an optimal nutritional strategy would be one in which very large differences in the f-Trp/BCAA ratio could be achieved without the potential negative consequences of ammonia buildup and the associated problems with palatability (especially if mixed with drinks taken during exercise). We reasoned that the well-known effects of carbohydrate feedings on free fatty acid mobilization could produce large reductions in plasma f-Trp while having very little effect on plasma BCAA during prolonged exercise. It seemed reasonable that some of the well-known benefits of carbohydrate feedings on endurance performance might involve central as well as peripheral mechanisms of fatigue (22). The benefits of carbohydrate feedings on peripheral mechanisms of fatigue are already well documented (20).

This hypothesis was tested in a double-blind, placebo-controlled laboratory study in which subjects drank either a water placebo, a 6% carbohydrate-electrolyte drink, or a 12% carbohydrate-electrolyte drink on three occasions. We found that prolonged cycling at 70% $\dot{V}O_2$max increased plasma f-Trp by approximately sevenfold (in direct proportion to plasma free fatty acids), while total Trp and BCAA changed very little. When subjects consumed either a 6% or a 12% carbohydrate-electrolyte solution (5 ml · kg⁻¹ · h⁻¹), the increase in plasma f-Trp was blocked in roughly a dose-response manner, and fatigue was delayed by approximately 1 h. The carbohydrate feedings caused a slight reduction in plasma BCAA (approximately 19% and 31% in the 6% and 12% carbohydrate groups, respectively), but this decrease was probably inconsequential with respect to the very large attenuation (five- to sevenfold) of plasma f-Trp (22). Although it was not possible to distinguish between the beneficial effects of carbohydrate feedings on central versus peripheral mechanisms of fatigue in this study, it is interesting that fatigue in this study that occurred after 3 to 4 h could not be explained by typical markers of peripheral fatigue, including cardiovascular, thermoregulatory, and metabolic function.

Conclusions

Fatigue during prolonged exercise has traditionally been associated with mechanisms that result in dysfunction of the contractile process within muscle. More recently, however, interest in possible central nervous system mechanisms of fatigue has grown as our understanding of the physiological workings of the nervous system has improved. Unfortunately, progress in this area has been hampered by a lack of good methodologies to distinguish central from peripheral mechanisms of fatigue during dynamic whole-body exercise.

Good evidence is beginning to accumulate in support of a role of brain 5-HT in central fatigue during prolonged exercise. For example, increases in 5-HT and 5-HIAA occur in various brain regions during prolonged exercise; the increase in 5-HT metabolism appears to peak as fatigue develops; and administration of 5-HT agonist and antagonist drugs increase and decrease fatigue in a predictable manner. Furthermore, in most studies of this kind, there is little if any support for a role of peripheral mechanisms in fatigue associated with increased 5-HT activity.

Although there is good reason to believe that nutrition might play a role in fatigue induced by brain 5-HT, the evidence in this area is very tenuous. Studies on the proposed role of branched-chain amino acid supplementation are limited, and there are reasons to think that this approach may not be a viable one. Carbohydrate supplementation, on the other hand, is associated with large decreases in the f-Trp/BCAA ratio (marker of Trp availability and 5-HT synthesis), and fatigue is clearly delayed by this nutritional strategy. However, it is still not possible to distinguish with any certainty between the proposed effects on central mechanisms of fatigue and those well-known effects on peripheral mechanisms involving the muscle itself.

References

1. Ahlborn, E.N.; Davis, J.M.; Bailey, S.P. Effects of ammonia on endurance performance in the rat. Med. Sci. Sports Exercise 24(5):S50; 1992.
2. Akil, H.; Liebeskind, J.C. Monoaminergic mechanisms of stimulation-produced analgesia. Brain Res. 94:279-296; 1975.
3. Alper, R.H. Evidence for central and peripheral serotonergic control of corticosterone secretion in the conscious rat. Neuroendocrinology 51:255-260; 1990.
4. Asmussen, E. Muscle fatigue. Med. Sci. Sports 11(4):313-321; 1979.

5. Bailey, S.P.; Davis, J.M.; Ahlborn, E.N. Serotonergic agonists and antagonists affect endurance performance in the rat. Int. J. Sports Med. 6:330-333; 1993.

6. Bailey, S.P.; Davis, J.M.; Ahlborn, E.N. Effect of increased brain serotonergic (5-HT$_{1C}$) activity on endurance performance in the rat. Acta Physiol. Scand. 145(1):75-76; 1992.

7. Bailey, S.P.; Davis, J.M.; Ahlborn, E.N. Neuroendocrine and substrate responses to altered brain 5-HT activity during prolonged exercise to fatigue. J. Appl. Physiol. 74(6):3006-3012; 1993.

8. Banister, E.W.; Cameron, B.J.C. Exercise-induced hyperammonemia: Peripheral and central effects. Int. J. Sports Med. 11 (suppl. 2):S129-S142; 1990.

9. Bhagat, B.; Wheeler, N. Effect of amphetamine on the swimming endurance of rats. Neuropharmacology 12:711-713; 1973.

10. Bigland-Ritchie, B.; Furbush, F.; Woods, J.J. Fatigue of intermittent submaximal voluntary contractions: Central and peripheral factors. J. Appl. Physiol. 61(2): 421-429; 1986.

11. Blomstrand, E.; Celsing, F.; Newsholme, E.A. Changes in plasma concentrations of aromatic and branch-chain amino acids during sustained exercise in man and their possible role in fatigue. Acta Physiol. Scand. 133:115-121; 1988.

12. Blomstrand, E.; Hassmén, P.; Ekblom, B.; Newsholme, E.A. Administration of branched-chain amino acids during sustained exercise—Effects on performance and on plasma concentration of some amino acids. Eur. J. Appl. Physiol. 63:83-88; 1991.

13. Blomstrand, E.; Hassmén, P.; Newsholme, E.A. Effect of branched-chain amino acid supplementation on mental performance. Acta Physiol. Scand. 136:473-481; 1991.

14. Blomstrand, E.; Perrett, D.; Parry-Billings, M.; Newsholme, E.A. Effect of sustained exercise on plasma amino acid concentrations and on 5-hydroxytryptamine metabolism in six different brain regions in the rat. Acta Physiol. Scand. 136:473-481; 1989.

15. Chaouloff, F. Physical exercise and brain monoamines: A review. Acta Physiol. Scand. 137:1-13; 1989.

16. Chaouloff, F.; Elghozi, J.L.; Guezennec, Y.; Laude, D. Effects of conditioned running on plasma, liver and brain tryptophan and on brain 5-hydroxytryptamine metabolism of the rat. Br. J. Pharmacol. 86:33-41; 1985.

17. Chaouloff, F.; Laude, D.; Elghozi, J.L. Physical exercise: Evidence for differential consequences of tryptophan on 5-HT synthesis and metabolism in central serotonergic cell bodies and terminals. J. Neural Trans. 78:121-130; 1989.

18. Chaouloff, F.; Laude, D.; Guezennec, Y.; Elghozi, J.L. Motor activity increases tryptophan, 5-hydroxyindoleacetic acid, and homovanillic acid in ventricular cerebrospinal fluid of the conscious rat. J. Neurochem. 46:1313-1316; 1986.

19. Chaouloff, F.; Laude, D.; Merino, D.; Serrurier, B.; Guezennec, Y.; Elghozi, J.L. Amphetamine and alpha-methyl-p-tyrosine affect the exercise induced imbalance between the availability of tryptophan and synthesis of serotonin in the brain of the rat. Neuropharmacology 26:1099-1106; 1987.

20. Coggan, A.R.; Coyle, E.F. Carbohydrate ingestion during prolonged exercise: Effects on metabolism and performance. Exercise Sport Sci. Rev. 19:1-40; 1991.

21. Davis, J.M.; Bailey, S.P.; Jackson, D.A.; Strasner, A.B.; Morehouse, S.L. Effects of a serotonin (5-HT) agonist during prolonged exercise to fatigue in humans. Med. Sci. Sports Exercise 25(5):S78; 1993.

22. Davis, J.M.; Bailey, S.P.; Woods, J.A.; Galiano, F.J.; Hamilton, M.; Bartoli, W.P. Effects of carbohydrate feedings on plasma free-tryptophan and branched-chain amino acids during prolonged cycling. Eur. J. Appl. Physiol. 65:513-519; 1992.

23. Enoka, R.M.; Stuart, D.G. Neurobiology of muscle fatigue. J. Appl. Physiol. 72(5):1631-1648; 1992.

24. Feldberg, W.; Myers, R.D. Effects of temperature of amines injected into the cerebral ventricles: A new concept of temperature regulation. J. Physiol. (London) 173:226-237; 1964.

25. Fernstrom, J.D. Dietary amino acids and brain function. J. Am. Diet. Assoc. 94:71-77; 1994.

26. Fitts, R.H.; Metzger, J.M. Mechanisms of muscular fatigue. In: Poortmans, J.R., ed. Principles of exercise biochemistry. 2nd ed. Vol. 38. Karger: Basel; 1993:248-268.

27. Freed, C.R.; Yamamoto, B.K. Regional brain dopamine metabolism: A marker for speed, direction, and posture of moving animals. Science 229:62-65; 1985.

28. Galiano, F.J.; Davis, J.M.; Bailey, S.P.; Woods, J.A.; Hamilton, M. Physiologic, endocrine and performance effects of adding branch chain amino acids to a 6% carbohydrate-electrolyte beverage during prolonged cycling. Med. Sci. Sports Exercise 23(4):S14; 1991.

29. Gerald, M.C. Effect of (+)-amphetamine on the treadmill endurance performance of rats. Neuropharmacology 17:703-704; 1978.

30. Green, H.J. Neuromuscular aspects of fatigue. Can. J. Sport Sci. 12 (suppl. 1):7s-19s; 1987.

31. Heyes, M.P.; Garnett, E.S.; Coates, G. Nigrostriatal dopaminergic activity is increased during exhaustive exercise stress in rats. Life Sci. 42:1537-1542; 1988.

32. Jauvet, M.; Pujol, J.-F. Effects of central alterations of serotonergic neurons upon the sleep-waking cycle. Adv. Biochem. Psychopharmacol. 11:199-209; 1974.

33. Leathwood, P.D.; Fernstrom, J.D. Effect of an oral tryptophan/carbohydrate load on tryptophan, large neutral amino acid, and serotonin and 5-hydroxyindoleacetic acid levels in monkey brain. J. Neural Trans. 79:25-34; 1990.

34. Newsholme, E.A.; Acworth, I.N.; Blomstrand, E. Amino acids, brain neurotransmitters and a functional link between muscle and brain that is important in sustained exercise. In: Benzi, G., ed. Advances in myochemistry. London: John Libbey Eurotext Ltd.; 1987:127-133.

35. Secher, N.H. Central nervous influence on fatigue. In: Shephard, R.J.; Astrand, P.-O., eds. Endurance in sport. Boston: Blackwell Scientific Publications; 1992:96-106.

36. Sjøgaard, G. Muscle fatigue. Med. Sport Sci. 26:98-109; 1987.

37. Varnier, M.; Sarto, P.; Martines, D.; Lora, L.; Carmignoto, F.; Leese, G.; Naccarato, R. Effect of infusing branched-chain amino acid during incremental exercise with reduced muscle glycogen content. Eur. J. Appl. Physiol. 69:26-31; 1994.

38. Verger, P.H.; Aymard, P.; Cynobert, L.; Anton, G.; Luigi, R. Effects of administration of branched-chain amino acids vs. glucose during acute exercise in the rat. Physiol. Behav. 55(3):523-526; 1994.

39. Vøllestad, N.K.; Sejersted, O.M. Biochemical correlates of fatigue. Eur. J. Appl. Physiol. 57:336-347; 1988.

40. Wagenmakers, A.J.M.; Bechers, E.J.; Brouns, F.; Kuipers, H.; Soeters, P.B.; Van der Vusse, G.J.; Saris, W.H.M. Carbohydrate supplementation, glycogen

depletion, and amino acid metabolism during exercise. Am. J. Physiol. 260: E883-E890; 1991.

41. Wagenmakers, A.J.M.; Coakley, J.H.; Edwards, R.H.T. Metabolism of branched-chain amino acids and ammonia during exercise: Clues from McArdle's disease. Int. J. Sports Med. 11:S101-S113; 1990.

42. Wilson, W.M.; Maughan, R.J. Evidence for a possible role of 5-hydroxytryptamine in the genesis of fatigue in man: Administration of paroxetine, a 5-HT re-uptake inhibitor, reduces the capacity to perform prolonged exercise. Exp. Physiol. 77:921-924; 1992.

43. Young, S.N. The clinical psychopharmacology of tryptophan. In: Wurtman, R.J.; Wurtman, J.J., eds. Nutrition and the brain. Vol. 7. New York: Raven; 1986:49-88.

PART X

Free Radicals in Exercise and Health

CHAPTER 36

Free Radicals, Exercise, and Health

Malcolm J. Jackson
University of Liverpool, Liverpool, England

Numerous studies have indicated the beneficial effects of a moderate amount of exercise on cardiovascular health, but the effects of many years of sustained exercise training and competition on susceptibility to disease in later life or on life-span have not been evaluated. Recent data have indicated that an overproduction of oxygen free radicals may be associated with exercise (5, 6) and other workers have proposed that increased free radical activity may be the cause of aging (10) and pathogenic for many of the common disorders of old age (9). Taken together, these data may imply that increased free radical activity during exercise leads to premature aging and an increased incidence of age-related disorders. It is therefore important to clarify whether free radicals are produced in excess during exercise and to determine the effects and importance of this to the casual and regular athlete.

This short review will examine a number of key questions concerning the role of free radicals in exercise. A considerable amount of work has been undertaken in this area, but basic data are still not available to fully answer these questions:

- Are free radical species produced in excess during exercise?
- Is any excess free radical production during exercise damaging or beneficial to tissues?
- Is the tissue antioxidant capacity modified by exercise?
- Does antioxidant supplementation reduce free radical activity during exercise?
- Does antioxidant supplementation during exercise have beneficial effects on tissues?

Are Free Radicals Produced in Excess During Exercise?

The unequivocal demonstration of increased free radical activity in complex biological tissues is difficult and is usually only accepted if a variety of indicators provide supportive evidence. This evidence can be in the form of measurements of indirect indicators of free radical activity (products of lipid peroxidation, DNA oxidation, protein oxidation), direct detection of free radicals (electron spin resonance techniques), or prevention of the putative free radical–mediated effect by supplementation with relatively specific antioxidants.

Initial suggestions that free radical processes, such as lipid peroxidation, were elevated during exercise came from studies of whole-body exercise in humans (6) and rats (3, 7). These were rapidly followed by studies of the products of free radical reactions within the tissues of exercising animals (5). These data indicated that exercise to exhaustion in rats resulted in decreased mitochondrial respiratory control, loss of sarcoplasmic reticulum integrity, increased lipid peroxidation, and increased free radical generation as shown by electron spin resonance (ESR) studies. This is perhaps the most widely quoted data in support of a role for free radical species in exercise-induced damage to skeletal muscle (and other tissues). It is notable that the exercise regime used was an endurance protocol in which the muscles were primarily contracting in a concentric manner.

Similar ESR studies undertaken by our group have also demonstrated an increased "stable" free radical signal in response to excess contractile activity of muscle (13), although our interpretation of these results was somewhat different from that of Davies et al. (5). In particular, we have studied the possibility that the increased ESR-visible free radical signal occurs following an exercise-induced accumulation of calcium (17) within the muscle cells (16) and is therefore a secondary consequence of alternative damaging processes (19).

Of particular relevance in this area are the possible effects on free radical production of the manner in which the muscle is used. Muscle may contract in a concentric manner (where the active muscle is allowed to shorten), an eccentric manner (where the muscle is lengthened), or an isometric manner (where the muscle remains at a fixed length). Eccentric contractions are considerably more damaging to muscle (21-23), but the different types of exercise have been relatively infrequently studied for their influences on free radical production (12).

Is Any Excess Free Radical Production During Exercise Damaging or Beneficial to Tissues?

It is generally assumed that excess free radical production is damaging to tissues, and the described association between excessive free radical production during exercise and tissue damage (5, 13) has supported this. However, it should be noted that at the current stage this has only been shown to be an association rather than a cause-and-effect relationship (12), and further work is required in this area.

A small amount of work has examined the possibility that beneficial effects may derive from free radicals produced during exercise. Salo et al. (30) reported that oxygen radicals stimulate the production of stress proteins in exercising muscle. These proteins may play a role in mitochondrial biogenesis and the training response to exercise. Free radicals may therefore be playing an important second messenger role in this situation.

Is the Tissue Antioxidant Capacity Modified by Exercise?

Exercise training is recognized to be an efficient way of reducing the susceptibility of muscles to exercise-induced muscle damage, and several studies have investigated the possibility that this may be associated with an increase in the tissue's defenses against free radicals. Exercise training in rats appears to be associated with an increase in the activity of muscle superoxide dismutase (11), and modifications in the concentration of antioxidants and in the activity of antioxidant enzymes have also been reported in humans (29).

Does Antioxidant Supplementation Reduce Free Radical Activity During Exercise?

There is considerable evidence that supplementation with specific antioxidants may reduce indicators of increased exercise-induced free radical activity in muscle or the circulation (5, 6, 13, 20, 32), although this alone is clearly insufficient evidence to advocate antioxidant supplements for athletes.

Does Antioxidant Supplementation During Exercise Have Beneficial Effects on Tissues?

This is perhaps the most important question for which an answer is required. Vitamin E is the antioxidant that has received most attention in this area. Davies et al. (5) originally found that vitamin E–depleted animals had a reduced exercise endurance. These effects were confirmed by further studies from the same group (24), and exacerbating effects of vitamin E deficiency on other models of exercise-induced muscle damage were reported by Jackson, Jones, and Edwards (14) and Amelink (1).

Our group has specifically examined the effects of vitamin E on damage processes in isolated skeletal muscle. These studies have demonstrated that vitamin E has protective effects against contractile activity–induced (14, 18) and calcium ionophore–induced (26-28) damage to skeletal muscle in vitro, but the mechanisms by which this protective effect occurs do not appear to be as clear-cut as some workers have proposed. Although the protective effects are apparent in animals fed diets rich in polyunsaturated fatty acids but not in animals fed a diet rich in saturated fatty acids (S. O'Farrell and M.J. Jackson, unpublished observations), in general agreement with the concept that the excess vitamin E is preventing free radical–mediated peroxidation of membrane polyunsaturated fatty acids, the protective effects also appear to be mimicked by phytol, isophytol, and a number of other lipophilic, non-antioxidant substances having long hydrocarbon side chains (26, 28). It is therefore clear that further work is required in this area to clarify the nature of the protection offered by vitamin E.

All of the preceding studies were undertaken in exercise models in which the predominant form of muscle activity was not specified or in which it was entirely isometric. Eccentric exercise has been infrequently studied from the point of view of free radical processes, but where damage to skeletal muscle specifically induced by eccentric contractions has been studied, conflicting data have been reported. In a detailed study of damage to mouse extensor digitorum longus muscle induced by eccentric contraction, Zerba, Komorowski, and Faulkner (33) found that treatment of animals with polyethylene glycol–superoxide dismutase significantly reduced the amount of injury that was present 3 d postexercise in mice of various ages. However, in a study of animals that undertook lengthening contractions during downhill walking, Warren et al. (32) could show no protective effect of vitamin E supplementation. Nevertheless, studies of human subjects undertaking eccentric exercise have reported changes in blood parameters indicative of increased free radical activity (25). Cannon and co-workers have also examined subjects undertaking downhill running. They found no protective effects of vitamin E supplementation against muscle damage (4), although the supplements did appear to reduce oxidative stress (20); these authors suggest that their data support a role for oxidants in the delayed-onset muscle damage.

Other antioxidants have been studied only infrequently as potential inhibitors of the deleterious effects of exercise, but the data that has been presented is inconclusive concerning possible protective effects of these substances (2, 8, 31). However, Jakeman and Maxwell (15) recently have studied the effects of vitamin C supplementation on eccentric exercise in humans and reported a smaller fall in muscle force production postexercise in the treated subjects than in untreated controls or a vitamin E–treated group.

Conclusion

In conclusion, it appears that there is substantial evidence in support of an increased production of free radical species during exercise, but the evidence that these species are responsible for any skeletal muscle damage that occurs as a result of the exercise is much less conclusive. It is clear that training enhances the antioxidant capacity of muscle, but whether antioxidant nutrient supplements are beneficial to subjects undertaking excessive or unaccustomed exercise is still not established.

References

1. Amelink, G.J. Exercise induced muscle damage. Utrecht, Netherlands: Univ. of Utrecht; 1990. PhD thesis.
2. Bendich, A. Exercise and free radicals: Effects of antioxidant vitamins. Med. Sport Sci. 32:59-78; 1991.
3. Brady, P.S.; Brady, L.J.; Ulrey, D.E. Selenium, vitamin E and the response to swimming stress in the rat. J. Nutr. 109:1103-1109; 1979.
4. Cannon, J.G.; Orencole, S.F.; Fielding, R.A.; Meydani, M.; Meydani, S.N.; Fiatarone, M.A.; Blumberg, J.B.; Evans, W.J. Acute phase response in exercise: Interaction of age and vitamin E on neutrophils and muscle enzyme release. Am. J. Physiol. 259:R1214-R1219; 1990.
5. Davies, K.J.A.; Quintanilha, A.T.; Brooks, G.A.; Packer, L. Free radicals and tissue damage produced by exercise. Biochem. Biophys. Res. Commun. 107: 1198-1205; 1982.

6. Dillard, C.J.; Litov, R.E.; Savin, W.M.; Tappel, A.L. Effects of exercise, vitamin E and ozone on pulmonary function and lipid peroxidation. J. Appl. Physiol. 45:927-932; 1978.

7. Gee, D.L.; Tappel, A.L. The effect of exhaustive exercise on expired pentane as a measure of *in vivo* lipid peroxidation in the rat. Life Sci. 28:2425-2429; 1981.

8. Gerster, H. The role of vitamin C in athletic performance. J. Am. Coll. Nutr. 8:636-643; 1989.

9. Halliwell, B.; Gutteridge, J.M.C. Free radicals in biology and medicine. Oxford: Clarendon; 1989.

10. Harman, D. A theory of ageing based on free radicals and radiation chemistry. J. Gerontol. 11:298-305; 1956.

11. Higuchi, M.; Cartier, L.J.; Chen, M.; Holloszy, J.O. Superoxide dismutase and catalase in skeletal muscle: Adaptive response to exercise. J. Gerontol. 40:281-286; 1985.

12. Jackson, M.J. Exercise and oxygen radical production by muscle. In: Sen, C.K.; Packer, L.; Hanninan, O., eds. Exercise and oxygen toxicity. London: Elsevier; 1994:49-57.

13. Jackson, M.J.; Edwards, R.H.T.; Symons, M.R.C. Electron spin resonance studies of intact mammalian skeletal muscle. Biochim. Biophys. Acta 847:185-190; 1985.

14. Jackson, M.J.; Jones, D.A.; Edwards, R.H.T. Vitamin E and skeletal muscle. In: Porter, R.; Whelan, J., eds. Biology of vitamin E. London: Pitman; 1983:224-239. (Ciba Foundation Symposium Series No. 101).

15. Jakeman, P.; Maxwell, S. Effect of antioxidant vitamin supplementation on muscle function after eccentric exercise. Eur. J. Appl. Physiol. 67:426-430; 1993.

16. Johnson, K.M.; Sutcliffe, L.H.; Edwards, R.H.T.; Jackson, M.J. Calcium ionophore enhances the electron spin resonance signal from isolated skeletal muscle. Biochim. Biophys. Acta 964:285-288; 1988.

17. Jones, D.A.; Jackson, M.J.; McPhail, G.; Edwards, R.H.T. Experimental muscle damage: The importance of external calcium. Clin. Sci. 66:317-322; 1984.

18. McArdle, A.; Edwards, R.H.T.; Jackson, M.J. Calcium homeostasis during contractile activity of vitamin E–deficient skeletal muscle. Proc. Nutr. Soc. 52:83A; 1993.

19. McArdle, A.; Jackson, M.J. Intracellular mechanisms involved in damage to skeletal muscle. Basic Appl. Myol. 4:43-50; 1994.

20. Meydani, M.; Evans, W.J.; Handelman, G.; Biddle, L.; Fielding, R.A.; Meydani, S.N.; Burrill, J.; Fiatarone, M.A.; Blumberg, J.B.; Cannon, J.G. Protective effect of vitamin E on exercise-induced oxidative damage in young and older adults. Am. J. Physiol. 264:R992-R998; 1994.

21. Newham, D.J.; Jones, D.A.; Edwards, R.H.T. Plasma creatine kinase changes after eccentric and concentric contractions. Muscle Nerve 9:59-63; 1986.

22. Newham, D.J.; Jones, D.A.; Tolfree, S.E.J.; Edwards, R.H.T. Skeletal muscle damage: A study of isotope uptake, enzyme efflux and pain after stepping. Eur. J. Appl. Physiol. 55:106-112; 1986.

23. Newham, D.J.; Mills, K.R.; Quigley, B.M.; Edwards, R.H.T. Pain and fatigue after concentric and eccentric muscle contractions. Clin. Sci. 64:55-62; 1983.

24. Packer, L. Vitamin E, physical exercise and tissue damage in animals. Med. Biol. 62:105-109; 1984.

25. Packer, L.; Viguie, C. Human exercise: Oxidative stress and antioxidant therapy. In: Benzi, G., ed. Advances in biochemistry 2. London: John Libbey Eurotext; 1989:1-17.

26. Phoenix, J.; Edwards, R.H.T.; Jackson, M.J. The effect of vitamin E analogues and long hydrocarbon chain compounds on calcium-induced muscle damage: A novel role for α-tocopherol. Biochim. Biophys. Acta 1097:212-218; 1991.

27. Phoenix, J.; Edwards, R.H.T.; Jackson, M.J. Effects of calcium ionophore on vitamin E deficient rat muscle. Br. J. Nutr. 64:245-256; 1990.

28. Phoenix, J.; Edwards, R.H.T.; Jackson, M.J. Inhibition of calcium-induced cytosolic enzyme efflux from skeletal muscle by vitamin E and related compounds. Biochem. J. 257:207-213; 1989.

29. Robertson, J.D.; Maughan, R.J.; Duthie, G.G.; Morrice, P.C. Increased blood antioxidant systems of runners in response to training load. Clin. Sci. 80:611-618; 1991.

30. Salo, D.C.; Donovan, C.M.; Davies, K.J.A. HSP70 and other possible heat shock or oxidative stress proteins are induced in skeletal muscle, heart and liver during exercise. Free Rad. Biol. Med. 11:239-246; 1991.

31. Sastre, J.; Asensi, M.; Gasco, E.; Pallardo, F.V.; Ferrero, J.A.; Furakawa, T.; Vira, J. Exhaustive physical exercise causes oxidation of glutathione status in blood: Prevention by antioxidant administration. Am. J. Physiol. 263:R992-R995; 1992.

32. Warren, J.A.; Jenkins, R.R.; Packer, L.; Witt, E.H.; Armstrong, P.B. Elevated muscle vitamin E does not attenuate eccentric exercise–induced muscle injury. J. Appl. Physiol. 72:2168-2175; 1992.

33. Zerba, E.; Komorowski, T.E.; Faulkner, J.A. Free radical injury to skeletal muscles of young adult and old mice. Am. J. Physiol. 258:C429-C435; 1990.

CHAPTER 37

Antioxidant Adaptations to Exercise

Garry G. Duthie, Alison McE. Jenkinson, Philip C. Morrice, John R. Arthur
Rowett Research Institute, Aberdeen, Scotland

Participation in regular exercise decreases morbidity. Apparent health benefits from a regular exercise program include improved psychological well-being and decreased risk of coronary heart disease through favorable modification of obesity, hypertension, and blood lipid profiles (3). However, exercise may also produce adverse effects, particularly in untrained individuals; these include postexercise muscle soreness and injury. The mechanisms underlying exercise-induced muscle damage are unclear but have been variously ascribed to mechanical tearing of fibers, macrophage invasion contributing to increased lysosomal enzyme activity, structural and metabolic alterations in muscle caused by high local temperatures, and impaired mitochondrial respiration (2).

Reactive oxygen species (ROS) have also been implicated in exercise-induced muscle damage. During mitochondrial oxidative phosphorylation, superoxide radicals (O_2^-) are produced when single electrons react with molecular oxygen. During basal metabolism, 1% to 4% of O_2^- originating in the mitochondria may leak into the cytosol, where iron or copper catalysis can promote the formation of highly reactive hydroxyl [OH^-]-like radicals. Moreover, in the respiratory chain during univalent reduction of oxygen, a semiquinone radical in the presence of hydrogen peroxide and high hydrogen ion concentration may propagate the formation of OH^- (14). Aerobic metabolic rate increases up to 10-fold during physical exercise, enhancing leakage of O_2^- from the mitochondria to the cytosol. This rise in oxygen free radical concentration could exceed the protective capacity of the cell's antioxidant defense mechanisms and lead to the abstraction of hydrogen atoms from a wide range of biomolecules, including the polyunsaturated fatty acids of cell and organelle membranes. This is corroborated by studies that have detected elevated indices of lipid peroxidation in plasma and tissues of humans and animals subjected to various types of exercise activity (1, 4, 6, 7, 16, 19, 20; table 37.1). Such peroxidation of the lipid and protein components of biological membranes may result in loss of membrane integrity and tissue damage. Moreover, ROS can also disrupt cellular calcium (Ca^{2+}) homeostasis by inactivating regulatory mechanisms such as Ca^{2+}-ATPase pumps, Na^+-Ca^{2+} exchange mechanisms, and the voltage-sensitive ryanodine receptor. The resulting loss of control of the asymmetric movement of Ca^{2+} across the cellular membranes can then precipitate the death of the

Table 37.1   Studies Indicating Elevated Indices of Lipid Peroxidation After Exercise

Type of exercise	Observation	Reference
20 min treadmill running by rats	↑in muscle and liver malonaldehyde	1
Exhaustive treadmill running by rats	↑in free radical adducts in muscle and liver	6
Untrained rats swimming to fatigue	↑in muscle thiobarbituric acid reactive substances (TBARS)	16
Cycling at 100% V̇O₂max	↑in plasma TBARS	19
Cycling at 75% V̇O₂max	↑in expired pentane	7
Cycling at 50% V̇O₂max	↑in expired pentane	4
45 min downhill running	↑in serum TBARS	20

cell by activation of potentially destructive biochemical pathways involving phospholipase A_2, neutral proteases, and lysosomal acid hydrolases (10).

An elaborate antioxidant defense system protects living organisms from oxidative stress. Damage to muscle cells after physical exercise is most severe when the individual is unaccustomed to the activity, suggesting that the antioxidant defense system of primarily sedentary subjects is unable to accommodate the exercise-induced enhanced free radical load. Training appears to decrease the damaging effects of exercise on skeletal muscle. Consequently, this brief review discusses whether the moderation of exercise-induced muscle damage and soreness resulting from training reflects an adaptive up-regulation of the antioxidant defense system. The possibility that individuals who exercise extensively may benefit from increased intakes of antioxidants is also discussed.

Modulation of Antioxidant Defense Systems

An antioxidant defense system protects cells from the potentially injurious effects of free radicals (9). Antioxidants are substances that, when present at much lower concentrations than an oxidizable substrate, significantly delay or prevent its oxidation. Certain essential antioxidants need to be taken up from the diet. Vitamin E is a major lipid soluble antioxidant that breaks the chain of free radical–mediated lipid peroxidation of polyunsaturated fatty acids in cell membranes. β-Carotene and other carotenoids may have a similar function, particularly in tissues with a low partial pressure of oxygen. Vitamin C scavenges free radicals in the water-soluble compartment of the cell and may regenerate vitamin E. In addition, several antioxidant enzymes, such as glutathione peroxidase, catalase, and superoxide dismutase, remove the toxic intermediates produced on oxidation of biological material. These enzymes require metal cofactors (selenium for glutathione peroxidase; iron for catalase; copper, zinc, and manganese for superoxide dismutase).

Thus, the efficiency of the antioxidant defense system depends in part on an adequate intake of foods containing nutrients such as vitamin E, vitamin C, ubiquinone, carotenoids, and the trace element cofactors for the antioxidant enzymes. Additionally, increased synthesis of endogenous antioxidants such as glutathione may occur in response to oxidative loads arising from genetic disorders, nutritional antioxidant deficiency, and smoking (21), whereas hormones, cytokines, and the metal cofactors impose pre- and posttranslational control over the genetic expression of antioxidant enzymes (13).

Antioxidant Adaptation to Exercise

Acute, submaximal exercise by moderately trained, healthy individuals produces few changes in the blood antioxidant defense system (28). For example, there were no changes in the activities of catalase, glutathione peroxidase, superoxide dismutase, and glucose-6-phosphate dehydrogenase in moderately trained athletes following completion of a half-marathon (11). However, alterations in blood antioxidant vitamin concentrations occurred that cannot be ascribed solely to fluid shifts from plasma to tissues. For example, post-race increases in plasma vitamin C concentrations have been ascribed to the efflux of ascorbate from the adrenal gland mediated by postexercise increases in plasma cortisol (12). Moreover, immediate post-race elevations in plasma uric acid, a potent antioxidant in plasma, may be due to enhanced purine oxidation in muscle with subsequent diffusion of hypoxanthine and uric acid into the bloodstream (11). Increases in erythrocyte vitamin E content also occur after both short-term and prolonged intensive exercise (11), which indicates mobilization of the antioxidant from tissues and plasma.

There are marked differences in blood antioxidant concentrations and antioxidant enzyme activities when subjects with sedentary lifestyles are compared with those who train regularly. Erythrocyte glutathione peroxidase and catalase activities rise in proportion to weekly training distance, although superoxide dismutase activity remains unaltered (24). Similarly, exercise training of rats causes proportionate enhancement of muscle mitochondrial and cytosolic glutathione peroxidase (17), and catalase is reported to increase in human skeletal muscle after training (15). Such adaptive responses to oxidative stress are contradicted by a study with female rats (27) that indicated that vitamin E deficiency, endurance training, or a combination of both failed to induce elevations in a range of antioxidant enzymes in skeletal muscle, heart, and liver. Such discrepancies between studies may indicate that exercise-induced changes in muscle antioxidant enzymes are muscle specific. For example, following treadwheel training of female rats at three levels of exercise intensity for 10 wk, glutathione peroxidase activity increased only in red gastrocnemius muscle, whereas superoxide dismutase activity was elevated in soleus muscle (23). Moreover, although observed changes in antioxidant enzymes may be associated with physical training, they may also be attributed in part to the confounding effects of altered food intakes. Daily energy intake is strongly related to the amount of physical training, and therefore increased antioxidant enzyme activities may reflect greater intakes of foods containing the enzyme cofactors.

Some experiments (reviewed in 18) with rats and human subjects suggest that following acute exercise there is an increase in plasma concentrations of both oxidized (GSSG) and reduced (GSH) glutathione; this may reflect a vasopressin-induced release of glutathione from the liver in an attempt to deliver GSH to the skeletal muscle, where it may be undergoing rapid oxidation. However, decreased plasma GSH has been observed in dogs after prolonged running on a treadmill. It is possible that the concentration of GSH in plasma depends on the training status of the exercising subject. For example, increased plasma GSH in trained subjects may arise because adapted skeletal muscle may deliver GSH into the circulation. Decreased plasma GSH following exercise by untrained individuals may reflect increased GSH consumption by muscle resulting in decreased export of GSH to plasma (18). Training also induces marked increases in erythrocyte GSH concentrations (24), which, in addition to enhancing the antioxidant capacity of the red cell, may contribute to vitamin E recycling and to the restoration of the activity of thiol-dependent enzymes after exercise-induced inactivation.

Antioxidant Supplementation and Exercise

Increases in antioxidant enzyme activities in trained athletes compared with sedentary individuals indicate adaptive up-regulation of the antioxidant defense system in response to enhanced, persistent oxidative loads arising from sustained exercise. Although increased blood GSSG concentrations and creatine kinase activities occur in dedicated athletes who run 80 to 147 km/wk (24), such adaptations may be insufficient to protect individuals who train extensively. Consequently, numerous studies (5, 7, 22, 25, 26) have assessed the benefits of augmenting the antioxidant defense system by supplementation with antioxidants such as vitamin E. Despite differences in exercise protocols, supplementation periods, and training status of subjects, most studies with human subjects indicate that increased vitamin E intake lowers indices of lipid peroxidation following exercise when compared with subjects on placebo (table 37.2). Because elevated indices of lipid peroxidation have been

Table 37.2   Studies on Vitamin E Supplementation and Lipid Peroxidation in Exercising Human Subjects

Type of exercise	Supplementation prior to exercise	Observation	Reference
Downhill running	48 d, 800 I.U. dlα-tocopherol/d	↓plasma creatine kinase in < 30-yr-olds	5
Cycling at 20%, 50%, and 75% V̇O₂max	2 wk, 1,200 I.U. dlα-tocopherol/d	↓expired pentane	7
Downhill running	48 d, 800 I.U. dlα-tocopherol/d	↓in urinary TBARS	22
Mountain climbing	10 wk, 400 mg dlα-tocopherol/d	↓exhaled pentane	25
Exhaustive cycling	4 wk, 300 mg dlα-tocopherol/d	↓serum TBARS	26

implicated in the pathogenesis of many diseases (8), individuals who train excessively should consider increasing their intakes of nutritional antioxidants.

Acknowledgments

Funding is appreciated from the Scottish Office Agriculture and Fisheries Department (SOAFD) and the University of Bristol.

References

1. Allessio, H.M.; Goldfarb, A.H. Lipid peroxidation and scavenger enzymes during exercise: Adaptive response to training. J. Appl. Physiol. 6:1333-1336; 1988.
2. Armstrong, R.B.; Warren, G.L.; Warren, J.A. Mechanisms of exercise-induced muscle fibre injury. Sports Med. 12:184-207; 1991.
3. Astrand, P. Why exercise? Med. Sci. Sports Exercise 24:153-162; 1992.
4. Balke, P.-O.; Snider, M.T.; Bull, A.P. Evidence for lipid peroxidation during moderate exercise in man. Med. Sci. Sports Exercise 16:181; 1984.
5. Cannon, J.G.; Orencole, S.F.; Fielding, R.A.; Meydani, M.; Meydani, S.N.; Fiatarone, M.A.; Blumberg, J.B.; Evans, W.J. Acute phase response in exercise: Interaction of age and vitamin E on neutrophils and muscle enzyme release. Am. J. Physiol. 259:R1214-R1219; 1990.
6. Davies, K.J.A.; Quintanilha, A.T.; Brooks, G.A.; Packer, L. Free radicals and tissue damage produced by exercise. Biochem. Biophys. Res. Commun. 107:1198-1205; 1982.
7. Dillard, C.J.; Litov, R.E.; Savin, W.M.; Dumelin, E.E.; Tappel, A.L. Effects of exercise, vitamin E, and ozone on pulmonary function and lipid peroxidation. J. Appl. Physiol. 45:927-932; 1978.
8. Duthie, G.G. Lipid peroxidation. Eur. J. Clin. Nutr. 47:759-764; 1993.
9. Duthie, G.G. Vitamin E and antioxidants. Chem. Ind. 2:42-44; 1991.
10. Duthie, G.G.; Arthur, J.R. Free radicals and calcium homeostasis: Relevance to malignant hyperthermia. Free Rad. Biol. Med. 14:435-442; 1993.
11. Duthie, G.G.; Robertson, J.R.; Maughan, R.J.; Morrice, P.C. Blood antioxidant status and erythrocyte lipid peroxidation following distance running. Arch. Biochem. Biophys. 262:78-83; 1990.
12. Gleeson, M.; Robertson, J.D.; Maughan, R.J. Influence of exercise on ascorbic acid status in man. Clin. Sci. 73:501-505; 1987.
13. Harris, E.D. Regulation of antioxidant enzymes. FASEB J. 6:2675-2683; 1992.
14. Jenkins, R.R. Free radical chemistry: Relationship to exercise. Sports Med. 5:156-170; 1988.
15. Jenkins, R.R.; Friendland, R.; Howard, H. The relationship of oxygen uptake to superoxide dismutase and catalase activity in human muscle. Int. J. Sports Med. 5:11-14; 1984.
16. Jenkins, R.R.; Martin, D.; Goldberg, E. Lipid peroxidation in skeletal muscle during atrophy and acute exercise. Med. Sci. Sports Exercise 15:93H; 1983.

17. Ji, L.L.; Stratman, F.W.; Lardy, H.A. Antioxidant enzyme systems in rat liver and muscle. Arch. Biochem. Biophys. 263:150-160; 1988.
18. Kretzschmar, M.; Muller, D. Aging, training and exercise. A review of effects on plasma glutathione and lipid peroxides. Sports Med. 15:196-209; 1993.
19. Lovlin, R.; Cottle, W.; Pyke, I.; Kavanagh, M.; Belcastro, A.N. Are indices of free radical damage related to exercise intensity? Eur. J. Appl. Physiol. 56:313-316; 1987.
20. Maughan, R.J.; Donnelly, A.E.; Gleeson, M.; Whiting, P.H.; Walker, K.A.; Clough, P.J. Delayed-onset muscle damage and lipid peroxidation in man after a downhill run. Muscle Nerve 12:332-336; 1989.
21. McPhail, D.B.; Morrice, P.C.; Duthie, G.G. Adaptation of the blood antioxidant defence mechanisms of sheep with a genetic lesion resulting in low red cell glutathione concentrations. Free Rad. Res. Commun. 18:177-181; 1993.
22. Meydani, M.; Evans, W.J.; Handelman, G.; Biddle, L.; Fielding, R.A.; Meydani, S.N.; Burrill, J.; Fiatarone, M.A.; Blumberg, J.B.; Cannon, J.G. Protective effect of vitamin E on exercise-induced oxidative damage in young and older adults. Am. J. Physiol. 264:R992-R998; 1993.
23. Powers, S.K.; Criswell, D.; Lawler, J.; Ji, L.L.; Martin, D.; Herb, R.A.; Dudley, G. Influence of exercise and fiber type on antioxidant enzyme activity in rat skeletal muscle. Am. J. Physiol. 266:R375-R380; 1994.
24. Robertson, J.D.; Maughan, R.J.; Duthie, G.G.; Morrice, P.C. Increased blood antioxidant systems of runners in response to training load. Clin. Sci. 80:611-618; 1991.
25. Simon-Schnass, I.; Pabst, H. Influence of vitamin E on physical performance. Int. J. Vit. Nutr. Res. 58:49-54; 1988.
26. Sumida, S.; Tanaka, K.; Kitao, H.; Nakadomo, F. Exercise-induced lipid peroxidation and leakage of enzymes before and after vitamin E supplementation. Int. J. Biochem. 21:835-838; 1989.
27. Tiidus, P.M.; Houston, M.E. Antioxidant and oxidative enzyme adaptations to vitamin E and training. Med. Sci. Sports Exercise 26:354-359; 1994.
28. Viguie, C.A.; Frei, B.; Shinenga, M.K.; Ames, B.N.; Packer, L.; Brooks, G.A. Antioxidant status and indices of oxidative stress during consecutive days of exercise. J. Appl. Physiol. 75:566-572; 1993.

CHAPTER 38

Tissue Iron and Reactive Oxygen: It's Not All Bad

Robert R. Jenkins
Ithaca College, Ithaca, New York, U.S.A.

The original report of Dillard et al. (11) that radical production was increased by exercise has been corroborated by several electron paramagnetic resonance (EPR) studies (10, 18). Those direct (EPR) measurements of radicals, combined with a host of other indirect approaches, have been the subject of recent reviews (19, 50) and confirm that radical production is increased by exercise. Since radicals have been implicated in pathologies such as Alzheimer's and Parkinson's disease (1), cancer (5), and vascular disease (14), they have been looked upon with disdain. That negative view of radicals was increased by the recent report that transgenic *Drosophila* equipped to overexpress the antioxidant enzymes superoxide dismutase and catalase experienced a slowed loss in physical performance and an increased life span. This provided the first direct support for the free radical hypothesis of aging (33). Barja (6) has recently challenged us to reexamine our myopic view of radicals as enemies and question whether oxygen radicals are actually a success of evolution. I shall contend that radicals bring both bad and good news.

The Bad News

Inorganic substances from across the periodic table play a variety of roles in essential biochemical mechanisms. For instance, phosphate, on the right, and calcium, on the left, modify regulatory enzymes. The transition metals, in the center, mediate electron transport. Iron, a member of this latter group, has received abundant attention by those interested in exercise biochemistry. Although full-blown anemia appears to be rare in athletes of either gender (15, 34) and endurance training benefits can accrue even during iron deficiency (9, 57) the interest of many sports medicine professionals continues to focus on iron supplementation. At the same time, interest in the general medical community has turned to the potential role of iron in disease. As early as 1981, Sullivan (52) called attention to the lower rate of coronary disease in premenopausal women as compared with postmenopausal women or with women who had undergone hysterectomy. Though the Finnish report of Salonen et al. (42) that supported Sullivan's contention has recently been countered by the prospective study of Sempos and colleagues (46), the issue has hardly been settled. Ascherio and Willett (4) have provided a brief critique on the status of the problem. Additionally, the epidemiological studies of Selby and Friedman (45) and Stevens et al. (51) have implicated elevated tissue iron stores with increased risk for certain cancers. Additionally, in developed countries, the genetic tendency to develop hemochromatosis, an iron-loading disorder, may exceed the tendency for clinically significant iron deficiency by a factor of two (17). For these reasons, warnings against the injudicious use of iron supplements are beginning to appear.

It is now widely accepted by workers in the field of free radical chemistry that transition metals play a pivotal role in the initiation of deleterious radical reactions. A reaction involving the Fenton reagent is typically suggested. In this case hydrogen peroxide, which is normally produced in cells, reacts with ferrous salts. This is outlined in reaction [1], where $-L$ represents ligand(s).

$$H_2O_2 + Fe^{2+} + -L \rightarrow HO^. + OH^- + Fe^{3+} + -L \qquad (1)$$

Alternatively the Fe-catalyzed Haber-Weiss reaction may be employed. Here the hydroxyl radical is produced when superoxide reacts with hydrogen peroxide in the presence of iron.

$$O_2^- + H_2O_2 + Fe^{2+} \rightarrow O_2 + OH^. + OH^- + Fe^{3+} \qquad (2)$$

Living organisms employ an elaborate system of protein transport and storage molecules to maintain tight control over transition metals. Within the cell, a utilization pool of iron bound to a low molecular mass must be available. This low–molecular mass *chelatable* or *transit* iron pool is normally held at or below detection limits.

Various biochemical events related to exercise may free iron from the high–molecular mass complexes, thus making it available to participate in free radical chemistry. For instance, Bralet, Schreiber, and Bouvier (7) have shown that acidosis results in an increased delocalization of iron in brain homogenates. We have employed the bleomycin assay to fractions of soleus muscle homogenates and recorded similar results. The assay is specific for low–molecular mass iron. Homogenates of soleus mitochondria were incubated at a pH of 5, 6, or 7. When iron was assayed as previously described (21), the results depicted in figure 38.1 were obtained. As pH declined, a greater amount of the total iron appeared in the low molecular mass form.

Serbinova and colleagues (47) have shown that exercise imposed on iron-loaded rats potentiated oxidative stress. When they loaded rats with an intramuscular injection of ferrum Hausmann and swam them to exhaustion, lipid peroxidation was significantly increased. Vitamin E and cytochrome P450 content decreased. We trained rats at 70% peak oxygen consumption and after 6 wk ran them to exhaustion (21). The exhausting exercise resulted in a significantly greater tissue iron level and susceptibility to tert-butyl hydroperoxide–stimulated oxidative stress in the nontrained animals.

Those working in the area of free radical chemistry and exercise typically have studied endurance exercise. It has been assumed that since such exercise delivers more oxygen to the tissue, more radicals would be formed. That idea must be reexamined. Figure 38.2 illustrates the rate of chemiluminescence of soleus muscle

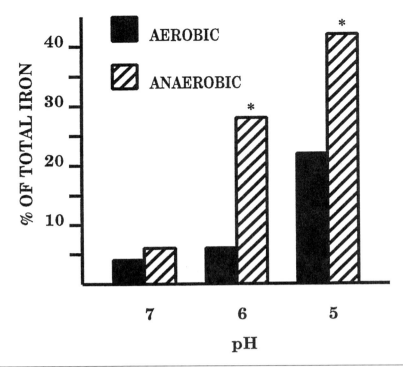

Figure 38.1 Influence of pH on release of low–molecular mass iron from soleus muscle total iron pool. Mitochondria separated from soleus homogenates were incubated under aerobic (95%, O_2/5% CO_2) and anaerobic (argon) conditions for 1 h in Krebs-Ringer buffer. *Significantly different from pH 7; $p < .05$.

homogenates incubated in the presence of 10 μM $FeSO_4$ and varying concentrations of oxygen. Surprisingly, the reaction was greatest at 20% oxygen and diminished as the concentration of oxygen increased. These results are in agreement with those of workers who have studied microsomes (35) or pure fatty acids (54). Thom and Elkbuken (54) have provided evidence that elevated oxygen concentrations increase termination reactions among hydroperoxyl, organic radicals, and hydrogen peroxide. Additionally, lactic acid has been shown to stimulate lipid peroxidation through a process that causes iron to dissociate from proteins (12). These results may explain why radical production has been shown to relate to the duration of ischemia (16) and call attention to the need for more studies of the potential for oxidative stress resultant from anaerobic exercise.

Muscle injury itself may provide a source of iron. Proteolysis is known to increase especially after eccentric exercise (23), and Maughan and colleagues (30) have shown that 45 min of downhill running resulted in both increased lipid peroxides and muscle enzyme release. Certainly, the leakage of myoglobin from muscle cells affords another potential source of iron (40).

Muscle wasting also results in the availability of iron in a form capable of stimulating oxidative stress. Kondo and co-workers (28) have conducted a series of studies on disuse atrophy. In their work, one ankle of a rat is immobilized in

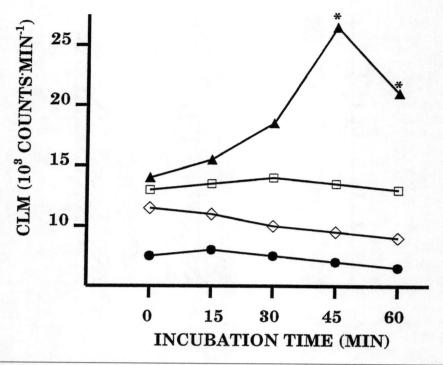

Figure 38.2   Influence of oxygen concentration on iron-stimulated chemiluminescence (CLM). Soleus muscle homogenates (10% wt./vol.) were incubated in Chelex 100–treated phosphate buffered saline (pH 7.4) gassed with 0% (circles), 20% (triangles), 50% (squares), or 100% (diamonds) oxygen/argon. Oxidative stress was stimulated with 10 μM $FeSO_4$ at time 0. *Significantly different from other concentrations; $p < .05$.

plantar flexion for 4, 8, or 12 d. They had previously shown that soleus muscle contained greater amounts of the transition metals iron, copper, zinc, and manganese than type II muscles (26). Immobilization resulted in a significant rise in soleus iron content, which was located in the microsomal fraction (27). The increased iron content was related to an increased susceptibility to oxidative stress as measured by increasing thiobarbituric acid–reactive substances and glutathione disulfide. The fact that deferoxamine suppressed the increase of those markers provided evidence that iron was directly involved (28).

There is now little doubt that oxygen radical production of muscles is increased during use and disuse. However, we must not assume that such radical production is always an adverse reaction.

The Good News

If we were to focus on the various intermediates of the citric acid cycle with the overriding thought that pH is one of the most closely regulated parameters in living organisms, it would be difficult to appreciate the value of the acids. Although radicals in general have long been known to play an important role in organic chemistry, until recently oxygen-centered radicals have, for the most part, been considered deleterious. That view is changing as the beneficial roles of oxygen-centered radicals or their reaction products are beginning to be elucidated. Additionally, the regulatory role of inorganic substances known to be initiators of radical chemistry have begun to be enumerated. In fact, O'Halloran (32) has recently reviewed the expanding literature involving transition metals in the control of gene expression. For instance, iron metabolism itself seems to be regulated by iron-sulfur clusters (25). The potential role of exercise in the involvement of transition metals and metal-binding agents in the initiation of radical chemistry has recently been reviewed (20).

Second Messengers

When one has the habit of thinking of radicals as ''bad guys,'' the notion that they may perform a beneficial second messenger role at first seems farfetched (31, 43). That difficulty persists despite the fact that there is now abundant evidence that nitric oxide serves in such a capacity (29, 55). That radical, like most others, can be both a friend or foe (13). There is growing evidence that exercise is capable of enhancing the vasodilatory influence of this molecule (22, 48). The concept that radicals and reactive oxygen species may serve in vasoregulatory control systems has broadened beyond nitric oxide. For instance, superoxide and hydrogen peroxide when administered alone resulted in vasoconstriction of pulmonary arterial smooth muscle (39). However, when hydrogen peroxide was administered in combination with nitric oxide, a relaxation of rabbit aorta was shown (58).

In addition to the evidence that oxygen-centered radicals are involved in regulation of blood flow, there is an impressive array of studies that implicate radicals in various aspects of neural transmission (2) and especially in gene regulation.

Gene Regulation

Shibanuma and co-workers (49) have provided evidence that active oxygens are involved in one of the earliest positive control events of cell growth in response to growth factors. They demonstrated that 0.1 to 0.2 mM hydrogen peroxide in combination with insulin stimulated the expression of mRNA for c-*fos*, KC, and JE, as well as the phosphorylation of a 78-kDa protein in quiescent Balb/3T3 clone cells. Hydrogen peroxide has also been shown to stimulate the transcription of c-*jun*, an early response gene required for mitogen-stimulated cell growth (36). The induction by hydrogen peroxide seemed to operate through protein kinase C and a product of the arachidonic acid cascade. Arachidonic acid has been shown to down-regulate the glucose transporter gene (GLUT4) by inhibiting transcription and increasing mRNA turnover (53). It is possible that the well-known enhancement of glucose transport by exercise results from a well-controlled production of oxygen-centered radicals that reduce the down-regulation by attacking arachidonic acid. For instance, arachidonic acid is readily attacked when hydrogen peroxide is produced in the presence of an iron source such as myoglobin (24).

The evidence for oxygen radicals serving as gene-activating second messengers is especially strong for genes regulated by the NF-$_\kappa$B transcription factor (44). The fact that the NF-$_\kappa$B factors seem to be especially important in regulation of immune system functions should be of special note to exercise scientists, since exercise has often been likened to the acute phase response (8, 56).

The potential role of exercise in the induction of heat-shock/stress proteins has aroused great interest. For instance, there were nine posters devoted to this topic at the recent American College of Sports Medicine meeting. Salo, Donovan, and Davies (41) were among the first to investigate the role of exercise in inducing these stress proteins. They have provided evidence that oxygen radicals may be linked to the induction of the hsp70 proteins, which are believed to be important in processing polypeptides in the mitochondria.

Obligatory Requirement?

Reid and colleagues (38) have shown that controlled production of hydrogen peroxide may actually be a friend to muscular contraction. Their work with diaphragm bundles demonstrated that an obligatory requirement for a low concentration of reactive oxygen may exist in unfatigued skeletal muscle. However, they also showed that increased levels of reactive species were related to the onset of fatigue (37). We have found that hydrogen peroxide also altered contractile force characteristics of rat epitrochlearis muscle and enhanced glycogen supercompensation. These data are shown in figure 38.3.

Aruoma et al. (3) have pointed out the potential inadequacy of statistical analysis of pooled data from large numbers of subjects in the identification of deficiencies in individuals. The results of free radical research in the past 10 years has clearly demonstrated the vast array of protective and adaptive mechanisms available to living organisms. Yet, genetic faults in normal defenses have been linked to disease. We need to develop the reflex of considering outlying data points not just as aberrant values but as potential clues to genetic variants.

Summary

1. There is now little doubt that both use and disuse result in an increased production of free radicals in muscle and other tissues. In most instances the tissues' defense systems are able to cope with the rate of radical production.
2. The potential for oxidative stress increases when loosely bound transition metals become available.
3. There is now a growing literature that demonstrates the beneficial role of radicals and reactive species in normal biological control.

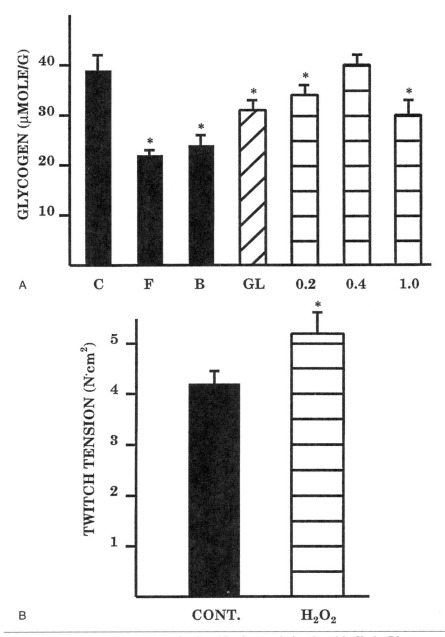

Figure 38.3 (A) Twitch tension of epitrochlearis muscle incubated in Krebs-Ringer buffer equilibrated with 95% O_2/5% CO_2. Muscles received either distilled H_2O (CONT.) or hydrogen peroxide (10^{-2} M). *Significantly different from control; $p < .05$. (B) Epitrochlearis muscles were incubated as in A. C = control, F = fatigued (50 twitches/min), B = buffer minus glucose, GL = with glucose (5.5 mM), and either 0.2, 0.4, or 1 mM hydrogen peroxide. *Significantly different from control; $p < .05$.

References

1. Adams, J.D.; Odunze, I.N. Oxygen free radicals and Parkinson's disease. Free Rad. Biol. Med. 10:161-169; 1991.
2. Aizenman, E.; Hartnett, K.A.; Reynolds, I.J. Oxygen free radicals regulate NMDA receptor function via a redox modulatory site. Neuron 5:841-846; 1990.
3. Aruoma, O.I.; Reilly, T.; MacLaren, D.; Halliwell, B. Iron, copper and zinc concentrations in human sweat and plasma. The effect of exercise. Clin. Chim. Acta 177:81-88; 1988.
4. Ascherio, A.; Willett, W.C. Are body iron stores related to the risk of coronary heart disease? N. Engl. J. Med. 330:1152-1153; 1994.
5. Bandy, B.; Davison, A.J. Mitochondrial mutations may increase oxidative stress: Implications for carcinogenesis and aging? Free Rad. Biol. Med. 8:523-539; 1990.
6. Barja, G. Oxygen radicals, a failure or a success of evolution? Free Rad. Commun. 18:63-70; 1993.
7. Bralet, J.; Schreiber, L.; Bouvier, C. Effects of acidosis and anoxia on iron delocalization from brain homogenates. Biochem. Pharmacol. 43:979-983; 1992.
8. Camus, G.; Deby-Dupont, G.; Deby, C.; Juchmes-Ferir, A.; Pincemail, J.; Lamy, M. Inflammatory response to strenuous muscular exercise in man. Mediat. Inflamm. 2:335-342; 1993.
9. Celsing, F.; Blomstrand, E.; Werner, B.; Pihlstedt, P.; Ekblom, B. Effects of iron deficiency on endurance and muscle enzyme activity in man. Med. Sci. Sports Exercise 18:156-161; 1986.
10. Davies, K.J.A.; Quintanilha, A.T.; Brooks, G.A.; Packer, L. Free radicals and tissue damage produced by exercise. Biochem. Biophys. Res. Commun. 107:1198-1205; 1982.
11. Dillard, C.J.; Litov, R.E.; Savin, W.M.; Dumelin, E.E.; Tappel, A.L. Effects of exercise, vitamin E and ozone on pulmonary function and lipid peroxidation. J. Appl. Physiol. 45:927-932; 1978.
12. Fauconneau, B.; Tallineau, C.; Hugnet, F.; Pontcharraudm, R.; Pirou, A. Evidence of lipoperoxidation induced by lactic acid on kidney homogenates. Toxicology 77:249-258; 1993.
13. Halliwell, B. Reactive oxygen species and the central nervous system. J. Neurochem. 59:1609-1623; 1992.
14. Halliwell, B. The role of oxygen radicals in human disease, with particular reference to the vascular system. Haemostasis 23:118-126; 1993.
15. Haymes, E.M.; Lamanca, J.J. Iron loss in runners during exercise implications and recommendations. Sports Med. 7:277-285; 1989.
16. Henry, T.D.; Archer, S.L.; Nelson, D.; Weir, E.K.; From, A.H.L. Postischemic oxygen radical production varies with duration of ischemia. Am. J. Physiol. 33:H1478-H1484; 1993.
17. Herbert, V. Prevalence of abnormalities of iron metabolism in the USA. In: Serum ferritin: A technical monograph. La Jolla, CA: National Health Laboratories; 1989:3-8.
18. Jackson, M.J.; Edwards, R.H.T.; Symons, M.C.R. Electron spin resonance studies of intact mammalian skeletal muscle. Biochim. Biophys. Acta 847:185-190; 1985.

19. Jenkins, R.R. Exercise, oxidative stress, and antioxidants: A review. Int. J. Sport Nutr. 3:356-375; 1993.

20. Jenkins, R.R.; Halliwell, B. Iron and metal binding agents: Possible role in exercise. In: Sen, C.K.; Packer, L.; Hänninen, O., eds. Exercise and oxygen toxicity. Amsterdam: Elsevier Science Pub.; 1994.

21. Jenkins, R.R.; Krause, K.; Schofield, L.S. Influence of exercise on clearance of oxidant stress products and loosely bound iron. Med. Sci. Sports Exercise 25:213-217; 1993.

22. Kane, D.W.; Tesauro, T.; Koizum, T.; Gupta, R.; Newman, J.H. Exercise-induced pulmonary vasoconstriction during combined blockade of nitric oxide synthase and beta adrenergic receptors. J. Clin. Invest. 93:677-683; 1994.

23. Kasperek, G.J.; Snider, R.D. Increased protein degradation after eccentric exercise. Eur. J. Appl. Physiol. 54:30-34; 1985.

24. Kelman, D.J.; DeGray, J.A.; Mason, R.P. Reaction of myoglobin with hydrogen peroxide forms a peroxyl radical which oxidizes substrates. J. Biol. Chem. 269:7458-7463; 1994.

25. Klausner, R.D.; Rouault, T.A.; Harford, J.B. Regulating the fate of mRNA: The control of cellular iron metabolism. Cell 72:19-28; 1993.

26. Kondo, H.; Kimura, M.; Itokawa, Y. Manganese, copper, zinc, and iron concentrations and subcellular distribution in two types of skeletal muscle. Proc. Soc. Exp. Biol. Med. 196:83-88; 1991.

27. Kondo, H.; Miura, M.; Kodama, J.; Ahmed, S.M.; Itokawa, Y. Role of iron in oxidative stress in skeletal muscle atrophied by immobilization. Pflügers Arch. 421:295-297; 1992.

28. Kondo, H.; Miura, M; Nakagaki, I.; Sasaki, S.; Itokawa, Y. Trace element movement and oxidative stress in skeletal muscle atrophied by immobilization. Am. J. Physiol. 262:E583-E590; 1992.

29. Lowenstein, C.J.; Dinerman, J.L.; Snyder, S.H. Nitric oxide: A physiologic messenger. Ann. Intern. Med. 120:227-237; 1994.

30. Maughan, R.J.; Donnelly, A.E.; Gleeson, M.; Whiting, P.H.; Walker, K.A.; Clough, P.J. Delayed-onset muscle damage and lipid peroxidation in man following a downhill run. Muscle Nerve 12:332-336; 1989.

31. Mosmann, B.T.; Marsh, J.P.; Shatos, M.A.; Doherty, J.; Gilbert, R.; Hill, S. Implication of active oxygen species as second messengers of asbestos toxicity. Drug Chem. Toxicol. 10:157-180; 1987.

32. O'Halloran, T.V. Transition metals in control of gene expression. Science 261:715-725; 1993.

33. Orr, W.C.; Sohal, R.S. Extension of life-span by overexpression of superoxide dismutase and catalase in *Drosophila melanogaster*. Science 263:1128-1130; 1994.

34. Pate, R.R.; Miller, B.J.; Davis, M.; Slentz, C.A.; Klingshirn, L.A. Iron status of female runners. Int. J. Sport Nutr. 3:222-231; 1993.

35. Puntarulo, S.; Turrens, J.F.; Cederbaum, A.I. Oxygen-concentration dependence of microsomal chemiluminescence. Free Rad. Biol. Med. 7:269-273; 1989.

36. Rao, G.N.; Lassegue, B.; Griendling, K.K.; Alexander, R.W. Hydrogen peroxide stimulates transcription of c-*jun* in vascular smooth muscle cells: Role of arachidonic acid. Oncogene 8:2759-2764; 1993.

37. Reid, M.B.; Haack, K.E.; Franchek, K.M.; Valberg, P.A.; Kobzik, L.; West, M.S. Reactive oxygen in skeletal muscle I. Intracellular oxidant kinetics and fatigue in vitro. J. Appl. Physiol. 73:1797-1804; 1992.

38. Reid, M.B.; Khawli, F.A.; Moody, M.R. Reactive oxygen in skeletal muscle III. Contractility of unfatigued muscle. J. Appl. Physiol. 75:1081-1087; 1993.

39. Rhoades, R.A.; Packer, C.S.; Roepke, D.A.; Jin, N.; Meiss, R.A. Reactive oxygen species alter contractile properties of pulmonary arterial smooth muscle. Can. J. Physiol. Pharmacol. 68:1581-1589; 1990.

40. Roxin, L.E.; Hedin, G.; Venge, P. Muscle cell leakage of myoglobin after long-term exercise and relation to the individual performances. Int. J. Sports Med. 7:259-263; 1986.

41. Salo, D.C.; Donovan, C.M.; Davies, K.J.A. HSP70 and other possible heat shock or oxidative stress proteins are induced in skeletal muscle, heart, and liver during exercise. Free Rad. Biol. Med. 11:239-246; 1991.

42. Salonen, J.T.; Nyyssonen, K.; Korpela, H.; Tuomilehto, J.; Seppanen, R.; Salonen, R. High stored iron levels are associated with excess risk of myocardial infarction in eastern Finnish men. Circulation 86:803-811; 1992.

43. Saran, M.; Bors, W. Oxygen radicals acting as chemical messengers: A hypothesis. Free Rad. Res. Commun. 7:213-220; 1989.

44. Schreck, R.; Reiber, P.; Baeuerle, P.A. Reactive oxygen intermediates as apparently widely used messengers in the activation of the NF-$_\kappa$B transcription factor and HIV-1. EMBO J. 10:2247-2258; 1991.

45. Selby, J.V.; Friedman, G.D. Epidemiologic evidence of an association between body iron stores and risk of cancer. Int. J. Cancer 41:677-682; 1988.

46. Sempos, C.T.; Looker, A.C.; Gillum, R.F.; Makuc, D.M. Body iron stores and the risk of coronary heart disease. N. Engl. J. Med. 330:1119-1124; 1994.

47. Serbinova, E.A.; Kadiiska, M.B.; Bakalova, R.A.; Koynova, G.M.; Stoyanovsky, D.A.; Karakashev, P.C.; Stoytchev, T.S.; Wolinsky, I.; Kagan, V.E. Lipid peroxidation activation and cytochrome P-450 decrease in rat liver endoplasmic reticulum under oxidative stress. Toxicol. Lett. 47:119-123; 1989.

48. Sessa, W.C.; Pritchard, K.; Seyedi, N.; Wang, J.; Hintze, T.H. Chronic exercise in dogs increases coronary vascular nitric oxide production and endothelial cell nitric oxide synthase. Circ. Res. 74:349-353; 1994.

49. Shibanuma, M.; Kuroki, T.; Nose, K. Stimulation by hydrogen peroxide of DNA synthesis, competence family gene expression and phosphorylation of a specific protein in quiescent Balb/3T3 cells. Oncogene 5:1025-1032, 1990.

50. Sjodin, B.; Hellsten Westling, Y.; Apple, F.S. Biochemical mechanisms for oxygen free radical formation during exercise. Sports Med. 10:236-254; 1990.

51. Stevens, R.G.; Graubard, B.I.; Micozzi, M.S.; Neriishi, K.; Blumberg, B.S. Moderate elevation of body iron level and increased risk of cancer occurrence and death. Int. J. Cancer 56:364-369; 1994.

52. Sullivan, J.L. Iron and the sex difference in heart disease risk. Lancet 1:1293-1294; 1981.

53. Tebbey, P.W.; McGowan, K.M.; Stephens, J.M.; Buttke, T.M.; Pekala, P.H. Arachidonic acid down-regulates the insulin-dependent glucose transporter gene (GLUT4) in 3T3-L1 adipocytes by inhibiting transcription and enhancing mRNA turnover. J. Biol. Chem. 269:639-644; 1994.

54. Thom, S.R.; Elkbuken, M.E. Oxygen-dependent antagonism of lipid peroxidation. Free Rad. Biol. Med. 10:413-426; 1991.

55. Warren, J.B.; Pons, F.; Brady, A.J. Nitric oxide biology: Implications for cardiovascular therapeutics. Cardiovasc. Res. 28:25-30; 1994.

56. Weight, L.M.; Alexander, D.; Jacobs, P. Strenuous exercise: Analogous to the acute-phase response? Clin. Sci. 81:677-683; 1991.

57. Willis, W.T.; Dallman, P.R.; Brooks, G.A. Physiological and biochemical corre-
    lates of increased work in trained iron-deficient rats. J. Appl. Physiol. 65:256-
    263; 1988.
58. Zembowicz, A.; Hatchett, R.J.; Jakubowski, A.M.; Gryglewski, R.J. Involve-
    ment of nitric oxide in the endothelium-dependent relaxation induced by hydro-
    gen peroxide in the rabbit aorta. Br. J. Pharmacol. 110:151-158; 1993.

PART XI

Ammonia Metabolism in Muscle

CHAPTER 39

Ammonia Metabolism in Muscle

Ronald L. Terjung
State University of New York, Syracuse, New York, U.S.A.

Extensive ammonia accumulation in blood can occur during very intense short-term exercise. Recent evidence demonstrates that substantial ammonia production also occurs during moderately intense but prolonged exercise. While there is no definitive evidence to indicate that this ammonia production is harmful, it is clear that exercise prompts significant challenges to ammonia metabolism in normal individuals. By way of introduction, this chapter is intended to identify the important ammonia-producing reactions, the ammonia-consuming reactions, and reactions involving amine nitrogen that are related to ammonia metabolism.

Ammonia-Producing Reactions

AMP Deaminase

By far the best-characterized and most understood reaction that produces ammonia in muscle during exercise is the entry reaction of the purine nucleotide cycle, AMP deaminase (figure 39.1). AMP deaminase (EC 3.5.4.6) is a highly controlled enzyme that is relatively inactive in resting muscle but that becomes highly active during contractions when there is an energy imbalance (10, 30, 38). How specific factors known to modulate AMP deaminase activity account for this exquisite control is unclear but must be related to changes established within the muscle during contractions. Factors likely to contribute to the control of AMP deaminase in contracting muscle in vivo include a change in substrate concentration, since the available AMP concentration in resting muscle is well below the K_m for AMP deaminase (24, 25); allosteric activation by an increase in ADP concentration; relief from inhibition by orthophosphate (24, 25); activation by a decrease in pH; and activation by AMP deaminase binding to myosin evident at low AMP concentrations (34, 35). There are likely to be other yet unrecognized influences.

Even though of secondary importance, the absolute rate of ammonia production within a muscle fiber could also be influenced by the enzymatic capacity of AMP

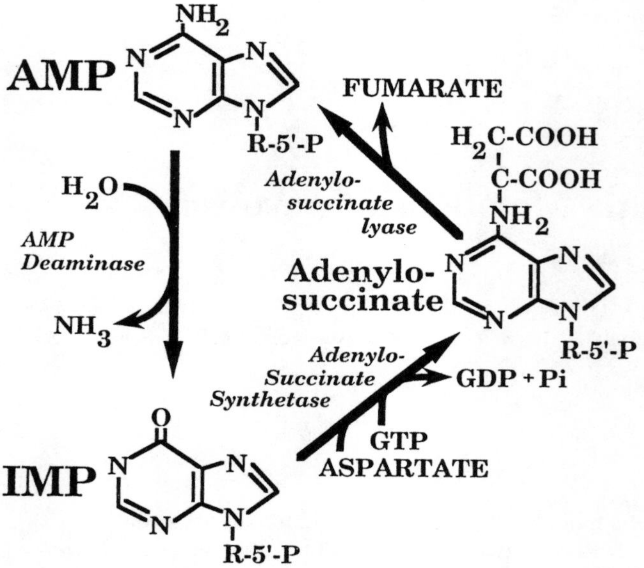

Figure 39.1   Reactions of the purine nucleotide cycle.

deaminase. The relatively high AMP deaminase activities in fast-twitch fibers, compared with relatively low activity in slow-twitch fibers of rats (35, 46), may contribute to the differences in IMP accumulation observed. However, the differences in IMP accumulation between type I and type II fibers observed in humans during exercise (20) occur even though the enzymatic capacity of AMP deaminase is apparently the same (32). Although the severe acidosis that is typical within muscle during very intense exercise should enhance enzymatic activity by bringing the enzyme closer to optimal pH, it is not essential for high rates of ammonia and IMP production (9). Even though much is understood about specific factors that affect AMP deaminase activity, our understanding of how the complex events within the active muscle control the enzyme to prompt ammonia production is incomplete at the present time.

Glutamate Dehydrogenase

Glutamate dehydrogenase (EC 1.4.1.2) is found within the mitochondria of skeletal muscle at a relatively low activity (14, 18, 44).

$$\text{glutamate} + NAD^+ \leftrightarrow \text{2-oxoglutarate} + NADH + NH_4^+ \qquad [1]$$

As an equilibrium enzyme, glutamate dehydrogenase can function in the production of ammonia and 2-oxoglutarate and in the fixation of ammonia in the production of glutamate, depending upon the concentrations of reactants and products. At present, its role within muscle is unclear. However, it is important to recognize that a major substrate in this reaction, glutamate, is at the focal point of transamination reactions (glutamate-pyruvate transaminase and glutamate-oxaloacetate transaminase) among amino acids. Thus, the α-amine on glutamate can be derived from many other amino acids. This places the glutamate dehydrogenase reaction in the position of coupling amino acid and ammonia metabolism in muscle. Of interest is the possible coupling of the amine derived from the branched-chain amino acids (leucine, isoleucine, and valine) to ammonia production during exercise (discussed later).

Other Reactions

Although not established as important, there are a number of other reactions that could theoretically produce ammonia during exercise. Adenosine deaminase (EC 3.5.4.4), which is found in muscle tissue, is thought to be important in controlling adenosine concentration by its deamination to inosine and ammonia. Any increase in adenosine deamination could technically contribute to ammonia production during exercise; however, it is probably of very little importance quantitatively. Adenosine concentration is very low in muscle, approximately 500 to 1,000 times lower than the adenine nucleotide pool even in highly vascular red muscle (1). Since the adenosine production rate is also likely to be quantitatively small, the potential contribution to ammonia production should be negligible.

Glutaminase (EC 3.5.1.2) is an important enzyme in ammonia metabolism in liver, gut and kidney tissue.

$$\text{glutamine} + H_2O \rightarrow \text{glutamate} + NH_3 \qquad [2]$$

The activity of this enzyme in muscle, however, has been attributed to the presence of infiltrating inflammatory cells (22). Last, the action of γ-glutamyltransferase (EC 2.3.2.2) can produce ammonia; however, significant accumulation of ammonia in blood has been implicated during pathological situations of liver disease (6). Thus, it is unlikely that any of these reactions play a quantitatively important role in ammonia production during exercise in normal, healthy individuals.

Ammonia-Consuming Reactions

Glutamine Synthetase

The action of glutamine synthetase (EC 6.3.1.2) serves to keep the ammonia concentration low within tissues.

$$\text{glutamate} + NH_3 + ATP \rightarrow \text{glutamine} + ADP \qquad [3]$$

This enzyme is effective in skeletal muscle as evidenced by significant glutamine production during an ammonia or amino acid load (33). Glutamine release from muscle can represent a meaningful source of nitrogen exported from this tissue during exercise (11, 21, 37). The action of glutamine synthetase is involved if the muscle's pool of glutamine has not declined proportionally. The release of glutamine from muscle carries a dual implication for metabolism. First, there must be a source for the ammonia fixed in the amide position. Second, the loss of the 2-oxoglutarate could represent a drain of important carbon skeletons from the muscle (41-43).

Other Reactions

There are some reactions that could consume the nitrogen of ammonia once fixed to the amide position of glutamine through the glutamine synthetase reaction. These involve particular metabolic pathways that probably experience a relatively low flux rate. For example, there is an amide nitrogen transfer as part of purine nucleotide synthesis (amidophosphoribosyltransferase, EC 2.4.2.14). The rate of this de novo nucleotide synthesis, however, is far too small to even make a measurable contribution to ammonia metabolism in muscle during exercise (40). Therefore, the overall impact on ammonia metabolism during exercise is expected to be negligible.

It is worth noting again that the reversible enzyme action of glutamate dehydrogenase could consume ammonia, if the mass balance of reactants and products favors the fixation of ammonia and the consumption of reducing equivalents or protons (31). This possibility seems remote as a contributor to overall ammonia metabolism in active muscle. However, we lack sufficient information about this possibility to make definitive conclusions.

Ammonia Production During Exercise

Short-Term, Intense Exercise

Ammonia production during short-term, intense exercise is due to AMP deamination in the active muscles. This has been established by stoichiometric changes in the concentrations of substrate (adenine nucleotides) and products of the reaction (IMP and ammonia) in the muscle (7, 12, 14, 30, 38). Ammonia accumulation does not occur during short-term, easy- to moderate-intensity exercise. Rather, ammonia production is initiated within contracting muscle when the severity of exercise is fairly intense (10, 28). This is apparent in figure 39.2 by the increase in blood ammonia concentration as a function of exercise intensity, expressed as a percentage of maximal oxygen consumption.

The absolute intensity of exercise that prompts ammonia production cannot be identified a priori, since an imbalance between the energy demand and the energy supply appears to be the crucial precipitating condition (10). Thus, during running or cycling, a contractile effort demanding even relatively low energy can cause extensive ammonia production if there is a relatively poor ability of muscle to meet the energy demands (i.e., impaired metabolism, low aerobic capacity). An extreme is seen during ischemic exercise in patients in whom blood flow is obstructed. On the other hand, a relatively high contractile effort can be sustained without AMP deamination and ammonia production if the aerobic capacity of the muscle (and individual) is high enough. For example, ammonia accumulation in blood is less at

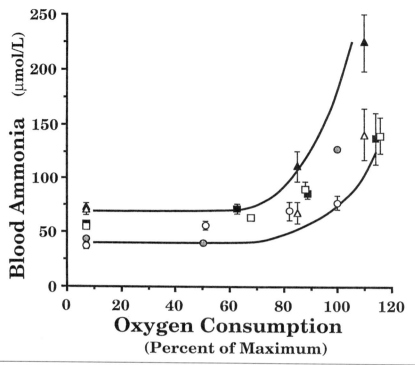

Figure 39.2   Changes in blood ammonia concentrations as a function of the intensity of short-term exercise, expressed as percentage of maximal oxygen consumption. The area between the two lines includes the response of normal individuals. Open circles: data from Wilkerson, Batterton, and Horvath 1977 (45); shaded circles: Babij, Matthews, and Rennie 1983 (2); triangles: Dudley et al. 1983 (8); squares: Lo and Dudley 1987 (23). Note that the response before (filled squares) and after (open squares) training are the same and that individuals with a high percentage of fast-twitch fiber population (filled triangles) exhibit higher blood ammonia than individuals with a high percentage of slow-twitch fiber population (open triangles) when exercising at the same percentage of maximal oxygen consumption.

the same absolute intensity of exercise after training than before training (23). However, if a higher absolute power output is required to achieve the same relative exercise intensity (i.e., approximately 115% $\dot{V}O_2$max) after training, blood ammonia concentrations reached the same high values (23). Another example of differences in ammonia accumulation is apparent among individuals differing in muscle fiber type populations. Individuals with a high fraction of fast-twitch fibers exhibit a much greater increase in blood ammonia than do individuals possessing a high fraction of slow-twitch fibers, even when exercising at the same demanding 110% $\dot{V}O_2$max (8). Although there can be variability among individuals, ammonia accumulation during short-term exercise, as illustrated in figure 39.2, becomes most exaggerated as the exercise intensity progresses beyond 70% to 80% $\dot{V}O_2$max up to supramaximal intensities.

Prolonged, Moderately Intense Exercise

Blood ammonia concentration increases during prolonged, moderately intense exercise that requires 70% to 80% of maximal oxygen consumption (5, 16, 26, 27, 37, 39, 42). Illustrated in the shaded area of figure 39.3 are characteristic changes in plasma ammonia concentrations while exercising for 60 min (at 70-75% $\dot{V}O_2$max). The processes accounting for this increase in the circulating ammonia pool are not clear. This is unfortunate, since the basis for this response is important to our understanding of muscle function and metabolism during prolonged exercise. Given the reasonable assumption that the ammonia is derived from the contracting muscula-ture, there are two possible sources: ammonia produced by the deamination of AMP to IMP via AMP deaminase and ammonia produced by the oxidative deamination of glutamate by glutamate dehydrogenase. The involvement of either or both of these pathways establishes a link among ammonia, the amine nitrogen of amino

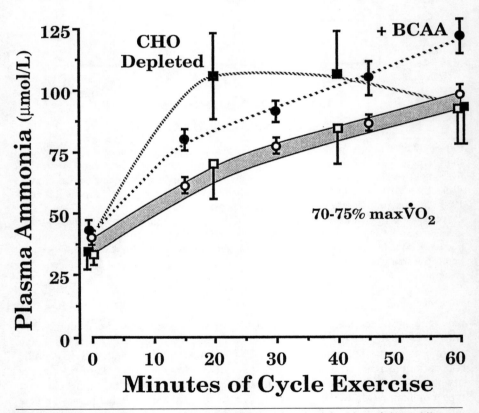

Figure 39.3   Changes in plasma ammonia concentrations as a function of time while per-forming cycle exercise at approximately 70% to 75% of maximal oxygen consumption. The shaded area is characteristic of the normal response. Data from MacLean and Graham 1993 (26) and Wagenmakers et al. 1991 (42). Also shown are increases in the blood am-monia response caused by carbohydrate depletion (filled squares, data from 42) and branched-chain amino acid loading (filled circles, data from 26).

acids, and energy demands in active muscle. Thus, it is important to consider the physiological responses and the reactions that couple these processes.

On one hand, the production of ammonia could simply be the consequence of muscle fiber recruitment necessary to sustain prolonged exercise at this intensity. Some muscle fibers that are initially recruited could become overtaxed energetically; an energy imbalance would prompt deamination of AMP to IMP and ammonia, coincident with fatigue of the fiber (motor unit). Overall exercise performance could continue without interruption as other motor units are recruited to achieve the necessary force development or shortening velocity (13). However, a progression in this process over time would lead to continued ammonia production until the available motor unit pool was recruited and the power output could no longer be sustained. There is evidence in support of this possibility. Experimental treatments that burden energy balance, fiber recruitment, or both—including hypoxia (36), glycogen depletion (4, 5, 42), β-sympathetic blockade (3, 17), and heat stress (39)—lead to exaggerated ammonia production during prolonged exercise. The example of carbohydrate depletion is illustrated in figure 39.3. Thus, in terms of ammonia metabolism, prolonged exercise (at 70-80% $\dot{V}O_2$max) may be as challenging to some of the muscle fibers as severe supramaximal exercise is to most of the active muscle. If this hypothesis is correct, then ammonia production during prolonged exercise becomes a simple consequence of the physiological events related to motor unit recruitment.

On the other hand, the production of ammonia could be purposeful in metabolic processes independently of the motor unit recruitment hypothesis previously developed. It could be related to unique reactions coupling amino acid, adenine nucleotide, and ammonia metabolism. Further, interesting results derived from experiments involving amino acid supplementation in patients (43) and normal individuals (26) raise intriguing possibilities. To consider these aspects further, it is important to review the pathways integrating amino acid and ammonia metabolism.

Interactions Among Amino Acid and Ammonia Metabolism

Illustrated in figure 39.4 are metabolic pathways that can exchange nitrogen among the amine of amino acids, the 6-amino position of the adenine nucleotides via the purine nucleotide cycle, and ammonia. The oxidation of amino acids first requires transamination to obtain the corresponding α-keto acid. This establishes an amine nitrogen load within the muscle that is normally handled by the release of alanine, obtained by transamination using pyruvate, or by glutamine efflux (cf. 19). There is little net benefit in energy supply to the muscle if the amino acid is oxidized to acetyl CoA (e.g., as with leucine), since an equivalent acetyl CoA could have been formed from the pyruvate used to carry the amine nitrogen out of the muscle. Two issues arise if glutamine efflux carries the amine nitrogen from the muscle: (a) the amine must first appear as ammonia (via which reaction?) to form the amide of glutamine and (b) the efflux of glutamine represents the loss of an important carbon skeleton. A potential advantage is achieved if these carbon sources can be retained within the cell while the amine nitrogen is metabolized and exported from the cell by other means, for example, as ammonia.

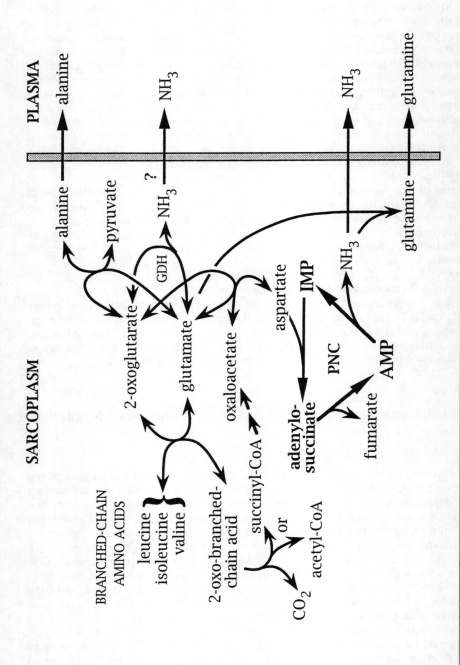

Figure 39.4   Metabolic reactions coupling amino acid amine, the purine nucleotide cycle, and ammonia metabolism in muscle.

Possible Role of the Purine Nucleotide Cycle

The reactions for direct ammonia production include AMP deaminase and possibly glutamate dehydrogenase. Production of ammonia via AMP deaminase will lead to the depletion of adenine nucleotides (AMP + ADP + ATP) if IMP accumulates and is not reaminated back to AMP, as occurs with intense, short-term exercise. On the other hand, if IMP is reaminated, the adenine nucleotide pool has recovered (14, 29) and becomes potentially available for subsequent repeat deamination. The reamination requires an amine source in the form of aspartate, which can ultimately be derived from other amino acids (e.g., leucine) via transamination (15). Thus, if the reactions of the purine nucleotide cycle function in concert, there could be a steady source of ammonia production without any large decline in nucleotide concentration. The net effect of the cycle would be to serve the deamination of amino acids. If the amino acid is leucine, further oxidation leads to acetyl CoA, a metabolite useful in energy provision via the TCA cycle. While this is probably of inconsequential benefit for energy supply during exercise (19), the metabolism of isoleucine and valine present special circumstances; as illustrated in figure 39.4, their metabolism leads to succinyl CoA, which in turn forms a TCA cycle intermediate. Wagenmakers (41) has raised the hypothesis that loss of TCA cycle intermediates impairs energy metabolism and contributes to muscle fatigue. Thus, the possible management of the amine nitrogen to form ammonia could be a consequence of metabolic processes important to energy metabolism in muscle during prolonged exercise (42).

Possible Role of Glutamate Dehydrogenase

The amine nitrogen load associated with the oxidation of amino acids (e.g., leucine, isoleucine, or valine) could be handled by the glutamate dehydrogenase reaction (see figure 39.4). Recall that the amine from one of the branched-chain amino acids is transaminated to form glutamate. The glutamate dehydrogenase reaction reforms the 2-oxoglutarate originally used to accept the amine during transamination from the branched-chain amino acid. Thus, this leads to the net deamination of the amino acid. As previously discussed, the most significant contribution that these amino acids may make toward energy metabolism is in the putative supply of TCA cycle intermediates and not simply as a carbon source for energy supply. While there is ample reason to question whether glutamate dehydrogenase serves a role in deamination (24, 25), critical experiments are needed to account for ammonia production in active muscle. In order to achieve definitive results in this inquiry, it will be essential to establish that AMP deaminase has not contributed to any observed effect.

Acknowledgment

Cited work by the author was supported by NIH grant AR 21617.

References

1. Arabadjis, P.G.; Tullson, P.C.; Terjung, R.L. Purine nucleoside formation in rat skeletal muscle. Am. J. Physiol. 264:C1246-C1251; 1993.

2. Babij, P.; Matthews, S.M.; Rennie, M.J. Changes in blood ammonia, lactate and amino acids in relation to workload during bicycle ergometer exercise in man. Eur. J. Appl. Physiol. 50:405-411; 1983.

3. Broberg, S.; Katz, A.; Sahlin, K. Propranolol enhances adenine nucleotide degradation in human muscle during exercise. J. Appl. Physiol. 65:2478-2483; 1988.

4. Broberg, S.; Sahlin, K. Hyperammoniemia during prolonged exercise: An effect of glycogen depletion? J. Appl. Physiol. 65:2475-2477; 1988.

5. Brouns, F.; Beckers, E.; Wagenmakers, A.J.M.; Saris, W.H.M. Ammonia accumulation during highly intensive long-lasting cycling: Individual observations. Int. J. Sports Med. 11:S78-S84; 1990.

6. Da Fonseca-Wollheim, F. Deamination of glutamine by increased plasma gamma-glutamyltransferase is a source of rapid ammonia formation in blood and plasma specimens. Clin. Chem. 36:1479-1482; 1990.

7. Driedzic, W.R.; Hochachka, P.W. Control of energy metabolism in fish white muscle. Am. J. Physiol. 230:579-582; 1976.

8. Dudley, G.A.; Staron, R.S.; Murray, T.F.; Hagerman, F.C.; Luginbuhl, A. Muscle fiber composition and blood ammonia levels after intense exercise in humans. J. Appl. Physiol. 54:582-586; 1983.

9. Dudley, G.A.; Terjung, R.L. Influence of acidosis on AMP deaminase activity in contracting fast-twitch muscle. Am. J. Physiol. 248:C43-C50; 1985.

10. Dudley, G.A.; Terjung, R.L. Influence of aerobic metabolism on IMP accumulation in fast-twitch muscle. Am. J. Physiol. 248:C37-C42; 1985.

11. Eriksson, L.S.; Broberg, S.; Björkman, O.; Wahren, J. Ammonia metabolism during exercise in man. Clin. Physiol. 5:325-336; 1985.

12. Gerez, C.; Kirsten, R. Untersuchungen uber Ammoniakbilding bei der Muskelarbeit. Biochem. Z. 341:534-542; 1965.

13. Gollnick, P.D.; Armstrong, R.B.; Saubert, C.W., IV; Sembrowich, W.L.; Shepherd, R.E.; Saltin, B. Glycogen depletion patterns in human skeletal muscle fibers during prolonged work. Pflügers Arch. 344:1-12; 1973.

14. Goodman, M.N.; Lowenstein, J.M. The purine nucleotide cycle. Studies of ammonia production by skeletal muscle in situ and in perfused preparations. J. Biol. Chem. 252:5054-5060; 1977.

15. Gorski, J.; Hood, D.A.; Brown, O.M.; Terjung, R.L. Incorporation of 15N-leucine amine into ATP of fast-twitch muscle following stimulation. Biochem. Biophys. Res. Commun. 128:1254-1260; 1985.

16. Graham, T.E.; Pedersen, P.K.; Saltin, B. Muscle and blood ammonia and lactate responses to prolonged exercise with hyperoxia. J. Appl. Physiol. 63:1457-1462; 1987.

17. Hall, P.E.; Smith, S.R.; Kendall, M.J. The effects of four β-adrenoceptor antagonists during modest exercise on plasma ammonia and heart rate. Clin. Sci. 72:679-682; 1987.

18. Holloszy, J.O.; Oscai, L.B.; Don, I.J.; Molé, P.A. Mitochondrial citric acid cycle and related enzymes: Adaptive response to exercise. Biochem. Biophys. Res. Commun. 40:1368-1373; 1970.

19. Hood, D.A.; Terjung, R.L. Amino acid metabolism during exercise and following endurance training. Sports Med. 9:23-35; 1990.

20. Jansson, E.; Dudley, G.; Norman, B.; Sollevi, A.; Tesch, P. ATP and IMP in single human muscle fibers. Clin. Physiol. 5 (suppl. 4):155; 1985.

21. Katz, A.; Broberg, S.; Sahlin, K.; Wahren, J. Muscle ammonia and amino acid metabolism during exercise in man. Clin. Physiol. 6:365-379; 1986.

22. Kelso, T.B.; Shear, C.R.; Max, S.R. Enzymes of glutamine metabolism in inflammation associated with skeletal muscle hypertrophy. Am. J. Physiol. 257:E885-E894; 1989.

23. Lo, P.Y.; Dudley, G.A. Endurance training reduces the magnitude of exercise-induced hyperammonemia in humans. J. Appl. Physiol. 62:1227-1230; 1987.

24. Lowenstein, J.M. Ammonia production in muscle and other tissues: The purine nucleotide cycle. Physiol. Rev. 52:384-414; 1972.

25. Lowenstein, J.M. The purine nucleotide cycle revised. Int. J. Sports Med. 11:S37-S46; 1990.

26. MacLean, D.A.; Graham, T.E. Branched-chain amino acid supplementation augments plasma ammonia responses during exercise in humans. J. Appl. Physiol. 74:2711-2717; 1993.

27. MacLean, D.A.; Spriet, L.L.; Hultman, E.; Graham, T.E. Plasma and muscle amino acid and ammonia responses during prolonged exercise in humans. J. Appl. Physiol. 70:2095-2103; 1991.

28. Meyer, R.A.; Dudley, G.A.; Terjung, R.L. Ammonia and IMP in the different skeletal muscle fibers after exercise in rats. J. Appl. Physiol. 49:1037-1041; 1980.

29. Meyer, R.A.; Terjung, R.L. AMP deamination and IMP reamination in working skeletal muscle. Am. J. Physiol. 239:C32-C38; 1980.

30. Meyer, R.A.; Terjung, R.L. Differences in ammonia and adenylate metabolism in contracting fast and slow muscle. Am. J. Physiol. 237:C111-C118; 1979.

31. Newsholme, E.A.; Leech, A.R. Biochemistry for the medical sciences. New York: Wiley & Sons; 1983.

32. Norman, B. IMP accumulation in energy deficient human skeletal muscle. Stockholm: Karolinska Institute; 1994. Dissertation.

33. Ruderman, N.B.; Berger, M. The formation of glutamine and alanine in skeletal muscle. J. Biol. Chem. 249:5500-5506; 1974.

34. Rundell, K.W.; Tullson, P.C.; Terjung, R.L. Altered kinetics of AMP deaminase by myosin binding. Am. J. Physiol. 263:C294-C299; 1992.

35. Rundell, K.W.; Tullson, P.C.; Terjung, R.L. AMP deaminase binding in contracting rat skeletal muscle. Am. J. Physiol. 263:C287-C293; 1992.

36. Sahlin, K.; Katz, A. Hypoxaemia increases the accumulation of inosine monophosphate (IMP) in human skeletal muscle during submaximal exercise. Acta Physiol. Scand. 136:377-382; 1989.

37. Sahlin, K.; Katz, A.; Broberg, S. Tricarboxylic acid cycle intermediates in human muscle during prolonged exercise. Am. J. Physiol. 259:C834-C841; 1990.

38. Sahlin, K.; Palmskog, G.; Hultman, E. Adenine nucleotide and IMP contents of the quadriceps muscle in man after exercise. Pflügers Arch. 374:193-198; 1978.

39. Snow, R.J.; Febbraio, M.A.; Carey, M.F.; Hargreaves, M. Heat stress increases ammonia accumulation during exercise in humans. Exp. Physiol. 78:847-850; 1993.

40. Terjung, R.L.; Tullson, P.C. Ammonia metabolism during exercise. In: Lamb, D.R.; Gisolfi, C.V., eds. Energy metabolism in exercise and sport. Indianapolis: Benchmark; 1992:235-268.

41. Wagenmakers, A.J.M. Role of amino acids and ammonia in mechanisms of fatigue. In: IVth Nice Symposium. Medicine and Sport. Basel: Karger; 1991.

42. Wagenmakers, A.J.M.; Beckers, E.J.; Brouns, F.; Kuipers, H.; Soeters, P.B.; van der Vusse, G.J.; Saris, W.H.M. Carbohydrate supplementation, glycogen

depletion and amino acid metabolism during exercise. Am. J. Physiol. 260:E883-E890; 1991.

43. Wagenmakers, A.J.M.; Coakley, J.H.; Edwards, R.H.T. Metabolism of branched-chain amino acids and ammonia during exercise: Clues from McArdle's disease. Int. J. Sports Med. 11:S101-S113; 1990.

44. Wibom, R.; Hultman, E. ATP production rate in mitochondria isolated from microsamples of human muscle. Am. J. Physiol. 259:E204-E209; 1990.

45. Wilkerson, J.E.; Batterton, D.L.; Horvath, S.M. Exercise-induced changes in blood ammonia levels in humans. Eur. J. Appl. Physiol. 37:255-263; 1977.

46. Winder, W.W.; Terjung, R.L.; Baldwin, K.M.; Holloszy, J.O. Effect of exercise on AMP deaminase and adenylosuccinase in rat skeletal muscle. Am. J. Physiol. 227:1411-1414; 1974.

CHAPTER 40

Ammonia Metabolism in Humans During Exercise

Kent Sahlin

Karolinska Institute and University College of Physical Education and Sports, Stockholm, Sweden

It has been known for a long time (28) that vigorously contracting muscle produces ammonia (ammonia in this chapter will be used synonymously for the sum of NH_3 + NH_4^+ = NH_3tot) and that this occurs in parallel to deamination of the adenine nucleotides. Due to the importance of ammonia formation in amino acid metabolism and in relation to fatigue, there has been a growing interest in ammonia metabolism during recent years. This short review will focus on ammonia metabolism in humans during exercise.

Concentration of Ammonia in Body Fluids and Transmembrane Transport

The concentration of ammonia in different body fluids at rest and during exercise is presented in table 40.1. At rest, the concentration of ammonia in blood is about four times higher than that in plasma, which means that erythrocyte concentration is about seven times higher than in plasma. Ammonia concentration in muscle at rest is fivefold higher than in plasma but lower than in erythrocytes. During exercise, ammonia is produced and released from the working muscle, and the concentration increases in the body fluids. Sweat has the highest ammonia concentration (9, 10), and during exercise at low temperature, ammonia in sweat can increase to more than 10 mmol/L (10), which is about 100 times higher than in plasma.

The differences in ammonia concentration between body fluids reflect in part the differences in H^+ concentration, where a high concentration of H^+ corresponds to a high ammonia concentration. The reason for this is that the membrane permeability in general is much higher for an uncharged molecule, such as NH_3, than for a charged molecule (NH_4^+). At a physiological pH, more than 98% of ammonia is present as NH_4^+ (pK = 9.25). However, due to the difference in permeability,

Table 40.1   Ammonia Concentration and pH of Various Tissues

	Plasma	Erythrocytes	Muscle cell	Sweat
Basal:				
Ammonia (μmol/L)	27 ± 3	194	140	827 ± 33
pH	7.4	7.2	7.0	4-6.8
Exercise at 75-80% $\dot{V}O_2$max to fatigue or for 30 min (sweat):				
Ammonia (μmol/L)	170 ± 29	337	566	7,140 ± 768
Exercise at 100% $\dot{V}O_2$max to fatigue:				
Ammonia	120 ± 18	392	1,354	—
pH	7.1	—	6.4	—

Ammonia concentration in erythrocytes has been calculated from values in whole blood and in plasma assuming hematocrits of 44% and 50% at rest and after exercise, respectively.

Presented values are expressed as μmol/L H_2O assuming 0.93 L H_2O/L plasma, 0.79 L H_2O/L erythrocytes, 3 L intracellular H_2O/kg dry muscle, 1 L H_2O/L sweat.

Values of ammonia concentration are calculated from data presented in 6, 9, 10, 17.

Values of pH are from 29 and scientific tables (erythrocyte pH).

transmembrane transport is considered to occur mainly in the form of NH_3 (5, 19), which is evidenced by the intracellular alkalization that occurs when extracellular ammonia concentration is increased experimentally (5). Ammonia is considered to be transported between body fluids by passive diffusion and will thus occur when a concentration gradient of NH_3 is present. After passage across the membrane, NH_3 will be converted to NH_4^+, and the degree of conversion will be related to the concentration of H^+. If transport of ammonia occurs solely as NH_3, the concentration ratio of ammonia (NH_3tot = NH_3 + NH_4^+ ≈ NH_4^+) between the intracellular (i) and extracellular (e) compartments at zero flux should be equal to the concentration ratio of H^+ [NH_3tot(i)/NH_3tot(e) = H^+(i)/H^+(e)]. Although the general pattern in table 40.1 demonstrates ammonia distribution according to differences in H^+ concentration, it cannot fully explain the differences in ammonia concentration between different compartments. For instance, at rest the muscle/plasma ratio is 4.5 for ammonia but only 2.5 for H^+. Consequently, at rest the gradient for NH_3 is directed outward, whereas the actual ammonia flux is inward (i.e., an uptake by the muscle). The discrepancy may be related to binding of ammonia to intracellular components, thus decreasing the free intracellular concentration, or alternatively to transmembrane ammonia flux as NH_4^+, for which the electrochemical gradient is directed inward. During exercise, there is an efflux of ammonia from muscle that is in accordance with the direction of the gradient for NH_3.

Ammonia Metabolism and Acid-Base Balance

Formation of ammonia by deamination of AMP or of amino acids (provided the carbon skeleton is oxidized to CO_2) corresponds to an uptake of protons (NH_3 +

$H^+ \rightarrow NH_4^+$) and could thus have implications for the acid-base balance. However, during high-intensity exercise, accumulation of ammonia in working muscle corresponds only to 3% of H^+ released through lactic acid accumulation (17), and the importance for acid-base balance will therefore be small. During prolonged exercise, there is a continuous release of ammonia from the muscle (discussed later), and the total release of base will be considerable. However, because formation, release, redistribution to other tissues, and metabolism of ammonia occur in the form of NH_3, the overall effect on acid-base balance will be small. At rest, the major route for disposal of ammonia and nitrogen in humans is excretion of urea. Protein catabolism and the further metabolism of ammonia in liver and kidney (excretion as urea or NH_4^+) have implications for the long-term, whole-body acid-base balance (2). A discussion of these aspects of ammonia metabolism, however, is beyond the scope of this chapter.

Sources of Ammonia in Skeletal Muscle

In skeletal muscle, ammonia can be formed through the reactions catalyzed by AMP deaminase and glutamate dehydrogenase (GDH; figure 40.1). Ammonia can also be formed through the glutaminase reaction by which glutamine is transformed

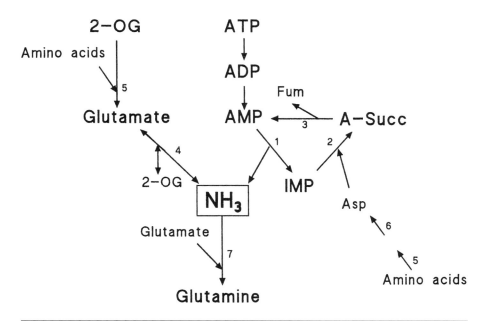

Figure 40.1   Metabolic processes related to ammonia metabolism in skeletal muscle. Numbers refer to the following enzymes: 1, AMP deaminase; 2, adenylosuccinate synthetase; 3, adenylosuccinase; 4, glutamate dehydrogenase; 5, amino transaminase; 6, glutamate oxaloacetate transaminase; 7, glutamine synthetase. Asp = aspartate; A-Succ = adenylosuccinate; Fum = fumarate; 2-OG = 2-oxoglutarate.

to glutamate and ammonia. This process is important in kidney, liver, and intestine and provides the basis for the function of glutamine as a nontoxic carrier of ammonia between organs. Glutaminase is not present in skeletal muscle, and therefore this process can be excluded as a mechanism of ammonia formation in the muscle cell.

AMP deaminase has a high activity in muscle (table 40.2) and catalyzes an irreversible reaction by which AMP is transformed to NH_3 and IMP. In human muscle, the in vitro activity of AMP deaminase in slow-twitch (ST) and fast-twitch (FT) fibers is similar (23, 25), whereas in rat muscle the activity is twofold higher in FT fibers (42). AMP deaminase is the first step in the purine nucleotide cycle (PNC) by which IMP can be transformed back to AMP. The PNC provides a route

Table 40.2   In Vitro Enzyme Activities of Potential Processes Involved in Ammonia Formation and In Vivo Rates of Ammonia Formation During Exercise

	Slow-twitch fibers	Fast-twitch fibers	Mixed muscle
Enzyme activities (mmol · kg⁻¹ dry wt. · min⁻¹):			
AMP deaminase	994[a]	958[a]	1,008[b]
Adenylosuccinase[c]	4.7	4.3	—
Glutamate dehydrogenase[d]	—	—	1.1-1.8
Rate of ammonia formation (mmol · kg⁻¹ dry wt. · min⁻¹):			
Static contraction[e]			2.8
Dynamic exercise at 100% V̇O₂max to fatigue[f]			0.7
Dynamic exercise at 70% V̇O₂max to fatigue[g]			0.05
Rate of ammonia formation in excess of IMP formation (mmol · kg⁻¹ dry wt. · min⁻¹):			
Static contraction[e]			0
Dynamic exercise at 100% V̇O₂max to fatigue[f]			0
Dynamic exercise at 70% V̇O₂max to fatigue[g]			0.02

Enzyme activities were measured at 35-37° C or converted to this temperature by using a Q_{10} of 2.

Rate of ammonia formation was calculated from the accumulation and release of ammonia.

[a]Human quadriceps femoris muscle. Norman 1994 (23).

[b]Human quadriceps femoris muscle. Norman, Hellsten-Westing, et al. 1994 (25).

[c]Rat soleus and quadriceps femoris muscle. Winder et al. 1974 (45).

[d]Human quadriceps femoris muscle. Wibom and Hultman 1990 (44).

[e]Katz et al. 1986 (18).

[f]Katz et al. 1986 (17).

[g]Broberg and Sahlin 1989 (7).

for amino acid deamination but also has other functions, such as maintenance of a high ATP/ADP ratio and replenishment of tricarboxylic acid intermediates (20).

GDH is a mitochondrial enzyme, and both $NAD^+/NADH$ and $NADP^+/NADPH$ can participate in the reaction. One of the proposed roles of this enzyme is to provide a link between these two redox systems (22). GDH catalyzes a reversible reaction and could thus function as both a source and a sink for ammonia, depending on the cellular concentration of reactants and products. The in vitro activity of GDH is much lower than for AMP deaminase (table 40.2), and the maximal activity is too small to sustain the high rates of ammonia formation during high-intensity exercise but sufficient to account for the ammonia formation that occurs in excess of adenine nucleotide breakdown during prolonged exercise (table 40.2). Since the optimal pH for this enzyme is about 8 and a rather high ADP concentration is required for attaining maximal activity, the quantitative role of this enzyme for ammonia formation in vivo has been questioned (1). Furthermore, it is at present not clear whether the GDH reaction functions as a source or as a sink for ammonia during exercise.

The source of ammonia in muscle could either be adenine nucleotides (through AMP deaminase) or amino acids (through PNC or GDH). Deamination of amino acids through PNC or GDH is preceded by a transamination reaction in which amino groups of the amino acids are diverted to glutamate, aspartate, or both (see figure 40.1). IMP can be degraded further to hypoxanthine and urate and excreted into blood. In a number of studies, it has been shown that the decrease in muscle content of adenine nucleotides (TAN) corresponds to a similar increase in IMP (16, 26, 31, 34-36) demonstrating that the further catabolism of IMP is small. Therefore, accumulation of IMP will, under most conditions, be a quantitative measure of ammonia formed through the net degradation of TAN. When ammonia formation exceeds the degradation of TAN (or accumulation of IMP), some of the ammonia originates from amino acid deamination.

Response During Short-Term Exercise

Ammonia Formation

At rest, there is a small uptake of ammonia by skeletal muscle, which during exercise changes to a release. The release of ammonia is dependent on the exercise intensity and duration. At intensities below 50% of $\dot{V}O_2$max, the muscle release of ammonia is small or negligible, but at higher work loads the release increases exponentially (figure 40.2). The increased release of ammonia corresponds to increases in muscle ammonia concentration. After short-term exercise at 50% of $\dot{V}O_2$max, muscle ammonia remained unchanged, whereas at 100% of $\dot{V}O_2$max muscle ammonia increased eightfold to 4.1 ± 0.5 mmol/kg dry mass (d.m.). A similar increase in muscle ammonia (3.6 mmol/kg d.m.; 18) was observed after sustained isometric contraction to fatigue (duration about 50 s). During short-term, high-intensity exercise, the majority of the ammonia produced (≈ 90%) is retained within the muscle, and only a small part is released into the blood (17). Total ammonia production during short-term exercise corresponds to a similar or larger decrease in TAN (figure 40.3), and it is evident that the major source of ammonia during short-term, intense exercise is the breakdown of adenine nucleotides to IMP.

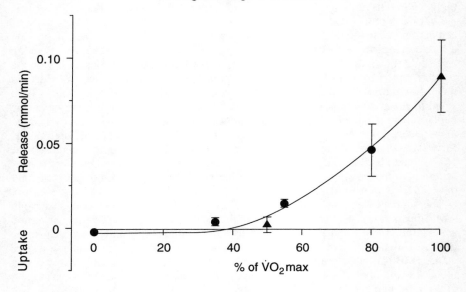

Figure 40.2   Leg exchange of plasma ammonia during short-term (< 15 min) cycling at different exercise intensities. Values are means ± *SE*. Circles: data from Eriksson et al. 1985 (12); triangles: data from Katz et al. 1986 (17).

These results in humans are in accordance with the results of a number of animal studies (for references see 41).

Importance of Muscle Fiber Type Composition and ATP Turnover for IMP Formation

Although the amount of ammonia accumulated in muscle after isometric contraction is similar to that after intensive cycling to fatigue (see figure 40.3), the rate of ammonia formation is much higher during isometric contraction due to the shorter duration of the exercise. The reason for the higher ammonia formation during static contraction than during cycling may be related to the twofold higher rate of ATP turnover or to the occlusion of muscle blood flow (and oxygen supply). The rate of AMP deamination during isometric contraction varies among subjects and is positively related to the ATP turnover rate (18), and it was concluded that activation of AMP deaminase occurred when energetic deficiency (signified by a low phosphocreatine level) was coupled with a high ATP turnover rate (18). The low rate of IMP formation during ischemic recovery (32) and during prolonged anoxia (24, 32) is consistent with the idea that a high ATP turnover rate is a prerequisite for attaining high rates of IMP formation.

Several findings suggest that ammonia formation is more pronounced in FT fibers than in ST fibers. Thus, after both intense (16, 31) and prolonged (26) exercise,

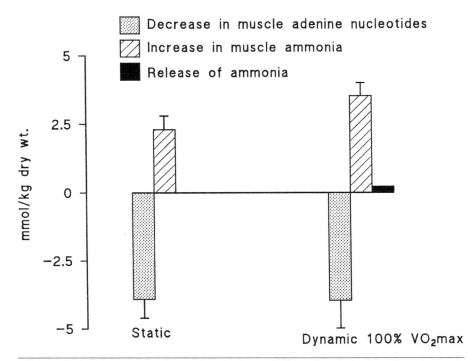

Figure 40.3 Decrease in muscle TAN and ammonia formation during high-intensity exercise to fatigue. Static exercise was sustained knee extension at 66% of maximum voluntary force to fatigue (18). Dynamic exercise was cycling to fatigue (17). The average duration of exercise was 52 s (static) and 5.2 min (dynamic). Release of ammonia was calculated from the femoral arteriovenous difference for plasma ammonia, plasma flow, and an estimated working muscle mass of 2 kg d.m. (one leg). Values are means ± *SE*.

IMP content was twofold higher in FT fibers than in ST fibers, and the blood ammonia reached during exercise was related to the relative amount of FT fibers in the quadriceps femoris muscle (11). Since the activity of AMP deaminase in humans is similar in FT and ST fibers (see table 40.2), factors other than the amount of enzyme must explain the heterogeneous response (e.g., differences in the metabolic state or in ATP turnover during exercise). The optimal pH for AMP deaminase is 6.2 to 6.5 (37), and differences in the metabolic characteristics between fiber types resulting in higher lactate and lower pH in FT fibers has been suggested to be the cause of the higher IMP formation rate in FT fibers (41). The hypothesis is supported by the positive relationship between ammonia and lactate in plasma, which has been observed in a number of studies after short-term exercise (12, 17, 21). However, during prolonged exercise and in patients with glycogen phosphorylase deficiency (McArdle's disease), a dissociation between ammonia and lactate levels occurs. The relationship between ammonia and lactate therefore may rather reflect an imbalance between utilization and regeneration of ATP (18), where the lactate level is related to the degree of metabolic stress. The higher ATP turnover rate in FT fibers (38) and the higher degree of metabolic stress may be the cause of the higher rate of IMP formation in FT fibers.

In contrast to human muscle where deamination of AMP to IMP occurs in both fiber types during exercise, stimulation of rat ST muscle (soleus) to fatigue resulted in no appreciable increase in IMP (41). The reason for the higher rate of IMP formation in the human ST fiber is not clear. Factors such as higher glycolytic capacity and higher rates of ATP turnover in the human versus rat ST fiber may be important.

Response During Prolonged Exercise

Ammonia Formation

During moderate-intensity exercise, there is a continuous increase in plasma ammonia with time, whereas plasma lactate remains relatively constant. The increase in plasma ammonia corresponds to an increased release of ammonia (7). Ammonia release was 2.5 times higher after 65 min of exercise than after 20 min of exercise (7). Muscle ammonia increased after prolonged exercise to fatigue and coincided with glycogen depletion (7). When calculated for the whole exercise period, formation of ammonia (accumulation + release) was about twofold higher than the decrease in TAN (figure 40.4). This suggests that the adenine nucleotide pool is not the only source of ammonia, but that deamination of amino acids also occurs. Deamination of amino acids could occur either by the PNC or by the GDH reaction (see figure 40.1). Considering the near-equilibrium nature of the GDH reaction, the decrease in substrate (glutamate), and the increase in the product (ammonia), one may question ammonia formation by this process during exercise. However, intramitochondrial concentration of the reactants may be different, and the GDH reaction as an ammonia-producing reaction cannot be ruled out.

During prolonged exercise, there is only a small increase in IMP during the first 30 min of exercise (27, 34), and in one study there was no increase of IMP at all (43), despite a large release of ammonia. Consequently, formation of ammonia during the initial period of exercise must be derived to a major extent from amino acid deamination. If ammonia formation during this period proceeds through the PNC, it must occur under conditions of only minor elevations in IMP.

The calculated ammonia formation (figure 40.4) is a minimal estimate, because some ammonia may be transferred to glutamate by the glutamine synthetase reaction and to 2-oxoglutarate by the GDH reaction if this functions as a sink of ammonia (as previously discussed). During prolonged exercise, there is a loss of nitrogen from the muscle in the form of ammonia, glutamine, and alanine. The net loss of nitrogen from each leg corresponds to about 0.2 mmol/min or about 6 mmol/kg d.m. during an exercise period of 60 min at 70% of $\dot{V}O_2$max (34). The nitrogen release may correspond to protein breakdown or to changes in the intracellular amino acid pool. Since the total amino acid content in muscle is large (about 104 mmol/kg d.m.; 4) a decrease of 6 mmol/kg d.m. is within the methodological error for the analysis. The relative importance of protein degradation and decrease in the intracellular amino acid pool for the nitrogen efflux is therefore unclear.

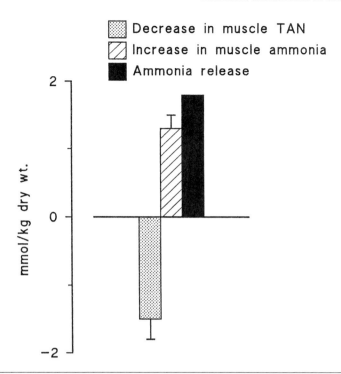

Figure 40.4   Decrease in muscle TAN and ammonia formation during prolonged exercise to fatigue at moderate intensity (70% V̇O₂max). Exercise duration was 65 min. Release of ammonia was calculated from the femoral arteriovenous difference for plasma ammonia, plasma flow, and an estimated working muscle mass of 2 kg d.m. (one leg) and was averaged over the whole exercise period. Values are means ± *SE* and are from Broberg and Sahlin 1989 (7).

Glycogen Depletion and IMP Formation

During prolonged exercise, deamination of AMP to IMP is closely associated with glycogen depletion. Thus, after prolonged exercise, accumulation of IMP occurs preferentially in fibers depleted of glycogen (26). Glycogen-depleted fibers (glycogen < 50 mmol/kg d.m.) contained two to three times (type I) or four to six times (type II) more IMP than did fibers with higher glycogen content (glycogen > 150 mmol/kg d.m.). The importance of low muscle glycogen for ammonia formation was further demonstrated by the augmented rate of ammonia and IMP formation during exercise with depleted muscle glycogen stores (7). Augmented plasma ammonia has also been observed in other studies during exercise with reduced initial muscle glycogen (8, 43) or CHO availability (14). In the study by Wagenmakers et al. (43), there was no increase in muscle IMP despite prolonged exercise at 70% to 75% of V̇O₂max, which was attributed to the high aerobic training status of the subjects. Supplementation with carbohydrates during prolonged exercise (40) or elevation of the initial glycogen level (39) has been shown to attenuate the increase in muscle IMP after similar periods of exercise, and supports the notion that a reduced availability of carbohydrates induces metabolic stress with a catabolism of the TAN pool.

Inter-Organ Ammonia Flux During Exercise

The efflux of ammonia from the muscle to the extracellular compartment increases with the duration and the intensity of the exercise (figure 40.5). During exercise at 70% $\dot{V}O_2$max, the average release of ammonia is 0.1 mmol/min (2 legs). The increased ammonia efflux results in an increased plasma ammonia concentration, and ammonia will be distributed in the body fluids (interstitial space, erythrocytes, resting muscle, CNS). Ammonia is extracted from blood by the liver (12), but the uptake is similar at rest and during exercise (about 0.01 mmol/min). The absence of increased splanchnic ammonia removal, despite large increases in arterial ammonia concentration, is probably a consequence of the decreased hepatic blood flow during exercise (12). Disposal of ammonia by the liver during exercise is thus relatively small.

A considerable amount of ammonia is excreted in sweat. The average excretion via sweat during 30 min of exercise at 40% and 80% of $\dot{V}O_2$max was 0.01 and 0.1 mmol/min, respectively (9). It has also been suggested that a considerable amount of ammonia is excreted through expired air (13). Assuming a similar partial pressure of NH_3 in alveolar air as in arterial blood (15), it can be calculated that the maximal rate of ammonia disposal by respiration is less than 0.01 mmol/min. The inter-organ flux of ammonia should also include glutamine, which is considered to be a carrier of ammonia. The release of glutamine from muscle increases during exercise and

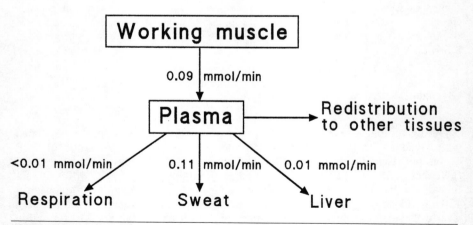

Figure 40.5 Inter-organ flux of ammonia during exercise at moderate intensity. The release of ammonia from working muscle (both legs) and the uptake by liver is after 15 min of exercise at 80% $\dot{V}O_2$max (12). Excretion of ammonia in the sweat is the average excretion during 30 min of exercise at 80% $\dot{V}O_2$max (9). Excretion of ammonia by respiration is calculated under the assumption that partial pressure of ammonia in alveolar air equals that in arterial blood. Leg glutamine release at 80% $\dot{V}O_2$max is 0.19 mmol/min (12) and may correspond to additional ammonia efflux from muscle.

is similar to (34) or higher than (12) the release of ammonia. However, since it is not clear whether this glutamine flux corresponds to a decrease in the intracellular glutamine pool or to a de novo glutamine formation from glutamate and ammonia, this potential flux of ammonia has not been included in figure 40.5.

Ammonia Formation and Muscle Fatigue

Muscle fatigue is a multifactorial phenomenon, and the importance of various factors will vary under different conditions. Under a number of conditions, muscle fatigue is associated with increased deamination of muscle adenine nucleotides. Thus there is an increased formation of IMP and ammonia at fatigue during both high-intensity exercise and prolonged exercise (previously discussed). Under conditions of reduced exercise capacity, as in patients with McArdle's disease (30) or in normal subjects during exercise under hypoxia (33) or beta-adrenoceptor blockade (6), there is an augmented rate of AMP deamination compared with control conditions. It has been suggested (18) that breakdown of TAN to IMP and ammonia reflects a condition of insufficient rate of ATP regeneration, resulting in transient increases in ADP and AMP (due to the adenylate kinase reaction) above that calculated from the creatine kinase and adenylate kinase equilibrium. An increase in AMP, due to the relative low affinity of AMP deaminase for AMP, will activate the enzyme and result in formation of IMP and ammonia. Muscle fatigue, according to this hypothesis, under some conditions may be related to energy deficiency.

There is also evidence that high plasma ammonia levels could affect the function of the nervous system and cause neurological disturbances (21). The exercise-induced increase in plasma ammonia has been implicated as a contributing factor in fatigue through an effect on the CNS causing convulsions and a loss of coordination (3, 21) and on the peripheral nervous system causing muscle cramps (8). Since ammonia is distributed between cellular compartments according to H^+ concentration, it is conceivable that high ammonia levels in the brain would be more prominent during prolonged exercise when plasma pH is close to normal than during high-intensity exercise.

Acknowledgments

The financial support from Swedish Medical Research Council (No 8671), Swedish Research Council of Sports Medicine, and Karolinska Institute is acknowledged.

References

1. Aragon, J.J.; Lowenstein, J.M. The purine-nucleotide cycle: Comparison of the levels of citric acid cycle intermediates with the operation of the purine nucleotide cycle in rat skeletal muscle during exercise and recovery from exercise. Eur. J. Biochem. 110:371-377; 1980.

2. Atkinson, D.E.; Bourke, E. Metabolic aspects of the regulation of systemic pH. Am. J. Physiol. 252:F947-F956; 1987.

3. Banister, E.W.; Cameron, B.J.C. Exercise-induced hyperammonemia: Peripheral and central effects. Int. J. Sports Med. 11:S129-S142; 1990.

4. Bergström, J.; Furst, P.; Noree, L.-O.; Vinnars, E. Intracellular free amino acid concentration in human muscle tissue. J. Appl. Physiol. 36:693-697; 1974.

5. Boron, W.F. Intracellular pH regulation. Curr. Top. Membrane Transp. 13:3-29; 1980.

6. Broberg, S.; Katz, A.; Sahlin, K. Propranolol enhances adenine nucleotide degradation in human muscle during exercise. J. Appl. Physiol. 65:2478-2483; 1988.

7. Broberg, S.; Sahlin, K. Adenine nucleotide degradation in human skeletal muscle during prolonged exercise. J. Appl. Physiol. 67:116-122; 1989.

8. Brouns, F.; Beckers, E.; Wagenmakers, A.J.M.; Saris, W.H.M. Ammonia accumulation during highly intensive long-lasting cycling: Individual observations. Int. J. Sports Med. 11:S78-S84; 1990.

9. Czarnowski, D.; Gorski, J. Sweat ammonia excretion during submaximal cycling exercise. J. Appl. Physiol. 70:371-374; 1991.

10. Czarnowski, D.; Gorski, J.; Jozwiuk, J.; Boron-Kaczmarska, A. Plasma ammonia is the principal source of ammonia in sweat. Eur. J. Appl. Physiol. 65:135-137; 1992.

11. Dudley, G.A.; Staron, R.S.; Murray, T.F.; Hagerman, R.C.; Luginbuhl, A. Muscle fiber composition and blood ammonia levels after intense exercise in humans. J. Appl. Physiol. 54:582-586; 1983.

12. Eriksson, L.S.; Broberg, S.; Björkman, O.; Wahren, J. Ammonia metabolism during exercise in man. Clin. Physiol. 5:325-336; 1985.

13. Graham, T.E.; MacLean, D.A. Ammonia and amino acid metabolism in human skeletal muscle. Can. J. Physiol. Pharmacol. 70:132-141; 1992.

14. Greenhaff, P.L.; Leiper, J.B.; Ball, D.; Maughan, R.J. The influence of dietary manipulation on plasma ammonia accumulation during incremental exercise in man. Eur. J. Appl. Physiol. 63:338-344; 1991.

15. Jacquez, J.A.; Poppell, J.W.; Jeltsch, R. Partial pressure of ammonia in alveolar air. Science 129:269-270; 1959.

16. Jansson, E.; Dudley, G.A.; Norman, B.; Tesch, P. ATP and IMP in single human muscle fibres after high intensity exercise. Clin. Physiol. 7:337-345; 1987.

17. Katz, A.; Broberg, S.; Sahlin, K.; Wahren, J. Muscle ammonia and amino acid metabolism during dynamic exercise in man. Clin. Physiol. 6:365-379; 1986.

18. Katz, A.; Sahlin, K.; Henriksson, J. Muscle ammonia metabolism during isometric contraction in humans. Am. J. Physiol. 250:C834-C840; 1986.

19. Kleiner, D. The transport of NH_3 and NH_4^+ across biological membranes. Biochim. Biophys. Acta 639:41-52; 1981.

20. Lowenstein, J.M. Ammonia production in muscle and other tissues: The purine nucleotide cycle. Physiol. Rev. 52:382-414; 1972.

21. Mutch, B.J.; Banister, E.W. Ammonia metabolism in exercise and fatigue: A review. Med. Sci. Sports Exercise 15:41-50; 1983.

22. Newsholme, E.A.; Leech, A.R. Biochemistry for the medical sciences. Chichester: John Wiley & Sons Ltd.; 1984.

23. Norman, B. IMP accumulation in energy deficient human skeletal muscle. With reference to substrate availability, fibre types and AMP deaminase activity. Stockholm: Karolinska Institute; 1994. Thesis.

24. Norman, B.; Heden, P.; Jansson, E. Small accumulation of inosine monophosphate (IMP) despite high lactate levels in latissimus dorsi. Clin. Physiol. 11:375-384; 1991.

25. Norman, B.; Hellsten-Westing, Y.; Sjödin, B.; Jansson, E. AMP deaminase in skeletal muscle of healthy males quantitatively determined by a new assay. Acta Physiol. Scand. 150:397-403; 1994.

26. Norman, B.; Sollevi, A.; Jansson, E. Increased IMP content in glycogen-depleted muscle fibres during submaximal exercise in man. Acta Physiol. Scand. 133:97-100; 1988.

27. Norman, B.; Sollevi, A.; Kaijser, L.; Jansson, E. ATP breakdown products in human skeletal muscle during prolonged exercise to exhaustion. Clin. Physiol. 7:503-510; 1987.

28. Parnas, J.K. Uber die Ammoniakbildung im Muskel un ihren Zusammhang mit Funktion und Zustandsänderung. 6. Der Zusammenhang der Ammoniakbildung und der Umwandlung des Adeninnucleotids zu Inosinsäure. Biochem. Z. 206:16-38; 1929.

29. Sahlin, K.; Alvestrand, A.; Brandt, R.; Hultman, E. Intracellular pH and bicarbonate concentration in human muscle during recovery from exercise. J. Appl. Physiol. 45:474-480; 1978.

30. Sahlin, K.; Areskog, N.-H.; Haller, P.G.; Henriksson, K.G.; Jorfeldt, L.; Lewis, S.F. Impaired oxidative metabolism increases adenine nucleotide breakdown in McArdle's disease. J. Appl. Physiol. 69:1231-1235; 1990.

31. Sahlin, K.; Broberg, S.; Ren, J.M. Formation of IMP in human skeletal muscle during incremental dynamic exercise. Acta Physiol. Scand. 136:193-198; 1989.

32. Sahlin, K.; Gorski, J.; Edström, L. Influence of ATP turnover and metabolite changes on IMP formation and glycolysis in rat skeletal muscle. Am. J. Physiol. 259:C409-C412; 1990.

33. Sahlin, K.; Katz, A. Hypoxemia increases the accumulation of IMP in human skeletal muscle during submaximal exercise. Acta Physiol. Scand. 136:199-203; 1989.

34. Sahlin, K.; Katz, A.; Broberg, S. Tricarboxylic acid cycle intermediates in human muscle during prolonged exercise. Am. J. Physiol. 259:C834-C841; 1990.

35. Sahlin, K.; Palmskog, G.; Hultman, E. Adenine nucleotide and IMP contents of the quadriceps muscle in man after exercise. Pflügers Arch. 374:193-198; 1978.

36. Sahlin, K.; Ren, J. Relationship of contraction capacity to metabolic changes during recovery from a fatiguing contraction. J. Appl. Physiol. 67:648-654; 1989.

37. Setlow, B.; Lowenstein, J.M. Adenylate deaminase. Purification and some regulatory properties of the enzyme from calf brain. J. Biol. Chem. 242:607-615; 1967.

38. Söderlund, K.; Hultman, E. ATP and phosphocreatine changes in single human muscle fibres following intense electrical stimulation. Am. J. Physiol. 261:E737-E741, 1991.

39. Spencer, M.K.; Katz, A. Role of glycogen in control of glycolysis and IMP formation in human muscle during exercise. Am. J. Physiol. 260:E859-E864; 1991.

40. Spencer, M.K.; Yan, Z.; Katz, A. Carbohydrate supplementation attenuates IMP accumulation in human muscle during prolonged exercise. Am. J. Physiol. 261:C71-C76; 1991.

41. Terjung, R.L.; Dudley, G.A.; Meyer, R.A.; Hood, D.A.; Gorski, J. Purine nucleotide cycle function in contracting muscle. In: Saltin, B., ed. Biochemistry of

exercise VI. Champaign, IL: Human Kinetics Publishers; 1986:131-147. (Int. Series Sport Sci.; vol. 16).

42. Tullson, P.C.; Terjung, R.L. Adenine nucleotide degradation in striated muscle. Int. J. Sports Med. 11:S47-S55; 1990.

43. Wagenmakers, A.J.M.; Beckers, E.J.; Brouns, F.; Kuipers, H.; Soeters, P.B.; van der Vusse, G.J.; Saris, W.H.M. Carbohydrate supplementation, glycogen depletion, and amino acid metabolism during exercise. Am. J. Physiol. 260: E883-E890; 1991.

44. Wibom, R.; Hultman, E. ATP production rate in mitochondria isolated from microsamples of human muscle. Am. J. Physiol. 259:E204-E209; 1990.

45. Winder, W.W.; Terjung, R.L.; Baldwin, K.M.; Holloszy, J.O. Effect of exercise on AMP deaminase in rat skeletal muscle. Am. J. Physiol. 227:1411-1414; 1974.

CHAPTER 41

Control of Skeletal Muscle AMP Deaminase During Exercise

Peter C. Tullson

State University of New York, Syracuse, New York, U.S.A.

Exercise increases the turnover rate of high-energy phosphates in skeletal muscle. At the limits of performance, this high turnover also leads to contractile failure when the means of maintaining a favorable intracellular milieu becomes exhausted. Phosphocreatine sustains a high phosphorylation potential at the onset of heavy exercise; with continued exercise, glycolysis and oxidative phosphorylation become increasingly important. When the capacity to provide ATP is insufficient, AMP deamination results. For example, depletion of phosphocreatine ($PCr + ADP_f \leftrightarrow Cr + ATP + H^+$) during conditions of intense exercise or muscle stimulation is usually associated with IMP formation. Deamination occurs more readily in muscles with a low or experimentally decreased ability to extract or use oxygen. Conversely, IMP formation occurs later or to a lesser extent in muscles with an improved mitochondrial content or oxygen delivery, for example, after endurance training (6). In a similar way, limitation of glycolysis due to lack of substrate (i.e., glycogen depletion) enhances AMP deamination, whereas complete inhibition of glycolysis by iodoacetic acid causes rapid and extensive IMP accumulation during muscle contraction (5).

A common feature of exercise-induced AMP deamination is an imbalance between ATP use and production, leading to an increase in free ADP (ADP_f). Forward flux through the near-equilibrium adenylate kinase reaction ($ADP_f + ADP_f \leftrightarrow AMP_f + ATP$) consequently increases; subsequent AMP deamination decreases the reverse reaction by mass action. Though this broad picture is consistent with experimental observations, the mechanism(s) coupling an imbalance between ATP use and formation with AMP deamination are unresolved. The nonequilibrium reaction catalyzed by AMP deaminase (AMPD) ($AMP \rightarrow IMP + NH_3$) probably serves to temper the rise in ADP_f, among other functions (see reviews 17, 42, 53). While the benefit of this cellular strategy is temporary, it is widely used in muscle fibers recruited during high-intensity exercise and probably allows force production to be sustained longer than would otherwise be the case. Up to half the total muscle adenylate pool may be deaminated when ATP use outstrips ATP replenishment via the creatine kinase reaction, glycolysis, and oxidative phosphorylation. Muscle oxidative capacity (reflected by both mitochondrial content and blood flow capacity), endurance training state, differences in the energy cost of contraction in slow- versus fast-twitch fibers, and different regulatory properties of AMPD isoforms all contribute to the observed differences in AMP deamination (52, 53).

Skeletal muscle fiber types also differ in their capacity to reaminate IMP. Reamination depends on metabolic energy (25, 53) and may be regulated by the ratio of guanosine triphosphate (GTP) to guanosine diphosphate (GDP), since the adenylosuccinate synthetase requires GTP and is inhibited by GDP (17; figure 41.1). This is consistent with the observation that deamination is more rapid in highly oxidative muscles (49). Reamination during contraction has been demonstrated in fast-twitch red muscle, especially during extended stimulation periods (13).

A great deal has been discovered about the effects of various small–molecular weight compounds on purified AMPD. In spite of this increased understanding, we still do not have a fully satisfactory picture of how AMPD is controlled in vivo. Hence, particular attention will be given to evaluate other possible means by which deamination may be regulated.

Regulation of AMP Deaminase

Notwithstanding the differences among fiber types (discussed later), the maximal activity of AMPD measured in vitro is extremely high in skeletal muscle. For example, rat fast-twitch white muscle has an in vitro AMPD activity of 350 to 400 $\mu mol \cdot min^{-1} \cdot g^{-1}$ wet mass (w.m.), while peak rates of AMP deamination have been estimated at only approximately 3 $\mu mol \cdot min^{-1} \cdot g^{-1}$ (6). Since AMPD catalyzes an irreversible reaction with a large decrease in free energy and since every IMP molecule formed obligates a high-energy phosphate (as GTP at the adenylosuccinate synthetase reaction; see figure 41.1) for reamination by the purine nucleotide cycle, an extremely effective means of inhibiting the enzyme is required (17). Unneeded cycling of IMP would impose an equivalent energetic cost.

Adenine nucleotide degradation and loss from skeletal muscle occur predominantly via the pathway AMP → IMP → inosine → hypoxanthine (figure 41.2). Because the adenylate pool (ATP + ADP + AMP) is constant in resting muscle, we can infer that the rates of synthesis and degradation are equal. The rate of de novo synthesis should be a fairly good estimate of flux through AMPD at rest as follows.

The de novo synthesis pathway builds on ribose-5-phosphate via a series of reactions that use the amino acids glutamine, glycine, and aspartate along with bicarbonate and formate to yield IMP. IMP is reaminated to AMP, which distributes to ATP and ADP via the myokinase reaction. Rates of de novo synthesis have been measured in different fiber sections of intact muscle using the rat hindquarter perfused with reconstituted blood containing [^{14}C]glycine as precursor. In fast-twitch white muscle, the rate was 26 nmol $\cdot g^{-1}$ w.m. $\cdot h^{-1}$ (51). This rate should approximate the rate of reamination because label reaching the adenine nucleotide pool must enter via IMP.

Assuming that all adenine nucleotide is lost via AMPD, the calculated upper rate of AMP deamination is 0.43 nmol $\cdot min^{-1} \cdot g^{-1}$ w.m., or only 1.2×10^{-4}% of the in vitro AMPD activity. During intense exercise, the measured peak rate of IMP formation is around 3,000 nmol $\cdot min^{-1} \cdot g^{-1}$ w.m. (5), or about a 7,000-fold increase.

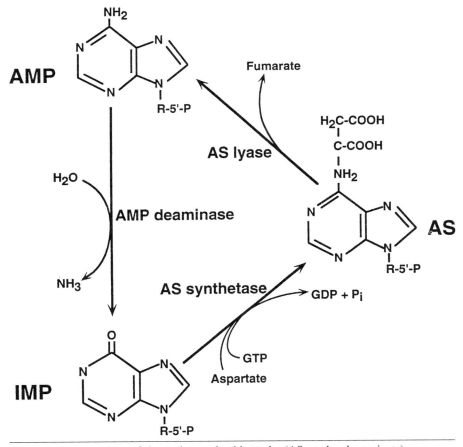

Figure 41.1   Reactions of the purine nucleotide cycle. (AS = adenylosuccinate).

To the degree that purine is lost through the 5'-AMP nucleotidase–initiated pathway (AMP → adenosine → inosine → hypoxanthine), we will overestimate resting flux through AMPD. For instance, if one-half of the purine degraded and lost from the muscle occurs via 5'-AMP nucleotidase, the increase in AMPD flux above that during rest would be 14,000-fold. How is AMPD flux maintained very low at rest, and what brings about the estimated 7,000-fold increase during intense exercise?

In vitro experiments utilizing purified enzyme have been a widely used approach to understand the regulation of AMPD. The substrate affinity of the enzyme has been determined in many studies; the K_m is usually reported to be 1 to 2 mM. This low substrate affinity contributes to the calculated low flux in resting muscle because the sarcoplasmic concentration of free AMP (AMP_f) is so much lower ($\approx 0.1 \ \mu M$) than the K_m. For this reason, any elevation in AMP_f via the adenylate kinase reaction should result in a proportionate increase in flux through AMPD and has been designated as a major factor stimulating AMP deamination during muscle contraction (5, 56). Inorganic phosphate (Pi) may also be important in maintaining a low AMPD flux, since its reported K_i toward deamination is 2 mM and is similar to the Pi

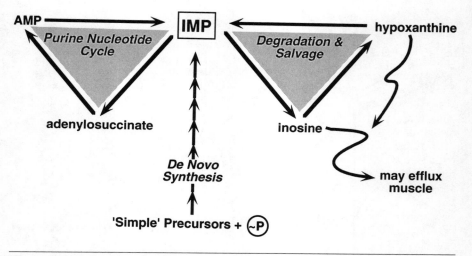

Figure 41.2   Integration of purine synthetic and degradative pathways.

concentration (2.5 mM) in resting rat skeletal muscle determined by phosphorus nuclear magnetic resonance (16). This inhibition must be overcome during exercise when Pi increases several-fold due to hydrolysis of PCr. Increases in ADP_f should act to lessen the Pi inhibition (56). Acidosis during intense exercise will bring the enzyme closer to its pH optima and lower the K_m of AMPD toward AMP (30).

Thus, one view of the control of AMPD relies on the concerted action of several metabolite effectors that are dependent on the myocyte energetic status to regulate AMPD flux over an estimated 7,000-fold range as needed. For the most part, physiological data from exercise studies in animals and humans are difficult to reconcile with this view for the following reasons. First, even when changes in metabolic effectors are in the appropriate direction, the magnitude of change is usually too small to account for the observed changes in the rate of deamination (5, 54). Most important, AMP deamination stops as contractile failure occurs, even though the cellular conditions (i.e., the concentrations of important modulators) are unchanged.

As described by Sahlin et al. (41), ATP turnover per se is necessary for deamination. They showed that 1 or 2 min of muscle stimulation without blood flow induced modest deamination. After that, if the muscle was kept anoxic during recovery for an additional 5 min, no further deamination took place, even though cellular conditions were energetically poised to stimulate IMP formation. Similarly, 4 h of anoxia at room temperature led to more severe energy depletion and an IMP accumulation that was no greater than that with 2 min of contractions.

How can this dependence of AMP deamination on ATP turnover be reconciled with simple allosteric control by metabolites? Three alternatives can be identified. First, an as yet unrecognized metabolite may be linked to ATP turnover and may activate AMPD when energy-depleted conditions exist. This may be a difficult hypothesis to evaluate without a serendipitous identification of such a compound, but there is some evidence that other activators or inhibitors exist. For example, a small–molecular weight inhibitor specific for skeletal muscle AMPD has been identified in serum (8). In addition, separation of skeletal muscle AMPD from small–molecular weight compounds in muscle extracts can result in an apparent activation of the enzyme, suggesting the presence of endogenous inhibitor(s) (11, 27).

Second, physical or kinetic compartmentalization of AMPD may occur, so that the true concentrations of effectors are actually an order of magnitude or more greater than are estimated with tissue measurements. To approach this alternative directly by positive experiment (i.e., to look for the compartment) may be technically infeasible at present. However, critical questions discussed later may help to establish the conditions necessary to demonstrate metabolite compartmentalization.

Third, AMPD may behave as a latent catalyst (terminology of Hochachka and Matheson [12]) that requires an activating signal(s) that acts as a switch to recruit functional enzyme activity as needed while preventing inappropriate expression of a potentially very high (and deleterious) activity. This switch might involve something like an enzyme-mediated covalent modification or protein-protein interaction. These latter two concepts of AMPD control, enzyme compartmentalization versus enzyme recruitment, will now be considered. Since they both may depend on the cellular localization of AMPD, the physical properties of the enzyme, what is known about the distribution of AMPD in skeletal muscle, and how it may change during exercise are summarized below.

Physical Properties

Purified skeletal muscle AMPD has a native monomeric molecular mass of 80 kDa (23, 32, 37); a range of lower molecular masses (66 to 79 kDa) has been reported for purified enzyme that has been attributed to a susceptibility toward proteolytic cleavage (18). The enzyme is thought to exist as a 270- to 320-kDa tetramer composed of identical subunits. Results obtained using enzyme purified from rat skeletal muscle show AMPD to be a Zn^{2+}-requiring enzyme (29).

AMPD is present in tissue-specific isoforms with unique chromatographic, electrophoretic, and immunological characteristics (23) that have recently been extended to the molecular level. All skeletal muscles, regardless of fiber type, possess a unique skeletal muscle isoform that is distinct from the enzyme present in other tissues. The genes from human and rat muscle AMPD share a high degree of structural and organizational homology (38). Nucleotide sequence homology was approximately 87% between the human and rat AMPD, with a deduced amino acid sequence homology of 92% (36). In light of this similarity, it is not surprising that AMPD from human and rat muscle also demonstrates immunological cross-reactivity with antisera prepared against the muscle enzyme from the other tissue (9, 24).

In addition, slow-twitch red skeletal muscle contains a second isoform, which in rabbit (24, 28), rat (9, 28), and mouse (9) is similar to the isoform isolated from heart. Curiously, the minor isoform in the cat soleus muscle (slow-twitch red) is immunologically similar to the enzyme isolated from erythrocytes (9). Human muscle AMPD has been chromatographically resolved into either one (24) or two species (28) and immunologically characterized as being more than 90% of the skeletal muscle isoform (9).

Distribution by Fiber Type

Muscle AMPD activity differs between fiber types. In all species examined thus far, including humans, the capacity for AMP deamination is higher in fast-twitch than in slow-twitch muscle. For instance, after intense treadmill running to fatigue, up to 50% of the ATP pool can be deaminated in fast-twitch fibers, while in the soleus, a predominantly slow-twitch muscle, no increase in IMP is seen (19, 22). In humans, the difference in IMP formation in fast-twitch (type II) versus slow-twitch (type I) fibers is not as great, being about twofold higher in fast-twitch fibers (14, 40). In animals possessing both fast-twitch red and white fibers, the low-oxidative white fibers have considerably greater AMPD activity assayed in vitro. In general, the differences in enzyme activity by fiber type are related to the peak rates of deamination among fiber types during brief, intense exercise. At the same time, it is important to keep in mind that the highest rates of AMP deamination measured during intense contractions could be accomplished with < 1% of the cell's enzymatic capacity (5), suggesting that (from the perspective of AMP deamination at least) the enzyme is present in considerable excess. In laboratory animals, muscle AMPD activity is quite consistent within species and fiber type. Humans are quite different in this regard; muscle AMPD activity varies widely among individuals and is related to fiber type composition (7). In a recent study, in vitro AMPD activity of vastus lateralis ranged from 50 to 160 $\mu mol \cdot min^{-1} \cdot g^{-1}$ (50). The extent of deamination seen during short-term, intense exercise seems to be closely related to the energetic imbalance and not closely coupled to the individual enzymatic capacity determined in vitro (50).

Cellular Localization

In rat muscle, the isoforms have been localized with immunofluorescence microscopy; the skeletal muscle isoform was concentrated subsarcolemmally and intermyofibrillarly, while the minor nonmuscle isoforms were localized to non-myocyte cells. Nearly one-third of the AMPD activity of rat soleus muscle was immunoprecipitated by antisera to the heart isoform; this isoform was prominently localized to blood vessels and capillary endothelial cells but was also present within myocytes (47).

In isolated chicken myofibrils and cultured chicken muscle fibers, AMPD was localized to the ends of the A-band (3). Longitudinal muscle sections analyzed by immunological or histochemical methods found AMPD in distinct cross-striations that corresponded with the A-band (20, 47). Cooper and Trinick (4) studied the localization of AMPD in rabbit myofibrils using electron microscopy and found that the enzyme was attached to the junction of the A- and I-bands but slightly further apart than the length of the A-band. They suggested that the enzyme was bound to end filaments extending out from the thick filaments. Recently, Koretz, Irving, and Wang (15) determined that AMPD could bind to native titin filaments, which are thought to be part of an elastic sarcomeric structure and to constitute the end filament.

Association With Myosin

During the preparation of purified myosin from rabbit muscle, it was observed that AMPD was a persistent minor contaminant; Ashby and Frieden (2) showed that AMPD could bind with myosin, heavy meromyosin, or subfragment-2 (S-2; the flexible α-helical hinge region of the myosin tail that connects with the globular head, which is termed subfragment-1 [S-1]) but did not bind with light meromyosin or S-1 (figure 41.3). The binding was fairly strong; it was not disrupted by 150 mM KCl, which would be expected to disrupt weak electrostatic binding. In vitro binding of purified proteins showed a stoichiometry of 2 AMPD:myosin, which was weakened by Pi. AMPD-myosin binding was specific; AMPD did not interact with phosphofructokinase or creatine kinase. Kinetic studies of AMPD performed by Ashby and Frieden (1) also showed that binding to S-2 myosin activated the enzyme slightly and reduced inhibition by GTP.

Studies using purified rat muscle AMPD also found specific tight binding, but kinetic studies suggested binding to light meromyosin with a stoichiometry of 1 AMPD:3 myosin; AMPD from heart did not associate with myosin (44). This binding resulted in changes of approximately 70% in activity with no change in myosin ATPase activity (45). Both the native 80-kDa AMPD monomer from rat skeletal muscle and the 66-kDa subunit formed by proteolysis were shown to bind to myosin heavy chain; binding of the 66-kDa species was reversed by 4 to 5 mM

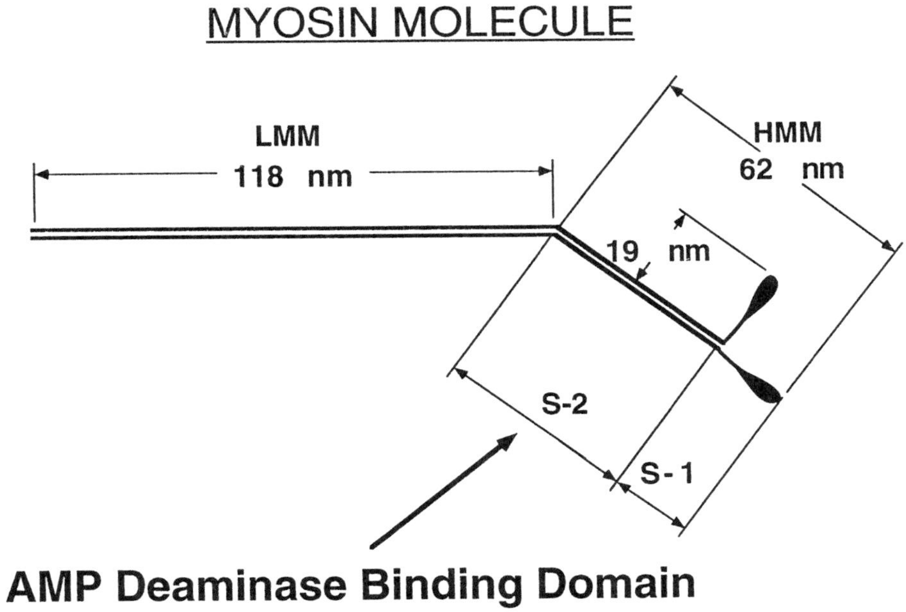

Figure 41.3 Diagram of myosin showing the putative AMP deaminase binding domain. (LMM = light meromyosin; HMM = heavy meromyosin; S-1 = subfragment 1; S-2 = subfragment 2).

ATP (18). Recently, the substrate affinities of rat muscle AMPD when either free or bound to myosin were compared. Myosin binding specifically alters the kinetic characteristics of AMPD such that a much higher affinity for AMP is observed (K_m bound ≈ 0.05 mM vs. K_m free ≈ 1.7 mM) at AMP concentrations below 0.15 mM; above this concentration free and myosin-bound AMPD display similar substrate affinities. This binding was also found to produce a marked resistance to inhibition by 10 mM Pi in the presence of 50 μM ADP (33). These kinetic effects were also observed using AMPD and S-2 myosin purified from rabbit muscle. Very similar negative cooperativity was observed by Ranieri-Raggi et al. (31) upon chemical modification of tyrosine residues of AMPD; this was interpreted as possibly deriving from a conformational change that influenced the binding properties of the activating site. While conjectural, myosin binding may induce a similar conformational change in AMPD.

Changes in AMPD-Myosin Binding With Exercise

Shiraki et al. (43) were first to show an influence of exercise on the distribution of AMPD. Using an in situ rat muscle preparation stimulated to promote deamination in mixed-fiber muscle, they determined that the fraction of AMPD in a soluble form after extraction in a low-salt buffer by centrifugation was decreased. The activity missing from the supernatant could be recovered from the pelleted fraction by reextraction with a buffer containing 300 mM KCl. Thus, the total AMPD activity was unchanged. This was interpreted operationally as myosin binding and was shown to be reversible; upon recovery from exercise, AMPD reverted to the soluble form. We recently confirmed and extended the observation of reversible binding of AMPD during exercise by showing that binding increased about fivefold over that found at rest (10-20%; 34). Binding was quite rapid and preceded IMP formation; it did not depend on cellular acidosis and could not be demonstrated unless energy utilization exceeded the aerobic capacity of specific fiber types. Dissociation was rapid (half time ≈ 15 s) and could be blocked by preventing metabolic recovery after exercise by ischemia. High-speed treadmill running to exhaustion by rats also induced AMPD binding in fast-twitch white fibers with coincident deamination; dissociation during recovery was an apparent first-order process that was slower (half time ≈ 50 s) than after in situ muscle stimulation. Recent studies in humans during prolonged moderate (35) and briefer intense cycling exercise (50) did not reveal any changes in AMPD distribution between the soluble and myosin pellet fractions.

AMPD-Myosin Binding and the Control of Deamination

Metabolite Microcompartmentalization

It has been proposed that localized increases in ADP_f and AMP_f that are not reflected in calculated estimates based on the creatine and adenylate kinase metabolites and equilibrium constants occur within muscle at sites of ATP utilization. It is argued that freeze-clamping cannot discern rapid changes in ADP_f and AMP_f and that metabolite measurements on tissue samples are averages that must obscure gradients within the myocyte (39, 41, 42). These putative localized increases in ADP_f and AMP_f have been suggested to account for the observed AMPD activation during intense exercise and could be the link connecting ATP turnover with deamination (42). Within this framework, binding of AMPD to myosin would place the enzyme near the site of the Ca^{2+}-activated actomyosin ATPase and near these presumed concentration transients.

The existence of ADP_f and AMP_f concentration transients has not been tested experimentally. Based on geometric and kinetic considerations, these concentration transients may be quite small and therefore difficult to detect.

The distance between thick and thin filaments is about 25 nm, while the axial distance between myosin heads in a thick filament is only 14.3 nm, a scale similar to the distance between the outer and inner mitochondrial membrane. We do not know precisely where AMPD binds on the S-2 myosin, but if we place the enzyme as close as possible to the myosin ATPase site (i.e., 20 nm, or the length of the myosin head), we can calculate the approximate volume of the sphere to which the ATPase supplies ADP_f as 3.35×10^{-17} cm^3 (see figure 41.3). With about 125 nmol of myosin per cubic centimeter of muscle (57), these spheres would have a combined volume of about 2.5 cm^3! This suggests that considerable overlap exists among myosin domains. Since individual myosin ATPases are regulated synchronously by increases in Ca^{2+}, each ATPase probably contributes to a "spatially averaged" ADP_f that demonstrates temporal oscillations (10).

For the location of AMPD at the S-2 region of myosin to be meaningful in terms of localizing the enzyme near the site of ATP utilization, there must be sufficient adenylate kinase activity present to transphosphorylate ADP to AMP and ATP. On the one hand, this intermediate step should tend to flatten temporal transients in AMP_f. In addition, if the adenylate kinase reaction is maintained near equilibrium, it should act to facilitate AMP diffusion and thus help diminish spatial AMP_f concentration transients, as is thought to be the case for creatine kinase (21). Both aspects of the adenylate kinase reaction should tend to lessen any ADP_f concentration transient.

Alternatively, one might imagine substrate channeling of ATP $\rightarrow$ ADP $\rightarrow$ AMP $\rightarrow$ IMP within a functional complex that could be formed under the appropriate energetic conditions. Examples of this are found in multienzyme complexes such as pyruvate dehydrogenase and may exist among enzymes of glycolysis (26). There is yet no evidence for a colocalization of AMPD and adenylate kinase, but it is an attractive hypothesis that may be testable. Thus far, available data suggest that adenylate kinase is restricted to the I-band and excluded from the A-band (55). It would be interesting to know whether the distribution of adenylate kinase is altered by muscle contraction.

Modification of AMPD

In addition to interpreting AMPD-myosin binding in terms of colocalization with the ATP utilization site, one could also view myosin binding as a switch that places the enzyme in a "high-gain" configuration, irrespective of location. As previously discussed, AMPD, when in a complex with myosin, has an approximately 20-fold greater affinity toward AMP and should be very effective at activating deamination at physiological concentrations of substrate. While theoretically attractive, the changes in distribution of AMPD induced by exercise leading to deamination have still only been characterized operationally. Positive evidence that AMPD associates with myosin under deaminating conditions and not some other cell constituent would strengthen the previously described kinetic activation of AMPD. The observation that AMPD can apparently diffuse away from its binding sites in glycerinated fibers (4) suggests that, although AMPD is localized near the A-band in resting muscle, the tightness of binding may be increased under deaminating conditions during exercise. In any event, it is clear that AMPD binding alone does not cause deamination, since ischemic postexercise muscle shows AMPD binding without further IMP accumulation (34).

A further conceptual difficulty is the 10% to 20% of AMPD that is found in the insoluble fraction at rest, since it would seem inconsistent to have this much enzyme poised to favor deamination. The recent conclusion by Koretz, Irving, and Wang (15) that AMPD is mainly bound to the elastic structural protein titin in situ may mean that AMPD in quiescent muscle could be mainly bound to titin and not myosin. Perhaps the clearance of AMPD from the soluble fraction is due to myosin binding, whereas AMPD-titin binding reflects a more permanent structural role.

Even if AMPD-myosin binding does act to switch AMPD to an activated form, the question remains, What brings about AMPD-myosin binding when metabolic conditions favor deamination? Might cross-bridge cycling in concert with the energetic state be necessary for AMPD-myosin binding and couple deamination with ATP turnover? In this regard, the observation that AMPD can undergo covalent modification by protein kinase C–mediated phosphorylation (46, 48) is particularly interesting. Could the phosphorylation state of AMPD change its affinity for myosin? If this were the case, the control of the involved kinase or phosphatase by cellular conditions related to an excessive ATP demand during exercise could be important.

Summary

AMPD activity can increase by as much as 7,000-fold. Control of deamination by nucleotides and inorganic phosphate, while important, is probably insufficient to account for the very low AMPD flux observed during rest or for the activation seen with intense exercise. One possibility is that other as yet unidentified compounds may contribute to AMPD regulation. Alternatively, a microenvironment of high substrate and activator concentration that activates deamination might exist near AMPD during high rates of ATP turnover; no evidence for this compartment has been identified thus far. Finally, it has been proposed that AMPD may act as a latent catalyst that is maintained in a relatively inactive state at rest and may be converted to an activated state when ATP use exceeds production. AMPD-myosin binding may be one part of such a recruitment scheme by increasing the responsiveness of AMPD to physiological concentrations of substrate. What controls the association of AMPD with myosin and whether it occurs under all circumstances where deamination takes place is not known.

References

1. Ashby, B.; Frieden, C. Adenylate deaminase. Kinetic and binding studies on the rabbit muscle enzyme. J. Biol. Chem. 253:8728-8735; 1978.
2. Ashby, B.; Frieden, C. Interaction of AMP-aminohydrolase with myosin and its subfragments. J. Biol. Chem. 252:1869-1872; 1977.
3. Ashby, B.; Frieden, C.; Bischoff, R. Immunofluorescent and histochemical localization of AMP deaminase in skeletal muscle. J. Cell Biol. 81:361-373; 1979.
4. Cooper, J.; Trinick, J. Binding and location of AMP deaminase in rabbit psoas muscle myofibrils. J. Mol. Biol. 177:137-152; 1984.
5. Dudley, G.A.; Terjung, R.L. Influence of acidosis on AMP deaminase activity in contracting fast-twitch muscle. Am. J. Physiol. 248:C43-C50; 1985.
6. Dudley, G.A.; Tullson, P.C.; Terjung, R.L. Influence of mitochondrial content on the sensitivity of respiratory control. J. Biol. Chem. 262:9109-9114; 1987.
7. Fishbein, W.N.; Armbrustmacher, V.W.; Griffin, J.L.; Davis, J.I.; Foster, W.D. Levels of adenylate deaminase, adenylate kinase, and creatine kinase in frozen human muscle biopsy specimens relative to type 1/type 2 fiber distribution: Evidence for a carrier state of myoadenylate deaminase deficiency. Ann. Neurol. 15:271-277; 1984.
8. Fishbein, W.N.; Davis, J.I.; Nagarajan, K.; Smith, M.J. Specific serum/plasma inhibitor of muscle adenylate deaminase. IRCS Med. Sci. Biochem. 9:178-179; 1981.
9. Fishbein, W.N.; Sabina, R.L.; Ogasawara, N.; Holmes, E.W. Immunologic evidence for three isoforms of AMP deaminase (AMPD) in mature skeletal muscle. Biochim. Biophys. Acta 1163:97-104; 1993.
10. Funk, C.; Clark, A.J.; Connett, R.J. How phosphocreatine buffers cyclic changes in ATP demand in working muscle. Adv. Exp. Med. Biol. 248:687-692; 1989.
11. Harmsen, E.; Verwoerd, T.C.; Achterberg, P.W.; De Jong, J.W. Regulation of porcine heart and skeletal muscle AMP-deaminase by adenylate energy charge. Comp. Biochem. 75:1-3; 1983.
12. Hochachka, P.W.; Matheson, G.O. Regulating ATP turnover rates over broad dynamic work ranges in skeletal muscles. J. Appl. Physiol. 73:1697-1703; 1992. (Review).
13. Hood, D.A.; Parent, G. Metabolic and contractile responses of rat fast-twitch muscle to 10-Hz stimulation. Am. J. Physiol. 260:C832-C840; 1991.
14. Jansson, E.; Dudley, G.A.; Norman, B.; Tesch, P.A. ATP and IMP in single human muscle fibres after high intensity exercise. Clin. Physiol. 7:337-345; 1987.
15. Koretz, J.F.; Irving, T.C.; Wang, K. Filamentous aggregates of native titin and binding of C-protein and AMP-deaminase. Arch. Biochem. Biophys. 304:305-309; 1993.
16. Kushmerick, M.J.; Meyer, R.A. Chemical changes in rat leg muscle by phosphorus nuclear magnetic resonance. Am. J. Physiol. 248:C542-C549; 1985.
17. Lowenstein, J.M. The purine nucleotide cycle revisited [corrected]. Int. J. Sports Med. 11 (suppl. 2):S37-S46; 1990. (Review; published erratum appears in Int. J. Sports Med. 11(5):411; 1990).

18. Marquetant, R.; Sabina, R.L.; Holmes, E.W. Identification of a noncatalytic domain in AMP deaminase that influences binding to myosin. Biochemistry 28:8744-8749; 1989.

19. Meyer, R.A.; Dudley, G.A.; Terjung, R.L. Ammonia and IMP in different skeletal muscle fibers after exercise in rats. J. Appl. Physiol. Resp. Environ. Exercise Physiol. 49:1037-1041; 1980.

20. Meyer, R.A.; Gilloteaux, J.; Terjung, R.L. Histochemical demonstration of differences in AMP deaminase activity in rat skeletal muscle-fibres. Experientia 36:676-677; 1980.

21. Meyer, R.A.; Sweeney, H.L.; Kushmerick, M.J. A simple analysis of the "phosphocreatine shuttle." Am. J. Physiol. 246:C365-C377; 1984. (Review).

22. Meyer, R.A.; Terjung, R.L. AMP deamination and IMP reamination in working skeletal muscle. Am. J. Physiol. 239:C32-C38; 1980.

23. Ogasawara, N.; Goto, H.; Yamada, Y. AMP deaminase isozymes in rabbit red and white muscles and heart. Comp. Biochem. 76:471-473; 1983.

24. Ogasawara, N.; Goto, H.; Yamada, Y.; Wantanabe, T.; Asano, T. AMP deaminase isoforms in human tissues. Biochim. Biophys. Acta 714:298-306; 1982.

25. Ogawa, H.; Shiraki, H.; Matsuda, Y.; Kakiuchi, K.; Nakagawa, H. Purification, crystallization, and properties of adenylosuccinate synthetase from rat skeletal muscle. J. Biochem. 81:859-869; 1977.

26. Pagliaro, L. Glycolysis revisited: A funny thing happened on the way to the Krebs cycle. News Physiol. Sci. 8:219-222; 1993.

27. Raffin, J.P.; Thebault, M.T. AMP deaminase from equine muscle: Purification and determination of regulatory properties. Int. J. Biochem. 23:1069-1078; 1991.

28. Raggi, A.; Bergamini, C.; Ronca, G. Isozymes of AMP deaminase in red and white skeletal muscles. FEBS Lett. 58:19-23; 1975.

29. Raggi, A.; Ranieri, M.; Taponeco, G.; Ronca-Testoni, S.; Ronca, G.; Rossi, C.A. Interaction of rat muscle AMP aminohydrolase with chelating agents and metal ions. FEBS Lett. 10:101-104; 1970.

30. Raggi, A.; Ranieri-Raggi, M. Regulatory properties of AMP deaminase isoenzymes from rabbit red muscle. Biochem. J. 242:875-879; 1987.

31. Ranieri-Raggi, M.; Bergamini, C.; Montali, U.; Raggi, A. Inactivation of rat muscle 5'-adenylate aminohydrolase by tyrosine nitration with tetranitromethane. Biochem. J. 193:853-859; 1981.

32. Ranieri-Raggi, M.; Raggi, A. pH-Dependent cold lability of rabbit skeletal muscle AMP deaminase. Biochim. Biophys. Acta 742:623-629; 1983.

33. Rundell, K.W.; Tullson, P.C.; Terjung, R.L. Altered kinetics of AMP deaminase by myosin binding. Am. J. Physiol. 263:C294-C299; 1992.

34. Rundell, K.W.; Tullson, P.C.; Terjung, R.L. AMP deaminase binding in contracting rat skeletal muscle. Am. J. Physiol. 263:C287-C293; 1992.

35. Rush, J.W.E.; MacLean, D.A.; Hultman, E.; Graham, T.E. Exercise causes branched-chain oxoacid dehydrogenase dephosphorylation but not AMP deaminase binding. J. Appl. Physiol. 78(6):2193-2200; 1995.

36. Sabina, R.L.; Fishbein, W.N.; Pezeshkpour, G.; Clarke, P.R.; Holmes, E.W. Molecular analysis of the myoadenylate deaminase deficiencies. Neurology 42:170-179; 1992.

37. Sabina, R.L.; Marquetant, R.; Desai, N.M.; Kaletha, K.; Holmes, E.W. Cloning and sequence of rat myoadenylate deaminase cDNA. Evidence for tissue-specific and developmental regulation. J. Biol. Chem. 262:12397-12400; 1987.

38. Sabina, R.L.; Morisaki, T.; Clarke, P.; Eddy, R.; Shows, T.B.; Morton, C.C.; Holmes, E.W. Characterization of the human and rat myoadenylate deaminase genes. J. Biol. Chem. 265:9423-9433; 1990.

39. Sahlin, K.; Broberg, S. Adenine nucleotide depletion in human muscle during exercise: Causality and significance of AMP deamination. Int. J. Sports Med. 11 (suppl. 2):S62-S67; 1990.

40. Sahlin, K.; Broberg, S.; Ren, J.M. Formation of inosine monophosphate (IMP) in human skeletal muscle during incremental dynamic exercise. Acta Physiol. Scand. 136:193-198; 1989.

41. Sahlin, K.; Gorski, J.; Edstrom, L. Influence of ATP turnover and metabolite changes on IMP formation and glycolysis in rat skeletal muscle. Am. J. Physiol. 259:C409-C412; 1990.

42. Sahlin, K.; Katz, A. Adenine nucleotide metabolism. Med. Sport Sci. 38:137-157; 1993. (Review).

43. Shiraki, H.; Miyamoto, S.; Matsuda, Y.; Momose, E.; Nakagawa, H. Possible correlation between binding of muscle type AMP deaminase to myofibrils and ammoniagenesis in rat skeletal muscle on electrical stimulation. Biochem. Biophys. Res. Commun. 100:1099-1103; 1981.

44. Shiraki, H.; Ogawa, H.; Matsuda, Y.; Nakagawa, H. Interaction of rat muscle AMP deaminase with myosin. I. Biochemical study of the interaction of AMP deaminase and myosin in rat muscle. Biochim. Biophys. Acta 566:335-344; 1979.

45. Shiraki, H.; Ogawa, H.; Matsuda, Y.; Nakagawa, H. Interaction of rat muscle AMP deaminase with myosin. II. Modification of the kinetic and regulatory properties of rat muscle AMP deaminase by myosin. Biochim. Biophys. Acta 566:345-352; 1979.

46. Thakkar, J.K.; Janero, D.R.; Yarwood, C.; Sharif, H.M. Modulation of mammalian cardiac AMP deaminase by protein kinase C–mediated phosphorylation. Biochem. J. 291 (pt. 2):523-527; 1993.

47. Thompson, J.L.; Sabina, R.L.; Ogasawara, N.; Riley, D.A. AMP deaminase histochemical activity and immunofluorescent isozyme localization in rat skeletal muscle. J. Histochem. Cytochem. 40:931-946; 1992.

48. Tovmasian, E.K.; Hairapetian, R.L.; Bykova, E.V.; Severin, S.E.J.; Haroutunian, A.V. Phosphorylation of the skeletal muscle AMP-deaminase by protein kinase C. FEBS Lett. 259:321-323; 1990.

49. Tullson, P.C.; Arabadjis, P.G.; Rundell, K.W.; Terjung, R.L. IMP reamination to AMP in rat skeletal muscle fiber types. Am. J. Physiol. 270:C1069-1074; 1996.

50. Tullson, P.C.; Bangsbo, J.; Hellsten, Y.; Richter, E.A. IMP metabolism in human skeletal muscle after exhaustive exercise. J. Appl. Physiol. 78(1):146-152; 1995.

51. Tullson, P.C.; John-Alder, H.B.; Hood, D.A.; Terjung, R.L. De novo synthesis of adenine nucleotides in different skeletal muscle fiber types. Am. J. Physiol. 255:C271-C277; 1988.

52. Tullson, P.C.; Terjung, R.L. Adenine nucleotide degradation in striated muscle. Int. J. Sports Med. 11 (suppl. 2):S47-S55; 1990. (Review).

53. Tullson, P.C.; Terjung, R.L. Adenine nucleotide metabolism in contracting skeletal muscle. Exercise Sport Sci. Rev. 19:507-537; 1991. (Review).

54. Tullson, P.C.; Whitlock, D.M.; Terjung, R.L. Adenine nucleotide degradation in slow-twitch red muscle. Am. J. Physiol. 258:C258-C265; 1990.

55. Wegmann, G.; Zanolla, E.; Eppenberger, H.M.; Wallimann, T. In situ compartmentation of creatine kinase in intact sarcomeric muscle: The acto-myosin overlap zone as a molecular sieve. J. Muscle Res. Cell Motil. 13:420-435; 1992.

56. Wheeler, T.J.; Lowenstein, J.M. Adenylate deaminase from rat muscle. Regulation by purine nucleotides and orthophosphate in the presence of 150 mM KCl. J. Biol. Chem. 254:8994-8999; 1979.

57. Woledge, R.C.; Curtin, N.A.; Homsher, E. Energetic aspects of muscle contraction. Monogr. Physiol. Soc. 41; 1985.

CHAPTER 42

Genetic Defects in Muscle That Affect Ammonia Metabolism: AMP Deaminase Deficiency

Richard L. Sabina

Medical College of Wisconsin, Milwaukee, Wisconsin, U.S.A.

Although many reactions produce ammonia, it is generated primarily by a hydrolytic deamination at the sixth position of the purine ring of 5'-adenylic acid (AMP) in exercising skeletal muscle (for a review, see 8). This reaction is catalyzed by AMP deaminase (EC 3.5.4.6) and also produces 5'-inosinic acid (IMP). Increased turnover of ATP during intense exercise disrupts equilibrium of the myokinase reaction and provides more substrate for the AMP deaminase (AMPD) reaction. AMP deamination, in turn, maintains the myokinase reaction towards ATP production:

$$2 \text{ ATP} \rightarrow (2 \text{ ADP} \leftrightarrow \text{ATP} + \text{AMP}) \rightarrow \text{IMP} + \text{NH}_3$$
$$\text{ATPase} \quad \text{Myokinase} \quad \quad \text{AMPD}$$

AMPD is a highly regulated enzyme and is synthesized in many different forms within and among various mammalian tissues and cells. In humans, inherited and acquired deficiencies of skeletal muscle AMPD, termed myoadenylate deaminase, have been described. Both forms are characterized by the lack of skeletal muscle ammonia production during exercise. This chapter covers the molecular biology of this purine catabolic activity, underlying abnormalities related to its deficiency in skeletal muscle, and available information regarding the experimental management of AMPD expression as it may pertain to phenotypic rescue of individuals exhibiting clinical symptoms attributed to myoadenylate deaminase deficiency.

Molecular Biology of AMP Deaminase Activity

Typically, information related to protein has preceded advances in the molecular biology of AMPD. Although many investigators have reported purifications of AMPD activities from a variety of mammalian tissues and cells, the most comprehensive is the work of Ogasawara and colleagues, who characterized three rat AMPD activities (16) and four from human tissues and cells (19). In the rat, isoform A is isolable from skeletal muscle, isoform B from kidney, and isoform C from heart. Each activity appears tetrameric and exhibits unique kinetic, chromatographic, and immunological behavior. In humans, isoform M is isolable from skeletal muscle, isoform L from liver, and isoforms E1 and E2 from erythrocytes. Isoforms E1 and E2 appear to be products of the same gene, as evidenced by their combined absence in an inherited deficiency of erythrocytes (18). Cross-species similarities have been noted between isoforms A and M and between B and L, whereas isoform C and the E isoforms appear distinct (19). Multiple AMPD activities can be found in most, if not all, mammalian tissues and cells, and five are chromatographically separable in rat brain, three of which appear to be heterotetrameric derivatives of isoforms B and C (17).

Using this information as a guide, three *AMPD* genes have been identified in rats and humans, and many corresponding cDNAs cloned, sequenced, and expressed. The *AMPD1* genes produce transcripts encoding isoforms A and M (21, 23). The human *AMPD2* gene produces transcripts encoding isoform L (1, 29). The human *AMPD3* gene produces transcripts encoding the E isoforms (9). The rat *AMPD2* gene is proposed to be specific for isoform B (1, 24), and the identification of a rat *AMPD3* gene (9) admits expression of the E isoforms in rat tissues and cells, a contention supported by immunocytochemical analyses.[1] Although a molecular explanation for isoform C is currently unavailable, immunocytochemical analyses indicate anti-C reactivity in human tissues[1], raising the possibility of a fourth mammalian *AMPD* gene.

Alignments among the human *AMPD* cDNAs predict conserved C-domains and divergent N-domains for each isoform (1, 9). Included in the predicted C-domain of all cloned forms of *AMPD* is the absolutely conserved motif, SLSTDDP. This sequence is highly similar to the SLNTDDP motif found in the biochemically related enzyme, adenosine deaminase (2). Crystallographic analysis has localized the consecutive aspartate residues of this latter motif in the catalytic site of murine adenosine deaminase (30), which has been taken to indicate their similar role in AMPD. Superimposed on predicted N-domain divergence, each mammalian *AMPD* gene characterized to date produces multiple transcripts differing at, or near, their 5' ends (9, 10, 12, 29). In many cases, these alternative transcripts are predicted to confer N-terminal variation to individual divergent N-domains. The functional significance of N-domain macrodivergence and N-terminal microdivergence across different AMPD activities is unknown. Proposed roles include contributions to kinetic properties, intracellular targeting through protein-protein interactions, and heterotetramer formation (1, 9).

Deficiency of AMP Deaminase in Skeletal Muscle

In 1978, Fishbein, Armbrustmacher, and Griffin published a study (4) of five unrelated individuals exhibiting an exercise-induced myopathy associated with severely reduced levels of skeletal muscle AMPD enzymatic activity, establishing myoadenylate deaminase deficiency as a "new" disease of muscle. There are now over 200 reported cases of myoadenylate deaminase deficiency, although the clinical picture is quite heterogeneous (for reviews, see 20 and 22). Based on a hypothesis put forth by Fishbein in 1985 (3) and on the identification of a common mutant *AMPD1* allele (13), clinical heterogeneity is currently explained by the following classes of deficient individuals (22): (a) homozygotes for the mutant *AMPD1* allele presenting with exercise-related myopathy only (symptomatic, inherited deficiency), (b) homozygotes for the mutant *AMPD1* allele with no apparent clinical symptoms (asymptomatic, inherited deficiency), and (c) homozygotes and heterozygotes for the mutant *AMPD1* allele coincidental with other neuromuscular disorders (acquired deficiency).

A mutant *AMPD1* allele has been identified in 11 unrelated, myopathic individuals and is characterized by double C → T transitions at nucleotides +34 and +143 (13). The latter point mutation results in a P48L substitution, yet catalytic activity is not detectably different from normal isoform M (13). The alteration at nucleotide +34, however, results in a Q12X nonsense mutation predicting a severely truncated polypeptide. This molecular explanation for inherited myoadenylate deaminase deficiency is consistent with data derived from analyses of biopsy material obtained from these and other patients (13, 21), that is, normal abundance of *AMPD1* transcript and no detectable cross-reactive protein.

Two additional features of the nonsense mutation affect the clinical picture of myoadenylate deaminase deficiency. First, nucleotide +34 is positioned at the 3' boundary of exon 2 (23), a 12 base pair miniexon in the *AMPD1* gene subject to an alternative splicing event that removes it from 0.6% to 2% of mature transcripts (12). This results in the production of an exon 1:exon 3 *AMPD1* transcript predicted to encode an isoform M variant containing a glutamic acid residue (E) in place of five amino acids (AEEKQ) near its N-terminus. The functional significance of this alternative splicing event is unknown, and the two rat *AMPD1* proteins are kinetically and immunologically similar (12). Exon 2–encoded residues are not predicted to alter potential posttranslational processing of myoadenylate deaminase (i.e., creation or elimination of potential modification sites). Nevertheless, the highly charged nature of this sequence indicates that it may be exposed where it could affect protein-protein or other interactions involving alternative forms of the protein.

Although functional ramifications of the alternative splicing event are unknown, its clinical consequences may be significant. Individuals homozygous for the mutant genotype are expected to produce low levels of catalytically active isoform M. This may explain why the "deficiency" is associated with only mild clinical symptoms. Furthermore, the variable nature of the alternative splicing event might provide a molecular explanation for symptomatic and asymptomatic inherited myoadenylate deaminase deficiency (12). Examination of relative alternative *AMPD1* transcript abundances in asymptomatic and symptomatic myoadenylate deaminase–deficient skeletal muscle would test this latter hypothesis.

Second, the nonsense mutation destroys a MaeII restriction endonuclease site (AC/gt → AT/gt) in the *AMPD1* gene, a feature that can be used to diagnose the mutant allele (13). In preliminary investigations, the mutant *AMPD1* allele has been detected in 12% of Caucasians and 19% of African-Americans (13), indicating a frequency sufficiently high to account for the reported 2% incidence of myoadenylate deaminase deficiency in muscle biopsies (20, 22). Moreover, these data indicate asymptomatic, deficient individuals far outnumber those with accompanying metabolic myopathy.

The molecular biology of an acquired myoadenylate deaminase deficiency is not as well understood. Clinically, this form of the disease is defined as secondary to a wide array of other neuromuscular complications (3) and is characterized by nonspecific decreases in skeletal muscle enzymatic activities (e.g. creatine kinase and myokinase), as well as in AMPD (3, 20). However, other activities are only partially depressed, while AMPD falls into the "deficient" range, that is, < 10% (3, 6, 20). While pathologies inherent to many associated neuromuscular diseases precipitate decreases in AMPD enzymatic activity (6, 15, 25) and *AMPD1* transcript abundance (25), a genetic component also seems likely. Prior to advances in the molecular biology of AMPD, Fishbein (3) had the insight to propose that while "muscle enzymes are lowered by pathologic damage," the simplest explanation for the disproportionate decrease in AMPD in acquired myoadenylate deaminase deficiency would be that "these patients are carriers of the enzyme-deficient trait, and subsequent disease has lowered their levels to the deficient state." The prevalence of the mutant *AMPD1* allele supports Fishbein's contention and its role in an acquired myoadenylate deaminase deficiency. Moreover, a coincidental homozygous geno-type for the mutant *AMPD1* allele might be anticipated in those cases of acquired myoadenylate deaminase deficiency in which the associated neuromuscular compli-cation does not exhibit significant pathology. Accordingly, an individual with a combined deficiency of McArdle's disease and myoadenylate deaminase deficiency has recently been diagnosed as homozygous for mutant alleles in both the myo-phosphorylase and *AMPD1* genes (28).

Other members of the *AMPD* multigene family may also affect the clinical picture of myoadenylate deaminase deficiency. Northern blot analysis of total cellular RNA isolated from adult human skeletal muscle demonstrates expression of the *AMPD3* gene, albeit at lower levels than the *AMPD1* gene (9). Immunocytochemical analysis of human skeletal muscle shows isoform E distributed in smooth muscle cells lining the vasculature, but also in skeletal myocytes, where it exhibits a similar cross-striation pattern to isoform M (7). However, isoform M is more prevalent in type II fibers, whereas isoform E is predominantly in type I fibers (7). Finally, isoform E comprises the majority of residual AMPD activity in myoadenylate deaminase–deficient skeletal muscle (5). Although relative *AMPD3* gene expression has not been analyzed across individuals, this combined information has been used to formulate a hypothesis that variable expression of isoform E may also play a role in the molecular distinction between symptomatic and asymptomatic inherited myoadenylate deami-nase deficiency (22).

Experimental Management of AMP Deaminase Expression

The estimated high frequency of the mutant *AMPD1* allele in the entire Caucasian and African-American populations predicts many asymptomatic myoadenylate deaminase–deficient individuals. The proposed molecular explanations for variable clinical symptoms imply a corollary that only a low level of enzymatic activity is required to alleviate myopathy inherent to the symptomatic population. If, as pro-posed, only a fine line of relative enzymatic activity separates these two deficient patient groups, then understanding how AMPD expression is regulated could lead to treatments designed to rescue symptomatic individuals.

Although relatively little is known, available molecular information indicates regulation of AMPD expression occurs at a number of levels. Availability of nucleic acid and immunological reagents for the various forms of AMPD has stimulated research in this area, such as (a) identification of two distinct cis-acting elements required for muscle-specific expression of the rat *AMPD1* gene that are located immediately upstream of the transcriptional start site (14), (b) regulation of the alternative splicing event involving the *AMPD1* primary transcript (discussed later), and (c) protein kinase C–mediated phosphorylation of AMPD (26, 27).

The following is known regarding factors proposed to be involved in determining asymptomatic and symptomatic inherited myoadenylate deaminase deficiency (i.e., relative levels of *AMPD1* alternative transcripts and total *AMPD3* gene expression):

1. Both are developmentally regulated in skeletal muscle: (a) relative abundance of exon 1:exon 3 *AMPD1* transcript increases during myogenesis, although its proportion compared to exon 1:exon 2:exon 3 transcript decreases (12, 24). These data indicate that factors controlling the alternative splicing event are more limiting later in development; (b) relative abundance of total *AMPD3* transcripts increase during in vitro myogenesis, yet their proportions remain the same.[2]

2. Alternative splicing of the primary *AMPD1* transcript is controlled by exon recognition and nucleocytoplasmic partitioning (11). Work performed in the rat indicates that exon 2 is intrinsically difficult to recognize, possibly due to its small size, and that intron 2 is removed from the primary transcript at a relatively slow rate. In addition, an RNA intermediate composed of exon 1:exon 2:intron 2:exon 3 is variably retained in the nucleus. Nuclear retention of this intermediate is associated with cytoplasmic accumulation of mature mRNA containing exon 2, while escape of the intermediate is associated with a reduction in the abundance of mature mRNA that retains exon 2.

3. Alternative splicing of the primary *AMPD1* transcript is differentially regulated in type I and type II fibers. The ratio of *AMPD1* mRNA that retains exon 2 (exon 1:exon 2:exon 3) to that which has exon 2 removed (exon 1:exon 3) is higher in a rat muscle group of predominantly type II fibers (i.e., extensor digitorum longus) compared with one with predominantly type I fibers (i.e., soleus; 10). In addition, suspended rat soleus muscle undergoes time-dependent conversions to type II fibers and higher ratios of *AMPD1* mRNA that retains exon 2.[3]

Building on these initial observations, additional work is needed to identify those factors involved in controlling the alternative splicing event of the primary *AMPD1* transcript and total *AMPD3* gene expression. Such knowledge may then be applied to controlling AMPD expression in symptomatic myoadenylate deaminase–deficient skeletal muscle with the prospect for phenotypic rescue of these individuals from their clinical complications.

Notes

1. Human and rat tissues and cells exhibit strong perinuclear reactivity with anti-E serum, which is also distributed along intercalated disks in the heart. Rat and human vascular elements, and erythrocytes contained therein, are strongly reactive with anti-C serum (R.L. Sabina, J.A. DeBruin, D.A. Riley, unpublished observations).

2. RNase protection analyses of total cellular RNA isolated from cultured human skeletal myocytes of low and high degrees of maturation demonstrate increased abundance of type 1a, 1b, and 1c *AMPD3* transcripts during myogenesis (R.L. Sabina, J.H. Veerkamp, manuscript in preparation).
3. Rat soleus muscle isolated from hindlimb suspended for 1, 3, and 7 d exhibits a gradual conversion of type I to type II fibers. RNase protection analysis of total cellular RNA isolated from the same muscles demonstrates a time-dependent increase in total *AMPD1* transcript, a greater proportion of which retains exon 2 (R.L. Sabina, D.A. Riley, unpublished observations).

References

1. Bausch-Jurken, M.T.; Mahnke-Zizelman, D.K.; Morisaki, T.; Sabina, R.L. Molecular cloning of AMP deaminase isoform L: Sequence and bacterial expression of human AMPD2 cDNA. J. Biol. Chem. 267:22407-22413; 1992.
2. Chang, Z.; Nygaard, P.; Chinault, A.C.; Kellems, R.E. Deduced amino acid sequence of *Escherichia coli* adenosine deaminase reveals evolutionarily conserved amino acid residues: Implications for catalytic function. Biochemistry 30:2273-2280; 1991.
3. Fishbein, W.N. Myoadenylate deaminase deficiency: Inherited and acquired forms. Biochem. Med. 33:158-169; 1985.
4. Fishbein, W.N.; Armbrustmacher, V.W.; Griffin, J.L. Myoadenylate deaminase deficiency: A new disease of muscle. Science 200:545-548; 1978.
5. Fishbein, W.N.; Sabina, R.L.; Ogasawara, N.; Holmes, E.W. Immunologic evidence for three isoforms of AMP deaminase (AMPD) in mature skeletal muscle. Biochim. Biophys. Acta 1163:97-104; 1993.
6. Kar, N.C.; Pearson, C.M. Muscle adenylic acid deaminase activity: Selective decrease in early-onset Duchenne muscular dystrophy. Neurology 23:478-482; 1973.
7. Kuppevelt, T.H.v.; Veerkamp, J.H.; Fishbein, W.N.; Ogasawara, N.; Sabina, R.L. Immunolocalization of AMP-deaminase isozymes in human skeletal muscle and cultured muscle cells: Concentration of isoform M at the neuromuscular junction. J. Histochem. Cytochem. 42:861-868; 1994.
8. Lowenstein, J.M. The purine nucleotide cycle revised. Int. J. Sports Med. 11:S37-S46; 1990.
9. Mahnke-Zizelman, D.K.; Sabina, R.L. Cloning of human AMP deaminase isoform E cDNAs: Evidence for a third AMPD gene exhibiting alternatively spliced 5'-exons. J. Biol. Chem. 267:20866-20877; 1992.
10. Mineo, I; Clarke, P.R.H.; Sabina, R.L.; Holmes, E.W. A novel pathway for alternative splicing: Identification of an RNA intermediate that generates an alternative 5' splice donor site not present in the primary transcript of AMPD1. Mol. Cell. Biol. 10:5271-5278; 1990.
11. Mineo, I; Holmes, E.W. Exon recognition and nucleocytoplasmic partitioning determine AMPD1 alternative transcript production. Mol. Cell. Biol. 11:5356-5363; 1991.
12. Morisaki, H.; Morisaki, T.; Newby, L.K.; Holmes, E.W. Alternative splicing: A mechanism for phenotypic rescue of a common inherited defect. J. Clin. Invest. 91:2275-2280; 1993.

13. Morisaki, T.; Gross, M.; Morisaki, H.; Pongratz, D.; Zollner, N.; Holmes, E.W. Molecular basis of AMP deaminase deficiency in skeletal muscle. Proc. Natl. Acad. Sci. USA 89:6457-6461; 1992.
14. Morisaki, T.; Holmes, E.W. Functionally distinct elements are required for expression of the AMPD1 gene in myocytes. Mol. Cell. Biol. 13:5854-5860; 1993.
15. Nagao, H.; Habara, S.; Morimoto, T.; Sano, N.; Takahashi, M.; Kida, K.; Matsuda, H. AMP deaminase activity of skeletal muscle in neuromuscular disorders in childhood: Histochemical and biochemical studies. Neuropediatrics 17:193-198; 1986.
16. Ogasawara, N.; Goto, H.; Watanabe, T. Isozymes of rat AMP deaminase. Biochim. Biophys. Acta 403:530-537; 1975.
17. Ogasawara, N.; Goto, H.; Watanabe, T. Isozymes of rat brain AMP deaminase: Developmental changes and characterizations of five forms. FEBS Lett. 58:245-248; 1975.
18. Ogasawara, N.; Goto, H.; Yamada, Y.; Nishigaki, I.; Itoh, T.; Hasegawa, I. Complete deficiency of AMP deaminase in human erythrocytes. Biochem. Biophys. Res. Commun. 122:1344-1349; 1984.
19. Ogasawara, N.; Goto, H.; Yamada, Y.; Watanabe, T.; Asano, T. AMP deaminase isozymes in human tissues. Biochim. Biophys. Acta 714:298-306; 1982.
20. Sabina, R.L. Myoadenylate deaminase deficiency. In: Rosenberg, R.N.; Prusiner, S.B.; DiMauro, S.; Barchi, R.L.; Kunkel, L.M., eds. The molecular and genetic basis of neurological disease. Boston: Butterworth-Heinemann; 1993:261-275.
21. Sabina, R.L.; Fishbein, W.N.; Pezeshkpour, G.; Clarke, P.R.H.; Holmes, E.W. Molecular analysis of the myoadenylate deaminase deficiencies. Neurology 42:170-179; 1992.
22. Sabina, R.L.; Holmes, E.W. Myoadenylate deaminase deficiency. In: Scriver, C.R.; Beaudet, A.L.; Sly, W.S.; Valle, D., eds. The metabolic and molecular bases of inherited disease. 7th ed. New York: McGraw-Hill; 1995:1769-1780.
23. Sabina, R.L.; Morisaki, T.; Clarke, P.; Eddy, R.; Shows, T.B.; Morton, C.C.; Holmes, E.W. Characterization of the human and rat myoadenylate deaminase genes. J. Biol. Chem. 265:9423-9433; 1990.
24. Sabina, R.L.; Ogasawara, N.; Holmes, E.W. Expression of three stage-specific transcripts of AMP deaminase during myogenesis. Mol. Cell. Biol. 9:2244-2246; 1989.
25. Sabina, R.L.; Sulaiman, A.R.; Wortmann, R.L. Molecular analysis of acquired myoadenylate deaminase deficiency in polymyositis (idiopathic inflammatory myopathy). Adv. Exp. Med. Biol. 309B:203-205; 1991.
26. Thakkar, J.K.; Janero, D.R.; Yarwood, C.; Sharif, H.M. Modulation of mammalian cardiac AMP deaminase by protein kinase C–mediated phosphorylation. Biochem. J. 291:523-527; 1993.
27. Tovmasian, E.K.; Hairapetain, R.L.; Bykova, E.V.; Severin, S.E.; Haroutunian, A.V. Phosphorylation of the skeletal muscle AMP-deaminase by protein kinase C. FEBS Lett. 259:321-323; 1990.
28. Tsujino, S.; Shanske, S.; Carroll, J.E.; Sabina, R.L.; DiMauro, S. Double trouble: Combined myophosphorylase and AMP deaminase deficiency in a child homozygous for nonsense mutations at both loci. Neuromusc. Disord. 5:263-266; 1995.

29. Van den Bergh, F.; Sabina, R.L. Characterization of human AMP deaminase 2 (AMPD2) gene expression reveals alternative transcripts encoding variable N-terminal extensions of isoform L. Biochem. J. 312:401-410; 1995.
30. Wilson, D.K.; Rudolph, F.B.; Quiocho, F.A. Atomic structure of adenosine deaminase complexed with a transition-state analog: Understanding catalysis and immunodeficiency mutations. Science 252:1278-1284; 1991.

PART XII

Exercise and Bone Metabolism

CHAPTER 43

Exercise and Bone Metabolism: An Overview

Everett L. Smith

University of Wisconsin, Madison, Wisconsin, U.S.A.

Skeletal modeling and remodeling processes depend on mechanical strain and systemic hormonal stimuli to maintain structural integrity (or strength) and serum calcium homeostasis, respectively. Bone strength or resistance to fracture is a function of bone mass or bone mineral density (BMD) and architecture (geometric and crystalline organization). The mechanical homeostatic mechanisms affect both quantity (BMD) and quality (architecture) of bones. For example, while the characteristic shape of a specific bone (such as the femur) is genetically determined, the organization of the trabeculae, osteons, and collagen fibers is biochemically and mechanically strain dependent. The loads applied to the skeleton in physical activities of daily living, primarily weight bearing and muscle contraction, provide a strain history and the minimal skeletal strength and protection against fracture from unexpected loads. Within a rather broad normal range for each individual, variation in the levels of mechanical loading through physical activity will not generate modeling or remodeling, and therefore BMD will not change. A strain threshold at the cellular level must be exceeded in order for an osteogenic response to be induced. This osteogenic response is related to strain-induced changes in the cell mechanosensor that trigger second messengers in bone metabolism. The osteogenic or resorptive response is specific and proportional to the strain at the cell membrane mechanosensor level. If change is to occur, the strain stimulus must be above the membrane normal range level or set point for the individual. Too great an increase in mechanical loading or physical activity, however, may cause fracture or fatigue damage rather than hypertrophy.

Effects of Exercise on Bone Mineral Density

Exercise intervention studies of sedentary subjects have usually shown a beneficial effect on BMD. Subjects in these studies have ranged from young men (26) to middle-aged and elderly osteoporotic women (8, 23). Bone loss was ameliorated or BMD increased for arm bone mineral content (BMC) (42, 44, 46, 47, 53), total body calcium (1), spine BMD (10, 14, 23), Calcium Bone Index (CaBI, a measurement of calcium content by neutron activation analysis of the central third of the body; 7, 8), tibia BMC (26), and femur BMD (29).

Femur BMD was positively affected in only one (29) of the intervention studies in which it was measured (29, 31, 43). The three studies differed in subject population and in the length and type of training protocols. Subject populations consisted of men aged 59 ± 2 (29), premenopausal women of mean age 38 (43), and post-menopausal women (31). Menkes et al. (29) and Rockwell et al. (43) used resistance training as the major exercise intervention, while Moroz, Sale, and Webber (31) included bicycle ergometer training and unilateral arm resistance training. The two resistance training studies differed in the resistance exercises used, exercise intensity, and number of repetitions. Assigning the variance in results to specific factors is therefore not feasible.

Although exercise intervention studies have demonstrated mixed results when the femur is measured, cross-sectional studies have shown significant correlations between femur BMD and muscular strength (6, 55) or work capacity (6, 38). Also, Heinrich et al. (15) found significantly higher femoral BMD in young female athletes who engaged in resistance training than in nonathletes, swimmers, or runners.

The optimal physical activity regimes and diet for increasing BMD have not yet been determined. Cross-sectional studies comparing BMD in dominant and nondominant arms in tennis players confirm a localized response to loading (19, 22, 30). Intervention studies incorporating upper-arm activities or movement against resistance (42, 44, 46, 47, 53) had a significant effect on arm BMD, while other exercise programs did not (1, 23). Bone hypertrophy was related to the apparent level of strain on the bone in cross-sectional studies comparing weight lifters (greatest hypertrophy), aerobic athletes, and swimmers (least hypertrophy; 2, 11, 15, 33). Most interventions in which the spine or hip were studied have consisted primarily of general weight-bearing aerobic exercise. When resistance training was added to a general exercise program (7, 42), groups that added the resistance training did not differ significantly in BMD or CaBI from the groups participating only in the general exercise program. Mixed results have been obtained in interventions consisting solely of resistance training. Two studies of postmenopausal women reported that resistance training increased spine BMD but not calcaneus, femur, or distal forearm BMD (14, 39). Other studies, however, found that resistance training did not affect vertebral BMD in postmenopausal women (34, 45) and that spine bone loss was increased in premenopausal women (43).

Mechanical Strain Homeostasis

Mechanical homeostasis optimizes skeletal strength by controlling the modeling and remodeling processes that maintain bone quantity and quality. In both soft and hard tissue, mechanical loading of the skeleton induces strain (change in length divided by length, $\Delta L/L$). Skeletal quantity, quality, and architecture are maintained by mechanical homeostatic mechanisms responsive to changes in strain relative to the strain history.

Bone is influenced by both strain magnitude and strain rate (25). Static strain has little effect on bone, while changes in dynamic strain relative to the strain history cause bone adaptation. Modeling and remodeling processes and cellular activity in response to mechanical loading are now being more clearly described. Osteoclast activity increases and osteoblast activity decreases with disuse, while osteoblastic formation increases and osteoclastic resorption decreases or does not change with mechanical loading above threshold levels. The intermediate steps between strain and bone cell response have not been clearly determined, but they appear to occur via second messenger pathways.

In order to more clearly understand the underlying control mechanisms at the cellular level, a number of in vitro models have been developed. In cell cultures, a variety of methods have been used to load osteoblasts. These include stretching thin sheets of tendon seeded with osteoblasts, using flexible culture dish floors that induce stretch on the cells when deformed, and creating flow chambers that provide strain by changes in flow pressures. In organ cultures, an extracted core of bone tissue is usually loaded with mechanically or hydraulically induced compression. In both cell and organ cultures, cellular responses are induced by directly straining the cultured cells, with the environment controlled for hormonal and mechanical stimuli. In organ culture, however, the living cells are maintained in a controlled environment that includes the calcified bone matrix.

Brighton et al. (3) used a specially constructed culture chamber where osteoblasts could be subjected to low-amplitude mechanical strain, while Reich and Frangos (40) used pressure to induce strain in cell cultures. In this controlled environment, the strain induced a significant increase in cell proliferation and levels of prostaglandin E_2 (PGE_2). Brighton et al. (3) hypothesized that the greater osteoblast proliferation was mediated in part by the increased levels of prostaglandin.

Regardless of the model used, the increased level of prostaglandin E_2 seems to be mediated by a receptor-triggered activation event from a mechanosensitive area of the cell membrane. The response is similar to that of hormonal receptor-triggered activation common to the second messenger pathways of adenylate cyclase and inositol phosphate cascades. In second messenger pathways, an extracellular stimulus is converted to an intracellular message without itself entering the cell. The cascade of events occurs in response to the mechanical stimulus and results in three intracellular messengers: adenosine 3',5'-monophosphate (cyclic AMP, cAMP), inositol 1,4,5-trisphospate (IP_3), and diacylglycerol (DAG; figure 43.1). IP_3 and DAG are formed by the cleavage of phosphatidyl inositol 4,5-bisphosphate (PIP_2). These two pathways are common to endothelial, muscle, fibroblast, and bone cells. The adenylate cyclase and inositol phosphate cascades are the hormonal receptor-triggered activation pathways for both calcitonin and parathyroid hormones.

The receptor-triggered activation converts an extracellular signal to an intracellular signal. In the inositol phosphate cascade, activation of phospholipase C, a membrane-bound enzyme, hydrolyzes PIP_2, a phospholipid in the cell membrane, into two intracellular messengers, IP_3 and DAG. IP_3 causes the rapid release of calcium (Ca^{2+}) from the endoplasmic reticulum, thereby activating many intracellular processes. IP_3 is also phosphorylated to inositol 1,3,4,5-tetrakisphosphate (IP_4), which further increases cytosolic Ca^{2+} by transiently opening calcium channels in the cell membrane. DAG-activated protein kinase C (PKC) is also a membrane-bound, calcium-dependent enzyme that phosphorylates cellular proteins and activates enzymes important in controlling cell division and proliferation. DAG is also degraded enzymatically to release arachidonic acid, which is required for the production of prostaglandins.

The adenylate cyclase cascade leads to increased levels of cAMP, which is universal in nearly all cell biochemical pathways as a second messenger. Cyclic

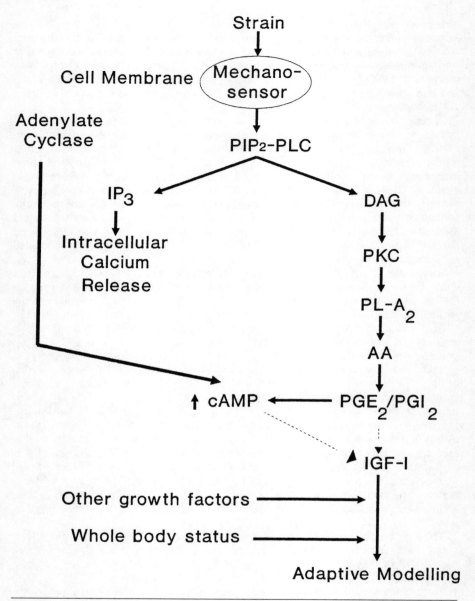

Figure 43.1   Proposed biochemical pathways following mechanical stimuli (24, 27). PIP_2 = phosphatidyl inositol 4,5-bisphosphate; PLC = phospholipase C; IP_3 = inositol 1,4,5-trisphosphate; DAG = diacylglycerol; PKC = protein kinase C; $PL-A_2$ = phospholipase A_2; AA = arachidonic acid; PGE_2 = prostaglandin E_2; PGI_2 = prostacyclin; cAMP = adenosine 3',5'-cyclic monophosphate; IGF-I = insulinlike growth factor.
Reprinted with permission of Everett L. Smith.

AMP is formed from ATP by the action of membrane-bound adenylate cyclase. This occurs in response to a membrane receptor-triggered activation by a hormonal, mechanical, or sensory stimulus to the membrane. Consequent to the activation of adenylate cyclase, cAMP is derived from ATP by the hydrolysis of pyrophosphate. The formation and release of cAMP into the cytosol results in the liberation of PKC and numerous other processes in cell metabolism.

The specific cells in the bone matrix that sense changes in strain and that control skeletal response have not been clearly determined. Lanyon (25) suggested that lining cells and osteocytes may be well situated morphologically to serve this role. Osteocytes and lining cells number as high as 20,000 cells per cubic millimeter and are interconnected via gap junctions (32, 36). In cell and organ cultures, these cells have shown responses to changes in mechanical strain. Both the lining cells and osteocytes have been shown to transduce mechanical strain into second messengers. Pead et al. (37) showed the transformation of quiescent lining cells to metabolically active osteoblasts 5 d after a single period of loading. El Haj et al. (13) observed significantly greater radioactive [^{3}H]uridine-labeled RNA in osteocytes 6 h after loading than in unloaded cores from the same dogs.

Membrane Mechanosensors

In the past few years, it has become clear that mechanical strain is transduced by mechanosensitive areas of the cell membrane to a biochemical signal in both animals and plants. The Venus flytrap and the Characeous alga are two plants that respond to mechanical stimuli by electrical charges and biochemical second messengers (17, 35, 52). The cellular response seems to correspond to the magnitude of the stimulus. In the skeletal system, mechanical loading that induces matrix strain is transduced into biochemical messages by receptor-triggered activation of osteoblasts, lining cells, and osteocytes. Many other cells in animals, such as capillary endothelial cells, muscle cells, and fibroblasts, have shown responses to mechanical stimuli. The stimulus may be the transduction of mechanical stress, pressure, or even possibly electrical charges into a biochemical signal that results in increased metabolic activity of the cell, inducing repair, proliferation, or hypertrophy.

Changes in cellular concentrations of prostaglandin E_2 (PGE_2) have been shown to mediate bone modeling and remodeling (41). When osteoblasts and osteocytes, in culture or bone matrix, are mechanically stimulated sufficiently to induce cellular strain, PGE_2 concentrations increase. Various bone preparations and methods of inducing strain—for example, compressive loads on bone biopsy core organ cultures, stretching, or increased fluid stress—have all increased prostaglandin PGE_2 synthesis (9, 12, 18, 24, 40, 41, 50, 54). Adenosine 3',5'-cyclic monophosphate (cAMP) and insulin-like growth factor (IGF-I) both increase subsequent to the rise in PGE_2. Hock, Centrella, and Canalis (16) reported that DNA synthesis increased in osteogenic periosteal cells proportionally to the increase in IGF-I.

Biochemical events and osteogenic responses have also been observed with doses of exogenous PGI_2, PGE_2, and estrogen in osteoblast organ culture. McCarthy et al. (28) observed an 8- to 54-fold increase in cAMP and a greater than 4-fold increase in prepro-IGF-I transcript levels when they dosed an osteoblast culture with .01 to 1 μM of PGE_2. Cheng, Zaman, and Lanyon (5) cultured the ulnar shafts from 110-g male rats and placed them in a loading chamber for 24 to 32 h. After a preincubation period of 5 h in the culture medium, one of each pair of ulnae was treated either by loading or perfusion with exogenous prostaglandins or estradiol. The ulnae were loaded cyclically with 500 g at 1 Hz for 8 min, providing −1,300 microstrain ($\mu\varepsilon$). The other ulnae were perfused with PGE_2 or PGI_2 (10 μM, 8 min) in the presence or absence of 17β-estradiol in the loading chamber. The 8-min exposure to either the mechanical strain or exogenous PGs plus estradiol produced an almost immediate increase in G6PD from osteoblasts and osteocytes. After sectioning and analyzing samples of the ulnae, it was found that the perfusion of the PGE_2 and PGI_2 had produced uniform distribution of G6PD in rat ulnae, while the cyclic loading resulted in a local G6PD distribution where the strain was concentrated in the osteocytes and osteoblasts. In addition to the G6PD response, Cheng, Zaman, and Lanyon (5) also reported significantly greater incorporation of [^{3}H]proline into collagen when the ulnae were either loaded or exposed to PGI_2 or PGE_2 for 8 min. Significantly greater alkaline phosphatase (ALP) activity was found only in the presence of loading or PGI_2. Estradiol exposure increased [^{3}H]proline incorporation into collagen, and either loading or PGI_2 magnified this response. Cheng, Zaman, and Lanyon (5) concluded that the osteogenic response of the cultured ulnae was enhanced by estrogen and loading together.

Jee et al. (20) used 5.5-month-old female rats to study the potential of PGE_2 to restore trabecular bone in the proximal tibia of ovariectomized (OX) rats. OX rats had 78% less bone after 5 mo when compared with control (sham-OX) rats. Thereafter, treatment with 6 mg/kg of PGE_2 was administered to the OX rats for 75 d. The PGE_2-treated rats increased bone formation rate and mineral apposition rate, and the ratio of formation to resorption increased from 0.6 to 5.8. The treated OX rats also had a significant decrease in percentage eroded surface and shortened bone resorption periods. While the treatment did not restore all of the bone that was lost in the OX animals, their bone mass increased to 47% that of the sham-OX control group. When PGE_2 treatment was withdrawn, however, resorption once again exceeded formation except when risedronate (a bisphosphonate) was used. This reduced osteoclastic resorption and resulted in a bone-sparing effect and maintenance of the trabecular bone gained by the PGE_2 treatment (49).

Carvalho et al. (4) investigated the regulation of the adenylate cyclase and the inositol phosphate pathways in osteoblast cell culture both with and without the addition of parathyroid hormone (PTH). Using the Flexercell system, mechanical strain was applied intermittently with 20 kPa of vacuum at 0.05 Hz for periods of 0.5, 1, 10, and 30 min and 1, 3, and 7 d. Increased levels of IP_3, PKC activity, and (within 10 min) cAMP were observed. These responses were enhanced with the addition of PTH during loading. Carvalho et al. (4) also noted that the cytoskeletal proteins vimentin, α-actinin, and focal contact protein vinculi showed a marked difference in alignment and orientation between strained and unstrained cultures. The re-alignment of cytoskeletal proteins along the lines of strain may be reflected in the orientation of collagen fibers in and architecture of the larger bone matrix.

It can be concluded from the studies reviewed that PGI_2, PGE_2, IGF-I, PTH, and estrogen are essential in the control and development of messages and the enhancement of those messages in skeletal modeling and remodeling.

While the sequence of biochemical events that leads to an osteogenic response from the osteoblast and osteocyte after mechanical loading are not entirely understood, a sequence of biochemical events may be suggested. Biochemical changes in the cell membrane have been observed within seconds after mechanical loading by strain or pressure. Following a load of 3,000 $\mu\epsilon$, Jones et al. (21) observed changes within milliseconds to 10 s in phosphoinositol, phospholipase C, and IP_3. Increased levels of IP_3 release calcium from the endoplasmic reticulum, resulting in the rapid rise in intracellular calcium. PKC and phospholipase A_2 activation also occur within 2 to 5 min after loading, both of which are important in the enzymatic degradation of DAG and the release of arachidonic acid required to synthesize PGE_2 and PGI_2 (21, 41, 51). A hypothesized sequence of events from the time of mechanical stimuli until the synthesis of IGF-I has been summarized from the literature (see figure 43.1). When this sequence is initiated (biochemically with PTH or mechanically), PGI_2, PGE_2, and IGF-I are produced and mediate bone modeling and remodeling.

References

1. Aloia, J.F.; Cohn, S.H.; Osuni, J.; Cane, R.; Ellis, K. Prevention of involutional bone loss by exercise. Ann. Intern. Med. 89:356-358; 1978.
2. Block, J.; Genant, H.K.; Black, D. Greater vertebral bone mineral in exercising young men. West. J. Med. 145:39-42; 1986.
3. Brighton, C.T.; Sennett, B.J.; Farmer, J.C.; Iannotti, J.P.; Hansen, C.A.; Williams, J.L.; Williamson, J. The inositol phosphate pathway as a mediator in the proliferative response of rat calvarial bone cells to cyclical biaxial mechanical strain. J. Orthoped. Res. 10:385-393; 1992.
4. Carvalho, R.S.; Scott, J.E.; Suga, D.M.; Yen, E.H.K. Stimulation of signal transduction pathways in osteoblasts by mechanical strain potentiated by parathyroid hormone. J. Bone Mineral Res. 9:999-1011; 1994.
5. Cheng, M.Z.; Zaman, G.; Lanyon, L.E. Oestrogen enhances the stimulation of bone collagen synthesis by loading and erogenous prostacyclin, but not prostaglandin E_2, in organ cultures of rat ulnae. J. Bone Mineral Res. 9:805-816; 1994.
6. Chow, R.K.; Harrison, J.E.; Brown, C.F.; Hajek, V. Physical fitness effect on bone mass in postmenopausal women. Arch. Phys. Med. Rehabil. 67:231-234; 1986.
7. Chow, R.K.; Harrison, J.E.; Notarius, C. Effect of two randomized exercise programmes on bone mass of healthy postmenopausal women. Br. Med. J. 292:607-610; 1987.
8. Chow, R.K.; Harrison, J.E.; Sturtbridge, W.; Josse, R.; Murray, T.M.; Bayley, A.; Dornan, J.; Hammond, T. The effect of exercise on bone mass of osteoporotic patients on fluoride treatment. Clin. Invest. Med. 10:59-63; 1987.
9. Dallas, S.L.; Zaman, G.; Pead, M.J.; Lanyon, L.E. Early strain-related changes in cultured embryonic chick tibiotarsi parallel those associated with adaptive modelling in vivo. J. Bone Mineral Res. 8:251-259; 1993.
10. Dalsky, G.P.; Stocke, K.S.; Ehsani, A.A.; Slatopolsky, E.; Lee, W.C.; Birge, S.J. Weight-bearing exercise training and lumbar bone mineral content in postmenopausal women. Ann. Intern. Med. 108:824-828; 1988.
11. Davee, A.M.; Rosen, C.J.; Adler, R.A. Exercise patterns and trabecular bone density in college women. J. Bone Mineral Res. 5:245-250; 1990.
12. Dodds, R.A.; Ali, N.; Pead, M.J.; Lanyon, L.E. Early loading-related changes in the activity of glucose 6-phosphate dehydrogenase and alkaline phosphatase in osteocytes and periosteal osteoblasts in rat fibulae in vivo. J. Bone Mineral Res. 8:261-267; 1993.

13. El Haj, A.J.; Minter, S.L.; Rawlinson, S.C.F.; Suswillo, R.; Lanyon, L.E. Cellular responses to mechanical loading in vitro. J. Bone Mineral Res. 5:923-932; 1990.
14. Gleeson, P.B.; Protas, E.J.; LeBlanc, A.D.; Schneider, V.S.; Evans, H.J. Effects of weight lifting on bone mineral density in premenopausal women. J. Bone Mineral Res. 5:153-158; 1990.
15. Heinrich, C.H.; Going, S.B.; Pamenter, R.W.; Perry, C.D.; Boyden, T.W.; Lohman, T.G. Bone mineral content of cyclically menstruating female resistance and endurance trained athletes. Med. Sci. Sports Exercise 22:558-563; 1990.
16. Hock, J.M.; Centrella, M.; Canalis, E. Insulin-like growth factor I (IGF-I) has independent effects on bone matrix formation and cell 14 replication. Endocrinology 122:254-260; 1988.
17. Hodick, D.; Sievers, A. On the mechanism of trap closure of Venus flytrap (*Dionaca mucipula ellis*). Planta 179:32-42; 1989.
18. Hsieh, H.-J.; Li, N.-Q.; Frangos, J.A. Shear stress increases endothelial platelet-derived growth factor mRNA levels. Am. J. Physiol. 260:H642-H646; 1991.
19. Huddleston, A.L.; Rockwell, D.; Kulund, D.N.; Harrison, R.B. Bone mass in lifetime tennis athletes. JAMA 244:1107-1109; 1980.
20. Jee, W.S.S.; Tang, L.; Ke, H.Z.; Setterberg, R.B.; Kimmel, D.B. Maintaining restored bone with bisphosphonate in the ovariectomized rat skeleton: Dynamic histomorphometry of changes in bone mass. Bone 14:493-498; 1993.
21. Jones, D.B.; Nolte, H.; Scholubbers, J.-G.; Turner, E.; Veltel, D. Biochemical signal transduction of mechanical strain in osteoblast-like cells. Biomaterials 12:101-110; 1991.
22. Jones, H.H.; Priest, J.D.; Hayes, W.C. Humeral hypertrophy in response to exercise. J. Bone Joint Surg. 59A:204-208; 1977.
23. Krolner, B.; Toft, B.; Nielsen, S.P.; Tondevold, E. Physical exercise as prophylaxis against involutional vertebral bone loss: A controlled trial. Clin. Sci. 64:541-546; 1983.
24. Lanyon, L.E. Control of bone architecture by functional load bearing. J. Bone Mineral Res. 7(S2):S369-S375; 1992.
25. Lanyon, L.E. Strain-related bone modelling and remodelling. Top. Geriatr. Rehabil. 4:13-24; 1989.
26. Margulies, J.Y.; Simkin, A.; Leichter, I.; Bivas, A.; Steinberg, R.; Giladi, M.; Stein, M.; Kashtan, H.; Milgrom, C. Effect of intense physical activity on the bone-mineral content in the lower limbs of young adults. J. Bone Joint Surg. 68(A):1090-1093; 1986.
27. Mayer, R.J.; Marshall, L.A. New insights on mammalian phospholipase A_2(s): Comparison of arachidonoyl-selective and nonselective enzymes. FASEB J. 7:339-348; 1993.
28. McCarthy, T.L.; Centrella, M.; Raisz, L.G.; Canalis, E. Prostaglandin E_2 stimulates insulin-like growth factor I synthesis in osteoblast-enriched cultures from fetal rat bone. Endocrinology 128:2895-2900; 1991.
29. Menkes, A.; Mazel, S.; Redmond, R.A.; Koffler, K.; Libanati, C.R.; Gundberg, C.M.; Zizic, T.M.; Hagberg, J.M.; Pratley, R.E.; Hurley, B.F. Strength training increases regional bone mineral density and bone remodelling in middle-aged and older men. J. Appl. Physiol. 74(5):2478-2484; 1993.
30. Montoye, H.J.; Smith, E.L.; Fardon, D.F.; Howley, E.T. Bone mineral in senior tennis players. Scand. J. Sports Sci. 2:26-32; 1980.
31. Moroz, D.; Sale, D.; Webber, C. The effect of intensive training on axial and appendicular bone mineral in normal postmenopausal women. J. Bone Mineral Res. 4:S233; 1989. (Abstract).

32. Mundy, G.R. Bone resorbing cells. In: Favus, M.J., ed. Primer on the metabolic bone diseases and disorders of mineral metabolism. Kelseyville, CA: American Society for Bone and Mineral Research; 1990:18-22.
33. Nilsson, B.E.; Westlin, N.E. Bone density in athletes. Clin. Orthoped. Relat. Res. 77:179-182; 1971.
34. Notelovitz, M.; Martin, D.; Tesar, R.; Khan, F.Y.; Probart, C.; Fields, C.; McKenzie, L. Oestrogen therapy and variable-resistance weight training increase bone mineral in surgically menopausal women. J. Bone Mineral Res. 6:583-590; 1991.
35. Okihara, K.; Ohkawa, T.; Tsutsui, I.; Kasai, M. A Ca^{2+} and voltage-dependent Cl-sensitive anion channel in the *Characea* plasmalemma: A patchclamp study. Plant Cell Physiol. 32:593-601; 1991.
36. Parfitt, A.M. The physiologic and clinical significance of bone histomorphometric data. In: Recker, R.R., ed. Bone histomorphometry: Techniques and interpretation. CRC Press: Boca Raton, FL; 1983:143.
37. Pead, M.J.; Suswillo, R.; Skerry, T.M.; Vedi, S.; Lanyon, L.E. Increased I [^{3}H]uridine levels in osteocytes following a single short period of dynamic bone loading in vivo. Calcif. Tissue Int. 45:647-656; 1988.
38. Pocock, N.A.; Eisman, J.A.; Yeates, M.G.; Sambrook, P.N.; Eberl, S. Physical fitness is a major determinant of femoral neck and lumbar spine bone mineral density. J. Clin. Inv. 78:618-621; 1986.
39. Pruitt, L.A.; Jackson, R.D.; Bartels, R.L.; Lehnard, H.J. Weighttraining effects on bone mineral density in early postmenopausal women. J. Bone Mineral Res. 7:179-185; 1992.
40. Reich, K.M.; Frangos, J.A. Effect of flow on prostaglandin E_2 and inositol trisphosphate levels in osteoblasts. Am. J. Physiol. 261:C428-C432; 1991.
41. Reich, K.M.; Frangos, J.A. Protein kinase c mediates flow-induced prostaglandin E_2 production in osteoblasts. Calcif. Tissue Int. 52:62-66; 1993.
42. Rikli, R.E.; McManis, B.G. Effects of exercise on bone mineral content in postmenopausal women. Res. Q. Exercise Sport 61:243-249; 1990.
43. Rockwell, J.C.; Sorenson, A.M.; Baker, S.; Leahey, D.; Stock, J.L.; Michaels, J.; Baran, D.T. Weight training decreases vertebral bone density in premenopausal women: A prospective study. J. Clin. Endocrinol. Metab. 71:988-993; 1990.
44. Simkin, A.; Ayalon, J.; Leichter, I. Increased trabecular bone density due to bone-loading exercises in postmenopausal osteoporotic women. Calcif. Tissue Int. 40:59-63; 1986.
45. Sinaki, M.; Wahner, H.W.; Offord, K.P.; Hodgson, S.F. Efficacy of nonloading exercises in prevention of vertebral bone loss in postmenopausal women: A controlled trial. Clin. Proc. 64:S762-S769; 1989.
46. Smith, E.L.; Gilligan, C.; Shea, M.M.; Ensign, P.; Smith, P.E. Exercise reduces bone involution in middle-aged women. Calcif. Tissue Int. 44:312-321; 1989.
47. Smith, E.L.; Reddan, W.; Smith, P.E. Physical activity and calcium modalities for bone mineral increase in aged women. Med. Sci. Sports Exercise 13:60-64; 1981.
48. Stryer, L. Biochemistry. 3rd ed. New York: W.H. Freeman and Co.; 1988.
49. Tang, L.Y.; Jee, W.S.S.; Ke, H.Z.; Kimmel, D.B. Restoring and maintaining bone in osteopenic female rat skeleton: I. Changes in bone mass and structure. J. Bone Mineral Res. 7:1093-1104; 1992.
50. Walsh, W.R.; Guzelsu, N. Ion concentration effects on bone streaming potentials and zeta potentials. Biomaterials 14:331-336; 1993.

51. Watson, P.A. Function follows form: Generation of intracellular signals by cell deformation. Fed. Am. Soc. Exp. Biol. J. 5:2013-2019; 1991.
52. Wayne, R. Excitability in plant cells. Am. Sci. 81:140-151; 1993.
53. White, M.K.; Martin, R.B.; Yeater, R.A.; Butcher, R.L.; Radin, E.L. The effects of exercise on the bones of postmenopausal women. Int. Orthoped. 7:209-214; 1984.
54. Zaman, G.; Dallas, S.L.; Lanyon, L.E. Cultured embryonic bone shafts show osteogenic responses to mechanical loading. Calcif. Tissue Int. 51:132-136; 1992.
55. Zimmerman, C.L.; Smidt, G.L.; Brooks, J.S.; Kensey, W.J.; Eekhoff, T.L. Relationship of extremity muscle torque and bone mineral density in post-menopausal women. Phys. Therapy 70:302-309; 1990.

CHAPTER 44

Mechanical Signal Transduction in Skeletal Tissues

David Jones, Gunnar Leivseth

Department of Experimental Orthopaedics and Biomechanics, Phillips University, Marburg, Germany; Department of Physiology, University of Tromso, Tromso, Norway

Nearly all types of cells, prokaryotic and eukaryotic, respond to the mechanical environment: environmental stresses (e.g., wind or activity), vibrations (e.g., sound), or self-induced stress. Self-induced stress is involved in cell division, for instance, and may be due to contractions of the actin cytoskeleton, which may cause motion or cell tension, but may also be due to the action of muscles on other tissues. Gravity is also thought to produce biological responses through mechanoreceptors. The specific cellular responses are certainly regulated by the amplitude of the mechanical loading and, to an extent, the frequency too. The response may be movement, synthesis of specific proteins, or cell division and is mainly regulated by second messenger systems. Self-induced mechanical stress is also thought to play a role in embryological development (2). One hypothesis holds that it is distortion of some cellular component that is transduced into a cell biological or electrophysiological response. Other hypotheses will be briefly treated later. In some single-cell organisms, organelles have adapted into vibration sensors and can elicit evasive or aggressive responses. In general, these organelles appear to be either based on the microtubule cytoskeleton system or on the actin cytoskeleton and perhaps are evolved from the two types of locomotor systems (microtubular-ciliary system or actin crawling system). The biochemistry of cilia has been recently reviewed by Satir, Barkalow, and Hamasaki (19), so cilia will not be discussed in further detail here except to note that they are used by many cells as fluid flow sensors and that mechanically loading a cilium results in changes to intracellular calcium, showing that the system can be driven in both ways. These two primitive patterns have been adapted in multicellular organisms for a variety of purposes; for instance, some light-sensing organelles, such as the rods of vertebrate eyes, are derived from cilia. It appears that, although the original function of the sensor has been changed, the biochemical transduction mechanism has been preserved. In cells that have to sense small deformations, some simple mechanisms have evolved that can amplify the movements. The most common is the lever, based on the cilium, which is connected to a membrane in which ion channels are located. Specialized organs, usually of this lever type, exist in animals to transduce small mechanical loads, such as vibrations, and link this transducer to the nervous system. Strains induced by stresses in the swim bladder of fish are detected and can aid in prey capture or predator evasion. The sensory hairs of vestibular ampullae and in the cochlea are examples of a ciliary mechanosensor where small vibrations are amplified by exploiting the production of shear between two surfaces (26).

Plants, too, can adapt to environmental wind forces and also to gravity (5). One of the biochemical transduction mechanisms involved, intracellular free calcium, appears to be identical to one of those that will be discussed later.

Apart from the sensing of mechanical deformations for sensing prey or predators and for defense, mechanical loading is also of great importance for multicellular organisms in maintaining tissue fitness. Most tissues model according to the mechanical loads put on them. They can be reduced in fitness if the loads are too low, be maintained or increased in fitness within a specific physiological range, and induce inflammation or fail when overloaded. Although it has been known since prehistory, most probably, that training increases fitness and although in the last century large programs of sport for health have been promoted in many countries, it is only within the last three years that medicine has placed a fundamental importance on exercise and training for general health, rehabilitation, and repair. This has come about through the ability to apply defined mechanical loads to cells and tissues and through advances in cellular and molecular biological techniques.

Having too much tissue in a high functional state is wasteful. Low-performance tissue means that the organism cannot meet the demands of the environment. This is especially so for skeletal and heart muscle, blood vessels, bone, skin, and lung epithelium. A sensing system with feedback operates in these tissues to maintain the optimal functionality of tissue, which is balanced between breakdown and buildup. For bone, this has been described as Wolff's law after Julius Wolff, who in 1882 postulated that bone adapts to mechanical loads to produce structures best fitted to withstand these forces. This principle is true of other tissues too. Whereas the mechanical loads on skin and muscle normally can result in strains of up to 120% on the cells, in bone the mechanical loading results in strains up to 0.5% (at which point bone begins to fracture), but more typically 0.3%. This places the strain-transducing mechanism(s) of bone cells at among the most sensitive, nearly equaling that of specialized organs such as the hearing apparatus. It is normal to describe changes in length using the dimensionless term *microstrain* (με). We can define strain (S) as the change in length (new length [l'] minus the original length [l]) divided by the original length, although there are other definitions that vary slightly:

$$S = (l' - l)/l$$

One unit of strain (in tension) is thus a doubling in length, so a 0.3% increase in length is 3,000 με. It is more convenient to use the term *microstrains* to avoid confusion between percentage change in tension and in compression.

The Role of the Strain Environment in Bone

The strains induced in bone by physical exercise were first measured accurately using strain gauges glued to bone by Lanyon (15). Lanyon and his colleagues established that in all weight-bearing bones so far studied, the maximal peak physiological strain is about 3,000 $\mu\epsilon$, and the lowest consistent with maintaining bone mass was 300 $\mu\epsilon$. Bone mass was maintained above 300 $\mu\epsilon$ and increased above 1,500 $\mu\epsilon$. Investigations into the rate at which strain was applied showed that the physiological effects of loading of bone were also frequency dependent (17). The word *peak* is emphasized here because, due to the shape and the way stresses are applied to the bone by the muscles, the surface strains vary in direction and amplitude at any one place. Depending on the species and the bone, bones generally bend in one major axis and twist slightly. Thus, one area of the surface has a peak tensile strain, and the opposite an area subjected to compressive strains. The neutral axis is in between and swings through about 40° as the bone twists. This means that not all the cells in bone experience the peak strains, and therefore their response must also be coordinated with those that receive the mechanical signal. If, however, the bone is loaded in an abnormal direction, say at right angles to the normal strain direction, a large amount of bone is produced in reaction to levels of strain that would normally just maintain bone mass. It can be hypothesized from these observations that the direction of strain is also sensed. Later we describe a mechanism that we hypothesize to link the strain-sensing transducer with the cytoskeleton and to allow the cell to relax in one direction and become amplitude sensitive in another. The strain response, however, is local to the bone that is loaded, and no significant systemic effects or effects on nearby bones have been detected.

Osteoporosis and Exercise

Osteoporosis is the clinical presentation of the consequences of loss of bone from various sites in the body (osteopenia), for which there are many causes. As pointed out by many reports in the literature and in the press, the fact that postmenopausal osteoporosis (PMO) is one of the major causes of death in women in the Western world indicates that at present there is too little knowledge about the cause of, possible therapies for, or the means to distinguish between the various manifestations of the disease. Osteoporosis has more than one cause, but the importance of inheritability and mechanical factors to skeletal mass cannot be overstated. Although the most serious of the osteoporotic diseases is PMO, osteoporosis also occurs with disuse, in ovariectomized women, in juveniles, and in elderly and alcoholic males. High turnover osteoporosis might be different from low turnover, and some rapidly developing osteoporoses might be a previously unrecognized type of osteogenesis imperfecta (24). Both male and female athletes can suffer from osteopenia; in females, osteopenia may be a consequence of hypothalamically induced amenorrhea (29).

It was recently suggested by Frost (4) that the sensitivity of the mechanotransducer in bone to mechanical loading, the mechanostat, is altered by the hormonal balance of the body; that is, the minimal effective level of strain needed to prevent disuse osteoporosis is altered by certain circulating factors. It is proposed that in osteopenia the level at which the mechanostat switches on is increased so that bone cannot maintain itself by normal loading; that is, the threshold found by Lanyon and Rubin (15, 17; previously discussed) is increased. There is some evidence to suggest that the change in mechanostat sensitivity is site specific, since cortical bone appears to be mechanically stimulated in some osteoporotic patients while the spongiosa continues to decline. Other factors that might affect the sensitivity of the mechanostat appear to be steroid hormones, especially estrogen in women. The mechanisms by which hormones, cytokines, and other factors interact with the mechanosensory apparatus has not yet really been investigated in bone or any other tissue. Some of the possible interactions and synergism between mechanical loading and cytokines, growth hormones, hormones, and other factors are discussed in more detail later. Exercise has been shown by a number of studies to be effective in increasing several parameters of bone mechanical properties. The studies of Smith et al. (23) and Simkin et al. (21, 22) were among the first undertaken.

A large number of investigations have been published on the effect of exercise on bone in animals and humans, measured in many different ways. More details about these are found in the review papers of Smith (chapter 43), Raab-Cullen (chapter 46), and Skerry (chapter 45).

Biophysical Mechanisms

Many theories have been advanced as to the mechanisms by which cells can sense mechanical loading. Some of these are listed in table 44.1. Electrical signals arising from piezoelectricity (especially in bone) and streaming potentials when tissue is deformed were proposed by Bassett and Becker (1) as the physiological trigger for Wolff's law. The hypothesis of strain-related potential has been supported by a large number of articles (e.g., 7) and by studies using direct current and alternating current electrodes placed in the bone. Although weak electrical fields have been shown conclusively to induce galvanotaxis, whether streaming potentials really play a role in bone or any other tissue is still debated.

We have performed experiments using a four-point bending apparatus (11), in which the amount of bending to produce a certain amplitude of strain depends on the thickness of the plate. A thin plate can be bent as much as a thick plate but does not develop a significant strain on the surface (12). In these experiments, the biological response was dependent on the strain amplitude and not on the streaming potential.

Table 44.1   Proposed Mechanisms of Mechanical Transduction

Strain-related potentials (SRP)

Activation of ion channels

Membrane tension

Cytoskeleton connected

Cytoskeleton-coupled PLC

Mechanical lever (primary cilium)

Stretch-Activated Ion Channels

Many investigators have found what appear to be stretch-activated potassium channels, and stretch-activated calcium channels have also been described by Duncan and Misler (3) in osteoblasts. Stretch-activated ion channels have also been suggested to play a role in the muscular response to stretch. Certainly, direct effects of mechanical loading on ion channels are more or less implicit in organs and organelles that sense vibrations, but it is difficult to suggest that the ion channels are activated by an indirect mechanism in this case. However, our studies indicate that this is indeed the case for osteoblastic ion channel activation. One of the ways to distinguish between direct and indirect effects is to measure the speed of the response. As discussed later, intracellular free calcium (IFC) is involved in the mechanotransduction mechanism in many cells, including osteoblasts. IFC activates the potassium channel, and there would therefore be a lag in time between the rise in IFC and the increase in membrane potential. However, if the K$^+$ channel is activated by strain directly, there might not be such a delay. Certainly, the subsequent depolarization of the cell is due to the entry of calcium ions following the hyperpolarization. This was shown recently by Jones and Bingmann (11) and has been confirmed by Duncan (1993, personal communication) using different cells and methodology. An indirect effect on potassium channels and calcium channels through IFC release is supported by our data, but this needs further investigation. Other data suggest that the ion channels in endothelial cells are directly activated by fluid flow before a change in phospholipase C (PLC) activity increases IFC (9).

Membrane Tension

Some authors have suggested that mechanotransduction occurs through applying tension to the membrane, which changes the activity of proteins such as ion channels directly inserted into it (16). However, the breaking tension of the cell membrane is in the order of 300 $\mu\varepsilon$, but many models suggest that during mechanical stretch the cell membrane unfolds; thus, stretches of 0.5 strain are possible before the membrane is damaged. Certainly, the mechanical properties of the cell membrane are very important for many cells, such as red blood cells, that have to pass through capillaries, but measurements of membrane stiffness are intimately connected to the mechanical properties of the cytoskeleton.

Cytoskeleton

Several studies have implicated the cytoskeleton as a site for the location of the nonciliary mechanosensor. Certainly, the cytoskeleton structure is involved in the regulation of adenylate cyclase, as studies with cytoskeleton disrupting agents have shown (27). Ingber (10) has suggested that the proteins involved in adhesion to matrix adhesion proteins and cell adhesion proteins—the integrins—are responsible for mechanotransduction. Integrins are a family of heterodimeric transmembrane proteins that can bind specific regions of matrix proteins, the most common region being defined by three amino acids: arginine, glycine, and aspartic acid (RGD). Without having cells fixed to the surface, strain in the material would not be transferred to the cell. The adhesion sites are also the sites at which cells generate tension. That cells themselves are under tension was perhaps first shown by Harris (8), who showed that cells could contract a thin layer (20 nm) of silicone in specific patterns. This tension has since been measured using a number of different methods in a number of different types of cells, and a general force of about 2 mN has been found (27). This force is in good agreement with the measured strength of adhesion molecule–matrix interactions and with the numbers of these molecules at the focal points of the attachment site.

Why do cells develop tension? The question might be partially answered by examination of Brownian motion, or thermal noise, in cells. Most cells display a flickering, which over an area of 250 nm has amplitudes of up to 300 nm and frequencies of between 1 and 25 Hz (and thus are not observable under the light microscope). Korenstein et al. (14) have investigated this phenomenon recently with more accurate equipment and have shown that these membrane fluctuations are modified by the state of the underlying cytoskeleton. The fluctuations were measured in all cell types investigated, including osteoblasts. These observations imply that, since the background fluctuations are of a larger scale than the applied strain (over a cell with a diameter of 40 μm, a 3,000-$\mu\varepsilon$ stretch is only 120 nm), a mechanosensor linked purely to the membrane will be in the noise of the background fluctuations. Thus, some membrane-only models for mechanotransduction might be incorrect, because local bending moments of the membrane exceed the physiological range. One function of cell tension could be to lift the mechanosensor out of the thermal noise. A tension of 2 pN across the cell probably reduces the thermal noise in the attachment site–cytoskeleton complex to less than 1%. This is further evidence that mechanoreceptors are located in the cytoskeleton rather than just in the membrane.

Relaxation and Directional Loading

Applying mechanical loading to many cell types in vitro often results in an orientation of the cells with respect to the direction of strain. This orientation is not observed in osteoblasts when strains of physiological amplitudes are applied, only at hyperphysiological strains, which are associated with other changes in the cells (discussed later). However, the stress fibers of the actin cytoskeleton when formed in older cultures do change direction at physiological amplitudes. When this occurs, it can be shown that the cells are more sensitive to strains in the axis of the orientation of the stress fibers and less sensitive at right angles to the cytoskeleton. It thus appears that cells relax in the direction of the normal strain. In osteoblasts, this process takes several days in vitro and is similar to effects induced by PLC activators such as parathyroid hormone (PTH) and prostaglandin; these have been shown in a number of studies to depolymerize the actin cytoskeleton. We have seen similar responses to mechanical loading. It could be hypothesized that the orientation is simply guided by the depolymerization of the cytoskeleton and repolymerization in the orientation of a less sensitive direction, which has the consequence that a greater biological response can be obtained by loading eccentrically. This seems to be true in bone—as shown by Simkin and Ayalon (21), who used small loads applied in abnormal directions for PMO exercises—and also in muscle.

Second Messengers

Mechanical signals received by the cell must somehow influence the biochemical machinery. Cells have a relatively small number (perhaps around 20) of distinct pathways that are used for self-regulation. The situation is complex because many of these pathways interact, either immediately or after a delay, and these interactions can be positive or negative. In table 44.2, the possible mechanisms of a signal transduction cascade in an actin-based mechanosensor are listed.

Effects Due to Release of Translated Genes (TGF-β, IGF)

As previously discussed, the exact nature of the transducer and whether there are more than one, linked to different biochemical pathways, are unknown. Molecular biological analysis of the pathways points to the possibility of more than one transducer in heart muscle, as will be discussed later.

Analysis of the second messenger pathways involved is complicated by the fact that many pathways interact and by the difficulty of analysis on an adequate time

Table 44.2 Signal Cascade in Mechanotransduction

Transducer
  One
  Multiple

Second messenger
  One
  Multiple (this is most likely)

Immediate effects (within 1 s)
  PLC activation
  Gap junction communication
  Ion channel activation

Release of signaling molecules

Intermediate effects (within 1-2 min)
  Arachidonic acid metabolism

Late effects (2 min-6 h)
  Gene activation

Secondary effects

base (i.e., in seconds rather than minutes). Jones et al. (11, 13) used imaging techniques to measure intracellular free calcium (IFC) and showed changes due to physiological strains within 160 ms. Membrane potentials can be measured under strain using classical electrophysiological techniques and also by newer imaging techniques. Fast imaging techniques are now also possible for cAMP, protein kinase C, and some phospholipases, requiring in some cases cell injection facilities. However, other second messengers require classical biochemical techniques, which at their quickest require several seconds and much expensive work to establish the kinetics. During activation of kinases, the maximum activity is detected (and measurable) after several minutes, but activation is thought to occur within several seconds. In many cases the possible chain of causality has been lost. Thus, the quickest measurable second messenger system so far measured is the release of IFC through the activation of a phospholipase C. This now classical pathway is found in nearly every cell and is involved at a very basic level of cellular control. The pathway is activated by a receptor coupled to a specific G-protein (Gp), which activates the phosphatidyl inositol–specific PLC. PLC splits the substrate—phosphatidyl inositol 4,5-bisphosphate (PIP_2)—into diacylglycerol (DAG) and inositol 1,4,5-trisphosphate (IP_3). IP_3 acts on intracellular calcium stores through a receptor to release stored calcium intracellularly, while DAG activates PKC. In osteoblasts, this PKC belongs to the calcium-modulated PKC family. Many factors affecting bone—PTH, epidermal growth factor (EGF), fragments of fibronectin that have EGF-like sequences, platelet-derived growth factor (PDGF), vasoactive intestinal peptide (VIP, found in the sympathetic nerves of the periosteum) substance P, ATP, and prostaglandins (PGs), to name just a few—also activate PLC. Some, such as EGF and PDGF, activate at the same time a tyrosine kinase; others, such as PTH, many of the PGs, and VIP, simultaneously stimulate adenylate cyclase and thus stimulate the cAMP-dependent protein kinase pathways (PKA). Although there are indications that multiple second messenger pathways might occur in osteoblasts, muscle cells, and endothelial cells, at present there is no direct evidence to support this, but it is quite likely in view of the biological responses. After the initial second messenger starts the cascade of reactions, the next step in the biochemical transduction chain can occur within a second. This appears to be the case with gap junction communication (20). Potassium channels are activated by the increased levels of IFC, followed within 500 ms by an influx of calcium from outside (11), due to the hyperpolarization of the cell. Since the gap junctions probably serve as a smoothing system rather than a signal transduction system per se, release of signaling molecules, as in smooth muscle cells and vascular endothelium, will occur after stretch (6, 25). A diagram of this mechanism is shown in figure 44.1.

Figure 44.1 shows the interrelationship between various agonists of PLC, IFC, calcium channels, and growth factors such as EGF and PDGF. Factors such as prostaglandins stimulate a receptor that is possibly linked to PLC. EGF and PDGF, as examples of tyrosine kinase–receptor growth factors, can activate PLC through a region of the receptor kinase complex when they are autophosphorylated (SH2 regions). Recently, Sadoshima and Izumo (18) investigated mechanical loading of heart muscle cells and showed the stimulation of multiple signaling pathways, including PLC and PKC, after applying physiological loads to heart muscle cells in the induction of c-fos. The c-fos gene is also stimulated in osteoblast-like cells 25 min after applying mechanical loading (L. Suva, personal communication). It seems possible that microgravitational forces are analogous to mechanical loading and that the effects are transduced through the mechanoreception system previously described.

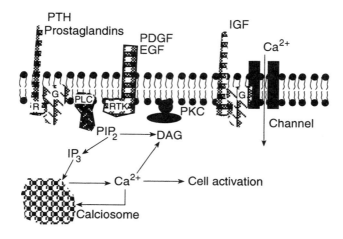

Figure 44.1   A diagram of the PLC-PKC-Ca^{2+} and Ca^{2+} channels activated by stretch, showing factors that possibly interact with the stretch sensor.

Strain Effects in Muscle

Strain effects in muscle appear to involve the same biochemical pathways as previously described for osteoblast and endothelial cells, although mechanically stimulated increases in IFC have not yet been measured in skeletal muscle and heart muscle. As for lung epithelial cells (28), the normal strain amplitudes are large (110-130%) in comparison with bone cells. As for all other cells so far investigated, prostaglandin synthesis is stimulated by physiological levels of strain. Much of what is known about regulation of genes by mechanical loading has been described using heart muscle cells, described later.

Gene Activation

The role of the second messengers is to activate some genes and to turn off others. Sadoshima and Izumo (18) investigated the control of c-*fos* expression and found that it is elevated by mechanical stretching of heart muscle cells. This work suggests the involvement of many pathways other than just PKC, Ca^{2+}, and PKA in strain transduction, but it is not known whether tyrosine kinases, for instance, are activated directly by the applied strain or are activated later in the cascade sequence.

Cell Communication

Not much attention has been directed to the importance of signaling molecules released immediately by strain in enabling communication with other cells in the tissue. This is important since tissue not only responds to the immediate strain environment, but can respond locally and as a whole organ. Gap junction communication in osteoblasts (20) does not appear to lead to any amplification mechanism of a signal, but rather a rectification of a hormonal or electrophysiological signal. The electrophysiological signal is degraded by 50% each time it passes through the junction. A consideration of the rate of diffusion, reduced by the viscosity of the cytoplasm and the small pores of the gap junctions, would also suggest that significant signals are perhaps not passed among cells this way. However, the gap junction network seems ideally suited for coordinating information about the distribution of strain within the tissue. The immediate release of signaling molecules might also play a significant role for short-term (minutes) modulation of the physiological response. Release of signaling molecules might be mediated by the depolarization of the membrane during calcium channel opening in a manner analogous to the mast cell degranulation. ATP is one of the many candidates, since osteoblasts possess ATP receptors linked to PLC, thus causing a positive feedback loop, a prerequisite for signal amplification. Factors other than PGE_2 might also be released from osteoblast membranes, which is a point for further investigation. Other growth factors, such as insulinlike growth factor II (IGF-II), could also be expected to be regulated by the strain-induced second messenger systems so far described. This process is dependent on mRNA synthesis, induced by the second messengers linked to the strain sensor.

Conclusions

Two general types of strain sensors appear to be present in nonnerve tissue: one based on the cilium and the other on an actin cytoskeleton–associated mechanism. The ciliary mechanism appears to be important to sense fluid flow. The cytoskeleton mechanism senses strain. In this sensor, intracellular calcium is increased first by PLC, and then a calcium channel is opened, due to cooperative effects of the increased calcium. A number of biochemical transduction mechanisms and intercellular messengers, similar in some respects to those stimulated by certain growth factors, lead to a coordinated tissue response. The sensor appears to be sensitive to the direction, frequency, and amplitude of the strain. Higher than normal strains lead to different cellular responses, undifferentiation of cells, and inflammation. Intelligent use of mechanical loading together with specific chemotherapies appears to hold much promise for the future.

References

1. Bassett, C.A.L.; Becker, R.O. Generation of electric potentials by bone in response to mechanical stress. Science 137:1063-1064; 1962.
2. Beloussov, L.V. The interplay of active forces and passive mechanical stresses in animal morphogenesis. In: Akkas, N., ed. Biomechanics of active movement and division of cells. Berlin, Heidelberg, New York, London, Paris, Tokyo: Springer-Verlag; 1994:369-392. (NATO ASI Ser. H. Cell Biol.).

3. Duncan, R.; Misler, S. Voltage-activated and stretch-activated Ba^{++} conducting channels in an osteoblast-like cell line (UMR 106). FEBS Lett. 251:17-21; 1989.
4. Frost, H. Vital biomechanics: Proposed general concepts for skeletal adaptations to mechanical usage. Calcif. Tissue Int. 42:145-156; 1988.
5. Gehring, C.A.; Williams, D.A.; Cody, S.H.; Parish, R.W. Phototropism and geotropism in maize coleoptiles are spatially correlated with increases in cytosolic free calcium. Nature 345:528-530; 1990.
6. Gibbons, G.H.; Dzau, V.J. The emerging concept of vascular remodelling. N. Engl. J. Med. 330:1431-1438; 1994.
7. Gjelsvik, A. Bone remodeling and piezoelectricity I. J. Biomech. 6:69-77; 1973.
8. Harris, A.K. Tissue culture cells on deformable substrata: Biomechanical implications. J. Biomech. Engin. 106:19-24; 1984.
9. Helminger, G.; Thoumine, O.; Wiesner, T.F.; Nerem, R.M. The active response of an endothelial cell to the onset of flow. In: Akkas, N., ed. Biomechanics of active movement and division of cells. Berlin, Heidelberg, New York, London, Paris, Tokyo: Springer-Verlag; 1994:369-392. (NATO ASI Ser. H. Cell Biol.).
10. Ingber, D. Integrins as mechanochemical transducers. Curr. Opin. Cell Biol. 3:841-848; 1991.
11. Jones, D.B.; Bingmann, D. How do osteoblasts respond to mechanical stimulation? Cells Methods 1:329-340; 1991.
12. Jones, D.B.; Leivseth, G.; Sawada, Y.; van der Sloten, J.; Bingmann, D. Application of homogenous, defined strains to cell cultures. In: Lyall, F.; El Haj, A.J., eds. Biomechanics and cells. Cambridge: Society for Experimental Biology/ Cambridge University Press; 1994:197-219.
13. Jones, D.B.; Nolte, H.; Scholübbers, J.-G.; Turner, E.; Veltel, D. Biochemical signal transduction of mechanical strain in osteoblast-like cells. Biomaterials 12:101-110; 1991.
14. Korenstein, R.; Tuvia, S.; Mittelman, L.; Levin, S. Local bending fluctuations of the cell membrane. In: Akkas, N., ed. Biomechanics of active movement and division of cells. Berlin, Heidelberg, New York, London, Paris, Tokyo: Springer-Verlag; 1994:369-392. (NATO ASI Ser. H. Cell Biol.).
15. Lanyon, L.E. In vivo bone strain recorded from thoracic vertebrae of sheep. J. Biomech. 5:277-281; 1972.
16. Petrov, A.G.; Usherwood, P.N.R. Mechanosensitivity of cell membranes. Ion channels, lipid matrix and cytoskeleton. Eur. Biophys. J. 23:1-19; 1994.
17. Rubin, C.T.; Lanyon, L.E. Regulation of bone mass by mechanical strain magnitude. Calcif. Tissue Int. 37:411-417; 1985.
18. Sadoshima, J.I.; Izumo, C. Mechanical stretch rapidly activates multiple signal transduction pathways in cardiac myocytes: Potential involvement of an autocrine/paracrine mechanism. EMBO J. 12:1681-1692; 1994.
19. Satir, P.; Barkalow, K.; Hamasaki, T. The control of ciliary beat frequency. Cell Biol. 3:409-412; 1993.
20. Schirrmacher, K.; Schmitz, I.; Winterhager, E.; Traub, O.; Bröummer, F.; Jones, D.B.; Bingmann, D. Characterisation of gap junctions between osteoblast-like cells in culture. Calcif. Tissue Int. 51:285-290; 1992.
21. Simkin, A.; Ayalon, J. Bone loading. London: Prion Multimedia Books, Ltd.; 1990.
22. Simkin, A.; Ayalon, J.; Leichter, I. Increased trabecular bone density due to bone-loading exercises in postmenopausal osteoporotic women. Calcif. Tissue Int. 40:59-63; 1987.

23. Smith, E.L.; Gilligan, C.; Mc Adam, M.; Ensign, C.P.; Smith, P.E. Deterring bone loss by exercise intervention in premenopausal and postmenopausal women. Calcif. Tissue Int. 44:312-321; 1989.

24. Spotila, L.D.; Constantinou, C.D.; Sereda, L. Mutation in a gene for type I procollagen (COLIA 2) in a woman with postmenopausal osteoporosis: Evidence for phenotypic and genotypic overlap with mild osteogenesis imperfecta. Proc. Natl. Acad. Sci. USA 88:5423-5427; 1994.

25. Sumpio, B.E.; Du, W.; Cohen, C.R.; Evans, L.; Isales, C.; Rosales, O.R.; Mills, I. Signal transduction pathways in vascular cells exposed to cyclic strain. In: Lyall, F.; El Haj, A.J. Biomechanics and cells. Cambridge: Cambridge University Press; 1994:3-22. (Soc. Exp. Biol. Ser. 54).

26. Thurm, U. Mechano-electric transduction. In: Hoppe, W.; Lohmann, W.; Markl, H.; Ziegler, H., eds. Biophysics. Berlin and Heidelberg: Springer-Verlag; 1983:666-671.

27. Watson, F.A. Function follows form: Generation of intracellular signals by cell deformation. FASEB J. 5:2013-2019; 1991.

28. Wirtz, H.R.W.; Dobbs, L.G. Calcium mobilisation and exocytosis after one mechanical stretch of lung epithelial cells. Science 298:1266-1269; 1990.

29. Wolman, R.L.; Faulmann, L.; Clark, P.T.I. Different training patterns and bone mineral density of the femoral shaft in elite female athletes. Ann. Rheum. Dis. 50:487-489; 1991.

CHAPTER 45

Morphological and Biochemical Responses of Bone to Mechanical Loading In Vitro

Timothy M. Skerry
University of Bristol, Bristol, United Kingdom

Mechanical loading is an important determinant of bone mass and is currently one of the least understood of the many osteotropic influences. There is little doubt that the mechanism by which mechanical events affect cell behavior to regulate the amount and distribution of the extracellular matrix involves the transduction of physical into biochemical events. Evidence exists to suggest that a sequence of changes occurs in the matrix and then in the cells of bone in a cascade of events that leads to a positive effect on bone balance in the case of increased loading and a negative effect in disuse.

The mechanism by which bone is lost or gained as a result of these two possibilities is complex, because the sum of all positive and negative osteotropic effects regulates the relative amounts of bone formation and resorption during the remodeling process. The effects of mechanical events on the skeleton therefore depend on their interactions with other local and systemic influences. In many circumstances, there will be no net loss or gain but rather maintenance of the tissue because it is adapted to the habitual activity of the individual. Although maintenance of mass may appear to be a passive process, the rapid and dramatic bone loss in disuse emphasizes that maintenance is the result of a continuing active requirement for the presence of load-bearing matrix.

Regulation of bone mass by mechanical loading is an important topic because of the prevalence of diseases such as postmenopausal osteoporosis and rheumatoid arthritis, in which functionally inappropriate bone loss occurs with consequent fracture and disability. Although there are differences between the bone loss due to estrogen deficiency and due to disuse, both are almost abolished in the absence of circulating parathyroid hormone, suggesting at least some common features. The study of mechanical effects on bone is therefore a valuable way to gain insights into the regulation of skeletal mass, and one which has direct clinical relevance. The main purpose of this chapter is to review in vitro explant models that have been used in the field. Such an account would be incomplete without reference to the mechanisms by which bone remodeling occurs and to cell culture and in vivo experiments in which similar findings validate results and put them into a physiological perspective. Finally, I wish to suggest possible new lines of inquiry combining existing and new techniques that will help to advance knowledge and increase understanding of the mechanisms of the response of bone to mechanical loading.

Among the many functions of the skeleton, the one that accounts predominantly for its shape, mass, and material properties is the requirement that it should bear loads. While mineral homeostasis or hematopoiesis could be achieved equally well or perhaps better by an amorphous mass of mineralized tissue rather than by a skeleton of highly organized compact and trabecular bone, the mechanical role is dependent on form.

Bone is unique among the tissues of the body in its level of resistance to mechanical forces, which results from the composition of the extracellular matrix. Since by definition this matrix is synthesized by bone cells, it is the actions of those cells that govern the mechanical properties of the bone and therefore the skeleton as a whole.

Since the mechanical demands placed on the skeleton are not static during life or even at different sites within a single individual, it follows that unless the skeleton is engineered to resist all foreseeable loads, there must be some regulation of its mass under different circumstances. The logic behind a dynamically regulated skeleton is clear. It is possible to hypothesize that during evolution, there were two diverging groups: those with overengineered skeletons that hardly ever failed and those with regulated bone mass, which may have fractured more frequently. As individuals, the fracture risk of the first group would have been low, but they would have carried a large mass of superfluous bone that would have made them less competitive as either predatory carnivores or herbivores trying to evade carnivores. The second group might have had slightly reduced survival possibilities as individuals but would have been more effective as a group in surviving to reproduce.

Such a hypothesis is attractive because the dynamically regulated skeleton is a feature of animals and humans. Increases in loading stimulate formation, while disuse or reduced activity causes bone loss. In order to understand the possible mechanisms for those changes, it is necessary to consider the general regulatory mechanisms in bone.

Local Cellular Interactions in Bone Remodeling

In order to understand the ways in which mechanical loading affects bone remodeling, it is necessary to examine the relevant cell types present in the locality of a bone surface, their interactions, and current perceptions of the mechanisms by which they are controlled (figure 45.1).

While many different cell types are involved in the processes that contribute to bone remodeling, it seems that the central role is played by bone-lining cells (BLC) or quiescent osteoblasts (34, 42). Bone-lining cells are thought to receive information from two sources. Osteocytes (OC) embedded within the matrix communicate with each other and with the lining cells (6, 9) and have been shown to respond to the levels of mechanical strain experienced by the bone (8, 20, 38). In addition, surface cells possess receptors for both systemic and local osteotropic agents such as parathyroid hormone (PTH), 1,25-dihydroxy vitamin D3 (1,25D) and numerous osteotropic cytokines (12, 13, 35). The lining cell therefore functions to integrate the effects of

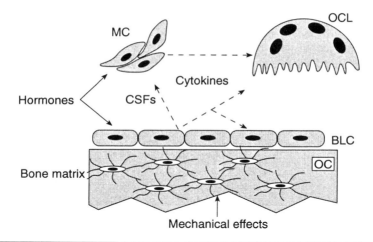

Figure 45.1   Local interactions at the bone surface. Osteocytes (OC) within the matrix are able to sense strain and communicate with bone-lining cells (BLC), which are also sensitive to both endocrine influences from circulating hormones and autocrine and paracrine cytokines. Colony stimulating factors (CSFs) act on marrow stromal cells (MC) to stimulate differentiation and activation of osteoclastic precursors, which fuse to form mature osteoclasts (OCL) capable of resorbing bone.

mechanical, endocrine, paracrine, and autocrine signals and provides an appropriate response to initiate formation or resorption.

The specific actions of the cells responsible for resorption and formation are under tight control by temporal and spatial expression of many different cytokines (24, 31, 43), but a detailed description of their actions is beyond the scope of this chapter. Osteotropic cytokines are produced by osteoblasts and marrow cells (MC) and are regulated globally by endocrine influences such as PTH, 1,25D, and estrogen. Locally, cell actions are controlled by paracrine and autocrine cytokines. Although there is little direct evidence to confirm the ability of mechanical loading to influence expression or actions of cytokines, such a mechanism would provide the link between deformation of the bone matrix and biochemical regulation of cell actions.

If there is a requirement for bone formation, then apposition may occur directly on the bone surface without previous resorption (28). In such a circumstance, there is recruitment of new osteoblast precursors, which proliferate and differentiate locally. Formation then occurs in which mature osteoblasts deposit new unmineralized matrix. Mineralization of the osteoid proceeds in a front from the existing bone surface. At the end of formation, a lining cell population is reestablished, and the surface becomes quiescent again. More usually, though, the effect of loading is to shift the balance during remodeling so that formation exceeds previous resorption.

Where there is insufficient mechanical stimulation to maintain bone mass, resorption occurs. Recruitment of osteoclast precursors in the marrow results from the expression of stimulators of differentiation and proliferation: colony stimulating factors (CSFs). Precursors are attracted to the specific site and fuse into activated, multinucleated osteoclasts (OCL), which are capable of resorption. At the same time, bone-lining cells change their shape to become more rounded so that mineralized matrix is exposed for resorption (1). Active resorption follows when osteoclasts bind to the bone surface by means of specific ligand-receptor interactions (47). Resorption occurs until some as yet unknown signaling process inhibits osteoclastic action. It has been suggested that elevation of extracellular calcium concentration or growth factors released from the bone matrix may be responsible (30). A role for the osteocytes within the bone in signaling the end of resorption is also possible.

The complexity of the relationships of bone cells and osteotropic agents often leads to conflicting or contradictory results (26). However, bone formation and resorption initiated by different stimuli appear to share common features. For example, bone resorption that occurs as a result of either disuse or estrogen withdrawal can be almost abolished by parathyroidectomy, suggesting a common mechanism (4, 15, 22). This shows that increased understanding of the effects of mechanical loading on bone has implications beyond recommendations for exercise regimes for osteoporotic women, since such knowledge also clarifies the pathology of bone loss in other conditions.

Effects of Mechanical Loading in Vivo

As a result of osteogenic loading of the skeleton in vivo, there are a number of possible outcomes. Where the bone being loaded is quiescent, new formation may occur (36). Where a strong drive toward resorption is present, such as in calcium-deficient animals, the effect of loading may be insufficient to stimulate formation, and it will only reduce the amount of resorption (21). If the loading stimulus is sufficiently osteogenic, however, it may completely inhibit resorption and stimulate formation (17). During growth, increased loading may enhance existing formation (41). In normal circumstances, though, the effect of habitual loading activity is to balance the effects of resorptive stimuli so that remodeling maintains bone mass at a constant level.

If formation is stimulated, there is a cascade of events that leads to the transformation of the resorbing or quiescent bone surface into a forming one. The earliest change detected in bone in vivo is the change in orientation of matrix proteoglycans (39, 40). This change is strain related but transient, returning to the previous state within 48 h if there is no further loading. It has been suggested that osteocytes perceive matrix deformation as a result of interactions with proteoglycans (27, 44), and rapid changes in osteocyte enzyme activity do accompany loading in vivo (8, 38). There is an increase in RNA synthesis by osteocytes 24 h after loading, as measured by uptake of [³H]uridine (29). Proliferative changes are visible on the bone surface within 48 h of loading, and these culminate in new bone formation within 5 d (28). The interaction of loading in vivo with other osteotropic influences is demonstrated by its ability to limit bone loss in ovariectomized animals and postmenopausal women (14, 32).

Limitations of Models of Mechanical Loading

Investigations of mechanical effects on bone fall into three categories: in vitro cell culture experiments, in vitro explant experiments, and in vivo studies.

Cell culture allows the use of sophisticated techniques to investigate the cellular and molecular biology of bone cells in a way that may be difficult or impossible in other systems. For example, it has been possible to clarify many of the intracellular consequences of loading by stretching cells cultured onto deformable substrates (19, 37, 45). One disadvantage of these techniques is that the cells are isolated from their matrix and are usually either osteoblast-derived primary cultures or some form of transformed cell line, which may respond differently from cells in situ. While such limitations apply to most cell culture experiments, the removal of cells from their matrix makes interpretation of results particularly difficult in a tissue where the mechanical properties of the matrix form the end point of physiological processes initiated by the deformation of the cells. In defense of these experiments, they do have a unique ability to provide very specific answers to questions that cannot be addressed by other means.

In vitro explant experiments allow examination of effects of loading on cells in their matrix. Clearly, it is necessary to devise an experimental system in which the explant is maintained in a viable state, which can be much harder than for cell culture experiments. In such experiments, the cells within the explant form all or most of the experimentally maintained population, so their actions and changes will provide the major influence on changes in soluble factors released into the medium, which can be assayed in a way not possible in vivo.

In vivo experiments can be divided into those in which there is a change in whole-body exercise and loading of much of the skeleton and those in which there is a change in the loading status of just one part of the skeleton. In the first case, there is the added complication of up-regulation of many other systemic responses to the exercise program, which would confound any search for soluble factors released into the circulation by the bones. Where there is regional loading or disuse, it is likely that any changes in circulating mediators will be obscured by the lack of change in the rest of the system. In addition, such studies are often slow, are complicated by greater biological variation than in vitro studies, and may require complex methods of analysis. However, in vivo experiments do have one feature that is denied to both of the in vitro methods of experimentation. This is that such experiments can be continued to observe the structural responses to the loading changes of the bone(s) in question. This in turn allows correlation of early changes with the ultimate goal of a putative osteoregulatory stimulus, namely, regulation of bone mass and strength.

This point highlights a major requirement of in vitro methods. They must be correlated with changes in vivo. Where direct comparisons are impossible, changes in vitro should be correlated with calibration studies that have some readily apparent parallel in vivo. Although many of the changes following loading have been demonstrated in vivo (table 45.1), it is often cumbersome and difficult to investigate very specific spatial and temporal changes, particularly in the early stages after loading. However, results that can be obtained from in vitro and in vivo methods can be used to demonstrate the physiological relevance of in vitro methods. For example, since loading has been shown to induce changes in gene and protein expression, to increase enzyme activity, and to stimulate cell proliferation, these effects can be used in vitro to validate the methods. If other changes can then be demonstrated that are not possible in vivo, they can then be seen in a physiological context.

Last, it is necessary that loading experiments take account of perhaps the most important single relevant variable, strain. Valid loading experiments should expose cells to strains similar to those that would initiate a physiological loading-related

Table 45.1   Effects of Loading In Vivo and In Vitro

Response	Cell culture	Explant	In vivo
Second messengers	+	+	−
Matrix interactions	−	+	+
Gene expression	+	+	+
Gene product	+	+	+
Enzyme activation	+	+	+
Cell proliferation	+	+	+
Resorption	−	+	+
Formation	−	−	+
Bone strength	−	−	+

Loading in vivo initiates a cascade of events that leads to bone formation, with an increase in strength. While in vitro methods cannot follow changes through to measure bone strength, they can be calibrated against known early changes in vivo.

+Can be investigated by this method; −cannot be investigated by this method.

response in their original location in vivo. For the most part, different locations within the skeleton receive broadly similar strains, but one significant exception is that calvarial cells receive strains that are very much lower than those in long bones (16). This finding calls into question the wisdom of using calvarial-derived cells or explants for in vitro experiments, as it is possible that such cells are very insensitive to the effects of low levels of strain. Neither is it clear whether they respond normally to elevated strains.

In Vitro Explant Studies

There have been a number of experiments designed to investigate the responses of bone to loading in vitro, and although each model has generated data that are consistent with future bone formation, many of them failed to address fully all of the requirements for a validated model.

The use of hydrostatic compression to apply forces to cells and explants has generated a large volume of data. This method was developed and used initially to apply compressive forces to cartilage cells (3), which experience a mixture of strain and hydrostatic forces in situ. The method has also been used in a number of experiments (reviewed in 2) to apply forces to fetal bone rudiments, which show increased growth and calcification compared with nonpressurized controls. However, since this model investigates what is essentially an endochondral ossification process, it is not truly a model for bone loading in vivo. Furthermore, the compressive forces applied via the gas phase above the culture medium do not generate strains within the explants that would have any osteogenic effect in vivo.

Lozupone, Favia, and Grimaldi (23) developed a model to load neonatal rat metatarsal bone explants in vitro and applied cyclical loads to the bones as they were cultured. The loads applied were calculated to engender double the force applied to the bone during standing in vivo. Preliminary findings suggested that five daily periods of loading were sufficient to increase the viability of osteocytes within the bones and to transform a quiescent periosteal surface into one in which there were more active osteoblasts. While the stimulation of periosteal proliferation is entirely consistent with loading-related changes, it is disturbing that osteocyte viability was affected so markedly in the nonloaded bones, particularly since death of osteocytes in vivo has been suggested to abrogate the remodeling response (10). Since their preliminary findings were published, the authors have moved to other (in vivo) experiments on bone remodeling.

In a series of experiments, Lanyon's group has developed three models to study mechanical loading of bone in vitro. The first of these models was one in which cylindrical cores of cancellous bone were removed from the distal femora of dogs (11). The cores of bone were washed and maintained in medium before being placed in the chamber of a loading device that allowed perfusion of medium during the experiment. Compressive loads applied to the samples were calculated to engender physiological strains within the tissues. The loading was shown to induce the same proteoglycan changes in the matrix and equivalent increases in enzyme activity and RNA synthesis in osteocytes as had been demonstrated previously in vivo (29, 38, 40). Furthermore, it was shown that loading increased release of prostaglandins E_2 and I_2 (measured as the metabolite 6-keto $PGF_{1\alpha}$). Histologically, the expression was localized in both osteoblasts and osteocytes. This model generated useful data on early changes following loading, but it has proved to be unsuitable for experiments with durations of several days.

In order to develop a model to overcome that problem and one in which measured rather than calculated strains could be applied, the same group developed a method to load embryonic chick tibiotarsal bones in vitro (7). Because the tibiotarsus is a cortical bone, it was possible to apply strain gauges to its surface and determine directly the loads needed to induce physiological strains.

Using some of the same calibration parameters as before, the model was validated by the same strain-related increases in RNA expression and G6PD activity in osteocytes and osteoblasts as before. It was also demonstrated by in situ hybridization that a single period of loading up-regulated gene expression for type 1 collagen (46).

The most recent model to be developed is one in which the ulnae are removed from young rats and loaded in vitro (5). This method allows direct measurement of strain and correlation of changes with the standard early loading-related activation of G6PD activity and [^{3}H]uridine uptake. A further advantage is that the same group has also developed a model for loading of the same bone in adult animals in vivo (41), so for the first time in vivo and in vitro experiments could be compared directly. At present, the experiments have been performed to investigate the interactions of estrogen and mechanical loading and have shown that the hormone potentiates the effect of loading, suggesting one possible mechanism for postmenopausal bone loss. Although the authors have only correlated their in vitro findings with bones of rather older rats in vivo, we have used the same methods to load smaller rat ulnae in vivo, so that there is now direct validation of that model (18).

In vitro explant experiments have therefore increased knowledge of the events that follow loading by demonstrating changes at intermediate time points between

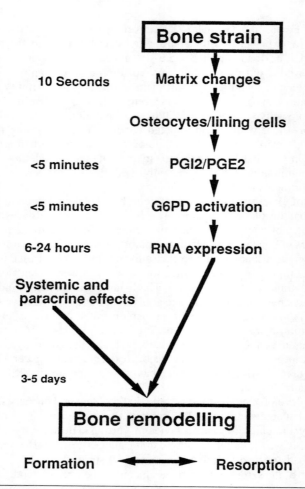

Figure 45.2   The sequence of changes following loading. Following loading of bone in vitro and in vivo, changes in matrix proteoglycans are the earliest detectable response. There is then a cascade of cellular events that leads after a number of days to stimulation of formation. Formation is not the inevitable consequence of loading though. Other influences, such as endocrine status, nutritional factors, or concurrent inflammation, may limit the osteogenic effect of loading to modulation or inhibition of existing resorption.

those investigated in vivo or in cell culture (figure 45.2). The importance of eicosanoid actions has been emphasized by the ability of indomethacin to block the changes seen. The ability of PGI_2 but not PGE_2 to induce equivalent changes to loading in vitro points to a specific prostaglandin-mediated step in the cascade of events (33).

Future Directions

While there has been a dramatic increase in understanding of bone biology generally as a result of the use of molecular biology techniques, there is as yet little information on the ability of mechanical loading to influence gene expression. It has proved difficult to demonstrate specific changes in gene expression in response to loading or disuse using RNA extraction/Northern blotting techniques, probably because of the heterogeneity of the tissues. In situ hybridization studies offer the benefits of localization of gene expression and correlation with other markers of formation and resorption in serial sections. However, the technique is not simple, and as a method of detecting a temporal sequence of changes in response to mechanical loading, either in vivo or in vitro, in situ hybridization is cumbersome.

Both Northern blotting and in situ hybridization also suffer from the drawback that they disclose the expression of known genes using specific probes. Since the questions that remain to be answered in relation to mechanical loading and bone are focused mainly on the role of the osteocyte and on the nature and timings of expression of as yet unidentified osteotropic cytokines by surface cells, the use of such specific techniques is a slow means of progressing.

With the advent of differential display techniques, it is possible to identify differences in gene expression between different samples and then to sequence those products. This approach has exciting possibilities because it allows searching for changes in unknown genes. Using the rat ulna model and reverse transcriptase–linked polymerase chain reaction (RTPCR) techniques with specific primers, we have identified a number of genes that are constitutively expressed by osteocytes and by periosteal cells on a resorbing bone surface (table 45.2; 25). To date, we have not found changes in any of those genes in response to loading of the bone that stimulates transformation of the resorbing surface into a forming one after 5 d (17). However, the use of differential display methods will undoubtedly prove informative in determining the temporal sequences of expression of genes in response to mechanical loading.

Table 45.2   Gene Expression in Osteocytes and Periosteal Cells

Gene	Osteocyte	Periosteum
β-Actin	+	+
Osteocalcin	+	+
Connexin 43	+	+
IL-1α	+	+
TNF-α	−	+
TRAP	−	+

Using RTPCR, RNA extracted from samples of periosteum on a resorbing surface and the underlying cortical bone were amplified using specific primers for the genes of interest. Osteocytes show clear evidence of expression of β-actin, osteocalcin, the gap junction protein connexin 43, and IL-1α, but not TNF-α and tartrate-resistant acid phosphatase (TRAP).

+ = mRNA expression detected; − = no mRNA expression detected.

Conclusions

There are still many unanswered questions regarding the specific events that occur in osteocytes and bone-lining cells in response to loading. The combination of in vitro and in vivo models with the power of molecular biology techniques has already advanced the study of mechanical loading in bone and will continue to do so. The increased understanding that accompanies those advances will have considerable significance in drug discovery and therefore in clinical treatments. The next few years will be exciting times as current understanding and knowledge is applied in the clinics and as new insights are gained to further advance this process.

Acknowledgments

I would like to thank Dr. Deborah Mason for the data for table 45.2 and the AFRC, ARC, MRC, and Wellcome Trust for funding the studies in which I have been involved.

References

1. Ali, N.N.; Melhuish, P.B.; Boyde, A.; Bennett, A.; Jones, S.J. Parathyroid hormone, but not prostaglandin E_2, changes the shape of osteoblasts maintained on bone in vitro. J. Bone Mineral Res. 5:115-121; 1990.
2. Berger, E.H.; Klein Nulend, J.; Veldhuijzen, J.P. Mechanical stress and osteogenesis in vitro. J. Bone Mineral Res. 7 (suppl. 2):397-401; 1992.
3. Bourret, L.A.; Rodan, G.A. The role of calcium in the inhibition of cAMP accumulation in epiphyseal cartilage cells exposed to physiological pressure. J. Cell. Physiol. 88:358-361; 1975.
4. Burkhart, J.M.; Jowsey, J. Parathyroid and thyroid hormones in the development of immobilization osteoporosis. Endocrinology 81:1053-1062; 1967.
5. Cheng, M.Z.; Zaman, G.; Lanyon, L.E. Estrogen enhances the osteogenic effects of mechanical loading and exogenous prostacyclin, but not prostaglandin-E_2. J. Bone Mineral Res. 8 (suppl. 1):151; 1993.
6. Curtis, T.A.; Ashrafi, S.H.; Weber, D.F. Canalicular communications in the cortices of human long bones. Anat. Rec. 212:336-344; 1985.
7. Dallas, S.L.; Zaman, G.; Pead, M.J.; Lanyon, L.E. Early strain-related changes in cultured embryonic chick tibiotarsi parallel those associated with adaptive modeling in vivo. J. Bone Mineral Res. 8:251-259; 1993.
8. Dodds, R.A.; Ali, N.N.; Pead, M.J.; Lanyon, L.E. Early loading-related changes in the activity of glucose 6-phosphate dehydrogenase and alkaline phosphatase in osteocytes and periosteal osteoblasts in rat fibulae in vivo. J. Bone Mineral Res. 8:261-267; 1993.
9. Doty, S.B. Morphological evidence of gap junctions between bone cells. Calcif. Tissue Int. 33:509-512; 1981.

10. Dunstan, C.R.; Somers, N.M.; Evans, R.A. Osteocyte death and hip fracture. Calcif. Tissue Int. 53 (suppl. 1):113-118; 1993.
11. El Haj, A.J.; Minter, S.L.; Rawlinson, S.C.F.; Suswillo, R.F.L.; Lanyon, L.E. Cellular responses to mechanical loading in vitro. J. Bone Mineral Res. 5(9): 1345-1351; 1990.
12. Eriksen, E.F.; Colvard, D.S.; Berg, N.J.; Graham, M.L.; Mann, K.G.; Spelsberg, T.C.; Riggs, B.L. Evidence of estrogen receptors in normal human osteoblast-like cells. Science 241:84-86; 1988.
13. Goldring, M.B.; Goldring, S.R. Skeletal tissue response to cytokines. Clin. Orthoped. Relat. Res. 258:245-278; 1990.
14. Hagino, H.; Raab, D.M.; Kimmel, D.B.; Akhter, M.P.; Recker, R.R. Effect of ovariectomy on bone response to in vivo external loading. J. Bone Mineral Res. 8:347-357; 1993.
15. Hillam, R.A.; Levi, A.J.; Skerry, T.M. Parathyroidectomy reduces trabecular bone loss and reduction of cortical bone strength after ovariectomy. Bone Mineral 25 (suppl. 1):44; 1994.
16. Hillam, R.A.; Mosley, J.M.; Skerry, T.M. Regional differences in bone strain. Bone Mineral 25 (suppl. 1):32; 1994.
17. Hillam, R.A.; Skerry, T.M. Inhibition of periosteal bone resorption and stimulation of formation by in vivo mechanical loading of the rat ulna in vivo. J. Bone Mineral Res. 10(5):683-689; 1995.
18. Hillam, R.A.; Skerry, T.M. Models for two phases of the bone remodelling cycle. Bone Mineral 25 (suppl. 1):44; 1994.
19. Jones, D.B.; Nolte, H.; Scholubbers, J.G.; Turner, E.; Veltel, D. Biochemical signal transduction of mechanical strain in osteoblast like cells. Biomaterials 12:101-110; 1991.
20. Lanyon, L.E. Osteocytes, strain detection, bone modeling and remodeling. Calcif. Tissue Int. 53 (suppl. 1):102-107; 1993.
21. Lanyon, L.E.; Rubin, C.T.; Baust, G. Modulation of bone during calcium insufficiency by controlled dynamic loading. Calcif. Tissue Int. 38:209-216; 1986.
22. Lindgren, J.U. The effect of thyro parathyroidectomy on the development of disuse osteoporosis in the rat. Clin. Orthoped. 118:251-255; 1976.
23. Lozupone, E.; Favia, A.; Grimaldi, A. Effect of intermittent mechanical force on bone tissue in vitro: Preliminary results. J. Bone Mineral Res. 7 (suppl. 2): 407-409; 1992.
24. MacDonald, B.R.; Gowen, M. The cell biology of bone. Bailliere's Clin. Rheumat. 7:421-443; 1993.
25. Mason, D.J.; Fermor, B.; Hillam, R.A.; Skerry, T.M. Investigation of osteocyte mRNA expression by RTPCR. Bone Mineral 25 (suppl. 1):34; 1994.
26. Nathan, C.F.; Sporn, M.B. Cytokines in context. J. Cell Biol. 113:981-986; 1991.
27. Palumbo, C.; Palazzini, S.; Zaffe, D.; Marotti, G. Osteocyte differentiation in the tibia of newborn rabbit: An ultrastructural study of the formation of cytoplasmic processes. Acta Anatom. 137:350-358; 1990.
28. Pead, M.J.; Skerry, T.M.; Lanyon, L.E. Direct transformation from quiescence to bone formation in the adult periosteum following a single brief period of bone loading. J. Bone Mineral Res. 3:647-656; 1988.
29. Pead, M.J.; Suswillo, R.F.L.; Skerry, T.M.; Vedi, S.; Lanyon, L.E. Increased ^{3}H-uridine levels in osteocytes following a single short period of dynamic bone loading in vivo. Calcif. Tissue Int. 43:92-96; 1988.

30. Pfeilschifter, J.; Seyedin, S.M.; Mundy, G.R. Transforming growth factor β inhibits bone resorption in fetal rat long bone cultures. J. Clin. Invest. 82:680-685; 1988.

31. Raisz, L.G. Bone cell biology: New approaches and unanswered questions. J. Bone Mineral Res. 8 (suppl. 1):457-465; 1993.

32. Ramsdale, S.J.; Bassey, E.J. Changes in femoral bone mineral density associated with impact exercise in postmenopausal women. J. Physiol. 467:313P; 1993.

33. Rawlinson, S.C.F.; Mohan, S.; Baylink, D.J.; Lanyon, L.E. Exogenous prostacyclin, but not prostaglandin E₂, produces similar responses in both G6PD activity and RNA production as mechanical loading, and increases IGF-II release, in adult cancellous bone in culture. Calcif. Tissue Int. 53:324-329; 1993.

34. Rodan, G.A.; Martin, J.J. The role of osteoblasts in hormonal control of bone resorption: A hypothesis. Calcif. Tissue Int. 33:349-351; 1981.

35. Rouleau, M.F.; Mitchell, J.; Goltzman, D. In vivo distribution of parathyroid hormone receptors in bone: Evidence that a predominant osseous target cell is not the mature osteoblast. Endocrinology 123:187-191; 1988.

36. Rubin, C.T.; Lanyon, L.E. Osteoregulatory nature of mechanical stimuli: Function as a determinant for adaptive remodeling in bone. J. Orthoped. Res. 5:300-310; 1987.

37. Sandy, J.R.; Meghji, S.; Farndale, R.W.; Meikle, M.C. Dual elevation of cyclic AMP and inositol phosphates in response to mechanical deformation of murine osteoblasts. Biochim. Biophys. Acta 1010:265-269; 1989.

38. Skerry, T.M.; Bitensky, L.; Chayen, J.; Lanyon, L.E. Early strain-related changes in enzyme activity in osteocytes following bone loading in vivo. J. Bone Mineral Res. 4:783-788; 1989.

39. Skerry, T.M.; Bitensky, L.; Chayen, J.; Lanyon, L.E. Loading-related reorientation of bone proteoglycan in vivo: Strain memory in bone tissue? J. Orthoped. Res. 6:547-551; 1988.

40. Skerry, T.M.; Suswillo, R.F.L.; El Haj, A.J.; Ali, N.N.; Dodds, R.A.; Lanyon, L.E. Load-induced proteoglycan orientation in bone tissue in vivo and in vitro. Calcif. Tissue Int. 46:318-326; 1990.

41. Torrance, A.G.; Mosley, J.M.; Suswillo, R.F.L.; Lanyon, L.E. Noninvasive loading of the rat ulna in vivo induces a strain related modeling response uncomplicated by trauma of periosteal pressure. Calcif. Tissue Int. 54:238-241; 1994.

42. Vaes, G. Cellular biology and biochemical mechanism of bone resorption. A review of recent developments on the formation, activation, and mode of action of osteoclasts. Clin. Orthoped. 231:239-271; 1988.

43. Wallach, S.; Avioli, L.V.; Feinblatt, J.D.; Carstens, J.H., Jr. Cytokines and bone metabolism. Calcif. Tissue Int. 53:293-296; 1993.

44. Weinbaum, S.; Cowin, S.C.; Zeng, Y. A model for the excitation of osteocytes by mechanical loading-induced bone fluid shear stresses. J. Biomech. 27:339-360; 1994.

45. Yeh, C.K.; Rodan, G.A. Tensile forces enhance prostaglandin E synthesis in osteoblastic cells grown on collagen ribbons. Calcif. Tissue Int. 36:S67-S71; 1984.

46. Zaman, G.; Dallas, S.L.; Lanyon, L.E. Cultured embryonic bone shafts show osteogenic responses to mechanical loading. Calcif. Tissue Int. 51:132-136; 1992.

47. Zambonin-Zallone, A.; Teti, A.; Gaboli, M.; Marchisio, P.C. Beta 3 subunit of vitronectin receptor is present in osteoclast adhesion structures and not in other monocyte-macrophage derived cells. Conn. Tissue Res. 20:143-149; 1989.

CHAPTER 46

In Vivo Bone Cell Histological and Biochemical Responses to Mechanical Loading

Diane M. Raab-Cullen

Creighton University, Omaha, Nebraska, U.S.A.

Bone mass and structure are regulated by daily mechanical loads that create bone deformation (microstrain, $\mu\varepsilon$). Bone cells detect aberrant loading patterns and immediately respond to mechanical challenges. The primary focus of this chapter is the skeletal response to increased mechanical loading. At the organ level, bone adapts to increased mechanical loads by increasing mass and altering shape to maintain an acceptable strain range during all loading activities. At the cellular level, adaptation occurs through the release of autocrine-paracrine signals, osteoblast proliferation and differentiation, and bone formation. Formation continues until adaptation is complete and strains return to "normal."

The skeleton is composed of cortical and cancellous bone. Although both types of bone have similar composition, their structural arrangements are different. In cortical bone, the cellular response to loading can be examined on three independent surfaces: periosteal, endocortical, and osteonal. Cancellous bone has an endosteal surface. Structural differences result in a different local environment for each surface during mechanical loading. Forces on bone produce regional differences in surface strains, fluid pressures, and streaming potentials. Since structural orientation determines the local strains and exposure to blood flow affects cell metabolism, each surface has a unique response to mechanical loads. Local biochemical signals can be generated from either osteoblasts lining the bone surfaces or from osteocytes contained within the bone matrix. Osteocytes may play a role in sensing strain, but it is the osteoblasts and precursor cells that ultimately proliferate, differentiate, and produce new matrix (21).

There are four types of in vivo models for mechanical loading: exercise, osteotomy, external loading through surgically implanted pins, and external loading through pads in contact with soft tissue. Each model has advantages and disadvantages, but together they offer an understanding of the in vivo skeletal system's response to mechanical loading.

Histologic Response to In Vivo Mechanical Loading

On the microscopic level, formation is usually quantified as extent of active mineralizing surface and the rate of mineral apposition (30). Formation is measured by injecting fluorescent calcium-binding labels at two time points and measuring the label length on the surface (mineralizing surface) and the distance between the two labels (mineral apposition rate). Bone formation rate is the product of active surface length and mineral apposition rate. The primary response to increased mechanical loading is de novo formation on the periosteal surface (modeling; 10, 34, 43). Periosteal expansion is the most efficient way to increase moment of inertia and thereby decrease strain during loading. Depending upon the strain created during loading, there can be endocortical formation and occasionally osteonal remodeling. Cancellous bone is not as well studied as cortical bone, because most exercise studies have not studied histology and most artificial loading experiments have focused on the bone diaphysis.

Exercise-Induced Bone Adaptation

In vivo, the primary cortical bone response to mechanical loading is increased periosteal formation. Extensive data on increased bone mass, size, and strength with exercise are available, but histological analysis of the response is fairly new. The surfaces involved and pattern of formation and resorption explain the more gross effects seen with mass and mechanical measurements. In a large animal model, the 3.5-yr-old sow, 20 wk of treadmill walking resulted in 27% greater periosteal surface activation in exercised than in control sows (34). Periosteal mineral apposition rate for the entire 20-wk period was 76% greater in exercised than in control sows. Endocortical formation and activation of osteonal remodeling were not different with exercise training. However, osteonal mineral apposition rate increased in the exercised sows, suggesting a general increase in osteoblast formation. Although walking is a low-intensity activity, it represented an increase in weight-bearing activity for the sows.

In thoroughbred horses, intense maximal exercise on a treadmill for 14 wk resulted in a 61% greater periosteal surface activation in exercised than in control horses (26). Periosteal mineral apposition rate was 22% higher in exercised than in control horses. These effects were localized to the dorsal surface where strains are estimated to reach 5,600 $\mu\varepsilon$ during this level of training. Endocortical surface activation in the exercised horses was 6.7 times higher than in controls. The greater response seen in the horses than in the sows may relate to the shorter study duration and to the greater strains created during more intense exercise in the horse than in the sow study. Intracortical porosity in the control horses was extensive compared with almost none in the exercised horses. This supports Frost's theory (14) that increased mechanical loading suppresses normal remodeling. The differences in porosity and increased periosteal formation support the noninvasive measurements of greater ultrasound velocity and bone mineral density in the trained than in the control horses.

In adult rats (14 mo) exercised on a treadmill for 9 wk, periosteal labeled surface and bone formation rate were two- to threefold greater than in controls (55). By 16 wk, bone formation rate was still elevated and cortical area was greater than in age-matched controls. The endocortical surface formation was not significantly higher than in controls at either time. In young, growing rats (6 wk), periosteal bone formation rate was similar to controls for the first 31 d, but remained high, while control formation rates decreased during days 32 to 41 of running (57). On the endocortical surface, there were no differences in formation due to exercise at 9 wk, and the exercised rats followed the same pattern of age-associated decrease in bone formation as controls at 16 wk. Endocortical formation responses to exercise are typically less common and not as intense as periosteal responses. Osteonal remodeling does not occur normally in the rat cortex.

The primary cancellous bone response to exercise in adult rats (14 mo) was a decrease in resorption surface (56). The ratio of resorption to formation was 70% lower in exercised than in control tibial metaphysis after 9 and 16 wk of moderate running exercise. Bone formation rate was elevated 42% at 16 wk of running. The net effect was a 5% increase in metaphyseal bone mineral density by 9 wk and 8.3% by 16 wk.

Exercise in animals is an excellent simulation of exercise in the human lower limbs. Unfortunately, exercise cannot be well controlled in terms of load magnitude, number of cycles, or frequency of application. Exercise loads have not been defined in terms of either local skeletal or systemic overload. Often intense exercise inhibits longitudinal growth, periosteal expansion, and cancellous bone formation in rapidly growing animals (2, 25). Studies are needed to examine the effects of various intensities of aerobic training on histomorphometric end points. A second problem with exercise studies, especially rat studies, is the lack of appropriate controls for either growth or altered mechanical loading. More data are needed on adult bone adaptation to a variety of loading conditions.

Mechanical Loading Through Osteotomy

Ulna osteotomy increases strains in the radius two- to fourfold. As an adaptation to the increased strains, the radius increases in size in proportion to the size of the missing ulna (7, 16, 22). Formation occurs on both the periosteum and the endosteum. In combination with the rapid increase in formation, resorption surfaces occur on periosteal and endocortical surfaces distant from the formation sites. The net effect is a reshaping of the bone through modeling and a change in the bending axis. In one study, periosteal expansion after osteotomy was due to an increase in length of active formation surface without an increase in mineral apposition rate (7).

Osteonal remodeling is common following osteotomy. It is elevated in the over-loaded limb and is localized primarily in areas of new bone formation where immature woven bone is remodeled into a more osteonal pattern. Although the activation frequency of remodeling is increased, as on the periosteum there is no increase in the rate of bone formation (7). This lack of change in apposition rate on both the periosteum and within the osteons conflicts with the large animal model exercise studies (26, 34).

External Loading With Implanted Pins and Wires

The implant models were the first to define mechanical variables that stimulate bone adaptation to loading. These models have the ability to control force magnitude, number of cycles, frequency, and pattern of force application. The major disadvantage is that surgical intervention on bone may stimulate bone formation (7, 10, 15). However, many of the early findings from these models have been confirmed in other models.

The early models found periosteal bone expansion was proportional to applied forces with cross-sectional area increasing up to 8.4% (10). In addition, formation was localized to periosteal surfaces under the highest strain during external loading (10, 18, 24). Endocortical formation was less than periosteal but was also observed in the areas of highest strain (18, 24). This is consistent with lower endocortical than periosteal strains during loading. Similar to the osteotomy models, patterns of osteonal activation have been seen in the regions of highest strains (10, 18, 23). In addition to strain magnitude, strain rate appears to be an important variable. Strain rate during load application explained up to 81% of the variance in periosteal expansion and 43% of the variance in osteonal remodeling (28).

Strain magnitude and number of loading cycles have been studied with the isolated turkey ulna model. This model applies external loads to a totally immobilized ulna. Loading at 36 cycles and 2,000 $\mu\epsilon$ or more with this model increases cortical area and bone mineral content up to 30% above control levels (43, 44). Daily application of 4 cycles maintained bone despite complete immobilization, and up to 3,600 cycles had no greater impact on formation than 36 cycles (43). There appears to be a threshold for stimulation that at high strains is reached with very few loading cycles. Cross-sectional area increases linearly with an increase in strain above 1,000 $\mu\epsilon$ (44). The increase is primarily periosteal and involves extensive woven bone formation at the higher loads. This model does not consistently find formation localized to regions of highest strain (33, 41, 43). Endocortical bone formation is seen in this model but is not well documented (43).

A new model involves implanting pins in 3-mo-old rat tail vertebrae (9). At 700 $\mu\epsilon$, this model stimulates periosteal woven bone and cancellous lamellar bone formation. After 8 d of loading, cancellous bone formation rate was 30 times greater than in nonloaded vertebrae. Both length of formation surface and mineral apposition rate increased. This model offers a unique opportunity to study cancellous bone response to loading.

External Loading With Pads

The rat tibia four-point bending model applies loads through pads that contact the medial and lateral lower leg surface (1, 35, 49). At moderate forces, the device creates strains of 1,200 to 1,700 $\mu\epsilon$ in 300-g female rats and stimulates periosteal formation in the regions of highest strain (17, 35-37). The typical response is an 80% increase in medial formation surface and a 53% increase in medial mineral apposition rate after 3 to 4 wk of loading. Although the lateral surface response is smaller and less consistent than the medial, formation surface increases 16% and mineral apposition rate increases 40%. The regional differences in response may relate to a 40% greater strain on the medial than on the lateral surface. With the four-point bending model, external loading on a typical exercise schedule of Monday-Wednesday-Friday is as effective at stimulating new bone formation as daily loading (34). At strains above 2,000 $\mu\epsilon$, the periosteal response is more robust and primarily woven bone (50, 51).

Forces in excess of 40 N create strains over 2,000 με on the periosteum and over 1,000 με on the endosteum. At these higher forces, it has been shown that the extent of endocortical lamellar bone formation increases linearly with strains above 1,050 με (50). This critical strain for activation of endocortical lamellar bone formation is similar to periosteal activation in the isolated ulna loading model (44).

A new rat ulna model has been developed that applies axial loads through the wrist and elbow joints to create compressive force in the ulna of young (230-g, male) rats (48). This model increases periosteal formation but decreases endocortical formation. Loads that create peak strains in excess of 3,000 με are required to initiate a periosteal formation response. Within stimulated ulna, regional periosteal formation was related to surface strain, with the intercept for formation at about 1,500 με. The relatively high strains required for stimulation in this model may result from a more physiological strain distribution during compression than other external loading models.

New Bone Structure

Periosteal and endocortical bone formation is typically in the form of lamellar bone: organized layers of compact bone. The cells are regularly spaced and the collagen is oriented in a consistent pattern alternating from layer to layer clearly visible under polarizing light (19). However, at sites of rapid formation, a fibrolamellar or more porous configuration of bone appears (12). The bone forms well-organized layers of tissue, but rather than concentric layers, the osteoblasts form large primary osteons. With exercise, the extent of forming surface and rate of formation increase. At the more rapid rates of formation, fibrolamellar bone is seen (34). With intense exercise, periosteal formations of bone extending perpendicular from the surface have been reported (26). These could be the beginning of either fibrolamellar bone or woven bone. Woven bone is disorganized, porous bone that forms with no obvious pattern (19). It usually occurs during rapid growth or during fracture and injury repair.

With artificially induced mechanical loading, woven bone formation is seen after ulna osteotomy (6, 16, 22), after loading through implanted pins (9, 43, 44), and after loading through external pads (48, 50, 51). In these models, the unique forces create nonphysiological patterns of strain within bone and stimulate bone formation at peak strains as low as 1,000 με, well below peak physiological strains that range from 2,100 to 3,200 με (42). At higher strains, they stimulate even greater bone formation, and eventually all stimulate woven bone formation. However, woven bone is not limited to artificial loading conditions. It was also observed in dog metacarpals with a return to normal weight-bearing activities following an extended period of immobilization (52).

Although stress fractures and microdamage may stimulate woven bone formation, microdamage is difficult to create in bone. At strains below 2,000 με, over a million cycles would be required to create fatigue damage (8). Even with osteotomy, woven bone formation is related to increased loads rather than to the surgical removal of the ulna (6). With intense mechanical loading, woven bone may simply be a rapid bone formation process that quickly adapts bone to dramatic increases in strain. Woven bone formed in response to external loading has been shown to remodel into dense, compact bone (51).

The Biological Response to Mechanical Signals

The actual signals and pathways involved in the transduction of mechanical loads into biological responses are still undefined. Scientists are diligently studying the initiation of bone cell response with in vitro and organ culture experiments. The in vivo studies of acute responses to loading have looked at proteoglycan and prostaglandin changes, total RNA production, mRNA expression, and osteoblast recruitment. Although these studies are primarily exploratory, they are a basis for applying in vitro knowledge to the intact system.

Acute Biochemical Markers of Mechanical Loading

Within bone, there is an immediate biochemical change in cell activity with mechanical loading. In the isolated turkey ulna, a brief loading session stimulated glucose-6-phosphate dehydrogenase (G6PD) activity within 6 min after loading (46). The increase in activity was proportional to the applied strains and occurred in both osteocytes and periosteal tissue. This increase in G6PD may be associated with an increase in RNA production, which increases within the first 24 h after loading (33). A similar increase in G6PD activity 5 min after loading in both osteocytes and periosteal tissue was found in an in vivo rat fibula compressive model (13). However, at 24 h, G6PD activity remained elevated only in the periosteal cells and had returned to control level in the osteocytes. Based upon in vitro work, the immediate increase in G6PD activity may be dependent upon prostaglandin release (39). Alkaline phosphatase activity was also examined 5 min and 24 h after loading and was elevated only at 24 h in the periosteal cells. The delayed periosteal increase in alkaline phosphatase activity corresponds to delayed increases in mRNA expression (3, 4, 38).

Prostaglandins are an important messenger in the transduction of mechanical signal to biologic response in vitro (5, 27, 40). An in vivo study with the isolated turkey ulna has shown some prostaglandin involvement in the response to loading (31). One hour after a single large dose of indomethacin (40 mg/kg) to inhibit prostaglandin synthesis, the ulna was externally loaded, and the periosteum was examined 5 d later. The indomethacin treatment depressed but did not prevent the increase in periosteal tissue thickness and new periosteal bone formation typically seen at that stage. Prostaglandins are probably important in the mechanical response pathway, and further study is necessary to clearly demonstrate their role. The initial release of PGE_2 with loading may be from cell stores rather than from rapid synthesis. Future studies need to pretreat the animals with indomethacin and examine the dose response.

Within bone, there appears to be some "memory" that immediately records mechanical loading and stores that record for a brief period. This memory allows sporadically applied, unique mechanical loads to result in bone formation. In the rat four-point bending model, formation increases similarly whether loading is performed every 24 h or 48 h (35). A possible mechanism for tissue memory might be proteoglycan arrangement in the bone matrix. Although collagen orientation does not change with loading in the isolated turkey ulna model, proteoglycan birefringence is altered (47). The optical path difference of polarized light was 36% greater immediately after loading compared with unloaded samples. The difference remained 25% greater 24 h after loading, but by 48 h there were no differences between loaded and unloaded ulna. This tissue memory may be an important mechanism for averaging daily strains and interpreting changes in strain energy density over several days (47).

Acute Changes in RNA Expression

Mechanical loading increases osteoblast proliferation and synthesis (3-5, 20). In vivo, it initiates a cascade of events that changes mRNA expression within 2 h (38) and increases RNA synthesis within 24 h (33). In vivo, c-*fos* mRNA expression is elevated fivefold 2 h after loading, remains elevated at 4 h, but returns to normal by 12 h after loading (38). The increase in c-*fos* message is also seen with in vitro studies that mechanically stimulate condylar (11) and cardiac tissue (45). The early c-*fos* expression is also consistent with periosteal cell proliferation following mechanical loading (32, 54). While the cell is expressing markers of proliferation, markers of osteoblast differentiation such as alkaline phosphatase and osteocalcin are depressed (38). In vitro, cell proliferation and alkaline phosphatase mRNA expression are mutually exclusive events, with the increase in osteoblast markers coupled to the down-regulation of proliferation (29). In vitro loading studies have found alkaline phosphatase depressed up to 24 h after loading (3, 4), while type I collagen mRNA expression is elevated by 18 h (58). The time at which mRNA expression for osteoblast markers increases in vivo has not been identified but probably occurs after 18 h. The present data suggest that mRNA expression is altered soon after mechanical loading and that the pattern of specific mRNA expression varies as the periosteal cell activity reflects cell proliferation and subsequently differentiation.

Similar to external loading models, mRNA expression increases with remobilization to normal weight-bearing activities after 9 d of skeletal unloading (53). Four hours after reloading, periosteal type I collagen and TGF-β were depressed 76% and 57%, respectively, while osteocalcin was 48% above control levels. Expression of all three mRNAs peaked at 24 h with levels 222% above controls. By 72 h after remobilization, osteocalcin and type I collagen were 57% and 68% below controls, respectively, but TGF-β remained 37% above control levels. The magnitude of the response was greater and the elevations in type I collagen and osteocalcin expression occurred much sooner with remobilization than with external loading. This variation in pattern may reflect sex- and age-related differences in skeletal growth rates. The unloaded rats were 6-wk-old males, while the externally loaded rats were 6-mo-old females. With reloading after immobilization, cancellous bone also showed increased mRNA expression for osteocalcin, TGF-β, and type I collagen, but the response was less dramatic and peaked at 4 h after reloading (53). The diminished response of cancellous bone relative to periosteal tissue may reflect the difference in cell populations. Cancellous bone contains osteocytes, osteoclasts, and marrow cells in addition to the osteoblast and preosteoblasts found in periosteal tissue.

Total RNA production is stimulated following external loading in the isolated turkey ulna (33). One day after loading, tritiated uridine incorporation in the ulnar cortical bone osteocytes was elevated sixfold in loaded versus control ulna. The tritiated uridine uptake was greatest in the ventral region, the area of typical bone formation with this model. The increase in total RNA is consistent with the increase in cell proliferation that occurs within the first 24 h after loading (32, 54).

Local Cellular Response

The time course of cell proliferation following force application in an orthodontic preparation was examined in rats injected with tritiated thymidine (54). The first labeled osteoblasts occurred 11 h after load application, and by 23 h there was a linear increase with time in number of labeled osteoblasts up to 71 h poststimulation. The primary source of these osteoblasts was believed to be connective tissue cells, in which tritiated thymidine labeling appeared within 5 h and peaked at 23 h after stimulation.

The periosteal bone formation that occurs with adaptation begins with osteoblast proliferation and differentiation. Within 5 to 6 d after a single loading session, the isolated turkey ulna shows a 2- to 14-fold thickening of the periosteal layer and a 2- to 6-fold increase in the number of osteogenic cell layers (32). The activation of quiescent cells within the osteogenic layer of the periosteum confirms observations made weeks after loading that bone formation occurs without prior resorption (modeling rather than remodeling).

Summary

The histological evidence of a consistent increase in periosteal formation and an occasional increase in endocortical formation explains the increases in bone mass seen with exercise training. The pattern of periosteal formation also explains the increase in moment of inertia and mechanical strength with loading. With histomorphometry, regional differences in formation and correlations with strain magnitude are possible. Microscopic examination has dispelled the notion that adult bones are incapable of modeling (formation without previous resorption) by demonstrating that modeling is the primary response to loading. The in vivo models are beginning to explore the immediate cellular messages and responses to mechanical loading. The early results from these models correlate well with the in vitro and organ culture results. The in vivo models serve an important role in validating in vitro findings and theories in the whole animal.

References

1. Akhter, M.P.; Raab, D.M.; Turner, C.H.; Kimmel, D.B.; Recker, R.R. Characterization of in vivo strain in the rat tibia during external application of a four-point bending load. J. Biomech. 25:1241-1246; 1992.
2. Bourrin, S.; Ghaemmaghami, F.; Vico, L.; Chappard, D.; Gharib, C.; Alexandre, C. Effect of a five-week swimming program on rat bone: A histomorphometric study. Calcif. Tissue Int. 51:137-142; 1992.

3. Brighton, C.; Strafford, B.; Gross, S.; Leatherwood, D.; Williams, J.; Pollack, S. The proliferative and synthetic response of isolated calvarial bone cells of rats to cyclic biaxial mechanical strain. J. Bone Joint Surg. 73A:320-331; 1991.
4. Buckley, M.; Banes, A.; Jordan, R. The effects of mechanical strain on osteoblasts in vitro. J. Oral Maxillofac. Surg. 48:276-282; 1990.
5. Buckley, M.; Banes, A.; Levin, L.; Sumpio, B.; Sato, M.; Jordan, R.; Gilbert, J.; Link, G.; Tran Son Tay, R. Osteoblasts increase their rate of division and align in response to cyclic, mechanical tension in vitro. Bone Mineral 4:225-236; 1988.
6. Burr, D.B.; Schaffler, M.B.; Yang, K.H.; Lukoschek, M.; Sivaneri, N.; Blaha, J.D.; Radin, E.L. Skeletal changes in response to altered strain environments: Is woven bone a response to elevated strain? Bone 10:223-233; 1989.
7. Burr, D.; Schaffler, M.; Yang, K.; Wu, D.; Lukoschek, M.; Kandzari, D.; Sivaneri, N.; Blaha, J.; Radin, E. The effects of altered strain environment on bone tissue kinetics. Bone 10:215-221; 1989.
8. Carter, D.; Caler, W.; Spengler, D.; Frankel, V. Fatigue behavior of adult cortical bone: The influence of mean strain and strain range. Acta Orthopaed. Scand. 52:481-490; 1981.
9. Chambers, T.; Evans, M.; Gardner, T.; Turner-Smith, A.; Chow, J. Induction of bone formation in rat tail vertebrae by mechanical loading. Bone Mineral 20:167-178; 1993.
10. Churches, A.E.; Howlett, C.R. Functional adaptation of bone in response to sinusoidally varying controlled compressive loading of the ovine metacarpus. Clin. Orthoped. Relat. Res. 168:265-280; 1982.
11. Closs, E.; Murray, A.; Schmidt, J.; Schon, A.; Erfle, V.; Strauss, P. c-*fos* Expression precedes osteogenic differentiation of cartilage cells in vitro. J. Cell Biol. 111:1313-1323; 1990.
12. Currey, J. The mechanical adaptations of bones. Princeton, NJ: Princeton University Press; 1984.
13. Dodds, R.; Ali, N.; Pead, M.; Lanyon, L. Early loading-related changes in the activity of glucose 6-phosphate dehydrogenase and alkaline phosphatase in osteocytes and periosteal osteoblasts in rat fibulae in vivo. J. Bone Mineral Res. 8:261-267; 1993.
14. Frost, H. Vital biomechanics: Proposed general concepts for skeletal adaptations to mechanical usage. Calcif. Tissue Int. 42:145-156; 1988.
15. Frost, H.M. Intermediary organization of the skeleton. Vol. 1. Boca Raton, FL: CRC Press; 1986:335-336.
16. Goodship, A.E.; Lanyon, L.E.; McFie, H. Functional adaptation of bone to increased stress. J. Bone Joint Surg. (Am.) 61:539-546; 1979.
17. Hagino, H.; Raab, D.; Kimmel, D.; Akhter, M.; Recker, R. The effects of ovariectomy on bone response to in vivo external loading. J. Bone Mineral Res. 8:347-357; 1993.
18. Hert, J.; Pribylova, E.; Liskova, M. Reaction of bone to mechanical stimuli: Part 3. Microstructure of compact bone of rabbit tibia after intermittent loading. Acta Anatom. 82:218-230; 1972.
19. Jee, W. The skeletal tissues. In: Weiss, L., ed. Histology cell and tissue biology. 5th ed. New York: Elsevier Biomedical; 1983:200-255.
20. Jones, H.H.; Priest, J.D.; Hayes, W.C.; Tichenor, C.C.; Nagel, D.A. Humeral hypertrophy in response to exercise. J. Bone Joint Surg. 59A:204-208; 1977.
21. Lanyon, L. Osteocytes, strain detection, bone modeling and remodeling. Calcif. Tissue Int. 53:S102-S107; 1993.

22. Lanyon, L.E.; Goodship, A.E.; Pye, C.J.; MacFie, J.H. Mechanically adaptive bone remodelling. J. Biomech. 15:141-154; 1982.
23. Lanyon, L.E.; Rubin, C.T. Static vs dynamic loads as an influence on bone remodelling. J. Biomech. 17:897-905; 1984.
24. Liskova, M.; Hert, J. Reaction of bone to mechanical factors: Part 2. Periosteal and endosteal bone apposition in the rabbit tibia due to intermittent stressing. Folia Morphol. (Prague) 19:301-317; 1971.
25. Matsuda, J.J.; Zernicke, R.K.; Vailas, A.C.; Pedrini, V.A.; Pedrini-Mille, A.; Maynard, J.A. Structural and mechanical adaptation of immature bone to strenuous exercise. J. Appl. Physiol. 60:2028-2034; 1986.
26. McCarthy, R.; Jeffcott, L. Effects of treadmill exercise on cortical bone in the third metacarpus of young horses. Res. Vet. Sci. 52:28-37; 1992.
27. Nishioka, S.; Fukada, K.; Tanaka, S. Cyclic stretch increases alkaline phosphatase activity of osteoblast-like cells: A role for prostaglandin E_2. Bone Mineral 21:141-150; 1993.
28. O'Connor, J.A.; Lanyon, L.E.; MacFie, H. The influence of strain rate on adaptive bone remodelling. J. Biomech. 15:767-781; 1982.
29. Owen, T.; Aronow, M.; Shalhoub, V.; Barone, L.; Wilming, L.; Tassinari, M.; Kennedy, M.; Pockwinse, S.; Lian, J.; Stein, G. Progressive development of the rat osteoblast phenotype in vitro: Reciprocal relationships in expression of genes associated with osteoblast proliferation and differentiation during formation of the bone extracellular matrix. J. Cell. Physiol. 143:420-430; 1990.
30. Parfitt, A.M.; Drezner, M.K.; Glorieux, F.H.; Kanis, J.A.; Malluche, H.; Meunier, P.J.; Ott, S.M.; Recker, R.R. Bone histomorphometry: Standardization of nomenclature, symbols, and units. J. Bone Mineral Res. 2:595-610; 1987.
31. Pead, M.; Lanyon, L. Indomethacin modulation of load-related stimulation of new bone formation in vivo. Calcif. Tissue Int. 45:34-40; 1989.
32. Pead, M.J.; Skerry, T.M.; Lanyon, L.E. Direct transformation from quiescence to bone formation in the adult periosteum following a single brief period of bone loading. J. Bone Mineral Res. 3:647-655; 1988.
33. Pead, M.J.; Suswillo, R.; Skerry, T.M.; Vedi, S.S.; Lanyon, L.E. Increased ^{3}H-uridine levels in osteocytes following a single short period of dynamic loading in vivo. Calcif. Tissue Int. 43:92-96; 1988.
34. Raab, D.M.; Crenshaw, T.D.; Kimmel, D.B.; Smith, E.L. A histomorphometric study of cortical bone activity during increased weight-bearing exercise. J. Bone Mineral Res. 6:741-749; 1991.
35. Raab-Cullen, D.; Akhter, M.; Kimmel, D.; Recker, R. Bone response to alternate day mechanical loading of the rat tibia. J. Bone Mineral Res. 9:203-211; 1994.
36. Raab-Cullen, D.; Akhter, M.; Kimmel, D.; Recker, R. Periosteal bone formation stimulated by externally induced bending strains. J. Bone Mineral Res. 9:1143-1152; 1994.
37. Raab-Cullen, D.; Kimmel, D.; Akhter, M.; Recker, R. Transient increase in bone formation after external mechanical loading. Transactions of 40th Annual Meeting of the Orthopedic Research Society 9:276; 1994. (Abstract).
38. Raab-Cullen, D.; Thiede, M.; Petersen, D.; Kimmel, D.; Recker, R. Mechanical loading stimulates rapid changes in periosteal gene expression. Calcif. Tissue Int. 55:473-478; 1994.
39. Rawlinson, S.; El Haj, A.; Minter, S.; Tavares, I.; Bennett, A.; Lanyon, L. Loading-related increases in prostaglandin production in cores of adult canine cancellous bone in vitro: A role for prostacyclin in adaptive bone remodeling? J. Bone Mineral Res. 6:1345-1351; 1991.

40. Rodan, G.; Mensi, T.; Harvey, A. A quantitative method for the application of compressive forces to bone tissue culture. Calcif. Tissue Res. 18:125-131; 1975.
41. Rubin, C.; Bain, S.; McLeod, K. Suppression of the osteogenic response in the aging skeleton. Calcif. Tissue Int. 50:306-313; 1992.
42. Rubin, C.; Lanyon, L. Dynamic strain similarity in vertebrates: An alternative to allometric limb bone scaling. J. Theor. Biol. 107:321-327; 1984.
43. Rubin, C.T.; Lanyon, L.E. Regulation of bone formation by applied dynamic loads. J. Bone Joint Surg. 66A:397-402; 1984.
44. Rubin, C.T.; Lanyon, L.E. Regulation of bone mass by mechanical strain magnitude. Calcif. Tissue Int. 37:411-417; 1985.
45. Sadoshima, J.; Izumo, S. Mechanical stretch rapidly activates multiple signal transduction pathways in cardiac myocytes: Potential involvement of an autocrine/paracrine mechanism. EMBO J. 12:1681-1692; 1993.
46. Skerry, T.M.; Bitensky, L.; Chayen, J.; Lanyon, L.E. Early strain-related changes in enzyme activity in osteocytes following bone loading in vivo. J. Bone Mineral Res. 4:783-788; 1989.
47. Skerry, T.M.; Bitensky, L.; Chayen, J.; Lanyon, L.E. Loading-related reorientation of bone proteoglycan in vivo. Strain memory in bone tissue. J. Orthoped. Res. 6:547-551; 1988.
48. Torrance, A.; Mosley, J.; Suswillo, R.; Lanyon, L. Noninvasive loading of the rat ulna in vivo induces a strain-related modeling response uncomplicated by trauma or periosteal pressure. Calcif. Tissue Int. 54:241-247; 1994.
49. Turner, C.H.; Akhter, M.P.; Raab, D.M.; Kimmel, D.B.; Recker, R.R. A noninvasive, in vivo model for studying strain adaptive bone modeling. Bone 12:73-79; 1991.
50. Turner, C.; Forwood, M.; Rho, J.; Yoshikawa, T. Mechanical thresholds for lamellar and woven bone formation. J. Bone Mineral Res. 9:878-897; 1994.
51. Turner, C.; Woltman, T.; Belongia, D. Structural changes in rat bone subjected to long-term, in vivo mechanical loading. Bone 13:417-422; 1992.
52. Uhthoff, H.K.; Jaworski, Z.F.G. Periosteal stress-induced reactions resembling stress fractures. A radiologic and histologic study in dogs. Clin. Orthoped. Relat. Res. 199:284-291; 1985.
53. Westerlind, K.; Morey-Holton, E.; Turner, R. The skeletal response to reloading following weightlessness. Transactions of 40th Annual Meeting of the Orthopedic Research Society 19:561; 1994. (Abstract).
54. Yee, J.A.; Kimmel, D.B.; Jee W.S.S. Periodontal ligament cell kinetics following orthodontic tooth movement. Cell Tissue Kinetics 9:293-302; 1976.
55. Yeh, J.; Aloia, J.; Chen, M. Growth hormone administration potentiates the effect of treadmill exercise on long bone formation but not on the vertebrae in middle-age rats. Calcif. Tissue Int. 54:38-43; 1994.
56. Yeh, J.; Aloia, J.; Chen, M.; Tierney, J.; Sprintz, S. Influence of exercise on cancellous bone of the aged female rat. J. Bone Mineral Res. 8:1117-1125; 1993.
57. Yeh, J.; Liu, C.; Aloia, J. Effects of exercise and immobilization on bone formation and resorption in young rats. Am. J. Physiol. 264:E182-E189; 1993.
58. Zaman, G.; Dallas, S.; Lanyon, L. Cultured embryonic bone shafts show osteogenic responses to mechanical loading. Calcif. Tissue Int. 51:132-136; 1992.

Related Books From HK

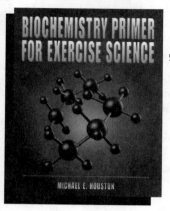

Michael E. Houston, PhD
1995 • Paper • 144 pp
Item BHOU0577
ISBN 0-87322-577-5
$22.00 ($32.95 Canadian)

Written by an exercise scientist with more than 25 years of experience teaching biochemistry, this book will appeal to even the most science-phobic exercise physiology student.

Designed for upper-level undergraduate and graduate students in exercise physiology with a limited background in biochemistry, it presents essential concepts of biochemistry—molecular biology, basic chemistry, metabolism, and transcription regulation—in a way that is easy to understand and relevant.

Concise yet comprehensive, this resource makes it easy for students to learn the background information necessary to understand the biochemistry of humans during physical activity. Readers will gain an understanding of human biochemistry as well as prepare themselves to understand the molecular developments that are at the forefront of exercise science. The book is also a valuable reference for individuals working in exercise physiology research.

Human Kinetics
The Information Leader in Physical Fitness
http://www.humankinetics.com/
2335

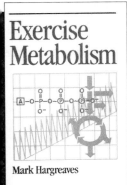